SMALL ANIMAL RADIOLOGY
AND ULTRASONOGRAPHY

Small Animal Radiology and Ultrasonography

A DIAGNOSTIC ATLAS AND TEXT

SECOND EDITION

RONALD L. BURK, DVM, MS

Diplomate, American College of Veterinary Radiology
(Radiology, Radiation Oncology)
Chief of Staff
Veterinary Specialists of South Florida
Cooper City, Florida

NORMAN ACKERMAN, DVM

Diplomate, American College of Veterinary Radiology
Kentucky Veterinary Specialists
Louisville, Kentucky

W. B. SAUNDERS COMPANY
A Division of Harcourt Brace & Company
PHILADELPHIA   LONDON   TORONTO   MONTREAL   SYDNEY   TOKYO

W.B. SAUNDERS COMPANY

A Division of Harcourt Brace Company

The Curtis Center
Independence Square West
Philadelphia, Pennsylvania 19106

Library of Congress Cataloging in Publication Data

Burk, Ronald L.
　　Small animal radiology and ultrasonography : a diagnostic atlas and text / Ronald L. Burk,
Norman Ackerman. — 2nd ed.
　　　p.　cm.
　　ISBN 0-7216-5270-0
　　1. Dogs—Diseases—Atlases.　2. Cats—Diseases—Atlases.　3. Dogs—Diseases—Diagnosis.
4. Cats—Diseases—Diagnosis.　I. Ackerman, Norman.　II. Title
SF991.B85　1996
636.7′089607572—dc20

95-42900

Companion animal practice is an ever-changing field. Standard safety precautions must be followed, but as new research and clinical experience grow, changes in treatment and drug therapy become necessary or appropriate. The authors and editors of this work have carefully checked the generic and trade drug names and verified drug dosages to assure that dosage information is precise and in accord with standards accepted at the time of publication. Readers are advised, however, to check the product information currently provided by the manufacturer of each drug to be administered to be certain that changes have not been made in the recommended dose or in the contraindications for administration. This is of particular importance in regard to new or infrequently used drugs. Recommended dosages for animals are sometimes based on adjustments in the dosage that would be suitable for humans. Some of the drugs mentioned here have been given experimentally by the authors. Others have been used in dosages greater than those recommended by the manufacturer. In these kinds of cases, the authors have reported on their own considerable experience. It is the responsibility of those administering a drug, relying on their professional skill and experience, to determine the dosages, the best treatment for the patient, and whether the benefits of giving a drug justify the attendant risk. The editors cannot be responsible for misuse or misapplication of the material in this work.

THE PUBLISHER

SMALL ANIMAL RADIOLOGY AND ULTRASONOGRAPHY:
A DIAGNOSTIC ATLAS AND TEXT

ISBN 0–7216–5270–0

PREFACE

This book continues with the goals stated in our first book, *Small Animal Radiology: A Diagnostic Atlas and Text*. We believe that the expanding interest in veterinary ultrasonography combined with continuing interest in veterinary radiology created a need for this book which presents diagnostic imaging in a pictorial format. We believe that radiography and ultrasonography are complementary imaging modalities. We have attempted to create a pictorial atlas which illustrates the radiographic and sonographic findings of most of the common (and some of the uncommon) diseases that affect dogs and cats. Normal studies have been included to provide a reference for appreciation of the pathologic. As with our first textbook, the intent of the text is to supplement the pictorial information.

We have again chosen to limit our images. Although we have not changed our opinion that at least two radiographic views and multiple ultrasonographic planes are needed for an accurate diagnosis, we have presented a single image for many of the lesions in order to present as many different lesions as possible. We also chose to exclude nuclear scintigrams, MRI and CT scans. We believe that these technologies will develop wider use in the future; however, for now, we feel our emphasis must be on radiography and ultrasonography.

As in our previous book, the author with primary responsibility for each chapter was accorded final discretion relative to the method of presentation and ultimate importance of specific material. Fortunately, disagreements were rare.

We would like express our appreciation for those who helped with this project. We are grateful to our colleagues whose many contributions to the veterinary literature have provided a basis for much of the information contained within the text. We are deeply indebted to the institutions and colleagues that have trained and supported us in the past (Henry Bergh Memorial Hospital of the ASPCA, University of Pennsylvania, University of Missouri, Columbia, and the University of California, Davis). We are especially grateful to our most recent institutional affiliations (The Animal Medical Center, Veterinary Specialists of South Florida and the University of Florida) for their moral and financial support as well as their case material. Finally, we are thankful for the patience, encouragement, and support (both collegial and emotional) of our spouses (Lisa Burk, VT, and Lourdes Corman, MD) as well as that of the children (Tiffany and Anthony Ackerman).

Ronald L. Burk, DVM, MS

Norman Ackerman, DVM

CONTENTS

Chapter One

INTRODUCTION

THE GENERAL CONTRIBUTION OF RADIOLOGY TO VETERINARY MEDICINE

The art and science of radiology became an integral part of veterinary medicine and surgery shortly after the exposure of the first radiographic films. This subsequently led to the publishing of the first English language text on the subject of radiology in canine practice.[1] Although many special radiographic procedures have been described since then, survey radiography remains the standard for the majority of antemortem anatomic diagnoses.

The computer's ability to manipulate data has been applied to various imaging technologies resulting in new images such as those seen with digital subtraction fluoroscopy, computerized tomography (CT), magnetic resonance imaging (MRI), nuclear scintigraphy, and diagnostic ultrasound. This technologic explosion has called for an expansion of veterinary expertise from just traditional diagnostic radiology to include all types of diagnostic imaging. Of these newer technologies, ultrasound has gained popularity most rapidly. While future developments in diagnostic imaging and the role for MRI, CT, and nuclear imaging remain to be defined, it is clear that diagnostic radiology and ultrasound will play an important and expanding role in the practice of small animal medicine and will contribute to improved health for pets.

THE ESSENTIALS OF RADIOGRAPHIC AND ULTRASOUND PHYSICS

The physics of radiology and ultrasound are complex, and merely mentioning the subject to some individuals elicits a response that ranges from fear to boredom. Several textbooks explain radiological and ultrasound physics in detail. Because our purpose is to emphasize radiographic and ultrasound diagnosis, these textbooks should be consulted if a more complete understanding of radiographic and ultrasound physics is desired.[2-7] A minimal knowledge of the physics of the processes involved is helpful to use radiology successfully. X-rays are electromagnetic radiations with very short wave lengths (high frequencies) and high energies. They are produced by bombarding a tungsten target with a stream of energetic electrons. The resulting x-ray beam is a collection of photons of different energies. These x-ray photons may pass through or be absorbed by a substance depending on their energy and the relative density, thickness, and atomic number of the substance. In medical radiology, after passing through body fluids, tissues, and/or organs, the photons ionize silver, which is contained in the emulsion of a photographic type of x-ray film. This may occur either directly, by interaction of the x-ray photon with the silver emulsion, or indirectly, by interaction of the x-ray photon with a fluorescent intensifying screen producing blue or green light which exposes the film. This pattern of ionized silver (the latent image) becomes visible after chemically developing and fixing the film. The visible image is a composite picture of the structures through which the x-rays passed before reaching the film. The radiograph is a 2-dimensional representation of 3-dimensional structures and represents the sum of their radiodensities and shapes.

Ultrasonography is based on the pulse echo principle. A pulse of high frequency sound (ultrasound) is transmitted into the body. This pulse travels through the body until it reaches a reflecting surface at which time a portion of the ultrasound pulse (the echo) is reflected back toward the source of the pulse. The transmitter keeps track of the time that elapses from the beginning of the pulse to the time the echo is received. This time is proportional to the distance the pulse traveled and allows for the determination of the reflecting surface's position and display of that position as a point on a cathode ray tube (CRT). The proportion of the pulse that is reflected is dependent upon the initial strength of the pulse, the ability of the reflecting surface to transmit sound (its acoustic properties), the angle at which the pulse strikes the reflecting surface, and the size of the reflecting surface relative to the size of the ultrasound beam. The amount of the ultrasound pulse that is reflected determines the brightness of the point produced on the CRT. If an adequate number of points can be transmitted and received, an image of the reflecting surfaces can be displayed on the CRT. This image is updated by sending multiple pulses and receiving multiple echoes in a relatively short period of time. The data are stored in a computer and transmitted to the CRT at a rate of 15 to 30 images per second. This produces a moving, flicker-free image on the CRT. This image is then recorded on video tape or on photographic film.

The echoes reflected from the body part being examined can also be displayed along a moving, time-oriented graph. This display is referred to as M-mode and is used most often in cardiology to display the motion of the ventricular walls, heart valves, and major vessels.

The transducer, which is used to both transmit and receive the ultrasound pulse, can vary in frequency. The higher the transducer frequency the greater the resolution and the lower the penetration of the sound beam. For most small animals, transducers in the 3 MHz to 7 MHz range are used. Ultrasound is subject to many artifacts. These have been described in detail and the physical principles governing their production have been explained.[2,3,5] Although we will discuss the effects of these artifacts on the image that is produced, these references should be consulted if a more complete understanding of the physical principles that produce these artifacts is desired.

RADIOGRAPHIC AND ULTRASOUND DIAGNOSIS

Several steps are required to obtain a radiographic diagnosis beginning with the patient's presentation and the recognition of the valuable information that radiography of a specific area may yield. Following this is the task of creating a diagnostic quality radiograph. The evaluation and interpretation of the radiograph are the next steps. Interpretation may lead to a specific diagnosis, but more often it leads to the development of a list of differential diagnoses based on the radiographic findings. Next, the clinician should compare the list of differential diagnoses with the possible diagnoses based on the patient's history and physical findings. The probability of a specific diagnosis should be factored into this evaluation. Finally, given all the data, a radiographic diagnosis or list of probable diagnoses should be developed. From this list, a plan for additional tests or further radiographic studies should be developed to confirm or deny the possible diagnoses or to establish a treatment plan.

Ultrasound diagnosis is also a multi-step process. In most cases the radiographic examination precedes the ultrasound examination. The size, shape, location, echo intensity, and homogeneity of the ultrasound images are evaluated. As in radiography, a list of differential diagnoses is developed and from this list a diagnostic or therapeutic plan is developed. Specific diagnoses may be determined; however, biopsy or needle aspirates are frequently required for a specific diagnosis and may be obtained with ultrasound guidance. Attempts to correlate echo intensity with tissue type have been unsuccessful. In many cases, a list of differential diagnoses will be developed based on the ultrasound findings.

INDICATIONS FOR RADIOGRAPHY AND ULTRASOUND

The indications for radiography are many. They range from recognition of specifically identifiable pathology (e.g., a palpable abdominal mass), to the evaluation for spread of disease (e.g., evaluating the lungs for metastasis from a tumor), to following the progression of either a disease or healing process, to the general evaluation of an area for any visible pathology. Radiographs provide excellent anatomic information but are limited in the evaluation of some tissues or organs. For example, the internal structure of the liver cannot be examined using non-contrast radiographs nor are radiographs useful for defining muscular anatomy.

Ultrasound is frequently performed in addition to radiography (e.g., for evaluation of the internal structure of an abdominal mass), but may be performed independent of the radiograph (e.g., for confirmation of a pregnancy). Ultrasound is superior to radiography in some circumstances but has limitations in other areas. Ultrasound provides information about size, shape, and location of structures; however, it also provides information about the architecture of the structure being examined. Ultrasound is best at distinguishing solid from cystic (fluid-filled) structures and provides internal detail not demonstrated radiographically. Abdominal masses should be evaluated to determine if they are solid or cystic and to determine if there are associated lesions in other areas (e.g., metastasis). Ultrasound is ideally suited for evaluation of animals with peritoneal fluid. In those patients with pleural fluid, mediastinal masses, or cardiac disease, ultrasound provides information that may not be evident on the radiograph. Pulmonary lesions are not usually accessible for ultrasound examination unless the area of lung involved is adjacent to the thoracic wall or surrounded by pleural fluid. Although ultrasound is not particularly useful for examination of the axial or appendicular skeleton or the skull, some information may be obtained from ultrasound evaluation of muscles, tendons, and the joints as well as examination of the orbit and brain (in animals with open fontanels).

Ultrasound is also extremely valuable for guiding fine needle aspirates or biopsies.[8] The needle can be observed as it passes through or into a lesion, and samples can be obtained from specific sites within an organ or mass (Fig. 1–1). When the needle cannot be identified, movement of the organ or lesion as the needle is moved can be used as indirect evidence of the needle's position. The individual performing the biopsy must be careful to ensure that the tip of the needle is identified. Air may be injected through the needle to identify the position of the tip of the needle. The tip of many biopsy needles has been roughened or coated to increase the intensity of the echo originating from it. Biopsy guides are helpful because they keep the needle in the plane of the transducer and often project the path of the needle onto the CRT. Biopsies may also be performed without the use of these guides with equal accuracy. Aspiration of fluid from cysts, abscesses, or hematomas can be performed to obtain samples for cytology or to reduce the size of the fluid-filled cavity. Ultrasound-guided biopsy is safe, with a serious complication rate of 1.2 percent in a review of 233 biopsies and 70 fine needle aspirates.[9] Major complications included perirenal hemorrhage and bile peritonitis. Minor local hemorrhage was identified in 5.6 percent of the patients in this study. Cats with hepatic lipidosis seem to be at greater risk for post-biopsy complications.

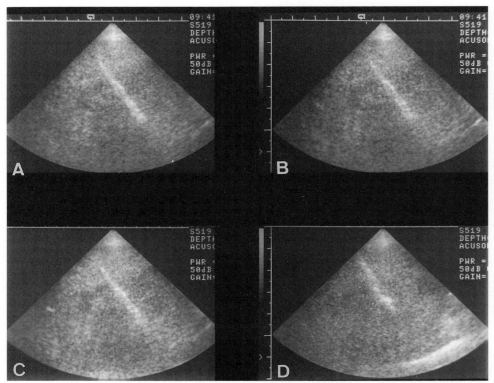

Figure 1–1. Transverse sonograms of the liver of a 10-year-old female mixed breed dog with a history of elevated liver enzymes and a mass arising from the lateral thoracic wall. A poorly defined hyperechoic lesion was noted in the ventral portion of the liver and a liver biopsy was performed to evaluate the lesion. The biopsy needle can be identified as a hyperechoic linear structure within the liver (A, B, & C). The hyperechoic line remains after the needle has been removed (D) because of the air that is injected at the time of the liver biopsy.

RADIOGRAPHIC AND ULTRASOUND TECHNIQUE

RADIOGRAPHIC TECHNIQUE

The overall radiographic technique must be correct or the radiograph should be repeated. Attempting to interpret an inferior radiograph will lead to an inferior diagnosis and may negatively impact the patient's care. The factors that must be considered in making diagnostic quality radiographs have been described in detail.[6,7] Using technique charts that change radiographic exposure with changes in patient size, and careful processing of the x-ray film using a time/temperature relationship, are strongly recommended. The factors that we would like to emphasize are the overall radiographic technique, patient preparation, and patient positioning for the particular study. Radiographic technique must be assessed for under- or overexposure as well as for inadequate penetration. Exposure is evaluated relatively easily because the exposed portion of the radiograph over which there was no animal (i.e., that part surrounding the animal's surface) should be completely blackened. Failure to accomplish this despite normal film processing indicates inadequate milliamp-seconds (mAs). If the film had adequate exposure but the area covered by the patient is still too light, then the kilovolt (peak) (kV(p)) should be increased. The standard increase in kV(p) to be able to visually detect a difference is 15 to 20 percent. If the overall film is too dark either the mAs or kV(p) should be reduced. Because it is difficult to discern which parameter should be adjusted, we recommend a decrease in mAs by reducing the exposure time. If this causes the radiograph to be light by virtue of inadequate radiation (i.e., too light in the areas not covered by the animal), the mAs should be restored and the kV(p) decreased. Inadequate penetration will result when the kV(p) is too low and the photon energy is insufficient to penetrate the subject. Increasing the kV(p) will produce more energetic photons, which will penetrate the subject. If this increase results in a radiograph that is too black (over exposed) the mAs must be decreased. As a general rule, a change in kV(p) of 15 to 20 percent is the equivalent of a two-fold change in mAs.

Proper patient preparation may be critical in discovering radiographic evidence of pathology. Although food restriction and enemas are not performed routinely prior to abdominal radiography, as a general rule the animal should not be fed and should be allowed to empty its bladder and colon if abdominal radiographs are anticipated. A stomach full of ingesta or a colon distended with feces may obscure an abdominal mass or interfere with evaluation of other organs. A long-haired animal that is wet may have the density of the hair superimposed over bone and this may mimic or obscure a fracture line.

Another critical factor to evaluate is the patient's positioning, which should be as perfect as possible. The oblique radiograph lends itself to misinterpretation, which may ultimately lead to decisions that harm the patient. Whenever an abnormality is detected, the possibility that it results from malpositioning must always be considered. Tracheal elevation, which may indicate cardiomegaly or a cranial mediastinal mass, may also be caused by failure to elevate the sternum or failure to extend the head and neck when positioning the animal for a lateral thoracic radiograph. Therefore, it is critical to insist on properly positioned radiographs and to require repeat radiographs and sedation or anesthesia, if necessary, to achieve proper positioning. Tranquilization or anesthesia may actually reduce the stress of radiography and may prove to be less dangerous than struggling with the animal to obtain a properly positioned radiograph. In addition, sedation may avoid the need for multiple attempts before obtaining a satisfactory radiograph.

At least two views taken at 90° angles to each other are almost always required. Without these it is impossible to create a mental image of the three dimensions of the structures of interest. Furthermore, some pathologies are more readily apparent on one view than the other, and if only one view is taken some diagnoses may be missed. In some circumstances two views taken at 180° to each other may be adequate. Comparison of right and left lateral recumbent radiographs of the abdomen may provide specific information about the gastrointestinal (GI) tract, because the air and fluid within the GI tract move with gravity. This may be adequate to identify gastric outflow obstruction or gastric dilatation volvulus in patients that are too sick for positioning in dorsal recumbency. Right and left lateral thoracic radiographs can provide information nearly equal to that obtained from a lateral and a ventrodorsal view.

ULTRASOUND TECHNIQUE

Ultrasound is both operator dependent and time consuming. The operator must be knowledgeable about normal anatomy, especially the positional relationships between anatomical structures such as abdominal organs and cardiac chambers. Familiarity with the artifacts commonly seen during an ultrasound examination is necessary. Because only a small area of the body is examined at one time and ultrasound does not produce the global image of anatomy provided by radiography, it is extremely important that the sonographer has a great deal of imaging experience. The images must be interpreted as they are acquired, and hard copies are usually made to document an observation rather than to produce something to be interpreted at a later date.

The quality of the ultrasound image is determined by the transducer selected, the gain settings on the machine, and the preparation of the patient. Patient preparation should include clipping the hair over the region of interest. Hair will trap air and this interferes with sound transmission. In areas with thin or fine hair, the air may be eliminated by wetting the hair with water or alcohol. After the hair has been clipped or dampened, ultrasound gel is used to ensure good contact and sound transmission from the transducer to the animal's tissues. If the ultrasound examination precedes the radiographic examination, the hair must be thoroughly cleaned after the ultrasound examination to avoid radiographic artifacts produced by wet or gel-contaminated hair.

A specific artifact often occurs at the point of contact between the transducer and the skin. This has been termed a reverberation artifact and produces a bright image area at the point of contact. The brightness of this artifact may vary with different ultrasound units, but in some units it interferes with examination of superficial structures.

The gain settings on the machine are used to vary the strength of the echo that returns from the structure of interest. Since the strength of the ultrasound beam decreases with increasing depth within the tissues, the machine can be adjusted to compensate for the loss of signal. In most machines this compensation is variable, with a slope that adjusts for the increasing loss of signal caused by sound reflection and refraction from tissues interposed between the transducer and the deepest structure to be imaged. The transducer should be selected based upon the thickness of the area that is being examined. Decreasing transducer frequency correlates with increased depth of ultrasound penetration with an accompanying loss of resolution. The transducer that is selected should be of a frequency that adequately penetrates the subject without having to set the gain too high. If the signal is not strong enough (e.g., the image is too black), the gain setting should be increased or a lower frequency transducer selected. If the signal is too bright, the gain should be decreased or a higher frequency transducer selected. The use of a high frequency transducer at high gain settings to compensate for lack of ultrasound penetration produces artifacts that may result in incorrect interpretation. Because air and bone reflect a large percentage of the ultrasound beam, the direction from which the organ is being imaged may be altered to avoid imaging through them. This is important when imaging the heart (e.g., the cardiac window is selected because of the absence of lung at the cardiac notch on the right side; the patient is imaged from below to take advantage of lung atelectasis on the recumbent side) and is also important when imaging the abdomen (e.g., the liver may be imaged through the intercostal spaces if the stomach is full of air and located between the usual position of the transducer caudal to the costochondral junctions; the liver and the air-filled bowel may be displaced away from the examination area by pushing on the abdominal wall using the transducer).

Patient positioning for ultrasound varies with the examination being performed. Many ultrasonographers prefer to examine the abdomen with the patient in dorsal recumbency. Most of the examination is performed from the ventral abdominal wall with some areas, such as the liver and gall bladder, examined through an intercostal space. Some individuals prefer to examine the abdomen with the patient in lateral recumbency. Much of this preference is a matter of training and experience, because a satisfactory examination can be performed from either position. If an animal cannot be restrained in either position, the examination may be accomplished with the patient standing. For cardiac examination, most individuals prefer to position the animal in lateral recumbency with the examination performed from the dependent side. This produces a larger air free cardiac window. The examination may be performed from the up side; however, inflation of the lung can reduce the size of the cardiac window. For examining most other body areas, the position that is most comfortable for the operator and the patient should be satisfactory.

SYSTEMATIC EVALUATION FOR RADIOGRAPHIC AND ULTRASOUND PATHOLOGY

The importance of systematically evaluating a radiograph needs to be emphasized repeatedly. The tendency to rely on inspiration and first impressions in evaluating radiographs is a poor practice that will result in diagnostic errors. It is difficult to ignore the presenting signs and concentrate solely on the radiographic information, especially when the clinician and radiographer are one and the same person; however, this should be attempted. Ideally, the radiographs should first be evaluated without knowledge or consideration of the animal's history or clinical signs. Then, the radiographs should be reevaluated in light of the patient's history and clinical signs for the purpose of answering those questions raised by the animal's presenting findings. There are several systems for radiographic evaluation including the inside-out method (i.e., beginning at the center of the radiograph and observing structures in ever enlarging concentric circles), the outside-in method (i.e., the opposite of the inside-out method), and the inventory method (i.e., evaluating each organ according to a predetermined list of those structures that should be present in any given area). The method used is a matter of personal preference and training experience; however, once adopted the method should be used consistently.

Ultrasound examinations should proceed in an orderly fashion with each organ or area of the animal being evaluated completely. Most organs should be evaluated in at least two planes. In some areas, such as cardiac ultrasound, these planes have been very well defined and should be adhered to strictly so that artifacts which mask or mimic disease are not created. In other areas, the planes are less well-defined and oblique or off axis views may be as valuable as the standard examination planes. Ultrasound is usually performed with some specific area of interest (e.g., evaluation of a mass in the region of the spleen). This area should be carefully evaluated, but other structures may be important in determining a final diagnosis and these should also be examined (e.g., presence of focal abnormalities within the liver in a patient with a splenic mass). The ultrasound examination of specific organs or anatomical regions must be approached from more than one angle or direction. For example, when examining the kidney the transducer should be moved from the cranial to the caudal pole in the transverse plane and from both medial to lateral and dorsal to ventral in the longitudinal plane. Each organ or region is examined carefully with attention being paid to the pattern of echoes produced as well as to the brightness of the echoes when compared to adjacent structures. The size of many structures can be measured precisely using calipers that are coupled to the computer and CRT. The examination must be complete.

RADIOGRAPHIC CHARACTERISTICS

The identity of any structure can be deduced from its radiographic appearance. Normal radiographic anatomy is learned from evaluating a large number of normal studies. This is particularly true for recognizing the normal anatomical variants that occur in different breeds. The comparison between the observed image and the expected normal appearance provides data upon which deductive reasoning is applied to form the basis for a radiographic diagnosis.

Certain radiographic features are used to determine the nature of an object seen on the x-ray film. These features are used to determine both normal anatomy as well as pathologic alterations and should be evaluated for every structure examined on the radiograph. These characteristics include size, shape, density, position, and architecture. In addition to these characteristics, some functional information can be derived from the radiograph.

SIZE

The size of an object can be determined directly by measuring the object as it appears on the radiograph, by comparing the object of interest to some adjacent normal structure, or by use of a non-specific term which reflects a subjective impression of relative size. Measurement of objects directly from the x-ray film image ignores the distortion that results from magnification of the image due to the distance from the object to the film. It also ignores geometric distortion which may occur because of x-ray beam divergence. The object may not be parallel to the film plane and may therefore be unevenly magnified. Thus, the size of a bone pin required to repair a fracture may be overestimated, because the femur is separated from the film by the thigh muscles and therefore the medullary diameter is actually less than that measured on the radiograph. One femur may appear shorter than the other in a ventrodorsal pelvic radiograph if the animal is experiencing pain and the affected hip cannot be extended to the same extent as the normal leg. To compensate for geometric distortion and to permit comparison between animals of greatly different sizes, comparison to some adjacent normal structure is often used. Thus, the length of the kidney is often compared to that of the second lumbar vertebra. Normal ranges for such comparisons have been established. Subjective impressions of organ size may also be made, and these are usually based on previous experience. Enlargement of the spleen, heart, and prostate, for example, are often diagnosed based on a subjective opinion of how big that structure has appeared on other radiographs of similar size animals.

SHAPE

Objects may be distinguished on the radiograph according to their shape. Distinction can be made between solid and hollow objects, spheres, cylinders and cubes, and flat or curved surfaces. Each produces a specific image. The image that is produced on the x-ray film differs from the patient's anatomy, because the radiograph is a 2-dimensional representation of a 3-dimensional structure. Overlapping of different structures as well as photographic and visual illusions may produce apparent images that do not truly represent normal anatomy. When the shape of a density does not conform to that of any normal anatomic structure or to any described pathology, the probability of a radiographic artifact is high. These may be readily apparent, because they occur infrequently and are so different from previously observed anatomy. However, some may mimic pathologic processes and must be recognized. A subjective contour artifact in which a geometric contour can be constructed from partial lines has been described (Fig. 1–2). This artifact often appears brighter or more prominent and appears to be closer to the viewer than normal structures. The artifact will disappear on closer examination.

DENSITY

Density is the mass of a structure per unit volume. It is a major factor in determining the amount of radiation that various objects absorb. Objects that absorb most or all of the radiation impinging upon them are termed *radiopaque*. The photons do not pass through these objects and therefore neither reach nor expose the x-ray film. These structures produce a clear area on the film which appears white or light gray when viewed. Objects that permit most of the radiation to pass through them are termed *radiolucent* and produce a black or dark gray image on the x-ray film.

Relative Density versus Absolute Density

The density of objects relative to one another determines their apparent shade of black, white, or gray on the x-ray film. Therefore, an understanding of relative subject densities is essential to the interpretation of a radiographic image. In terms of radiographic density, the animal may be considered as being composed of five components: (1) air (in the respiratory or GI tracts); (2) fat or cartilage (both have the same radiographic density); (3) tissue (including blood, body fluids, muscle, and various parenchymal organs); (4) bone; and (5) metal (usually because of ingestion or introduction through accident or surgery). These elements can easily be ranked in order of decreasing subject density when their composition is considered. Metallic objects, the most dense, have a high atomic number and absorb nearly all of the x-ray photons; this prevents the ionization of the silver in the photographic emulsion and causes a white image on the radiographic film. Various metallic foreign ob-

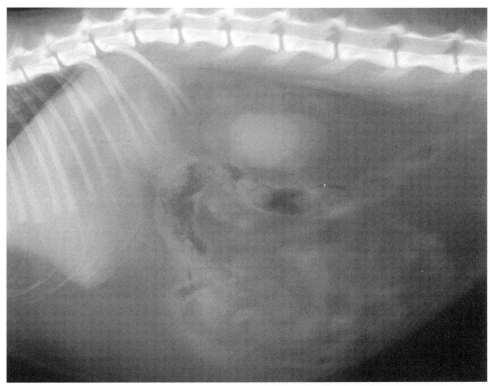

Figure 1–2. Lateral abdominal radiograph of a mature cat. The caudal pole of the right kidney and the cranial pole of the left kidney overlap producing a subjective contour artifact. This artifact appears brighter than the real shadows of the kidneys.

jects produce this radiographic density: surgical devices such as intramedullary pins, metallic sutures or hemostatic clips, minerals such as stones, or barium containing compounds. Bone, which is composed of elements having a somewhat lower atomic number and an organic matrix which absorbs less radiation, produces a nearly white or light gray image. Muscles, blood, and various organs, which are composed predominately of water and absorb approximately equal amounts of radiation, produce comparable shades of gray on the film. Therefore, these objects are described as fluid- or tissue-dense. This shade of gray is darker than that of bone. Fat and cartilage absorb even less radiation than the fluid- or tissue-dense elements and produce a darker gray image on the film. Air or gas absorbs the least amount of radiation and produces a black image. Therefore, the usual components of an animal being radiographed in order of decreasing subject densities are metal, bone, tissue, fat or cartilage, and air.

The density of an object may appear to change when it is surrounded by an object of different density. This is an optical illusion and can be observed when a dense cystic calculus, which appears white on a non-contrast radiograph, is surrounded by dense iodine-containing contrast material during a contrast cystogram. The white cystic calculus appears gray when surrounded by the more opaque (denser) contrast (Fig. 1–3). When tissue-dense structures, such as the prepuce or a nipple, which are surrounded by air, are seen on a ventrodorsal radiograph superimposed on the remaining abdominal structures they often appear to be bone dense.

Another visual illusion that results from density differences is the Mach band effect.[10] In this phenomenon, either a bright or a dark line may occur at borders of structures. The Mach band effect is caused by a specific physiologic process in the normal eye. This may be readily observed in the hind limb where the fibula crosses the tibia producing an apparent dark line which might be mistaken for a fracture

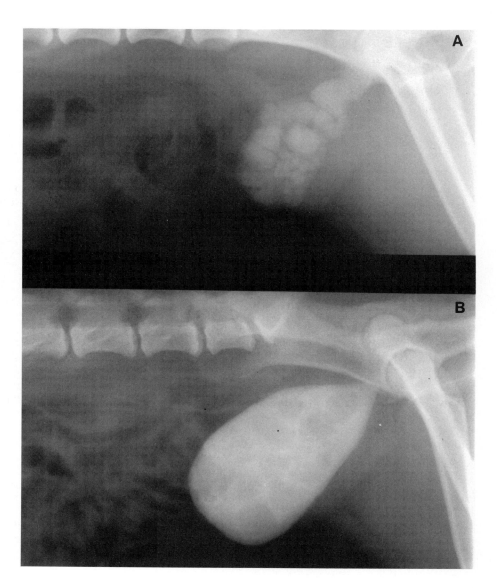

Figure 1–3. Close-up views of lateral abdominal radiographs of a mature dog before (A) and after (B) the intravenous administration of water soluble iodinated contrast material. The radiopaque cystic calculi appear white (dense) on the non-contrast radiograph (A) and appear gray (less dense) when surrounded by the more opaque contrast material (B). This is an optical illusion and if measured by means of a densitometer the opacity of the calculi would be identical in both images.

(Fig. 1–4). This effect may be seen in any area in which two objects of different density are adjacent to one another.

The thickness of a structure is also important in determining the relative subject density evident on an x-ray film. Thicker or larger volumes of the same material will absorb more radiation and produce an image that is whiter; however, the effect is less than that resulting from an inherent density difference. Therefore, the size of the structure must also be considered when its composition is being deduced from its radiographic appearance.

The size and shape of objects are perceived by visual definition of their external borders. The ability to perceive these borders requires that objects be adjacent to something of a different density. For example, some species of jellyfish are nearly invisible in water because they contain so much water themselves. Yet a fish, such as a tuna, is readily apparent in water and easily described by size and shape. To discriminate between objects on a radiograph, they must be of different subject densities. Whenever an object of one density lies against an object of a different density, a margin will be evident. The greater the difference between the densities of the two objects, the sharper the margin will appear on the radiographic film. Conversely, whenever two objects of the same density lie in contact with each other, their margins will not be visible. In the abdomen, for example, the presence of abdominal fat

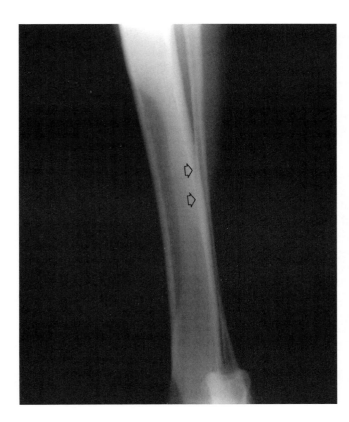

Figure 1–4. Close up view of a cranial-caudal radiograph of the tibia and fibula of a mature dog. A radiolucent (dark) line is visible in the mid-tibia at the point where the fibula crosses the tibia (*arrows*). This is a Mach line and should not be confused with a fracture.

outlines the tissue-dense abdominal organs, and the inner surface of the stomach and intestines can often be identified because they contain air. Evaluation of the bowel wall will demonstrate that the inner wall, which is in contact with the lumenal gas, is better defined than the outer wall, which is in contact with the surrounding abdominal fat. This is because of the greater difference in subject density between the air and tissue-dense structures when compared to the fat and tissue-dense structures.

POSITION

The position of objects on a radiograph is also used to establish their identity. The object must be identified on two views to establish its location. For example, certain abdominal organs will normally be found in specific areas within the abdominal cavity. An ovoid tissue-dense mass in the caudal ventral abdomen would most likely be the urinary bladder or associated with the male or female reproductive tract (i.e., prostate, retained testicle, uterine body, or cervical mass). Abdominal organs may also displace other structures from their normal position. Thus, enlargement of the spleen will displace the intestines caudally, dorsally, and to the right. The displacement of the intestines indicates that the mass is originating from the cranial, ventral, left abdomen and is therefore associated with the spleen. Some diseases produce lesions that may be seen radiographically in specific locations. For example, primary tumors of long bones are usually metaphyseal in location while metastatic tumors are more frequently diaphyseal. The lesion's location may therefore help discriminate between these two conditions, which might otherwise have similar radiographic features. In some circumstances, failure to identify an abnormality on a second view will help to establish its location. For example, identification of a mass in the hilar region of the lung on a lateral radiograph and inability to identify the mass on a ventrodorsal radiograph helps to localize the mass to the mediastinum or hilus and, therefore, indicates that the mass is not located in the lung.

ARCHITECTURE

The term "architecture" is used to describe the internal structure (when visible) of an object and is stated in terms of homogeneity, granularity, or irregularity. Architecture may also refer to the definition of the object or extent to which its margins are definable. Thus, the trabeculation of a bone may be evaluated and alterations from stress remodeling, tumor destruction, or osteopenia may be recognized. Food or fecal material may also be recognized as a granular mixture of air, soft tissue, and bone.

FUNCTION

Contrast radiography is usually required in order to obtain functional information. Even with contrast studies, evaluation of physiologic levels of function is not usually possible. However, it is possible to recognize some anatomic changes on non-contrast radiographs that indicate abnormal function. An example would be colonic distension with granular material suggesting difficulty or interference with defecation. Another example is the dilation of the small intestine to a greater than normal diameter, which may indicate interference with peristalsis or obstruction to normal flow of ingesta. Identification of an enlarged caudal vena cava and hepatomegaly in a dog with right heart disease may indicate that right heart failure rather than merely right heart disease is present.

ULTRASOUND CHARACTERISTICS

Certain features should also be evaluated during an ultrasound examination. These include size, shape, echo intensity, position, and architecture.

SIZE

Most structures can be directly measured using the calipers, which are integrated with the software used in the ultrasound machine. These calipers are very accurate and specific measurements can be made. Very large organs, such as the liver, are difficult to measure as the extent of the organ is rarely imaged in a single frame. In these cases, a subjective impression of the organ size is obtained by estimating the amount of the external body surface that is covered while the entire organ is examined. The operator should be careful when making the measurements to ensure that the angle at which the measurement is being made corresponds to some established standard. For example, specific values have been established for measurement of the cardiac chambers, however oblique off-axis measurements may obscure or mimic disease.

SHAPE

As in evaluation of size, the shape of an object can be distorted if an off-axis view is obtained. Ultrasound is sensitive to alterations in shape of structures. These abnormalities are easily and accurately demonstrated provided the organ is imaged from some standard position. In order to obtain good transducer skin contact, pressure is often applied to the abdomen when performing an abdominal ultrasound examination. This can distort the shape of structures, and is usually most apparent in examination of the urinary bladder. The bladder shape can be distorted because of transducer pressure.

ECHO INTENSITY

The echo intensity of an organ is usually specific to that organ, however it may be altered by machine settings, the transducer selected, patient preparation, the angle with which the sound beam strikes the organ, and the nature of the tissue that surrounds the organ of interest. Poor contact between the transducer and the skin may cause structures to appear hypoechoic. Increased gain settings or lower frequency transducers may make deeper structures appear more echogenic. The echo intensity of abdominal organs is usually compared to other abdominal organs. Thus, the kidney is described as being hypoechoic (blacker) and the spleen is described as being hyperechoic (whiter) relative to the liver. Ultrasound artifacts also affect an organ's echointensity. In the presence of peritoneal fluid, the abdominal organs may appear to be more echogenic. The portion of the liver that is imaged through the gall bladder may appear more echogenic (brighter) than the portion away from the gall bladder. Angling the transducer away from the perpendicular during examination of a tendon will decrease the echointensity of the tendon.

POSITION

An organ's position can be readily detected with ultrasound. Both abdominal masses and normal structures may be displaced from their natural position by transducer manipulation. This can make it difficult to determine the origin of the mass. Displacement from normal position can be recognized when the architecture of the organ is normal. For example, displacement of the kidney from its usual position may create some confusion, especially if the architecture is altered and recognition of the structure as a kidney is difficult.

ARCHITECTURE

The echo pattern of normal organs is usually specific. The structure may be anechoic (lacking internal echoes), uniformly echogenic, or may be of mixed echogenicity. Some organs can be recognized because of their specific echo pattern. The liver can be identified because of the bright parallel echoes produced by the portal veins, and the spleen can be recognized because of the pattern of vessels entering the hilus.

RADIOGRAPHIC AND ULTRASOUND ABNORMALITIES

When an abnormality is detected on a radiograph, the possibilities that must be considered are: (1) the radiographic change was caused by a specific disease, (2) the radiographic change represents a normal anatomic variant, or (3) the radiographic change is the result of a technical or physical artifact. In most instances, when the radiographic abnormality is identified on only one view or is the only change identified despite the fact that the expected disease almost always presents with several different radiographic changes, it is highly likely that the change represents a normal anatomic variant or radiographic artifact.

Although a radiograph should be evaluated initially without consideration of the patient's history or clinical signs, it should then be reevaluated after these facts have been determined. This "second look" should detect any abnormalities that are expected based upon the presumptive diagnosis. For example, if a dog is radiographed for evaluation of urinary tract disease, the original viewing should evaluate the entire abdomen. The "second look" should concentrate upon the urinary tract. This may be helpful in deciding that densities originally ascribed to ingested matter in the intestinal tract are actually calcification in the kidneys or ureters, or perhaps that renal shadows were difficult to define. If this patient were being radiographed for a dystocia, this condition might be overlooked or considered insignificant because of normal decrease in abdominal fat in a heavily lactating bitch; however, this new information may be extremely important in a dog with polyuria, polydipsia, and vomiting. Additional radiographs obtained after administration of enemas or laxatives, extra views, selective abdominal compression, or radiographic contrast studies may be necessary to completely or properly evaluate the patient.

This "second look" often helps put the radiographic findings in their proper perspective. For example, a narrowed intervertebral disc space may indicate acute or previous disc prolapse and only the patient's clinical signs can establish if the disc prolapse is acute. Shoulder osteochondrosis and panosteitis may be identified on radiographs of the shoulder of a young, large breed dog. Only a careful physical examination will determine which of the two lesions is responsible for the dog's acute lameness. If the radiographic changes do not fit the animal's clinical signs, either the radiographic changes, the clinical signs, or both should be reevaluated.

Generally, a single disease produces several recognizable radiographic changes. The more of these radiographic changes present on a single study, the more reliable the radiographic diagnosis becomes. Thus, the radiologist should be aware of the possible variations that may occur with a disease and not rely on the presence or absence of a single, falsely labeled "pathognomonic" radiographic change.

Similar considerations accompany ultrasound abnormalities. Artifacts are a greater problem in ultrasound than in radiography, because the technique is extremely operator dependent. Artifacts frequently seen during ultrasound exams include shadowing, distant enhancement, reverberation, beam width, and section thickness. Shadowing is a frequently observed acoustic artifact which results in a decrease or absence of signal in areas that should contain echoes (Figs. 1–5 and 1–6). It results from attenuation or reflection of the sound beam from a highly reflecting surface. Because of this, the pulse is almost completely reflected and is unable to reach deeper structures, producing a black area deep to the reflecting surface. Shadowing is most often observed beneath bone or air but may also be seen deep to catheters, drains, or vascular clips. The shadow will hide the underlying anatomy. This is frequently seen when the air-filled stomach or the ribs hide portions of the liver. The presence of a shadow also provides useful information. It indicates the presence of a highly reflective surface and helps the operator recognize the presence of gas or mineral. Not all mineral materials shadow completely, therefore, the absence of shadowing does not rule out the presence of mineralization.

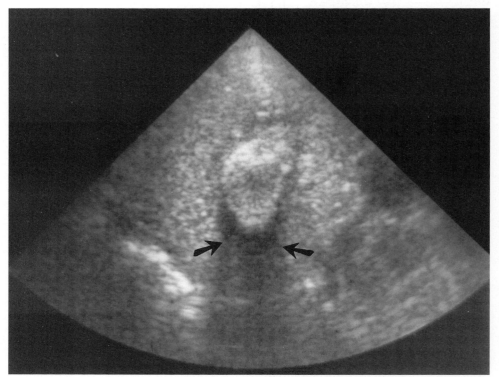

Figure 1–5. Transverse sonogram of the left kidney of a mature dog. There is a hypoechoic (black) band (*arrows*) extending deep to the renal pelvis. This decrease in signal is a shadowing artifact which results from reflection or attenuation of the ultrasound beam by renal pelvic mineralization. Although the renal pelvis is slightly hyperechoic the shadowing helps to confirm that renal pelvic mineralization is present.

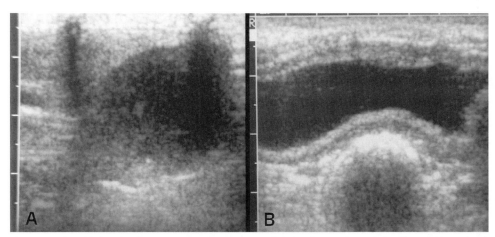

Figure 1–6. Abdominal sonograms of a mature dog in the region of the liver (A) and urinary bladder (B). The ribs produce hypoechoic (black) bands (*arrows*) which extend deep to their position (A). The colon also produces a hypoechoic band (*arrows*) deep to its position (B). Shadowing may be due to the presence of bone (A) or gas (B). Also note the distortion of the bladder due to transducer pressure.

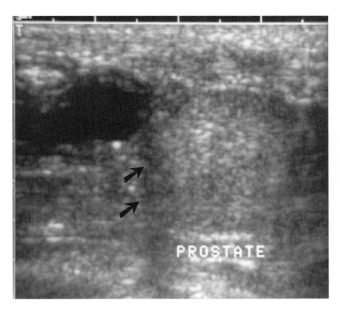

Figure 1–7. Longitudinal sonogram of the caudal abdomen of a mature male dog. The anechoic urinary bladder and prostate are visible. A hypoechoic (black) band can be seen cranial to the margin of the prostate (*arrows*). This is a refraction artifact.

Refraction, or bending, of the ultrasound beam can produce an artifact similar to a shadowing artifact (Fig. 1–7). This occurs when the ultrasound beam passes through a highly echogenic interface. A decrease in the intensity of the ultrasound beam results, and there may be no sound left to produce echoes from the structures deep to the interface. This may occur beneath the walls of fluid-filled structures such as cysts. The area beneath the structure causing the acoustic shadow may have some echoes because of reverberation, beam width, or slice thickness artifacts.

Acoustic enhancement results in stronger signals deep to fluid-filled structures (Fig. 1–8). These structures have no internal echoes to reduce the amount of sound transmitted across them, resulting in increased echoes from the underlying structures. This enhancement artifact is used as one of the criteria which helps to identify the presence of fluid within a structure.

Reverberation occurs when the sound beam is bounced back and forth between the transducer and a highly reflective interface within the patient (Figs. 1–9 and 1–10). The computer interprets each reverberation as a separate signal, placing the

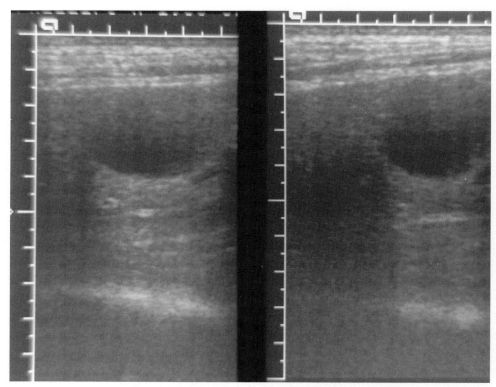

Figure 1–8. Longitudinal sonograms of the cranial abdomen of a dog. The liver and gall bladder are visible. The portion of the liver deep to the gall bladder appears more echogenic (brighter) than the area cranial and caudal to the gall bladder. This is because of acoustic enhancement. The fluid within the gall bladder does not attenuate the ultrasound to the same extent as the liver thereby increasing the strength of the echoes from that portion of the liver deep to the gall bladder.

source of the signal at a distance corresponding to the time elapsed from signal transmission to echo reception. Comet tail and ring down artifacts are forms of reverberation artifacts (Fig. 1–11). The comet tail artifact may originate at a highly reflective surface, such as a fluid:gas interface, and is helpful in indicating the presence of air. The ring down artifact commonly occurs within metals and is often observed in association with biopsy needles or metallic foreign objects. Reverberations are more likely to occur when the interface is close to the transducer, at highly reflecting surfaces, and when high gain settings are used. Reverberations can also occur within a structure such as a cyst, in which the echoes may be reflected off the far wall of the cyst back toward the near wall and then toward the far wall again. Thus, the signal resulting from reverberations may be impossible to distinguish from real echoes. Air and bone are the most common sources of reverberation artifacts. Increasing the gain only increases the intensity of the reverberations; therefore, echoes that are observed beyond bone and gas interfaces are artifacts.

A mirror-image artifact is also a form of reverberation artifact (Fig. 1–12). This is observed most often when examining the liver, and produces an image of the liver on the thoracic side of the diaphragm. The image is a mirror of that seen on the abdominal side of the diaphragm.

The ultrasound beam has a finite dimension, consequently echoes that originate from structures within the center as well as from the edges of the beam are included in the image. These produce beam width or section thickness artifacts and can be responsible for adding echoes to an anechoic structure or subtracting echoes from a hyperechoic structure (Figs. 1–13 and 1–14). This can result in the false presence of echogenic material within the urinary or gall bladder. Electronic noise may also add echoes to an anechoic structure.

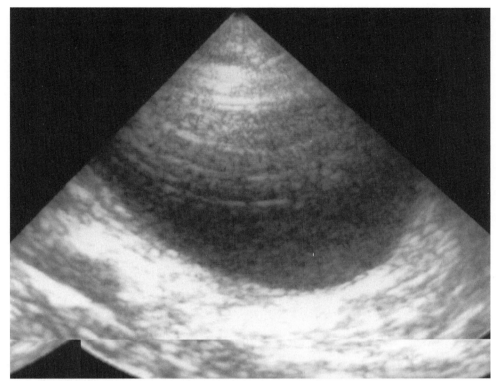

Figure 1–9. Longitudinal sonogram of the urinary bladder of a dog. A series of echogenic (bright) parallel lines can be seen within the superficial portion of the urinary bladder. These are reverberation artifacts. They may be originating at the skin surface or from the dorsal bladder wall. They are accentuated by the high-gain setting that was used to obtain this image.

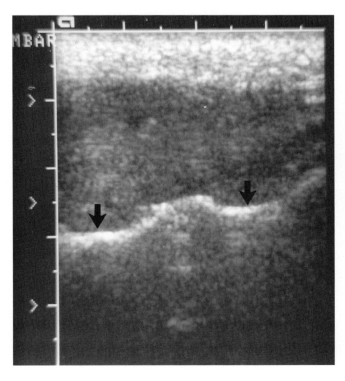

Figure 1–10. Longitudinal sonogram of the caudal lumbar region of a dog. The ventral surface of the lumbar vertebra is visible as a highly echogenic curved line (*arrows*). The echoes that are visible deep to the vertebral bodies are reverberation artifacts. The heteroechoic mass ventral to the vertebral bodies represents enlarged sublumbar lymph nodes.

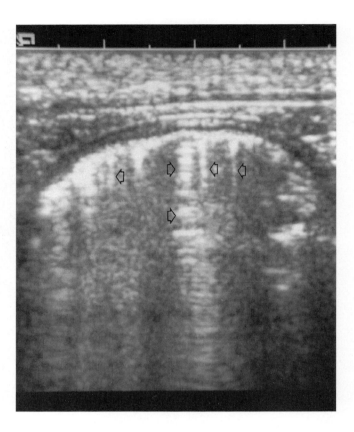

Figure 1–11. Transverse sonogram of the stomach of a dog. The echogenic bands (*arrows*) extending deep to the gastric wall represent comet tail and ring down reverberation artifacts. These result from the highly reflective interface between the gastric wall and intraluminal air. All the echoes within the gastric lumen are artifacts.

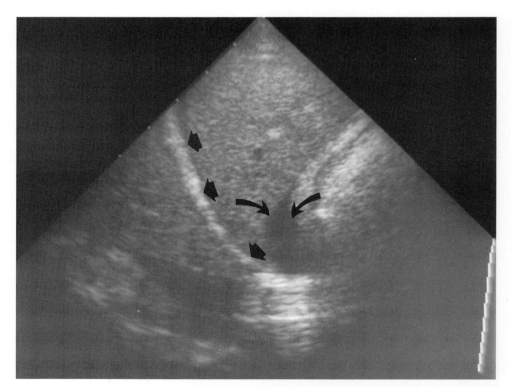

Figure 1–12. Longitudinal sonogram of the cranial abdomen of a cat. The diaphragm is evident as an echogenic (bright) curved line (*arrows*). The normal liver can be seen adjacent and caudal to the diaphragm and a mirror image of the liver can also be identified deep and cranial to the diaphragm. There is a small amount of anechoic peritoneal fluid (*curved arrows*) in the dorsal abdomen between the liver and stomach.

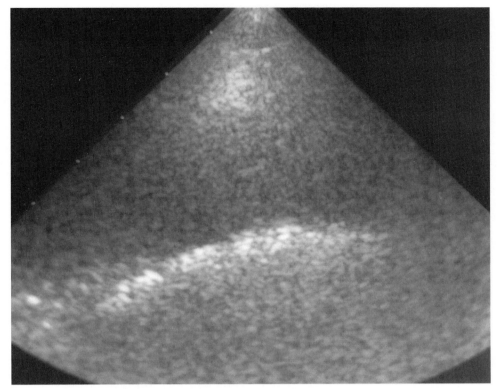

Figure 1–13. Longitudinal sonogram of the urinary bladder of a dog. There are many echoes within the bladder lumen. These are the result of reverberation or electronic noise artifacts. These artifacts add echoes to the normally anechoic urine and could be misinterpreted as echogenic cellular material within the urinary bladder.

Because of the number of artifacts that occur during an ultrasound examination, when an abnormality is observed it must be evaluated carefully to determine that it is not an artifact. The ultrasound lesion must fit the patient's clinical signs. Lesions detected that are not consistent with those signs should be suspect. The ultrasonographer must be aware of the lesions that may accompany the presumptive diagnosis. If an area in which a lesion would be anticipated (based on the presumptive diagnosis) cannot be thoroughly evaluated because of poor patient cooperation or interference from overlying gas or bone, the sonographer should be prepared to repeat the ultrasound examination or to suggest alternative diagnostic techniques or additional patient preparation, anesthesia, or sedation. As with radiographs, rarely is the ultrasound diagnosis specific, and additional studies, such as aspiration or biopsy, are frequently required for a specific anatomic diagnosis. Difficulty in examining certain patients adds to the problem in determining a specific ultrasound diagnosis.

DEVELOPING A DIFFERENTIAL DIAGNOSIS

After an abnormality has been identified radiographically or ultrasonographically using the features described in this chapter, a list of differential diagnoses should be established. This list should include all possible causes of the described radiographic or ultrasound abnormalities. Diagnoses should include all possible etiologies: toxic, infectious, metabolic, nutritional, degenerative, neoplastic, iatrogenic, immune, idiopathic, and developmental. The probable diagnosis is usually based on determining which of the differential diagnoses can produce all of the radiographic or ultrasonographic abnormalities observed. This probable diagnosis may be specific (e.g.,

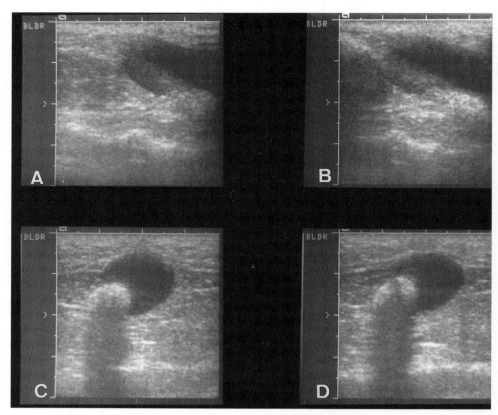

Figure 1–14. Longitudinal (A & B) and transverse (C & D) sonograms of the urinary bladder of a 4-year-old female mixed breed dog with a 2-week history of vomiting and diarrhea. In the longitudinal sonograms (A & B) there is a hyperechoic area that appears to be within the dorsal aspect of the urinary bladder. In the transverse sonograms (C & D) this hyperechoic area is identified as the colon, which is indenting the dorsal lateral aspect of the bladder. This creates a beam-width or slice-thickness artifact because, due to the width of the ultrasound beam, a portion of the colon is included along with the urinary bladder when the longitudinal sonogram was obtained.

osteosarcoma in the case of a bone tumor with a sunburst pattern in the distal radius of a 9-year-old male Saint Bernard; renal cyst in the case of a focal anechoic area within the kidney) or general (e.g., an enlarged kidney in a 5-year-old mixed breed female dog; increased echogenicity of the liver in a cat with hepatomegaly).

RECOMMENDATION FOR FURTHER DIAGNOSTICS OR THERAPY

Once a radiographic or ultrasound diagnosis is reached, a program for confirmation of the diagnosis or for treatment of the problem should be developed. This step is the result to which the radiograph or ultrasound examination is properly oriented. Further diagnostics that might be indicated include additional diagnostic imaging procedures, blood tests, endoscopy, aspiration, ultrasound-guided biopsy, or surgical exploration. Treatment plans might include pharmacologic therapies (e.g., antibiotics for pneumonia) or surgical treatments (e.g., partial ligation of porto-systemic shunts).

REFERENCES

1. Schnelle GB. Radiology in canine practice. Evanston, IL: The North American Veterinarian, Inc, 1945.
2. Bartrum RJ, Crow HC. Real time ultrasound. 2nd ed. Philadelphia: WB Saunders Co, 1983.

3. Curry TS, Dowdey JE, Murry RC. Christensen's physics of diagnostic radiology. 4th ed. Philadelphia: Lea & Febiger, 1990.
4. Herring DS, Bjornton G. Physics, facts, and artifacts of diagnostic ultrasound. Vet Clin North Am 1985;15(6):1107–1122.
5. Kremkau FW. Diagnostic ultrasound: Principles, instruments and exercises. 3rd ed. Philadelphia: WB Saunders Co, 1989.
6. Morgan JP, Silverman S. Techniques of veterinary radiography. 4th ed. Ames, IA: Iowa State Press, 1987.
7. Ticer JW. Radiographic technique in veterinary practice. 2nd ed. Philadelphia: WB Saunders Co, 1984.
8. Hager DA, Nyland TG, Fisher P. Ultrasound-guided biopsy of the canine liver, kidney and prostate. Vet Rad 1985;26:82.
9. Leveille R, Partington BP, Biller DS, Miyabayashi T. Complications after ultrasound-guided biopsy of abdominal structures in dogs and cats: 246 cases (1984–1991). JAVMA 1993;203:413.
10. Papageorges M, Sande RD. The Mach phenomenon. Vet Rad 1990;31(6):274–280.

Chapter Two ▨▨▨▨▨▨▨▨▨▨▨▨▨▨▨▨▨▨▨▨

THE THORAX

Diagnostic images of the thorax are important when evaluating patients with known or suspected thoracic disease. The images can confirm or deny a diagnosis that is suspected on the basis of the history or physical examination. They can also reveal information not otherwise detectable, suggest a diagnosis not previously considered, and provide baseline information on the patient's condition for evaluation of disease progression or regression. The images can provide specific information after formulating a tentative clinical diagnosis or list of differential diagnoses; however, evaluating the images only to consider these diagnoses is a serious error. The choice of imaging modality (radiography, ultrasonography, computed tomography, etc.) will vary with the disease process that is most likely. In many cases, the use of more than one modality will be totally appropriate and frequently necessary. The entire imaging study should be evaluated systematically without consideration of the tentative diagnoses so that unsuspected conditions are not overlooked. The images should then be re-examined paying special attention to those areas in which, because of the patient's history or physical examination, abnormalities may be present.

TECHNICAL QUALITY—RADIOGRAPHIC

The technical quality of a thoracic radiograph is extremely important, because radiographic changes of disease can be masked or mimicked by inappropriate radiographic technique. The patient's position, respiratory phase, exposure factors, beam restricting devices, darkroom procedures, and viewing conditions are all important aspects of the thoracic radiographic evaluation. All of these factors alter the radiograph's technical quality, and their effects must be recognized so that technical errors neither obscure nor are mistaken for disease.

PATIENT'S POSITION

A minimum of a lateral recumbent radiograph (either right or left lateral) and either a dorsoventral (sternal recumbent) or ventrodorsal (dorsal recumbent) radiograph should be obtained. In certain situations (especially when evaluating for the presence of metastatic tumors of the lungs), the use of both lateral views and either a dorsoventral or ventrodorsal views have been recommended.[1-4] It appears that the use of two views is statistically adequate in these situations.[5] However, some radiologists continue to recommend taking the opposite lateral view when evaluating a patient for pulmonary metastasis.

The appearance of the thorax varies depending on the position of the patient when radiographed, because the dependent lung lobes partially collapse, even in an unanesthetized animal.[6-9] Consistent positioning with each radiograph is more important than the position in which the patient is placed. Comparison with previous

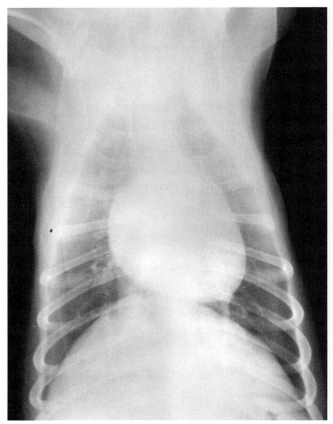

A

Figure 2–1. (A&B) A 12-year-old male Labrador retriever was presented for evaluation of a large mass in the caudal abdomen. The cardiac silhouette appears shorter and more round when (A) the dorsoventral radiograph is compared to (B) the ventrodorsal radiograph. **Diagnosis:** Normal thorax.

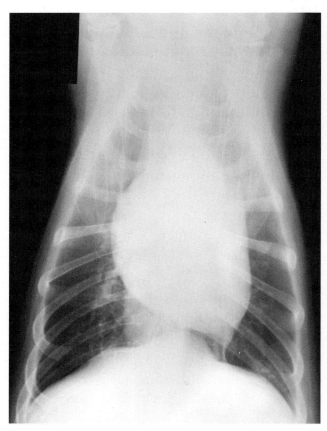

B

radiographs and recognition of radiographic abnormalities will be facilitated if the same position is used each time that the animal is examined.

In lateral recumbency, the dependent diaphragmatic crus is usually cranial to the opposite crus, and the cranial lung lobe bronchus on the dependent side is usually dorsal to the opposite cranial lobe bronchus.[10] The cardiac silhouette appears longer from apex to base in the right lateral recumbent when compared to the left lateral recumbent radiograph.[1,11,12] In left lateral recumbency, the cardiac silhouette may fall away from the sternum and the right middle lung lobe inflates. This produces a radiolucency that separates the heart from the sternum. In right lateral recumbency, contact between the heart and sternum is usually maintained. In the ventrodorsal radiograph, the cardiac silhouette appears longer and narrower, the accessory lung lobe appears larger, and the caudal vena cava appears longer than in the dorsoventral radiograph (Fig. 2–1).[13,14]

The x-ray beam should be centered over the thorax, because geometric distortion of the thoracic structures will occur, especially when larger films are used (Fig. 2–2). The x-ray beam should be centered just behind and between the caudal scapular borders in the dorsoventral or ventrodorsal radiograph and at the 4th to 5th intercostal space in the lateral radiograph. The forelimbs should be pulled cranially and fully extended on both views.

In order to obtain a properly positioned lateral thoracic radiograph, especially in dogs with narrow and deep thoracic conformation, the sternum must be mildly elevated from the x-ray table by a foam sponge or other radiolucent device. Proper lateral positioning can be recognized on a radiograph when the dorsal rib arches are

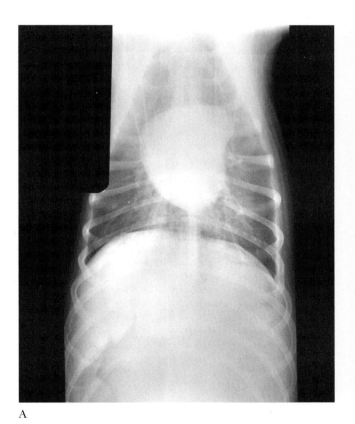
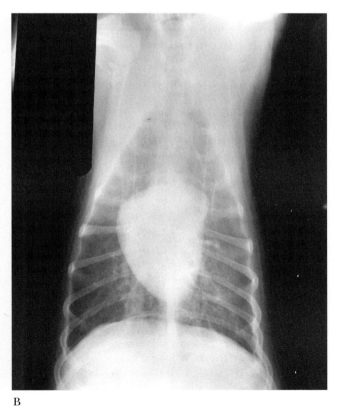

A   B

Figure 2–2. (A&B) A 5-year-old spayed German shepherd dog was presented for evaluation of the thorax prior to treatment for heartworm disease. (A) In the initial ventrodorsal thoracic radiograph the cardiac silhouette appears short. There is a prominent pulmonary knob. (B) The thoracic radiograph was repeated. The prominent pulmonary knob is again seen. The cardiac silhouette appears longer. The difference in cardiac silhouette length is due to geometric distortion resulting from malpositioning of the dog relative to the x-ray beam. In (A) the x-ray beam is incorrectly centered over the diaphragm, while in (B) the x-ray beam is centered behind the scapulae. There are incidental findings of old fractured ribs on both the right and left side. **Diagnosis:** Enlarged pulmonary artery segment due to heartworm disease.

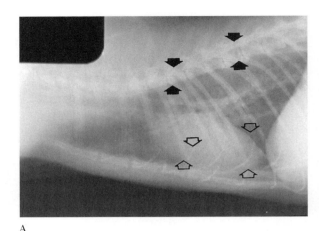

Figure 2–3. (A&B) A 2-year-old female Persian cat presented with an anterior uveitis. Thoracic radiographs were obtained to evaluate the cat for systemic involvement. (A) In the initial lateral thoracic radiograph the thorax is markedly rotated. The dorsal arches of the ribs are separated (*closed arrows*). The costochondral junctions are at widely different levels (*open arrows*). (B) An additional lateral thoracic radiograph was obtained. The ribs are superimposed, and the costochondral junctions are at the same level. The thoracic rotation moves the trachea closer to the thoracic spine and creates an apparent cardiomegaly. **Diagnosis:** Normal thorax.

A

B

Figure 2–4. (A&B) A 2-year-old female Persian cat presented with anterior uveitis. (A) In the initial ventrodorsal thoracic radiograph the cardiac silhouette is shifted into the left hemithorax. This is due to malpositioning with rotation of the sternum to the left. Note that the dorsal spinous processes are angled to the right (*arrows*). (B) The ventrodorsal thoracic radiograph was repeated. The cardiac silhouette is in its normal position. The dorsal spinous processes are centered on the thoracic vertebrae (*arrows*). **Diagnosis:** Normal thorax.

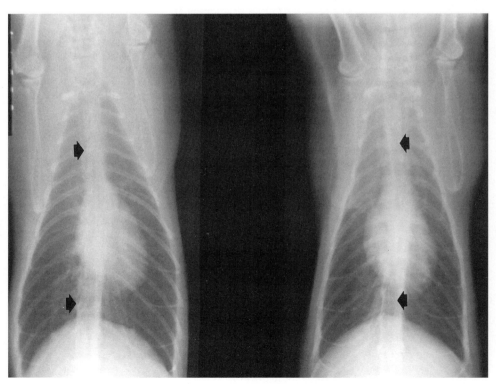

A   B

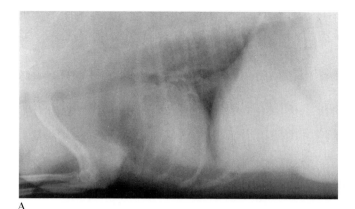

A

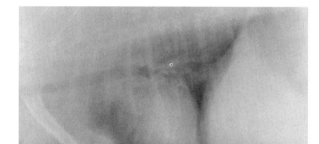

B

Figure 2–5. (A&B) A 5-year-old male mixed breed dog presented with a 5-month history of cervical pain. Thoracic radiographs were obtained prior to anesthesia. The density of the cranial mediastinum appears to be increased in the initial lateral radiograph (A). This is due to positioning of the right forelimb over the cranial thorax. The cranial thorax is normal in density in a repeat lateral thoracic radiograph (B). The forelimb has been extended. **Diagnosis:** Normal thorax.

superimposed and the costochondral junctions are at the same horizontal level (Fig. 2–3). In a ventrodorsal or dorsoventral thoracic radiograph, the sternum and vertebral column should be superimposed and the distance from the center of the vertebral bodies to the lateral thoracic wall should be equal on both the right and left sides (Fig. 2–4).

In the lateral radiograph, malpositioning may produce artifactual tracheal elevation and/or splitting of the main stem bronchi (see Fig. 2–3). Malpositioning also alters the shape of the cardiac silhouette and can create or obscure the impression of cardiomegaly or cardiac chamber enlargement. The cardiac apex always shifts in the same direction as the sternum. An apex shift to the right will accentuate or mimic an apparent right heart enlargement; a shift to the left will minimize the apparent size of the right ventricle.[15]

The forelimbs should be pulled cranially to avoid superimposition of their density over the cranial lung lobes, which will increase cranial lung lobe and mediastinal densities. This can create or obscure pulmonary or mediastinal lesions (Fig. 2–5).

The best radiographs for thoracic evaluation are those in which the animal is most comfortable and therefore can be symmetrically positioned. Once right or left lateral, ventrodorsal, or dorsoventral radiographs are obtained, those positions should be repeated on all subsequent examinations.

RESPIRATORY PHASE

Obtaining a radiograph at peak inspiration provides optimum contrast, detail, and visibility of thoracic structures. While many animals will spontaneously inspire maximally, some will not. It may be necessary to interfere with respiration momentarily by obstructing the animal's nares and closing its mouth. This forces a deep inspiration when the obstruction is removed.

The increased pulmonary density seen at expiration can mimic the appearance of pulmonary disease. The pulmonary vessels are shorter, wider, and less sharply defined at expiration than at inspiration. The cardiac silhouette appears relatively larger at expiration because it is surrounded by less aerated lung. The caudal vena cava may appear wider and be less clearly defined at expiration (Fig. 2–6).

The difference between inspiration and expiration must be recognized due to the artifacts created by an expiratory radiograph.[16] Compared to the lateral radiograph exposed at full expiration, the lateral radiograph exposed at full inspiration has:

1. Increased size of the lung lobes cranial to the cardiac silhouette.
2. Slight elevation of the cardiac silhouette from the sternum.

Figure 2–6. (A&B) A 12-year-old male Pekingese presented with a single acute episode of collapse. (A) In the initial lateral thoracic radiograph there is an apparent increase in pulmonary density. The right diaphragmatic crus overlaps the cardiac silhouette. The diaphragm is located at the level of T–11. These findings indicate that this radiograph was obtained at expiration. (B) A second lateral thoracic radiograph was obtained. The right diaphragmatic crus is positioned more caudally. The size of the right cranial lung lobe is increased. The diaphragm is positioned caudally to the level of T–13. The overall pulmonary density appears normal. The pulmonary vascular structures are more clearly defined. **Diagnosis:** Normal thorax. The apparent increase in pulmonary density on (A) was due to expiration. This can mimic pulmonary disease and obscure pulmonary vascular structures and can create the appearance of mild cardiomegaly.

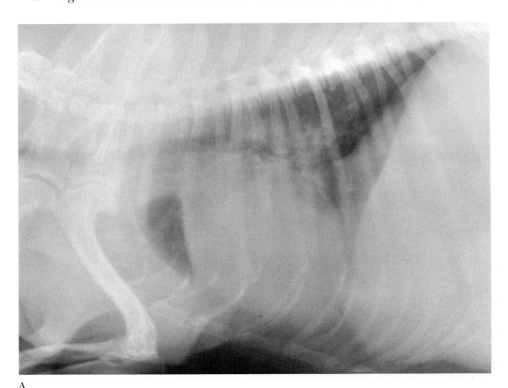

A

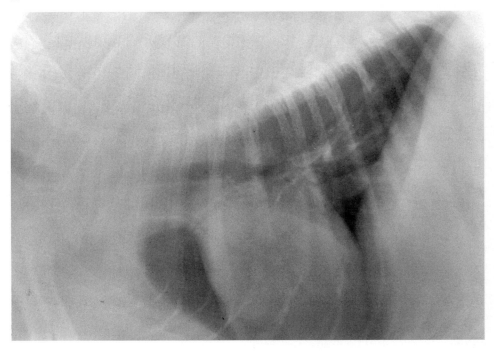

B

3. Extension of the pulmonary cupula cranial to the first rib.

4. Increased ventral angulation of the trachea.

5. A flatter diaphragm.

6. Greater separation of the diaphragm from the caudal cardiac margin.

7. A more ventral position of the point at which the diaphragm contacts the cardiac silhouette.

8. A lumbodiaphragmatic angle caudal to T–12 (compared to T–11 at expiration).

9. A wider lumbodiaphragmatic angle.

10. An increased size and lucency of the accessory lung lobe.

11. A caudal vena cava that is more parallel to the vertebral column and appears more elongated, distinct, and thinner.

When compared to the ventrodorsal expiratory radiograph, the inspiratory radiograph has:

1. A smaller cardiac silhouette (this is more apparent than real due to a decreased cardiothoracic ratio).

2. An increased thoracic width (most obvious caudal to the 6th rib).

3. An increased thoracic cavity length.

4. The diaphragmatic dome positioned caudal to mid-T–8.

5. A wider cardiodiaphragmatic angle.

6. Decreased cardiodiaphragmatic contact.

7. A more distinct, less blunted cardiac apex.

8. A costodiaphragmatic angle caudal to T–10.

Most radiographs are exposed between full expiration and full inspiration; therefore, it is unlikely that all of these changes will be seen in any one radiograph. The changes should be used as guides for recognizing the expiratory radiograph and are most obvious when an inspiratory and expiratory radiograph are placed side by side.

EXPOSURE FACTORS

A properly exposed radiograph is essential to be able to evaluate pulmonary disease correctly. For this reason, a technique chart based upon the patient's greatest thoracic dimension (usually measured at the level of the xiphoid cartilage for the ventrodorsal view and at the "spring of the ribs" for the lateral view), along with measuring all patients at the same anatomic site, ensures the reproducible radiographic exposure of different patients or of the same individual on repeat exam. Exposure factors used should be recorded so that follow-up examinations may be made using the identical technique. Unfortunately, technique charts are designed for the average individual, and the patient's physical status and conformation must be considered when selecting a technique. An emaciated Afghan hound will require less exposure than an average conditioned German shepherd or an obese cocker spaniel, even though their lateral thoracic measurements may be identical. A radiographic technique that is ideal for the German shepherd will overexpose the Afghan hound and underexpose the cocker spaniel. This occurs because the Afghan hound's thorax is mostly air-dense lung while the cocker spaniel's thorax is mostly fat- and tissue-density. Overexposure of the radiograph may hide intrapulmonary disease, while underexposure may mimic the appearance of a pulmonary infiltrate (Fig. 2–7).

Selection of specific kilovolt (peak) (kV(p)) and milliamp-second (mAs) settings is a matter of personal preference. As a general rule, the highest mA setting, shortest exposure time, and a high kV(p) setting are preferred for thoracic radiography. The technique selected depends on machine capability and the x-ray film and

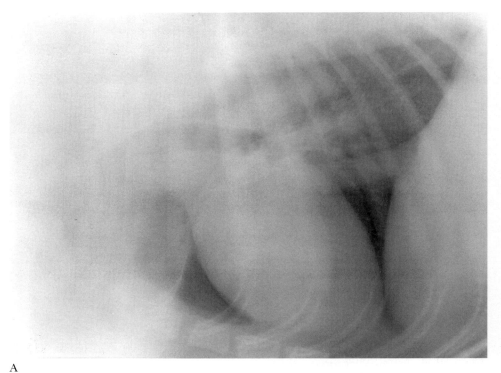

A

B

Figure 2–7. (A&B) A 2-year-old male Labrador retriever presented with an acute onset of vomiting, nystagmus, and ataxia. (A) In the initial lateral thoracic radiograph the increased density of the thorax is the result of underexposure. (B) A second lateral thoracic radiograph was obtained using the proper radiographic technique. The pulmonary structures and airways are much more clearly defined in the second radiograph. Underexposure of the radiograph can mimic a pulmonary infiltrate. **Diagnosis:** Normal thorax.

screens used. Exposure time is extremely important, since exposures of $^1/_{30}$ second or less are essential in order to minimize respiratory motion; longer exposure times may result in apparent motion causing blurring of pulmonary vessels, bronchi, interstitial structures, and overlying bony structures. This can create the appearance of a pulmonary infiltrate or obscure pulmonary lesions. If motion is suspected, the bony structures should be evaluated closely, since loss of definition of ribs or bony structures can be readily detected.

GRIDS

A fixed or moveable grid should be used for thoracic radiographs of those patients whose thoracic dimension exceeds 10 cm. A fine line grid is best. The machine's capability must be considered when selecting a grid. Scatter radiation will cause film fog, which produces a resultant overall increase in pulmonary density and loss of structural detail. In general, the use of a grid is recommended for patients whose chest measurement is greater than 10 cm; however, the patient's conformation must be considered when grids are employed. Since less scatter radiation occurs in a 10-cm wide, thin dog than in a 10-cm wide, obese dog, use of a grid is recommended in obese dogs that are 8 cm or greater.

BEAM RESTRICTING DEVICES

Beam restricting devices (collimators) are designed to precisely limit the x-ray exposure to the area being radiographed. This reduces patient and technologist exposure and improves the quality of the radiographic image by reducing the amount of scatter radiation. Close collimation with beam restriction to the thoracic area is ideal.

DARKROOM PROCEDURES

Many excellent radiographs are ruined in the darkroom during processing. Careful handling of the x-ray film before, during, and after processing is essential. A standard time/temperature film developing protocol is extremely important, because thoracic radiographic density is always compared to a mental standard established from previous cases and radiographs of the same patient at an earlier date. Underdeveloping will increase and overdeveloping will decrease the apparent thoracic density. Altering the processing time will not rescue an improperly exposed radiograph.

VIEWING CONDITIONS

The conditions in which the final product is evaluated are important. The radiograph should be completely fixed, washed, and dried before viewing. Because there is a natural impatience to determine the cause of a disease as soon as possible, many radiographs are examined while still wet. Some abnormalities will be a great deal more apparent after a film is dry. Therefore, it is imperative that the radiograph be re-examined after it is dry.

A quiet, darkened area with illumination provided by a light source designed for radiographic viewing is best. A high intensity beam or "hot-light" should be available and used to examine overexposed areas on the radiograph. Masks that block out the light from the unexposed edges of the radiograph are helpful.

Positioning the radiograph on the viewbox in a consistent manner will facilitate radiographic interpretation. By convention, lateral radiographs are placed with the animal's head to the viewer's left, and ventrodorsal or dorsoventral radiographs are placed with the animal's head up and its right side on the viewer's left. When this is done consistently, anatomic structures are seen at specific places on the radiograph and both normal and abnormal densities and shapes may be quickly recognized.

Proper thoracic radiographic interpretation results from the production of excellent, not merely acceptable, thoracic radiographs, from experience gained by careful systematic interpretation, and from the knowledge of various thoracic diseases and how they affect the appearance of a radiograph.

TECHNICAL QUALITY—SONOGRAPHIC

PATIENT PREPARATION

Proper patient preparation for sonography requires only a few steps. First, the site to be examined must be prepared so that good contact can be made between the transducer and the patient. Air cannot be tolerated at the transducer/skin interface because it blocks the transmission of the sound waves. The best way to prepare the site is to clip all hair from the area of interest. Then, liberally apply ultrasound contact gel to establish good surface contact between the probe and the patient. In dogs or cats with short or thin hair-coats or if hair clipping cannot be done, a thorough soaking of the patient's hair to remove all air from between the shafts of the hair may be adequate. Isopropyl alcohol works well for this purpose. Then, ultrasound gel should be liberally applied.

The proper patient positioning and probe orientation depend upon which anatomic structure is being imaged. Examination of the heart and mediastinum is facilitated by restraining the patient in lateral recumbency on a table or support constructed in such a manner that the probe can be applied to the area of interest from the dependent side. This is best accomplished with a table that has a cut-out in its surface so that the probe is readily moveable underneath the patient. This serves to maximize the size of the ultrasonographic window, because the dependent lung will collapse and the heart will move toward the dependent thoracic wall.

Manual restraint is adequate for most patients. Light sedation can be used if needed. Ketamine hydrochloride has been shown to have minimal effects on the feline heart.[17]

ULTRASOUND EQUIPMENT

Evaluation of thoracic anatomy is facilitated by using the highest frequency transducer that will adequately penetrate the structure.[18] Equipment used for echocardiography should be able to produce both M-mode and B-mode studies, should be able to measure the actual size of imaged structures in both modes, and should be able to simultaneously record an electrocardiogram. Ideally, the transducer head should be small enough to allow for positioning between ribs. For cardiac exams, a high frame rate is preferable to capture the instantaneous image of the moving structures. Evaluations of other thoracic structures (mediastinal masses, etc.) may be better performed using a low frame rate. Various combinations of contrast and post-processing functions are determined by the individual sonographers preference.

Sonography is best performed in a quiet room with subdued lighting. Excess ambient light makes evaluation of the images more difficult.

ECHOCARDIOGRAPHIC TECHNIQUE

A complete echocardiogram requires the use of at least B- and M-mode studies. B-mode (real-time, two-dimensional mode) reveals an image of cardiac anatomy in a manner that is clearly representative of the actual anatomy. The size, location, echogenicity, and motion of various structures can be evaluated. M-mode (TM mode, Time-motion mode, or motion mode) reveals a graphic representation of an isolated portion of the cardiac anatomy. This is the so-called "ice pick" view. This graphic representation continuously displays an isolated narrow line of structures over time so that the motion of the structures within the beam is clearly seen and recorded. M-mode is used for measuring cardiac chamber diameters and wall thickness as well as for observing the motion and physical relationships of structures to each other (e.g., the tip of the septal leaflet of the mitral valve in diastole to the interventricular septum).

Ideally, echocardiograms should be performed with a simultaneous recording of the electrocardiogram so that the mechanical and electrical activity of the heart can be correlated. Measurements of wall thicknesses and chamber diameters are made at either end-systole or end-diastole, as determined by electrical activity landmarks (e.g., end-diastole at the onset of the QRS complex). Simultaneous ECG is also used to ensure that the specific image chosen for measurement represents a part of a normally conducted cardiac cycle.

The methods of obtaining proper cardiac images have been well described.[18-20] The transducer location for the right parasternal views is between the right 3rd and 6th intercostal spaces between the sternum and costochondral junctions (Fig. 2–8). From this location, the long-axis 4-chamber view and the long-axis LV outflow view are obtained. Also obtained from this location are the short-axis views. Other images that can provide useful information include the left caudal parasternal long axis 2-chamber view, the long axis left ventricular outflow view, the 4-chamber view, and the 5-chamber view. The transducer location for the left caudal parasternal views is between the 5th and 7th intercostal spaces, as close to the sternum as possible. Left cranial parasternal views (both long axis and short axis) may also be helpful on occasion. The transducer location for these views is the left 3rd and 4th intercostal spaces between the sternum and the costochondral junctions.[20]

Specific positioning and images should be used for Doppler studies. The proper positioning aligns the ultrasound beam as parallel as possible to the direction of blood flow. This will minimize artifacts and optimize the Doppler signal.

THORACIC SONOGRAPHY TECHNIQUE

Thoracic structures other than the heart may also be studied. The use of a stand-off pad or fluid offset probe may be helpful in evaluating superficial structures that may be obscured by near-field artifact. The intercostal soft tissues may be visualized directly, and the subcutaneous fat and underlying muscles may be delineated clearly. The normal parietal pleura is thin and is not identified as a separate structure. Sonography may be a useful tool for evaluation of pleural disease, particularly if hydrothorax is present.[21] The cranial mediastinum may also be studied. This may be attempted by using the heart as an acoustic window. However, the normal left and right cranial lung lobes usually prevent visualization of normal mediastinal structures using this approach. If hydrothorax or a very large mass is present, the cranial mediastinum may also be scanned from other portals (thoracic inlet, directly over the mass). In normal studies, no structures will be clearly identified, because the lungs will nearly completely envelope the mediastinal structures. If pleural fluid is present, various normal cranial mediastinal structures may be identified.

Right Parasternal Window   **Left Parasternal Windows**

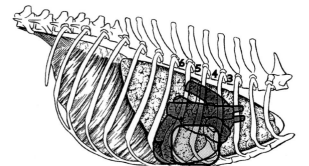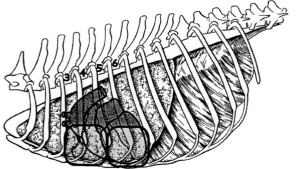

Figure 2–8. Diagrams of the thorax showing the proper transducer locations for the right and left parasternal echocardiographic views. (Reproduced with permission from Thomas WP, Gaber CE, Jacobs GJ, et al. Recommendation for standards in transthoracic two-dimensional echocardiography in the dog and cat. JVIM 1993;7:248.)

SYSTEMATIC IMAGE INTERPRETATION

Evaluation of the radiograph's technical quality is the first phase of radiographic interpretation. Although an imperfectly exposed and positioned radiograph may have to be examined because of the patient's clinical status, the effect of these factors on the radiograph must be considered during radiographic evaluation. Any observed "lesion," which could be caused by poor technique, must be evaluated critically. A systematic approach to interpretation will decrease the likelihood of overlooking an abnormality. The particular system used is less important than is its consistent application every time a radiograph is examined.

One system that may be used is the following:

1. Examine the soft tissue structures outside the thorax including the cervical soft tissues, soft tissues of the forelimbs, and that portion of the abdomen shown on the radiograph.

2. Examine the bony structures including the vertebral column, ribs, sternebrae, and long bones.

3. Examine the diaphragm including both crura and the cupula (dome).

4. Examine the pleural space (i.e., the potential space between the lungs and the thoracic wall and between the separate lung lobes).

5. Examine the mediastinum and all its reflections (i.e., cranially and ventrally between the right cranial and left cranial lung lobes, caudally between the accessory and left caudal lung lobe, and ventrally around the cardiac silhouette and diaphragm).

6. Examine the trachea and trace it to and beyond the bifurcation and as far down each of the bronchi as possible.

7. Examine the esophagus or the area through which it normally passes.

8. Examine the cardiac silhouette evaluating its size, shape, and position especially relative to the animal's thoracic conformation.

9. Examine the aorta tracing it as far caudally as possible.

10. Examine the caudal vena cava from heart to diaphragm.

11. Examine the lung. Look at its overall density, the size, shape and pattern of pulmonary arteries, veins, bronchial and interstitial structures.

12. Go back and re-examine anything that appeared abnormal on the first examination and interpret that abnormality in light of any other abnormality noted.

13. Combine all radiographic abnormalities into a list of possible diagnoses in order of probability or, when possible, make a specific diagnosis.

14. Re-evaluate the abnormalities noted in light of the clinical, historical, or physical findings and determine a radiographic diagnosis.

Evaluation of the sonogram should begin with an assessment of technical factors. Depth gain and overall power should be appropriate for the structures being examined. Alignment to a structure and symmetry of the cardiac chambers is critical in many cases.

The echocardiogram should follow a set course of study. The right parasternal long axis ventricular outflow study, followed by the right parasternal long axis 4-chamber view and then the right parasternal short axis views constitutes a routine, thorough study. Measurements should be made in the M-mode (but can be made in the B-mode if absolutely necessary) and should be timed to the ECG. Left-sided views should then be used if clinically indicated. Doppler studies should likewise follow a set protocol for evaluating the areas in question.

NORMAL RADIOGRAPHIC AND SONOGRAPHIC ANATOMY

SOFT TISSUES

The soft tissues surrounding the thorax should be evaluated. Fascial planes should be outlined by fat; soft tissues should have a uniform homogenous density. The position of the forelimbs should be noted because their superimposition over the cranial thorax adds to that region's density. Skin folds are created when patients are positioned for thoracic radiography and these can be identified as tissue-dense lines that have a distinct, dense margin. These lines can usually be traced beyond the thoracic margins (Fig. 2–9). The nipples and other cutaneous structures may be superimposed on the lung and mimic intrapulmonary nodules. In certain situations, the nipples may be coated with barium to positively identify them: however, in most cases, examining the patient and confirming the location of the nipples is enough. Pleural masses may extend into the external soft tissues; therefore, intercostal swellings should be evaluated critically. The hepatic and gastric shadows should be examined noting their position, size, shape, and density. If hepatic or gastric abnormalities are observed or suspected, an abdominal radiograph should be obtained.

The soft tissues surrounding the thorax do not have specific sonographic characteristics—they appear as any other soft tissue. The muscles are heteroechoic, and the

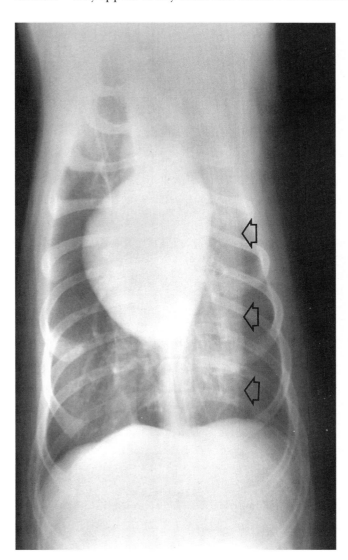

Figure 2–9. Ventrodorsal radiograph of a 6-year-old male Irish setter presented for evaluation of seizures. The thorax is normal. There is a skin fold present superimposed on the left side of the thorax (*arrows*). Note the sharply defined margin of this skin fold. The skin fold can be traced beyond the margins of the thoracic cavity. **Diagnosis:** Normal thorax.

fat tissue between fascia as well as the fibrous connective tissues are hyperechoic. The soft tissues of the thorax are not routinely evaluated by sonography.

BONY STRUCTURES

The vertebral column, ribs, sternebrae, and bones of the proximal forelimb are usually included on a thoracic radiograph. An exposure that is correct for thoracic viscera usually underexposes these bony structures. Positioning for thoracic radiographs is not ideal for evaluation of these bones; however, the vertebral column, ribs, sternebrae, scapulae, and long bones should still be examined. A radiograph, properly exposed for evaluation of bony structures, must be obtained if abnormalities are observed.

The vertebral column should have a smooth continuous contour. Disc spaces should be uniform, and rib articulations and joint spaces should be symmetrical. An apparent decrease in bone density will be observed along the ventral aspect of the vertebral bodies because of superimposition of the lung. The pattern within the lung may create the appearance of irregular vertebral body density; careful examination will identify the pattern as pulmonary in origin.

On the lateral radiograph, each pair of ribs should be superimposed where they articulate with the vertebrae; additionally, the costochondral junctions should appear at the same level. Because of the curvature and density of the ribs, abnormalities may be subtle. Tracing the ribs from right to left across the thorax on the ventrodorsal view facilitates lesion detection. The rib density should be uniform and a faint cortical shadow should be visible. A rib head, neck, and tubercle can be identified proximally; however, the size and shape of these structures are variable. The costochondral junctions are slightly widened, and the costal cartilages may calcify in a solid, irregular, granular or stippled pattern. Calcification may begin before 1 year of age, usually increases with age, and may appear irregular or even expansile. Malalignment or breaks in the costal cartilages are common and, although these may represent fractures, are usually normal aging changes and are without clinical significance.

In addition to the ribs and costal cartilages, the rib spacing should be evaluated and should show uniformity from side to side. Uneven spacing suggests uneven inflation of the lung and may reflect soft tissue, rib, pleural, pulmonary, or diaphragmatic pathology.

The ribs of certain breeds, such as the dachshund and basset hound, first curve outward then inward at or near the costochondral junction. This is followed by an outward then inward curve to their sternal attachment. In the ventrodorsal radiograph of these dogs, the thoracic wall conformation produces an extra density over the lung. This should not be mistaken for pleural or pulmonary disease (Fig. 2–10).

The sternebrae and their intersternebral cartilages should be evaluated. The amount of mineralization of the chondral and intersternebral cartilages usually increases with age and is greater in larger dogs. Malalignment of sternebrae is frequently observed and is insignificant unless accompanied by intra- or extrathoracic soft tissue swelling or clinical signs. Sternebral malformations are usually insignificant. Variation in the size and number of sternebrae and in the shape of the manubrium and xiphoid are common.

Thoracic conformation varies with breed and each variation influences the appearance of the thoracic viscera. It is important to note the animal's thoracic shape and evaluate the thoracic viscera accordingly. Three major categories may be observed:

1. Deep and narrow—such as doberman pinschers, Afghan hounds, collies, and whippets (Fig. 2–11).

2. Intermediate—such as German shepherd dogs, Labrador retrievers, and dalmatians (Fig. 2–12).

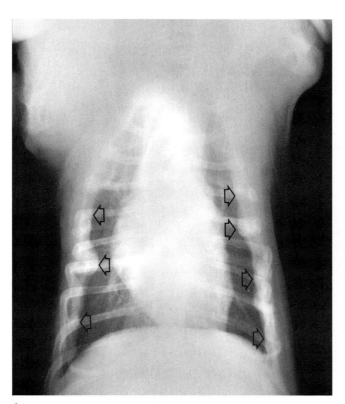

Figure 2–10. (A&B) An 11-year-old male basset hound presented with multiple cutaneous mastocytomas. The thorax was evaluated for intrathoracic metastases. The thorax is normal. The cardiac silhouette size and shape are normal for a dog of wide thoracic conformation. Note the soft tissue density that overlies the right and left sides of the lateral thoracic margin (*arrows*). This density is created by the configuration of the thoracic wall and does not represent pleural disease. The metallic density in the right cranial thorax represents a vascular clip, which was present in the soft tissues dorsal to the thoracic vertebral bodies. **Diagnosis:** Normal thorax.

A

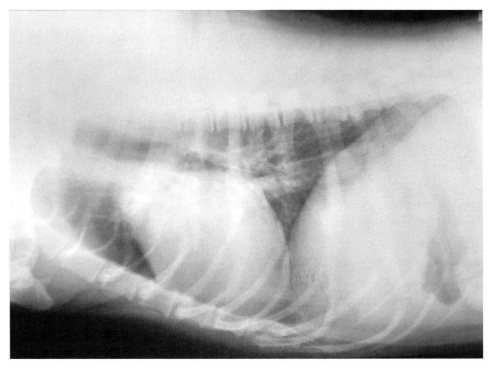

B

3. Shallow and wide—such as English bulldogs, basset hounds, and dachshunds (Fig. 2–13).

Some variation occurs even within the same breed; therefore, categorization should be based on each individual's conformation.

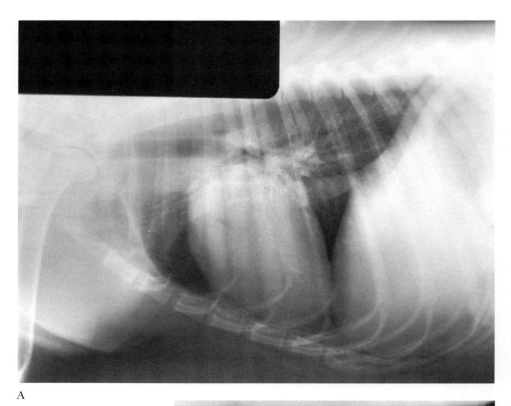

A

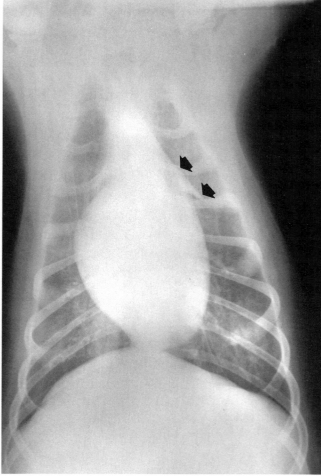

Figure 2–11. (A&B) A 2-year-old female Doberman pinscher presented for routine ovariohysterectomy. Thoracic radiographs were obtained at the owner's request. The thorax is normal. (A) On the lateral radiograph the cardiac size and shape are normal for a dog of narrow thoracic conformation. (B) on the ventrodorsal radiograph a soft tissue-dense triangular structure is present in the cranial left thorax on the ventrodorsal radiograph. This represents soft tissue and fat within the cranial mediastinum (*arrows*). In young dogs, the thymus may be identified in this location. **Diagnosis:** Normal thorax.

B

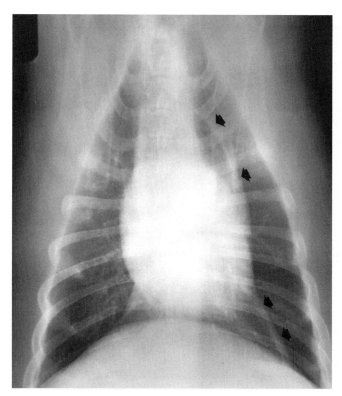

A

Figure 2–12. (A&B) An 11-year-old female German shepherd dog presented with a 2-month history of unilateral epistaxis. The thorax is normal. (A) On the ventrodorsal radiograph fat density can be seen in the cranial mediastinum (*arrows*) and also outlines the caudal mediastinum (*arrows*). (B) The density ventral to the cardiac silhouette on the lateral radiograph represents fat in the ventral mediastinum. There is an indentation in the cranial ventral margin of the cardiac silhouette at the site of the interventricular groove (*open arrow*). Pulmonary structures are easily identified with calcification present within some bronchial walls. This is most obvious on the lateral radiograph over the cardiac silhouette. The size and shape of the cardiac silhouette are normal for a dog with intermediate thoracic conformation. **Diagnosis:** Normal thorax.

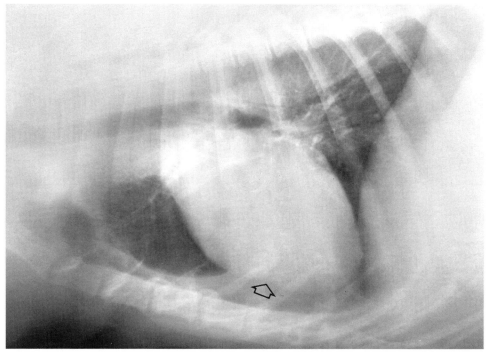

B

DIAPHRAGM

The diaphragm defines the caudal margin of the thoracic cavity. It is visible radiographically because the air-filled lung contacts its smooth cranial surface. With deep inspiratory efforts, the diaphragmatic attachments to the thoracic wall may appear on the ventrodorsal or dorsoventral views as peaks or scalloped margins

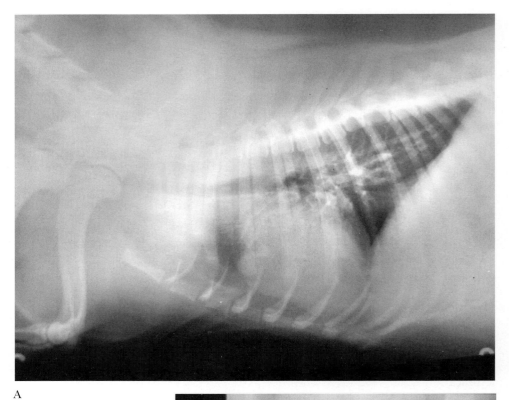

A

Figure 2–13. (A&B) A 7-month-old male English bulldog presented with a 1-month history of anorexia. The thorax is normal for a dog of this breed. The cardiac silhouette appears enlarged; however, it is normal for a dog of wide thoracic conformation. (A&B) The cranial mediastinum also appears widened; however, this dog is obese and the mediastinal widening represents an accumulation of fat. (B) On the ventrodorsal radiograph fat is also seen within the caudal mediastinum (*closed arrows*). The accumulation of fat is also responsible for the separation of the lungs from the thoracic wall in the caudal portion of the thorax (*open arrows*). **Diagnosis:** Normal thorax.

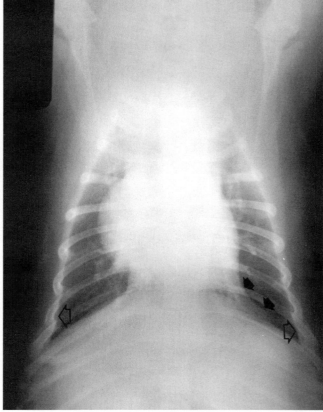

B

along the diaphragm margin. This has been referred to as "tenting" of the diaphragm. The caudal margin of the diaphragm blends with the shadows of the liver and stomach. The diaphragm is composed of a right and left crus in its dorsal aspect and a central cupula, or dome, in the ventral portion. There are three separate openings through the diaphragm for the aorta, esophagus, and caudal vena cava. Because of its curved shape, the diaphragmatic profile changes with the animal's position and the x-ray beam angle.[10] The diaphragm's shape is also influenced by respiratory phase, pressure from abdominal contents, breed, obesity, and age. Because of the diaphragm's complex shape, aerated lung will be superimposed over the liver and pulmonary pathology may be readily identified in those areas.

In the ventrodorsal and dorsoventral radiographs, the cranial peak of the cupula frequently lies to the right of the midline. The caudal vena cava interrupts the diaphragmatic outline at about this point. The crura may be identified as separate structures overlapping the cupula laterally, curving caudally toward the midline, and blending with the vertebral column at about T–10. The crura are more often evident on a ventrodorsal view; this varies between individuals and one, both, or neither crura may be seen. On the lateral radiograph, all three portions of the diaphragm are usually evident, with the dependent crus usually cranial to the opposite crus.[10] The margins of the caudal vena cava interrupt the outline of the right crus. When the animal is in right lateral recumbency, the air-filled gastric fundus may be identified caudal to the left crus. Fat within the falciform ligament ventral to the liver may outline the diaphragmatic cupula on the abdominal side. This may be a helpful finding in patients with pleural fluid in which diaphragmatic hernia is being considered as a possible diagnosis.

Sonographically, the diaphragm is not specifically identifiable. The interface of the diaphragm and the air-filled lung creates a hyperechoic line that has the shape of the normal diaphragm. This interface is frequently misidentified as the diaphragm. The caudal vena cava can usually be identified traversing the diaphragm. Identification of the esophagus at the esophageal hiatus is more difficult due to air in the stomach and lung.

PLEURAL SPACE

The pleural space is a potential space between the visceral and parietal pleura and between the visceral pleura of adjacent lung lobes. In normal animals, a small amount of serous fluid is present within this space; however, because of the size of this space and the small amount of fluid which it contains, it is not radiographically visible. Fluid or air accumulation within this potential space, or fibrosis, or calcification of the pleura will make the pleural space visible. When the direction of the x-ray beam is parallel to an interlobar fissure, it may be radiographically evident as a thin linear tissue density. The locations of the interlobar fissures within the thorax are fairly consistent and these should be specifically examined. Fat may accumulate beneath the parietal pleura in obese animals and be visible (see Fig. 2–13). The pleural space width may be accentuated on an expiratory radiograph in a normal animal.

The normal pleural space is not identifiable sonographically because it is so small. Pleural thickening or calcification is usually not identified. Air that is free in the pleural space is extremely difficult to differentiate from air that is within the lung. Pleural fluid is readily identifiable as a hypoechoic area between the thoracic wall and the lung.

MEDIASTINUM

The mediastinum separates the right and left hemithoraces into unequal portions and is formed by pleural reflections (mediastinal pleura), which are extensions of the parietal pleura and visceral pleura from both sides. The cranial mediastinum contains a number of vascular, lymphatic, and other structures (i.e., cranial vena cava; brachiocephalic, subclavian, and internal thoracic arteries; azygous vein; thoracic duct; phrenic, vagal, recurrent laryngeal, cardiosympathetic, and cardiovagal nerves; esophagus; trachea; sternal and cranial mediastinal lymph nodes). The right cranial lung lobe displaces the cranial ventral mediastinum to the left. The accessory lung lobe displaces the caudal ventral mediastinum into the left hemithorax. The mediastinum is fenestrated in the dog and does not prevent passage of fluid or air between the right and left hemithoraces. However, the mediastinum is usually complete (i.e., not fenestrated) in the cat. The mediastinum communicates cranially with the cervical fascia and caudally with the retroperitoneal space.

The dorsal mediastinum extends from the thoracic inlet to the diaphragm, but it is not radiographically identifiable. The ventral mediastinum is divided into pre- and post-cardiac portions by the heart. The pre-cardiac mediastinum contains a number of soft tissue-dense structures and is readily identified radiographically. On the ventrodorsal radiograph, it lies mostly on the midline; however, its ventral portion is displaced to the left by the right cranial lung lobe. On the lateral radiograph, the ventral pre-cardiac mediastinum may be identified from the trachea to the ventral margin of the cranial vena cava. Except for the tracheal lumen or calcified tracheal rings, the individual tissue-dense structures within the cranial mediastinum cannot usually be identified. The caudal ventral mediastinum (post-cardiac) casts a shadow on the ventrodorsal view only. It extends obliquely from the cardiac silhouette to the diaphragm and is displaced to the left by the accessory lung lobe.[22] The caudal mediastinal structures (i.e., caudal vena cava, aorta, esophagus) are discussed separately. In puppies and kittens, the thymus may produce a widened cranial ventral mediastinum. In older dogs and cats (especially obese individuals), the pre-cardiac and much less frequently the post-cardiac mediastinum may be quite wide. The fat may separate the cardiac silhouette and lung from the sternum on the lateral view mimicking pleural fluid (see Figs. 2–12 and 2-13). The fact that mediastinal fat is present should be recognized, because where the fat is contiguous with the heart the cardiac margins will remain apparent. This occurs because the fat is less dense than the heart. A mediastinum that is widened as a result of fat accumulation will not displace the trachea. This characteristic helps distinguish fat within the mediastinum from widening due to a mediastinal mass. Also, the lateral mediastinal margins are usually smooth and linear when widened due to fat accumulation, whereas masses usually cause the medial margin of the cranial lobes to be curvilinear. In obese animals, small volumes of pleural fluid and small mediastinal masses can be hidden within the mediastinal fat.

The mediastinum can be viewed using the heart as a sonographic window. Normal individual structures (other than the aorta and post cava) are not normally identified because the lung almost completely envelopes the heart and blocks transmission of the sound waves.

Computed tomography has been used to evaluate the mediastinum and the normal structures have been described.[23,24]

TRACHEA

The air-filled radiolucent trachea is easily identified in every thoracic radiograph. It is an important landmark for evaluating the mediastinum and the cardiac silhouette. The position of the trachea in the cranial thorax may vary depending on the position of the head and neck. When the head and neck are extended, the normal trachea is straight; head or neck flexion may produce a dorsal or rightward curve in the trachea (Fig. 2–14). The trachea usually has a mild ventral slope from the thoracic inlet to the tracheal bifurcation. The degree of ventral deviation varies with thoracic conformation and is greater in animals with deep and narrow thoracic dimensions when compared to those with shallow and wide conformation.

The tracheal diameter varies slightly with respiration in most animals. This variation may be increased in older small breed dogs, especially those with tracheal chondromalacia. The cervical trachea narrows slightly at inspiration and widens slightly at expiration, while the reverse happens in the intrathoracic trachea. Tracheal size should equal the internal laryngeal diameter measured at the cricoid cartilage or should be at least three times the diameter of the proximal third of the third rib; if the diameter is smaller, a diagnosis of tracheal hypoplasia may be made.[25]

The inner (mucosal) surface of the trachea should be smooth and well defined.

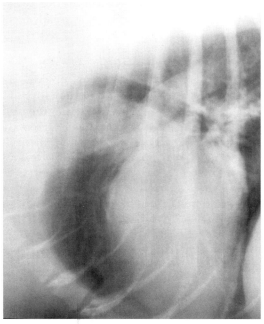 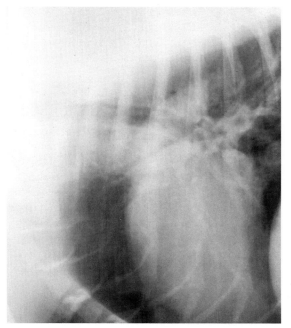

A   B

Figure 2–14. (A&B) A 4-year-old spayed Doberman pinscher with a mass in the oral cavity. The thorax was radiographed to evaluate the dog for the possibility of pulmonary metastases. (A) In the initial lateral radiograph the trachea appeared to be deviated dorsally, cranial to the cardiac silhouette. (B) A second lateral thoracic radiograph was obtained with the head and neck extended. The tracheal deviation is no longer identified. There was no evidence of pulmonary metastases. **Diagnosis:** Normal thorax.

On the lateral radiograph, the esophagus may overlap the trachea at the thoracic inlet and partially obscure its lumen. The significance of this overlap shadow is controversial and some radiologists consider it a sign of partial collapse of the dorsal trachealis muscle. Tracheal ring calcification varies but usually increases with advancing age.

The trachea branches into the bronchial tree caudal to the aortic arch at the 5th or 6th intercostal space. A ventrodorsal radiograph may need to be overexposed to demonstrate the trachea and bronchial branches because of the superimposed density of the sternum and spine. The angle at which the bronchi branch will vary, but it is usually 60 to 90 degrees. On the right lateral radiograph, a slight ventral deviation of the trachea occurs at the bifurcation followed by a dorsal deflection of the caudal main stem bronchi. The right cranial lobe bronchus is usually the most cranial bronchial branch with the left cranial lobe bronchus branching next from the ventral trachea.[26] The right middle lobe bronchus is rarely identified. The main stem bronchi to the caudal lung lobes continue caudally and dorsally.

In younger dogs, the larger bronchi can be traced only a short distance beyond the bifurcation. In older dogs, the bronchial walls may be traced more peripherally due to either bronchial or peribronchial fibrosis or calcification.

ESOPHAGUS

The normal esophagus is usually not visible because of the blending of its fluid density with that of other mediastinal structures. However, if the esophagus contains a swallowed bolus of air, it may be identified anywhere along its path. In some individuals, the normal esophagus can be seen on the lateral radiograph as a fluid-dense stripe dorsal to the caudal vena cava and extending caudally from the heart to the diaphragm.

The esophagus is located to the left of the trachea at the thoracic inlet, becomes dorsal to the trachea in the cranial mediastinum, and continues at that level to the diaphragm. The esophagus can become dilated when an animal is anesthetized or exhibit marked aerophagia associated with struggling during restraint. This dilation should not be misinterpreted as esophageal disease.

CARDIAC SILHOUETTE

Radiographic evaluation of the cardiac silhouette is complicated by the size and shape variations in different species, breeds, and individuals and by the effect of mal-positioning on its appearance. The cardiac silhouette is not a profile of the heart itself but is composed of the heart, pericardium, pericardial and mediastinal fat, and other structures at the hilus of the lung.

Cardiac size varies very slightly with respiration. A minimal increase in size at expiration is enhanced by a decreased lung volume and increased sternal contact.

The cardiac size and shape vary during the cardiac cycle.[27] This change is most noticeable in larger dogs and when short exposure times are used. Ventrodorsal radiographs of the heart during ventricular systole are characterized by a widened cranial portion, narrowed apex, and bulging or accentuation of the main pulmonary artery.

Since the angulation and position of the heart within the thorax vary depending on the animal's thoracic conformation, the cardiac shape also varies. Dogs with deep and narrow thoracic conformation have an elongated, thin, oval, or egg-shaped heart, which often seems relatively small when compared to the thoracic volume, and on the lateral radiograph, the heart is almost perpendicular with minimal sternal contact (see Figs. 2–11 and 2–14). The normal variation in cardiac shape, observed when comparing ventrodorsal and dorsoventral radiographs, is most apparent in dogs with this thoracic conformation. In these dogs, the cardiac apex is frequently positioned on the midline.

Dogs with intermediate thoracic conformation have a wider cardiac silhouette which, on the lateral radiograph, is inclined cranially within the thorax and has more sternal contact than dogs with deep, narrow conformation (see Figs. 2–7 and 2–12). The cardiac silhouette has a reverse "D" shape in the dorsoventral radiograph, and the cardiac apex is usually positioned slightly to the left of the midline.

Dogs with shallow, wide thoracic conformation have a short, round cardiac silhouette which, on the lateral radiograph, has a marked cranial inclination and a long area of sternal contact (see Figs. 2–10 and 2–13). On the ventrodorsal or dorsoventral radiograph, the cardiac apex is usually located to the left of the midline and is often difficult to identify because of its broad shape. This type of dog has a heart that always appears to be enlarged relative to the thoracic volume.

The size and shape of the feline heart is fairly uniform among different breeds and is similar to that of the dog, except that the apex is narrower when compared to the base or cranial cardiac margin.[28] In older cats, an increased sternal contact often occurs along with an elongated aortic arch.[29] Pericardial fat accumulation may create the appearance of cardiomegaly.

Sternal and thoracic wall deformities also affect the position and consequently the shape and relative size of the cardiac silhouette. Some consideration must be given when these deformities are present.

Variation in thoracic conformation and cardiac size among normal dogs and cats is a problem in recognizing cardiac disease; previous radiographs for comparison are always helpful. When these are not available, mild or sometimes moderate degrees of apparent cardiomegaly should be considered to be of questionable significance unless supported by clinical, electrocardiographic, or ultrasonographic evidence of cardiomegaly.

Several methods have been proposed for measuring cardiac silhouette size. A recently described system uses a vertebral scale methodology to measure heart size.[30] The overall heart size is measured and compared to the thoracic vertebrae (beginning at T4 and proceeding caudally). The vertebral heart size (VHS) is then expressed as total units of vertebral length to the nearest 0.1 vertebra. Using this system, the sum of the long and short axes of the heart, expressed as VHS, was 9.7 ±0.5 vertebrae. Exceptions were noted in dogs with a short thorax (e.g., miniature schnauzer) or a long thorax (e.g., dachshund). Since a diagnostic decision is rarely made based solely on cardiac size, these schemes may not add a great deal of advantage over a subjective evaluation.

The outline of the cardiac silhouette is a composite of different structures. Several schemes have been proposed for remembering which cardiac chamber or vessel forms each segment or portion of the cardiac outline. The simplest method divides the cardiac silhouette into four segments. On the lateral radiograph, the cranial dorsal segment is formed predominately by the right ventricle atrium (more specifically the right auricular appendage) and the cranial ventral segment by the right ventricle. The caudal dorsal segment is formed by the left atrium and the caudal ventral by the left ventricle. On the ventrodorsal radiograph, the cranial right segment is formed by the right ventricle atrium and the caudal right segment by the right ventricle. The cranial left segment is formed by the confluent shadows of the descending aorta, main pulmonary artery, and left auricular appendage. The caudal left segment is formed by the left ventricle.

Another scheme for describing the cardiac margins uses clock references. In the lateral radiograph, the left atrium occupies the twelve to two o'clock position, the left ventricle is found from two to five or six o'clock, the right ventricle from five or six to nine or ten, and the right auricular appendage from ten to eleven o'clock. The area from eleven to twelve o'clock is formed by the pulmonary artery and occasionally by the aorta; however, the cranial mediastinum obscures these structures. In the ventrodorsal radiograph, the main pulmonary artery is located from one to two o'clock, the left auricular appendage from two to three o'clock, left ventricle from three to five or six o'clock, the right ventricle from five or six to ten o'clock, and the right atrium from ten to eleven o'clock. The region from eleven to one o'clock is obscured by the cranial mediastinum and contains the cranial vena cava, right auricle, and aortic arch. The clock face model serves as a rough guide, but thoracic conformation and position of the cardiac apex will slightly alter these cardiac chamber positions.

On the lateral radiograph, the cardiac silhouette extends from the 3rd or 4th to the 7th or 8th rib and occupies roughly two-thirds of the thoracic height. It has a dorsal base, a rounded cranial border, and a slightly less rounded caudal border. The cardiac apex contacts or is slightly separated from the 7th sternebrae. The ventral margin of the cranial vena cava blends with the cranial cardiac margin and an indentation may be present at this point. This is the point of division between the right atrium and right ventricle. In obese dogs, another indentation (the interventricular groove) may be identified on the ventral cardiac margin (see Fig. 2–12). Ventral to the point where the caudal vena cava crosses the caudal cardiac margin, a third indentation may be identified. This is roughly the point of division between the left atrium and left ventricle. Identification of the cranial or caudal waist or interventricular groove is often difficult but can serve as useful landmarks.

The heart's appearance may vary between dorsoventral and ventrodorsal views and may also vary in consecutive dorsoventral or ventrodorsal views due to shifting of the cardiac apex. If the position of the apex is carefully noted, the changes that result should not be too confusing. On the ventrodorsal or dorsoventral radiograph, the cardiac silhouette in the average dog extends from the 3rd to the 8th or 9th rib. At its widest point, it occupies one-half to two-thirds of the thoracic width. The cranial margin of the heart blends with the mediastinal density. Contained within this area is the right auricle and aortic arch. The right lateral cardiac border is rounded. The apex is usually located to the left of the midline and has a somewhat blunted tip. The left lateral border, almost straight and free of bulges, produces a shape that has been described as a "lopsided egg" or reverse "D."

Normal echocardiographic anatomy has been well described.[17–20,31–35] The structures that are seen depend upon the view that is used. The most commonly used images are the right parasternal views. These are usually displayed with the cardiac apex to the left and the base to the right. All of the cardiac chambers are displayed on the

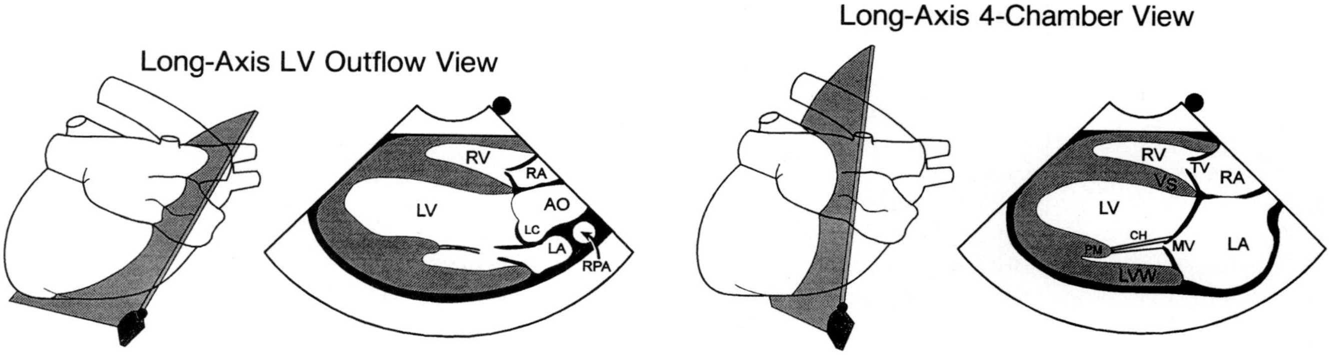

Long-Axis LV Outflow View

Long-Axis 4-Chamber View

Figure 2–15. Diagrammatic representations of the normal appearance of the right paraster-nal long axis 4-chamber view and long axis left ventricular outflow view: *RA*–right atrium, *TV*–tricuspid valves, *RV*–right ventricle, *LA*–left atrium, *MV*–mitral valves, *LV*–left ventricle, *CH*–chordae tendineae, *PM*–papillary muscle, *VS*–interventricular septum, *LVW*–left ventric-ular free wall, *AO*–aorta, *LC*–left coronary cusp, *RPA*–right pulmonary artery. (Reproduced with permission from Thomas WP, Gaber CE, Jacobs GJ, et al. Recommendation for standards in transthoracic two-dimensional echocardiography in the dog and cat. JVIM 1993;7:248.)

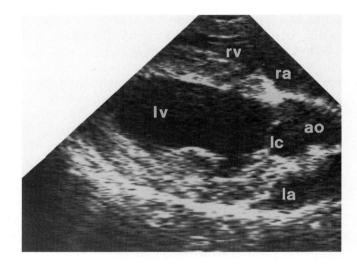

Figure 2–16. A right parasternal long-axis left ventricular outflow view of the heart showing the right atrium (*ra*), right ventricle (*rv*), aorta (*ao*), left cusp of the aortic valve (*lc*), left ventricle (*lv*), and left atrium (*la*). This view is taken at a slightly different angle than that shown in Figure 2–15. **Diag-nosis:** Normal heart.

right parasternal long axis left ventricular outflow view (Figs. 2–15 and 2–16). The size and relationship of the chambers and walls in this view have been measured.[31–33] The measurements are usually performed using the M-mode study (Figs. 2–17 and 2–18). The normal values for both dogs and cats have been described (Figs. 2–19, 2–20, 2–21, 2–22) (Table 2–1). These values must be applied carefully because there is some variation in the mean values among different breeds.[36] The normal values for cats show much less variation.[33] Also obtained from this site is the right paraster-nal, long axis, 4-chamber view, which is used to assess both the right and left heart (Figs. 2–15 and 2–23). The right parasternal short axis views can also be obtained from this window and can be used to evaluate the left ventricular (LV), left atrial (LA), and aortic (Ao) diameters and wall thicknesses (Figs. 2–24, 2–25, 2–26, 2–27, 2–28, 2–29). By taking measurements at a site just below the tips of the mitral valve leaflets between the papillary muscles, both fractional shortening and ejection frac-tions can be calculated. Fractional shortening is a commonly used index of cardiac performance and is calculated from the formula:

$$\frac{\text{LV end-diastolic dimension} - \text{LV end-systolic dimension}}{\text{LV end-diastolic dimension}} \times 100$$

Ejection fractions can be calculated from the fractional shortening, but because of their critical dependence on assumptions of ventricular shape, which are not always

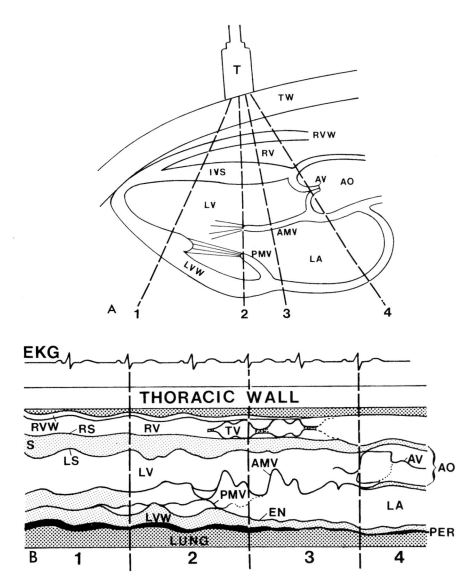

Figure 2–17. (A&B) Composite diagram showing the standard M-mode sites for cardiac mensuration using the right parasternal long-axis left ventricular outflow tract view: *T*–transducer, *TW*–thoracic wall, *RVW*–right ventricular wall, *RV*–right ventricle, *IVS*–interventricular septum, *LV*–left ventricle, *LVW*–left ventricular wall, *AV*–aortic valve, *AO*–aorta, *AMV*–anterior leaflet of the mitral valve, *PMV*–posterior leaflet of the mitral valve, *LA*–left atrium, *PER*–pericardium, *TV*–tricuspid valve, *EN*–endocardium. (Reproduced with permission from Bonagura JD, O'Grady MR, Herring DS. Echocardiography: Principles of interpretation. VCNA 1985;15:1177.)

accurate in the multiple breeds and sizes of animals examined, they are used infrequently in veterinary medicine. The structures at the heart base (e.g., pulmonic valve and pulmonary artery) are best observed with the right parasternal short-axis views of the heart base. Other views that may be helpful in specific cases include the left caudal (apical) parasternal 4-chamber and 5-chamber views (Figs. 2–30, 2–31, and 2–32), left caudal (apical) parasternal 2-chamber, and the left cranial parasternal long axis views.

The motion of the various cardiac components should be evaluated. Although motion of the left atrial wall is difficult to assess, the structure and motion of the mitral valve leaflets have been closely studied. The valve leaflets, anterior (septal) and posterior, should appear as slender, smoothly marginated, clearly delineated echogenic structures. The anterior leaflet is hinged to the atrium at the same level as the left coronary cusp of the aortic valve. The posterior is affixed at the junction of the atrial and ventricular myocardium. During early diastole (the passive stage of left ventricular filling) the mitral valve opens to its widest extent. The septal leaflet touches (in cats and small breed dogs) or nearly touches (large breed dogs) the interventricular septum. In an M-mode echocardiogram, the point of maximal excursion of the septal leaflet is referred to as the "E" point (see Fig. 2–18). The distance between the "E" point and septum is referred to as the E-point septal separation

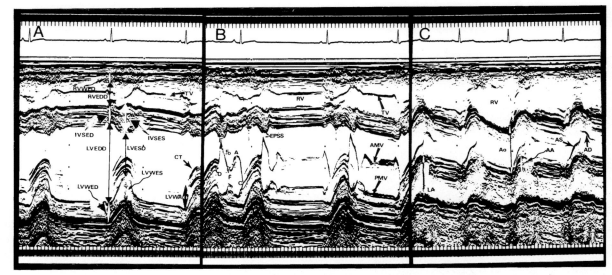

Figure 2–18. M-mode echocardiograms with simultaneous ECG tracing demonstrating structures that are routinely measured in a complete echocardiographic examination. Frame A: *RVWED*–right ventricular wall at end-diastole, *RVEDD*–right ventricular end-diastolic diameter, *TV*–tricuspid valve, *IVSED*–interventricular septum at end diastole, *IVSES*–interventricular septum at end systole, *LVEDD*–left ventricular end-diastolic diameter, *LVESD*–left ventricular end-systolic diameter, *LVWED*–left ventricular wall at end-diastole, *LVWES*–left ventricular wall at end-systole, *LVWA*–left ventricular wall amplitude. Frame B: *RV*–right ventricle, *D*–initial opening of the mitral valve, *E*–maximum early diastolic opening of the mitral valve, *F*–closure of leaflets after early diastolic filling (the slope from E to F is the velocity of diastolic closure) *C*–closure of mitral leaflets just before systole, *EPSS*–E point septal separation, *AMV*–anterior leaflet of the mitral valve, *PMV*–posterior leaflet of the mitral valve. Frame C: *RV*–right ventricle, *Ao*–aortic root, *AS*–aortic valve during systole, *AD*–aortic valve during diastole, *AA*–aortic amplitude, *LA*–left atrium. (Reproduced with permission from Moise NS. Echocardiography. In: Fox PR, ed. Canine and feline cardiology. New York:Churchill Livingstone Co, 1988;124.)

(EPSS). The posterior leaflet closely approaches the left ventricular free wall. As this stage ends, the leaflets begin to fall together. In later diastole, the left atrial contraction begins (the active stage of left ventricular filling) and the leaflets are again distracted. Their excursion is not as great as that seen with passive filling. The point of maximal excursion of the septal leaflet in this phase is referred to as the "A" point—this may not be apparent in views that are "off angle" or in patients with marked tachycardia. As ventricular systole begins, the valve leaflets close completely meeting in a straight line across the mitral valve orifice. The valve leaflets should not bulge nor displace into the left atrium.

The motion of the left ventricular free wall and interventricular septum should also be observed (see Fig. 2–18). During systole, these structures should approach each other symmetrically. A slight lag between the septum and free wall may be seen because the septum depolarizes a few milliseconds before the free wall, causing it to contract that much sooner. If there is a larger lag, this may represent an oblique angle through the ventricle. During diastole, the ventricular walls should move apart.

The aortic valve should be closed during diastole and open during systole. On the M-mode echocardiogram, the cusps of the aortic valve will appear as an open rectangle at the time the aortic valves are open. When closed, the cusps will appear as a single line (see Figs. 2–17 and 2–18).

Contrast echocardiographic studies use saline that has been well shaken with air so that it contains large numbers of microscopic bubbles. This is injected intravenously and the microbubbles are apparent as multiple, small, discrete hyperechoic foci as they pass through the right heart and into the pulmonary arteries. The bub-

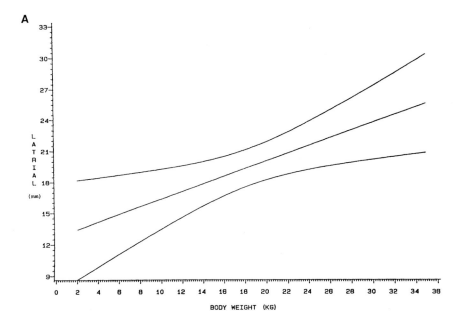

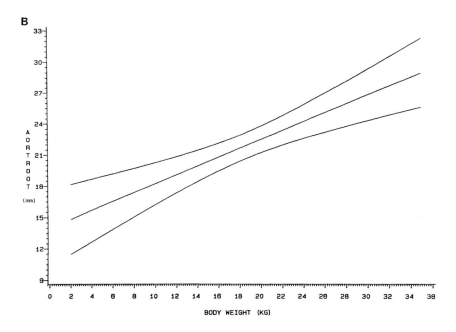

Figure 2–19. Graphs showing the normal values (predicted value ±95% confidence interval) of the left atrium (A) and aortic root (B). (Reproduced with permission from Bonagura JD, O'Grady MR, Herring DS. Echocardiography: Principles of interpretation. VCNA 1985;15:1191.)

bles are cleared by the alveolar capillaries and should not appear in the left heart. Special transducers (e.g., transesophageal transducers) have been used to obtain high resolution images of heart base structures. However, these transducers are expensive and not readily available.

Doppler echocardiography allows determination of the direction and velocity of blood flow by using information from the Doppler shift effect. This physical principle results from a shift in frequency of an echo that is induced by a change in position of the structure that is generating the echo. The shift will be to a higher frequency if the structure is moving toward the transducer and to a lower frequency if it is moving away from the transducer. The magnitude of the shift is related to the object's speed of movement. This Doppler shift can be used to assess hemodynamic

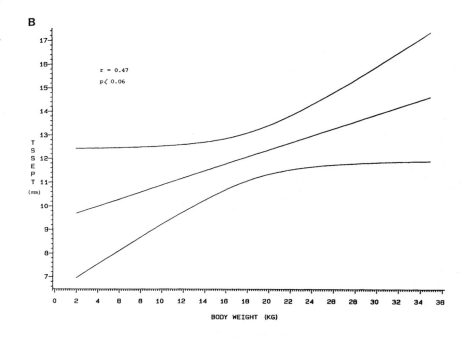

Figure 2–20. Graphs showing the normal values (predicted value ±95% confidence interval) of the normal ventricular septal thickness in diastole (A) and systole (B). (Reproduced with permission from Bonagura JD, O'Grady MR, Herring DS. Echocardiography: Principles of interpretation. VCNA 1985;15:1190.)

information. Conventionally, flow (or movement) away from the transducer is displayed below and flow toward the transducer is displayed above the baseline. The pressure is estimated by determining the red cell velocity, squaring that number, and multiplying the result by four.[18]

Machines that are capable of simultaneously displaying both a two-dimensional and a Doppler image (pulsed Doppler) are useful, because the site from which the Doppler signal originates is visible. In areas with high flow rates or in areas that are relatively distant from the transducer, a continuous Doppler (non-imaging) system is more accurate. As a general rule, lower frequency transducers are better for Doppler studies and higher frequency transducers produce better images (at the cost of less depth penetration). A compromise must often be made in transducer selection.

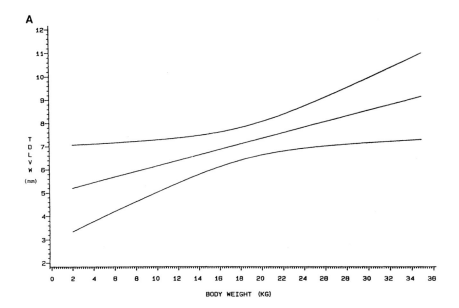

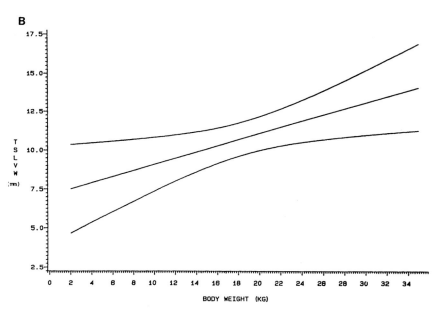

Figure 2–21. Graphs showing the normal values (predicted value ±95% confidence interval) of the normal left ventricular wall thickness during diastole (A) and systole (B). (Reproduced with permission from Bonagura JD, O'Grady MR, Herring DS. Echocardiography: Principles of interpretation. VCNA 1985;15:1189.)

Doppler studies may be performed to investigate blood flow characteristics at any site in the heart. Many of the common sites have been described (Fig. 2–33).[37,38] An example of the detailed information available using Doppler echocardiography can be seen in studies of the left atrium. Sampling is usually performed using a left caudal parasternal view (4-chamber inflow view). To evaluate mitral valve competency, the sample volume position should be in the left atrium one quarter of the distance between the mitral annulus and the dorsal wall. To evaluate the flow across the mitral valve, the sample volume is positioned in the left ventricle just distal to the mitral valve annulus at the point of maximal opening of the mitral valve.[37,38] Normal studies at heart rates less than approximately 125 beats per minute will clearly reveal separate flows during passive (E-wave) and active (A-wave) filling of the ventricle. With very slow rates, a separate L-wave associated with pulmonary vein inflow may be seen between the E-wave and A-wave. During systole, a 4th wave (S-wave) is seen, which is a low velocity positive turbulent flow signal and occurs after the A-wave. In heart rates greater than approximately 125 beats per minute, these flow phases begin

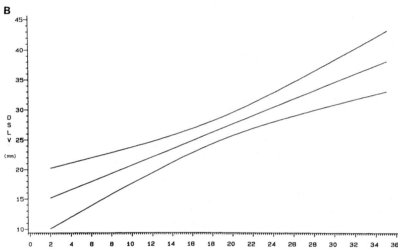

Figure 2–22. Graphs showing the normal values (predicted value ±95% confidence interval) of the left ventricular internal dimension during diastole (A) and systole (B). (Reproduced with permission from Bonagura JD, O'Grady MR, Herring DS. Echocardiography: Principles of interpretation. VCNA 1985;15:1188.)

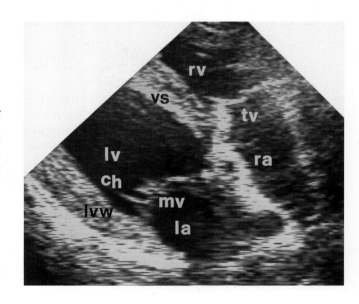

Figure 2–23. A right parasternal long-axis 4-chamber view of the heart showing the right atrium (*ra*), tricuspid valve (*tv*), right ventricle (*rv*), left atrium (*la*), mitral valve (*mv*), left ventricle (*lv*), chordae tendineae (*ch*), interventricular septum (*vs*), and left ventricular free wall (*lvw*). This view was taken at a slightly different angle than that shown in Figure 2–15. **Diagnosis:** Normal heart.

TABLE 2-1. Normal Echocardiographic Values in Cats

MENSURAL	(N = 11)[22]	(N = 25)[23]	(N = 30)[24]	NG[6]	(N = 30)[25,c]	(N = 16)[26,c]
LVEDD (cm)	1.51 ± 0.21[a]	1.48 ± 0.26[a]	1.59 ± 0.19[a]	1.10–1.60[b]	1.40 ± 0.13[a]	1.28 ± 0.17[a]
LVESD (cm)	0.69 ± 0.22	0.88 ± 0.24	0.80 ± 0.14	0.60–1.00	0.81 ± 0.16	0.83 ± 0.15
Ao (cm)	0.95 ± 0.15	0.75 ± 0.18	0.95 ± 0.11	0.65–1.10	0.94 ± 0.11	0.94 ± 0.14
LA (cm)	1.21 ± 0.18	0.74 ± 0.17	1.23 ± 0.14	0.85–1.25	1.03 ± 0.14	0.98 ± 0.17
LA/Ao (cm)	1.29 ± 0.23	—	1.30 ± 0.17	0.80–1.30	12.10 ± 0.18	—
IVSED (cm)	0.50 ± 0.07	0.45 ± 0.09	0.31 ± 0.04	0.25–0.50	0.36 ± 0.08	—
IVSES (cm)	0.76 ± 0.12	—	0.58 ± 0.06	0.50–0.90	—	—
LVWED (cm)	0.46 ± 0.05	0.37 ± 0.08	0.33 ± 0.06	0.25–0.50	0.35 ± 0.05	0.31 ± 0.11
LVWES (cm)	0.78 ± 0.10	—	0.68 ± 0.07	0.40–0.90	—	0.55 ± 0.88
RVED (cm)	0.54 ± 0.10	—	0.60 ± 0.15	—	0.50 ± 0.21	—
LVWA (cm)	0.50 ± 0.07	—	—	—	—	0.32 ± 0.11
EPSS (cm)	0.04 ± 0.07	—	0.02 ± 0.09	—	—	—
AA (cm)	0.36 ± 0.10	—	—	—	—	—
MVEFS (mm/sec)	54.4 ± 13.4	—	87.2 ± 25.9	—	—	83.78 ± 23.81
ΔD% (%)	55.0 ± 10.2	41.0 ± 7.3	49.3 ± 5.3	29–35	42.7 ± 8.1	34.5 ± 12.6
LVWT (%)	39.5 ± 7.6	—	—	—	—	—
IVST (%)	33.5 ± 8.2	—	—	—	—	—
HR (beats/min)	182 ± 22	167 ± 29	194 ± 23	—	255 ± 36	—
WT (kg)	4.3 ± 0.5	4.7 ± 1.2	4.1 ± 1.1	—	3.91 ± 1.2	—

[a]Mean ± SD.
[b]Usual range.
[c]Cats anesthetized with ketamine.

NG, information not given; LVEDD, left ventricular end-diastolic diameter; LVESD, left ventricular end-systolic diameter; Ao, aorta; LA, left atrium; LA/Ao, left atrium to aortic root ratio; IVSED, interventricular septum at end-diastole; IVSES, interventricular septum at end-systole; LVWED, left ventricular wall at end-diastole; LVWES, left ventricular wall at end-systole; RVED, right ventricular diameter at end-diastole; LVWA, left ventricular wall amplitude; EPSS, E-point-septal separation; AA, aortic amplitude; MVEFS, mitral valve E-F slope; ΔD%, fractional shortening; LVWT, left ventricular wall thickening; IVST, interventricular septal thickening; HR, heart rate; WT, weight.

Source: Reproduced with permission from Moise NS. Echocardiography. In: Fox PR, ed. Canine and feline cardiology. New York: Churchill Livingstone Co, 1988;27.

Short-Axis Views

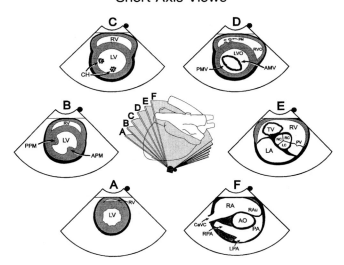

Figure 2–24. Diagrammatic representations of the normal appearance of the right parasternal short-axis views: *RA*–right atrium, *TV*–tricuspid valves, *RV*–right ventricle, *LA*–left atrium, *MV*–mitral valves, *LV*–left ventricle, *CH*–chordae tendineae, *APM*–anterior papillary muscle, *PPM*–posterior papillary muscle, *VS*–interventricular septum, *LVW*–left ventricular free wall, *AO*–aorta, *LC*–left coronary cusp, *RD*–right coronary cusp, *NC*–noncoronary cusp, *LPA*–left pulmonary artery, *RPA*–right pulmonary artery, *CaVC*–caudal vena cava. (Reproduced with permission from Thomas WP, Gaber CE, Jacobs GJ, et al. Recommendation for standards in transthoracic two-dimensional echocardiography in the dog and cat. JVIM 1993;7:250.)

to coalesce and at rates greater than 200 beats per minute, the E- and A-waves are no longer distinguishable.[37] Similar information may be obtained at multiple sites within the heart.

AORTA

The aortic arch and branches of the ascending aorta are obscured by the fluid density of the cranial mediastinum. On the lateral radiograph, the descending aorta can be identified crossing the trachea cranial to the tracheal bifurcation and continuing

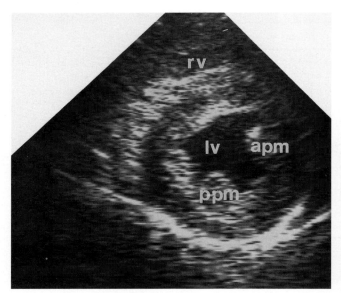

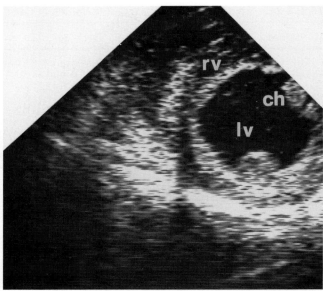

Figure 2–25. A right parasternal short-axis view of the heart at the level of the papillary muscles reveals the anterior papillary muscle (*apm*), posterior papillary muscle (*ppm*), left ventricle (*lv*), and the right ventricle (*rv*). **Diagnosis:** Normal heart.

Figure 2–26. A right parasternal short-axis view of the heart at the level of the chordae tendineae reveals the chordae tendineae (*ch*), left ventricle (*lv*), and the right ventricle (*rv*). **Diagnosis:** Normal heart.

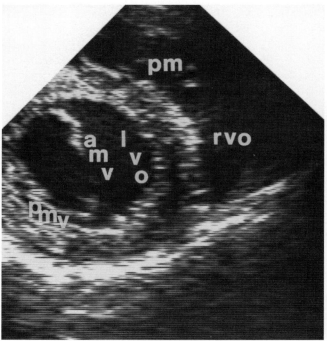

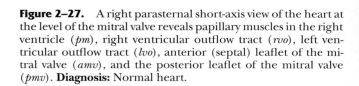

Figure 2–27. A right parasternal short-axis view of the heart at the level of the mitral valve reveals papillary muscles in the right ventricle (*pm*), right ventricular outflow tract (*rvo*), left ventricular outflow tract (*lvo*), anterior (septal) leaflet of the mitral valve (*amv*), and the posterior leaflet of the mitral valve (*pmv*). **Diagnosis:** Normal heart.

caudally and dorsally from that point. If a good inspiratory radiograph is obtained, the aorta may be traced to the diaphragm; however, in most normal animals, its smooth margin (especially the dorsal aspect) is obscured before reaching the diaphragm. The aorta tapers only slightly as it transits the caudal thorax.

In some older cats and dogs the aorta has an "S"-shaped or question mark (?) deformity across and dorsal to the trachea (Fig. 2–34). This deformity is without clinical significance.

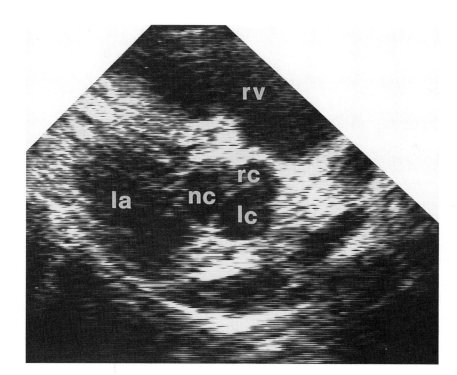

Figure 2–28. A right parasternal short-axis view of the heart at the level of the aortic valve reveals the right cusp of the aortic valve (*rc*), the left cusp of the aortic valve (*lc*), the noncoronary cusp of the aortic valve (*nc*), left atrium (*la*), and right ventricle (*rv*). **Diagnosis:** Normal heart.

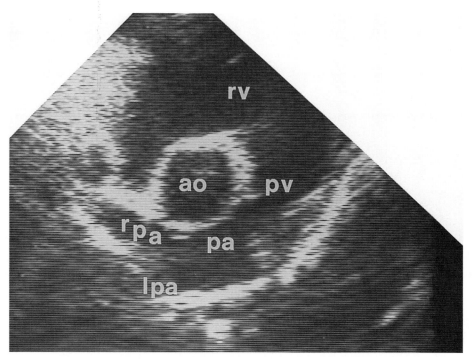

Figure 2–29. A right parasternal short-axis view of the heart at the level of the pulmonic valve reveals the right ventricle (*rv*), pulmonic valve (*pv*), main pulmonary artery (*pa*), left pulmonary artery (*lpa*), right pulmonary artery (*rpa*), and aorta (*ao*). **Diagnosis:** Normal heart.

In the ventrodorsal radiograph, the aortic arch can be detected as it crosses the left cranial aspect of the cardiac silhouette at about the one o'clock position. Proximal to this, the aorta is obscured by the cranial mediastinal density. The aorta usually can be followed caudally, but only its left margin is visible. This margin gradually approaches the midline and is lost at about the level of the cardiac apex or slightly caudal to the diaphragmatic cupula. A prominent cranial bulge may accompany the "S"-shaped curve that is observed on the lateral radiograph in older dogs and cats. Otherwise, the aortic margin should be smooth, tapering gradually as it progresses caudally.

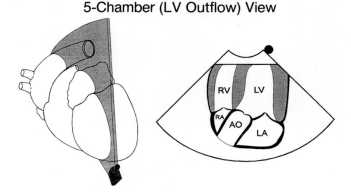

4-Chamber (Inflow) View

5-Chamber (LV Outflow) View

Figure 2–30. Diagrammatic representations of the normal appearance of the left caudal parasternal 4-chamber (inflow) and 5-chamber (LV outflow): *RA*–right atrium, *RV*–right ventricle, *LA*–left atrium, *LV*–left ventricle, *AS*–atrial septum, *AO*–aorta. (Reproduced with permission from Thomas WP, Gaber CE, Jacobs GJ, et al. Recommendation for standards in transthoracic two-dimensional echocardiography in the dog and cat. JVIM 1993;7:251.)

Figure 2–31. A left parasternal long-axis 4-chamber (inflow) view reveals left ventricle (*lv*), left atrium (*la*), atrial septum (*as*), right atrium (*ra*), and right ventricle (*rv*). **Diagnosis:** Normal heart.

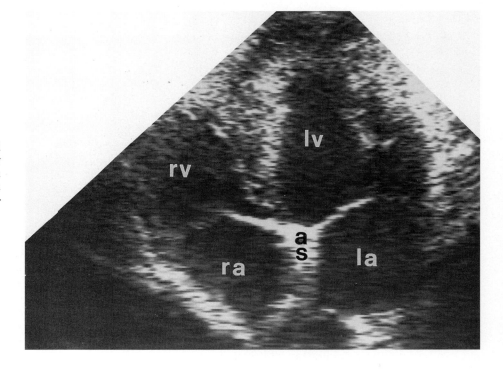

Radiographic guidelines have not been established for evaluation of aortic size; however, the aorta should be roughly equal to the caudal vena cava in width. The size of the caudal vena cava varies considerably with respiration and cardiac cycle. Echocardiography provides an excellent means to evaluate the aortic root and

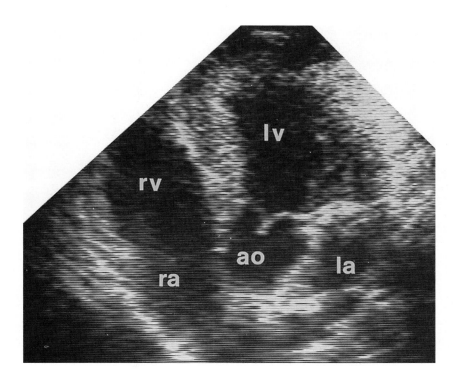

Figure 2–32. A left parasternal long-axis 5-chamber (LV outflow) view reveals the left ventricle (*lv*), left atrium (*la*), aorta (*ao*), right atrium (*ra*), and right ventricle (*rv*). **Diagnosis:** Normal heart.

portions of the ascending and descending aorta. The right parasternal, long-axis, left ventricular outflow view demonstrates the outflow tract, the valvular cusps, the aortic bulb (sinus of Valsalva), and a portion of the ascending aorta (see Figs. 2–15 and 2–16). With cranial positioning of the transducer, the majority of the aortic arch can be imaged in some individuals. The short axis view of the heart base also demonstrates the aorta and all three cusps of the aortic valve (see Figs. 2–24 and 2–28). The appearance of the aortic valves has been described as resembling the symbol for the Mercedes Benz automobile.

Doppler studies of the aorta can be performed using the left apical, long axis, left ventricular outflow tract view. However, the 5-chamber (left ventricular outflow) view is preferable.[37,38] The sample volume is placed in the middle of the aorta at the distal end of the aortic bulb. Normal studies reveal a rapid laminar acceleration phase (downstroke) followed by the deceleration phase (upstroke). A second, much smaller wave may be seen immediately after the dominant signal, which represents early diastolic flow.[37,38]

CAUDAL VENA CAVA

The caudal vena cava may be traced from the diaphragm to the point where it enters the right atrium cranial to the caudal margin of the cardiac silhouette. On the lateral radiograph, the caudal vena cava, located at about the midpoint of the thoracic height, tapers and slopes slightly downward from the diaphragm to the cardiac silhouette. The size of the caudal vena cava changes with respiration and phase of the cardiac cycle. It is larger and shorter at expiration and collapses slightly during diastole. The caudal vena cava has been reported to be equal to or smaller than the length of T5 or T6 in dogs.[30]

The caudal vena cava is more easily identified in the ventrodorsal when compared to the dorsoventral radiograph. It can be traced from the heart to the diaphragm along the right side of the vertebral column. The width of the caudal vena cava in the ventrodorsal view is usually uniform, and, although a mild even curvature is not abnormal, its margins should be smooth, straight, and parallel.

The visibility of the caudal vena cava depends on aeration of the accessory lung

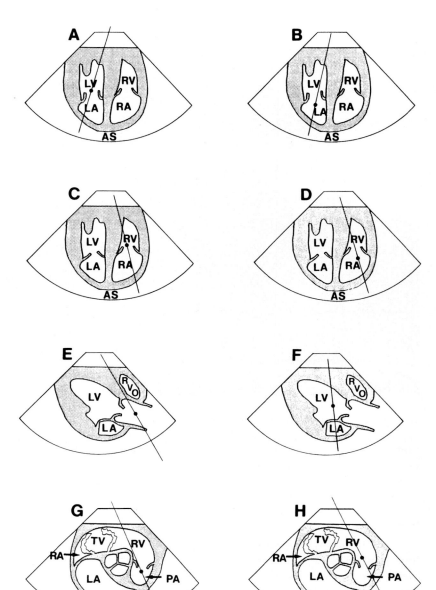

Figure 2–33. Diagrammatic demonstrations of the views and placement of sample volumes for Doppler echocardiographic studies of the (A) mitral valve, (B) left atrial flow, (C) tricuspid valve flow, (D) right atrial flow, (E) aortic valve flow, (F) left ventricular outflow tract flow, (G) pulmonary valve flow, (H) right ventricular outflow tract flow: *LA*–left atrium, *LV*–left ventricle, *RA*–right atrium, *RV*–right ventricle, *RVO*–right ventricular outflow tract, *TV*–tricuspid valve, *PA*–pulmonary artery, and *AS*–atrial septum. (Reproduced with permission from Kirberger RM, Bland-van den Berg P, Darazs B. Doppler echocardiography in the normal dog: Part I, velocity findings and flow patterns. Vet Radiol 1992;33:372.)

lobe. Poor margin definition may be observed on expiratory radiographs, dorsoventral radiographs, and in animals with accessory lung lobe infiltrates.

In general, the diameter of the caudal vena cava should be approximately equal to that of the aorta. The comparison can be unreliable because of the effects of the cardiac cycle. If the observed alteration in the size of the vena cava is confirmed by other thoracic pathology (i.e., small vena cava with small heart and pulmonary vessels; large vena cava with large right heart), or is consistent on sequential radiographs, it should be considered significant.

The vena cava is usually not identified on an echocardiogram. It is easily viewed in the cranial abdomen as it passes through the diaphragm and liver. The intrathoracic vena cava may be identified when hydrothorax is present. The normal size of the caudal vena cava has not been well defined. It is frequently evaluated when right heart failure is suspected, but the analysis is highly subjective and a diagnosis of right heart failure is usually suspected on distension of hepatic veins rather than caudal vena cava diameter.

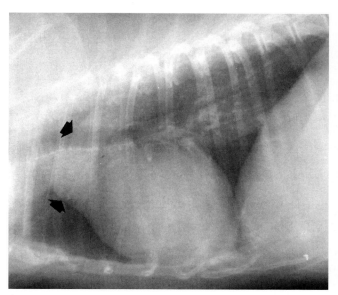

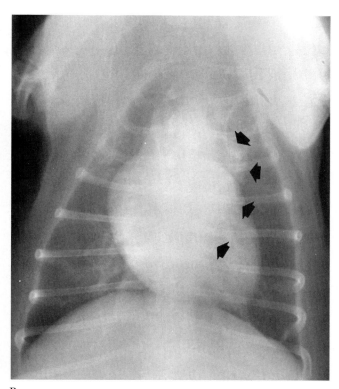

A

B

Figure 2–34. (A&B) A 14-year-old male Yorkshire terrier presented with nasal obstruction and dyspnea. The thorax is normal. (A) The aorta is redundant and extends cranial to the cardiac silhouette (*arrows*) on the lateral radiograph and (B) also extends into the left hemithorax (*arrows*) on the ventrodorsal radiograph. This elongation and redundancy of the aorta is often seen in normal, old dogs. There is no evidence of pulmonary metastases. The cardiac silhouette is normal size and shape. **Diagnosis:** Normal thorax.

LUNG

The air within the lung provides a natural contrast permitting identification of the fluid dense pulmonary vessels, bronchial walls, and pulmonary interstitium; therefore, radiographs are ideal for evaluating the lung's gross morphology. Evaluation of normal structures relies on the lung being well aerated so that structures stand out in contrast, and this must be considered anytime a thoracic radiograph is evaluated. The lung appearance dramatically changes during different phases of the respiratory cycle.

Limited functional information may be obtained by evaluating vascular size and distribution and by comparing inspiratory and expiratory radiographs. Fluoroscopy, serial radiography, and cineradiography or videoradiography are required to enable a better radiographic evaluation of functional pulmonary abnormalities. Preferred methods for such studies include scintigraphy or pulmonary function tests.[39,40] These techniques are beyond the scope of this text and will be mentioned briefly when appropriate to the disease being discussed.

The individual lung lobes are not identified on thoracic radiographs of normal animals; however, knowledge of the area that each lung lobe occupies and familiarity with the relationships between adjacent lung lobes and other thoracic organs are very important in understanding the radiographic appearance of most pulmonary abnormalities. The branching pattern of the major bronchi can be traced distally from the trachea, and this helps to locate specific pulmonary structures.

The right lung is divided into cranial, middle, caudal, and accessory lobes. The left lung is divided into cranial and caudal lung lobes with the left cranial lobe subdivided into cranial and caudal portions.

In the lateral radiograph the right cranial lung lobe occupies most of the cranial thorax from the tracheal bifurcation to the thoracic inlet. It extends cranial to the 1st or 2nd rib and wraps around the cranial aspect of the cardiac silhouette. The right middle lung lobe has a somewhat triangular shape; its apex extends dorsally to the tracheal bifurcation and its base extends along the sternum covering the area of the cardiac silhouette. The right caudal lung lobe contacts the right cranial lobe dorsal to the tracheal bifurcation and contacts the middle lung lobe ventral to this point. It extends caudally to the diaphragm and ventrally to the sternum. The accessory lung lobe is between the cardiac silhouette and the diaphragm and overlaps the cardiac border. It extends dorsally above the caudal vena cava to about the level of the esophagus and extends ventrally to the sternum.

The left cranial lung lobe occupies an area similar to that of the right cranial and middle lobes. It extends cranially to the cranial edge of the right cranial lobe, often extending beyond the first rib. Its tip may be identified as an oblong or oval lucency in the cranial thorax, since it extends from left to right across the midline at this point. The left caudal lung lobe occupies an area similar to that of the right.

The dependent lung collapses slightly in normal, conscious animals and, therefore, the "up" lung is best evaluated in a lateral thoracic radiograph.[9] Therefore, in right lateral recumbency, the normal structures and abnormalities in the left lung are most easily seen and in left lateral recumbency those in the right lung lobes are most apparent.

In the dorsoventral and ventrodorsal radiographs, the right cranial lung lobe occupies the right cranial thorax and extends across the midline cranial to the cardiac silhouette. The right middle lung lobe occupies the area lateral to the cardiac silhouette and overlaps a portion of the heart. The right caudal lung lobe occupies the right caudal thorax, extends to the midline dorsally, but is separated from it ventrally by the right middle and accessory lung lobes. The accessory lung lobe occupies the area between the heart and the diaphragm, wraps around the caudal vena cava, and extends across the midline displacing a fold of the caudal mediastinum to the left.

The left cranial lung lobe occupies the left cranial thorax extending across the midline at the level of, or slightly cranial to, the first rib. It extends to the midline dorsally and contacts the heart ventrally. The left caudal lung lobe occupies the left caudal thorax extending to the midline dorsally, but is displaced to the left away from the midline by the accessory lung lobe ventrally.

Dorsoventral and ventrodorsal radiographs present different profiles because of decreased inflation of the dependent portions of each lobe. The lung lobes overlap each other, the heart, and diaphragm. This factor must be remembered when evaluating and localizing lesions within the lung.

Pulmonary arteries, pulmonary veins, and the walls of the larger airways can be identified within the lung. Pulmonary vessels are fluid-dense, taper gradually, and branch as they are traced peripherally. When they branch perpendicular to the x-ray beam, the vessels produce a round density, which is denser but of the same size as the vessel from which it originates. The pulmonary arteries and veins may be identified only when their position relative to their accompanying bronchus can be established. On the lateral radiograph, the artery is dorsal and the vein is ventral to the bronchus. On the ventrodorsal radiograph, the artery is lateral and the vein medial to the bronchus. Pulmonary arteries will tend to converge toward their origin from the main pulmonary artery (i.e., cranial to the tracheal bifurcation), while pulmonary veins will converge around the left atrium (i.e., caudal to the tracheal bifurcation). Arteries are reportedly denser, more curved, and better delineated than veins; however, detection of this difference is difficult. Bronchial arteries cannot be identified. Vascular structures in the lung periphery cannot usually be classified as arterial or venous.

Evaluation of arterial and venous size is important in disease recognition. Arteries and their adjacent accompanying veins should be the same size. Unfortunately, the vessels may be superimposed on the lateral radiograph; therefore, identification and comparison can be difficult. Vascular size is evaluated subjectively and, although several standards have been proposed, none are completely reliable. Increased pulmonary perfusion is frequently accompanied or manifested by an increase in number of vascular structures.

The shape of the pulmonary vessels and manner in which they branch should also be evaluated. Smooth, gradual tapering is expected and alterations from this appearance are abnormal.

The bronchial walls are not normally visible beyond the main lobar bronchi. Calcification and fibrosis occur with advancing age and as a result of prior pulmonary disease, with the bronchial walls becoming more apparent (see Fig. 2–12). Longitudinally, bronchial walls appear as thin, parallel fluid-dense lines or, on cross section, as ring-like fluid densities. Often, the bronchial wall is obscured by the adjacent pulmonary vessel; however, the end-on pulmonary vessels may be identified as fluid-dense dots on either side of the ring-like bronchial density.

Additional fluid-dense lines may become apparent, especially in older animals.[41] Usually thinner than vascular shadows, these additional fluid-dense lines do not have the round shape or straight parallel line pattern of bronchial walls. They produce patterns that are often described as reticulated or net-like. They are generally referred to or classified as interstitial densities originating from the supporting connective tissue of the lung and from pulmonary lymphatics. They must be recognized because they will become accentuated in various pulmonary diseases.

Many artifactual shadows may be superimposed on and appear to be within the lung; however, these can often be identified on both views and their extrapulmonary origin established.

Ultrasonography has limited use within the lung because of the total inhibition of transmission of ultrasound through air. It can be used in those situations in which the pulmonary pathology is in contact with the pleura or thoracic wall, thus providing a sonographic window.

Computed tomography has many uses within the lung.[42] However, its utility is limited by the cost of the equipment and the need for general anesthesia during the study.

After all thoracic structures have been evaluated, the patient's history and clinical features should be reviewed and the radiograph re-evaluated. Unfortunately, the radiograph may not detect mild pathology, and many diseases produce no radiographic change. Therefore, a normal thoracic radiograph does not exclude a diagnosis of thoracic disease, and a repeat study after a period of time may be beneficial.

CERVICAL SOFT TISSUES

Abnormalities in the cervical soft tissues may be related to intra-thoracic lesions or may produce clinical signs similar to those of thoracic disease. Cervical lesions can extend into the thoracic cavity and some thoracic lesions can spread to the neck. A properly positioned thoracic radiograph should not include the cervical area. A separate radiograph of this area should be obtained. The oral and nasal pharynx, larynx, cervical tracheal, and cervical esophagus should be evaluated.

LARYNX AND PHARYNX

The larynx and cervical trachea should not be routinely included on thoracic radiographs. A symmetrically positioned lateral radiograph that is centered on the larynx is required to evaluate this area. Anesthesia or sedation is usually necessary, but an endotracheal tube may interfere with the examination. The ventrodorsal radiograph is rarely helpful, because superimposition of the larynx over the skull and cervical spine interferes with evaluation of most laryngeal structures. The radiograph should include the oral and nasal pharynx as well as the larynx.

The air within the pharynx and larynx outlines the soft tissue structures.[43] Swallowing, breathing, and changes in head and neck position will not only result in variation in the appearance of these structures, but may partially obscure them (Fig. 2–35).

The soft palate divides the oral and nasal pharynx. The margin of the soft palate should be smooth, and its width should taper slightly (i.e., it is thinner at its caudal tip). The caudal margin of the soft palate usually contacts the cranial tip of the epiglottis; this varies with head and neck position.

The laryngeal cartilages are visible in most dogs and may be calcified in older (especially larger) dogs (Fig. 2–36). The epiglottis is curvilinear, extending dorsally from the base of the larynx to the soft palate. The laryngeal saccules may be identified as somewhat thin, ovoid lucencies located caudal to and extending dorsally from

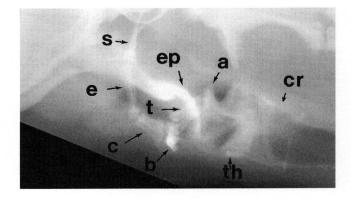

Figure 2–35. A 12-year-old spayed mixed breed dog presented with a 1-month history of coughing and gagging. A lateral radiograph of the larynx reveals mineralization of the epiglottis and arytenoid and cricoid cartilages. This is normal for a dog of this age. The stylohyoid bone (*s*), epihyoid bone (*e*), ceratohyoid bone (*c*), basihyoid bone (*b*), and thyrohyoid bone (*t*) can be identified. The epiglottis (*ep*), arytenoid cartilage (*a*), thyroid cartilage (*th*), and cricoid cartilage (*cr*) are also identified in this study. **Diagnosis:** Normal larynx.

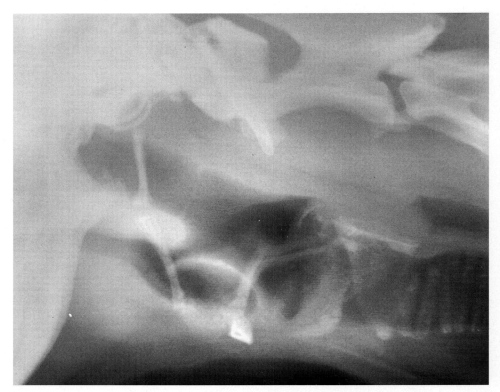

Figure 2–36. A 9-year-old male German shepherd dog presented with a 6-week history of difficulty breathing. A nasal cavity obstruction was suspected. In this lateral radiograph of the larynx, the larynx appears normal. There is marked calcification of the laryngeal cartilages and tracheal rings. **Diagnosis:** Normal larynx.

the base of the epiglottis. Their location varies with oblique patient positioning, although in many normal dogs they are not visible. The thyroid cartilage is a somewhat rectangular shaped density located caudal to the laryngeal saccule. The arytenoid cartilage extends rostrally from the apex of the thyroid cartilage. Its cuneiform process is usually seen as a blunt projection with its cranio-dorsally directed tip protruding into the pharynx. The cricoid cartilage is triangular with its base dorsal and apex ventral.

Identification of the hyoid bones depends upon proper radiographic exposure and correct symmetrical positioning. They are best evaluated on a lateral radiograph. The thyrohyoid bones extend ventrally from the cuneiform process of the arytenoid cartilage, cross the epiglottis at about its midpoint, and extend to the ventral floor of the oral pharynx. The basihyoid bone usually appears more dense than the other hyoid bones, because it is viewed end-on and therefore appears as a dense, somewhat triangular shaped structure. The ceratohyoid bones are the shortest of the paired hyoid bones. They extend rostrally from the basihyoid and are usually parallel to the soft palate. The epihyoid bones extend dorsally and rostrally from the ceratohyoid to the level of the soft palate. The stylohyoid bones extend dorsally and caudally from the epihyoid bones to the area caudal to the osseous bulla. The tympanohyoid cartilages attach to the stylohyoid bones and are not usually visible. All hyoid bones except the basihyoid are paired and should be symmetrical. Their symmetry depends on the accuracy with which the head and neck are positioned. In a well positioned lateral radiograph, these bones should be superimposed and their normal alignment should result in continuity from one bone to the next.

CERVICAL TRACHEA

The cervical trachea should be uniform in width throughout its length (Fig. 2–37). The individual tracheal rings may be identified if enough calcification is present. The inner (mucosal) surface should be intact and smooth. A slight dorsal indentation may be present immediately caudal to the cricoid cartilage, but, in general, the dorsoventral tracheal diameter should not be less than that of the larynx.[25] Flexion and extension of the head and neck will alter the position of the trachea.

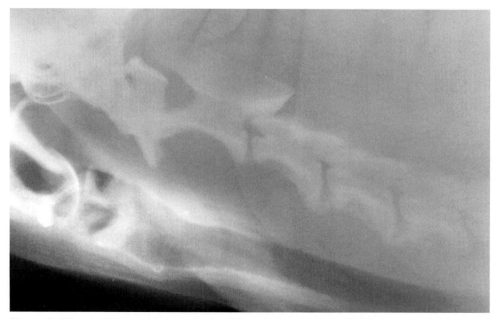

Figure 2–37. A 12-year-old spayed mixed breed dog presented with a 1-month history of coughing and gagging. A lateral radiograph of the cervical trachea was normal. The tracheal cartilages are faintly visible. The diameter of the cervical trachea is normal with a slight narrowing of the lumen caudal to the cricoid cartilage. **Diagnosis:** Normal cervical trachea.

Identification of the cervical trachea is difficult on the ventrodorsal radiograph due to superimposition of the vertebral column. Additionally, poor patient positioning will alter the trachea's location on this view.

CERVICAL ESOPHAGUS

The cervical esophagus should not be visible unless the animal swallows a bolus of air at the time of the radiographic exposure. The area through which the esophagus passes should be evaluated. The esophagus begins dorsal to the cricoid cartilage, remains dorsal to the trachea, and gradually moves laterally and to the left at the midcervical area. It continues to lie on the left side until it passes the thoracic inlet. The esophagus may be visible as a soft tissue density overlying the trachea through the midcervical area and beyond the thoracic inlet. This appearance may indicate tracheal collapse, chondromalacia of the tracheal cartilages, or a flaccid trachealis muscle.

RADIOGRAPHIC AND SONOGRAPHIC ABNORMALITIES

SOFT TISSUE ABNORMALITIES

Soft tissue abnormalities include soft tissue swelling and changes in density. The extent and location of the swelling are important. Localized or defined soft tissue swellings may be caused by tumors or localized infections (i.e., abscess, granuloma). Diffuse soft tissue swelling may result from subcutaneous fluid administration, edema, hemorrhage, or cellulitis (i.e., diffuse infection). Extension of the soft tissue swelling into the thoracic cavity or involvement of adjacent bone provide important clues to the radiographic diagnosis. Oblique radiographs may be necessary to detect pleural extension of an external mass.

Soft tissue masses that protrude from the thoracic wall and are surrounded by air often appear quite dense and may be mistaken for mineralized masses. Nipples are the most common of these masses and their location is an important distinguishing feature. Typically, three sides of these masses can be clearly identified, with the fourth side (where the mass is attached to the skin) blending with the underlying skin.

Alteration in soft tissue density may be the result of gas accumulation (subcutaneous emphysema), calcification, or foreign material. Subcutaneous emphysema usually results from puncture wounds or skin ulceration. It may also result from extension of pneumomediastinum, or from pharyngeal, tracheal, or esophageal perforation. A small amount of subcutaneous air may be present from subcutaneous injection of medication. Subcutaneous air usually produces a sharply marginated, linear radiolucency that outlines and dissects along fascial planes. The relative radiolucency of the lesion, despite its small volume, allows for differentiation between subcutaneous air and subcutaneous fat (Fig. 2–38). In animals with paracostal hernias, intestinal loops may be herniated subcutaneously along the thoracic wall. These gas-filled loops can usually be identified by their typical round or tubular shape.

Soft tissue calcification may occur within some mammary gland tumors or in tumors associated with the ribs or costal cartilages (Fig. 2–39). Linear cutaneous calcification may be seen with Cushing's syndrome. Foreign material on the skin or in the hair coat may mimic soft tissue calcification. In many cases, careful physical examination is necessary to identify the foreign material. Although linear or "plaque-like" calcified densities are more typical of Cushing's syndrome, the pattern of calcification is non-specific. Amorphous calcified masses may be malignant or benign neoplasms, abscesses, or hematomas.

Subcutaneous foreign bodies may be identified if they are radiopaque; however,

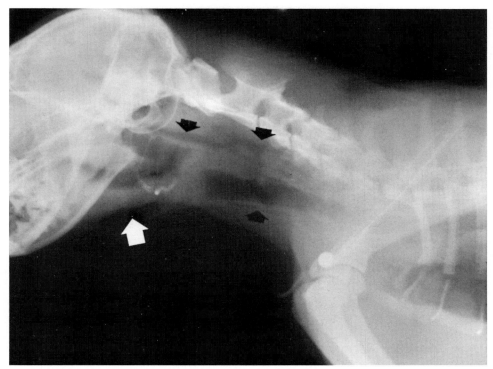

Figure 2–38. (A&B) A 4-year-old female cat presented with an acute onset of expiratory dyspnea. A foul odor was present in the oral cavity. Gas is noted in the retropharyngeal area, around the trachea, and ventral to the larynx (*arrows*). The larynx is indistinct and increased in density. The radiographic findings are indicative of laryngeal swelling with subcutaneous emphysema. The possibility of a radiolucent foreign body should be considered. **Diagnosis:** Laryngitis with necrosis of the laryngeal mucosa. The animal was endoscopically examined. The cause of the laryngitis and mucosal ulceration could not be determined.

tissue-dense foreign bodies will not be detected. Although fistulography has been recommended, it is rarely used because the loose subcutaneous tissue of the dog and cat allow contrast dissection along planes other than those associated with the foreign body or fistula.

Ultrasound can be utilized to determine the nature and extent of abnormalities in soft tissues. The size and shape of a lesion may be clearly delineated if surrounded by tissue of different echogenicity (e.g., a subcutaneous mass surrounded by fat). In cases where the lesion blends into similarly echogenic tissue, the delineation may not be so clear. The question of whether a mass is solid or cystic will be answered by the ultrasound examination. Cystic structures have few or no internal echoes, have a distinct wall, and show evidence of through transmission. Solid structures have internal echoes and less sharply defined walls. Hematomas and abscesses have similar internal structure with hypoechoic or anechoic cavities, while most tumors have a more uniform mixed echogenic appearance. Soft tissue mineralization (hyperechoic foci with shadowing) may be identified. The echogenicity of the mass should always be compared to the adjacent normal tissue. This can be useful in identifying a lipoma that is uniformly hyperechoic compared to the surrounding tissue. Ultrasonography is rarely tissue- or cell-specific. It is very useful in guiding a needle into a fluid-containing cavity for aspiration or biopsy.

BONY ABNORMALITIES

Abnormalities of the bony thorax are discussed in conjunction with evaluation of the specific portion of the axial skeleton (i.e., ribs, spine, sternum); however, those

Figure 2–39. (A&B) A 10-year-old spayed German shepherd dog presented with mammary tumors. There is a large soft tissue and mineralized density lesion located in the area of the caudal ventral right thorax. (A) This mass overlies the right caudal lung lobe (*arrows*) on the ventrodorsal radiograph and mimics an intrapulmonary lesion; (B) on the lateral radiograph, its position external to the thorax is clearly identified. Note that the cranial, dorsal, and ventral margins of this mass are distinctly outlined while the caudal margin is less distinct. This is due to air outlining the margins of the mass with its attachment caudally blending with the thoracic wall density. External thoracic masses may overlie the lung and mimic intrapulmonary disease; usually, their position can be accurately identified on one of the two radiographic projections. **Diagnosis:** Mammary gland mass on the right ventral caudal thoracic wall. There is no evidence of pulmonary metastases.

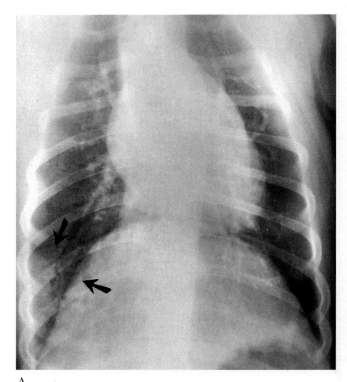

A

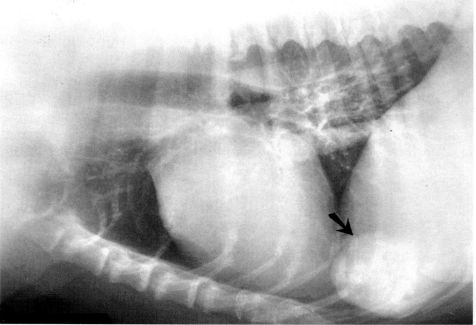

B

bony abnormalities that may be associated with intrathoracic pathology are briefly discussed.

VERTEBRAL LESIONS

Vertebral body fractures or dislocation may accompany thoracic trauma (Fig. 2–40). Malalignment of vertebral segments and collapse or shortening of a vertebral body may be observed. In order to detect pathological fractures, the density of the vertebral bodies should be evaluated carefully.

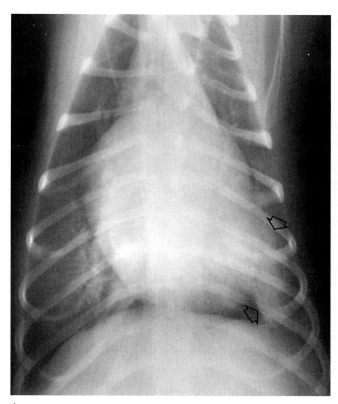

A

Figure 2–40. (A&B) A 1-year-old female toy poodle was presented following thoracic trauma. (A) On the ventrodorsal radiograph there is a soft tissue density present in the left caudal lung lobe (*open arrows*). This localized interstitial density is representative of pulmonary contusion. There are no rib fractures identified. (B) On the lateral radiograph there is ventral displacement of T–11 relative to T–10 (*closed arrows*). No evidence of displacement is seen on (A). The fracture of T–10 is easily identified on (B). Lesions such as this should not be overlooked in animals radiographed for evaluation of thoracic trauma. This dog exhibited pain without neurologic deficits. **Diagnosis:** Pulmonary contusion. Fracture of T–10.

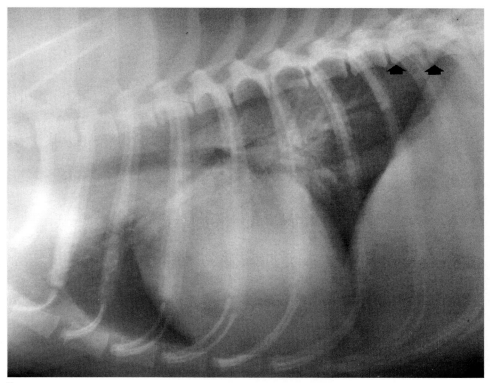

B

Primary or metastatic neoplasms may affect the ribs or vertebral bodies. These areas should be examined for productive, destructive, or mixed lesions, especially in patients radiographed for pulmonary metastasis (see Fig. 2–42). Mediastinal masses may invade adjacent vertebral bodies, and the bony lesion can indicate the etiology of these masses. Osteomyelitis or discospondylitis may be identified in a patient radiographed for other reasons.

RIB FRACTURES

Rib lesions may accompany thoracic abnormalities. Rib fractures often result from chest wall trauma. Pathologic rib fractures should be recognized. The interruption of the cortical margins, radiolucent fracture line, malalignment of fragments, or increased density from overlapping fracture ends may be observed when rib fractures occur. Chest wall asymmetry and uneven spacing of the ribs suggests rib fractures. Medially displaced rib fragments can penetrate the lung. Thoracic wall instability (flail chest) can result from adjacent segmental rib fractures. Fracture of several adjacent ribs at two or more sites can produce a thoracic wall that moves inward on inspiration and outward at expiration. This may markedly interfere with pulmonary function.[44] Thoracic radiographs exposed at both inspiration and expiration may document the extent of the instability.

Pathologic fractures should be suspected whenever a solitary rib fracture or fractures in nonadjacent ribs are detected. Bony proliferation or lysis of the rib will be seen if the rib is examined closely. A subcutaneous or pleural soft tissue mass may be detected if the rib area is examined carefully.

Tearing of the intercostal muscles will result in the space between two ribs being significantly larger on one side when compared to the other side (Fig. 2–41). This is commonly seen in small animals that have been bitten by a large dog. If the tear is extensive, the lack of chest wall continuity can result in paradoxical chest wall mo-

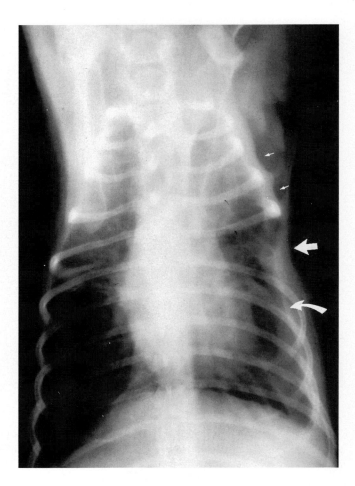

Figure 2–41. A 3-year-old male Yorkshire terrier that had been attacked by a larger dog presented in shock and with dyspnea. The ventrodorsal radiograph reveals an abnormal separation between the left 5th and 6th ribs (*large, straight arrow*). There is gas in the soft tissues around this area (*small arrows*). Pleural fluid density (presumably a blood clot) is present at the site (*large, curved arrow*). No evidence of pneumothorax is noted. **Diagnosis:** Intercostal tear of the left 5th intercostal space, pleural hematoma, subcutaneous emphysema.

tion and severely compromised respiratory function. Asymmetrical rib spacing may also occur in association with soft tissue trauma (bruising), previous thoracotomy, hemivertebra, and pulmonary or pleural disease.

Healed rib fractures should be recognized and not mistaken for more significant pathology such as metastatic tumor. Cortical malalignment or expansion of the bony margin will persist for years after the original injury. The bony trabecular pattern will be smooth and evenly mineralized, and soft tissue swelling will be absent or minimal. These features are useful in discriminating between healed fractures and rib metastasis.

RIB TUMOR AND INFECTION

Tumor and infection may involve the ribs, and both productive and destructive bony lesions may be identified. Infection may be hematogenous, may extend from the chest wall, or, less often, may extend from the pleural space. Osteomyelitis is usually proliferative with minimal amounts of bony destruction. Rib tumors may be primary or metastatic. Fibrosarcoma, chondrosarcoma, and osteosarcoma may arise from the rib or costal cartilage. These tumors may grow inward and produce large extrapleural masses (Fig. 2–42). Rib destruction and/or soft tissue calcification may be evident radiographically. Displacement or invasion of adjacent ribs may occur. Metastatic lesions are often small when detected and may be proliferative, destructive, or both. Cortical expansion, a soft tissue mass, or both may be identified. The cortical malalignment usually associated with rib fracture will not be present unless a pathologic fracture has occurred.

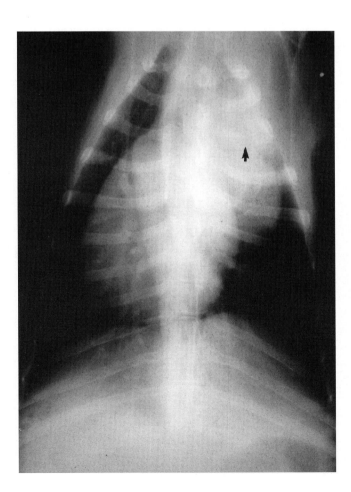

Figure 2–42. A 9-year-old male Old English sheepdog presented with a 2-month history of coughing. The ventrodorsal radiograph reveals a large tissue density mass in the area of the cranial portion of the left cranial lung lobe. Close examination reveals lysis of the left 3rd rib (*arrow*) suggesting the mass is arising from the rib and extending into the thoracic cavity. **Diagnosis:** Chondrosarcoma of the left 3rd rib.

THORACIC WALL ANOMALIES

Several types of chest wall deformity have been described. Pectus excavatum (funnel chest, chondrosternal depression) is a reduction in the dorsoventral thoracic diameter due to displacement of the sternum dorsally into the thorax (Fig. 2–43).[45] This usually displaces the cardiac silhouette to one side or the other and creates soft tissue shadows that overlie the lung and create difficulty in cardiac and pulmonary evaluations. In the lateral radiograph, the sternum may be superimposed on the cardiac silhouette and curvature of the ribs may be observed.

Pigeon breast, another chest wall deformity, may be acquired in dogs with cardiomegaly secondary to congenital heart disease (Fig. 2–44). It has no clinical significance. The sternum is angled excessively in a caudoventral direction producing a dorsoventral thoracic diameter, which is markedly increased at the xiphoid when compared to the manubrium.

Sternal abnormalities are frequent and usually without clinical significance. Soft tissue infection, tumors, and trauma may affect the sternebrae. Few sternal anomalies are significant. Absence, splitting, or malformation of the xiphoid cartilage has been associated with peritoneopericardial diaphragmatic hernia, and this can be a useful radiographic feature in distinguishing that condition from other pericardial diseases.[46]

An acute bony lesion rarely occurs without an associated soft tissue injury; consequently, the evaluation of the bony structures cannot be divorced from the evaluation of the adjacent soft tissues. In the absence of a soft tissue lesion most bony deformities can be ignored.

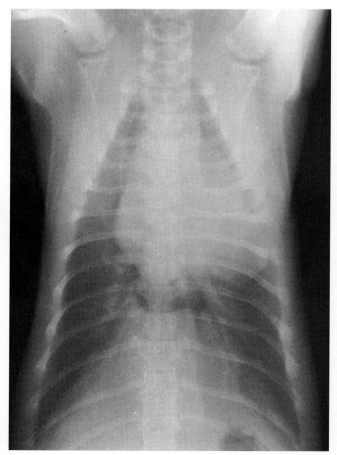

Figure 2–43. (A&B) A 9-month-old male Pekingese presented with a 3-month history of coughing. (A) On the lateral radiograph the thorax is compressed in a dorsoventral direction. The caudal sternebrae are elevated dorsally. There is a depression in the external thoracic wall at this point. The cardiac silhouette and trachea are displaced dorsally. (B) On the ventrodorsal radiograph, the cardiac silhouette is shifted into the left hemithorax. There is no evidence of pulmonary disease. **Diagnosis:** Pectus excavatum.

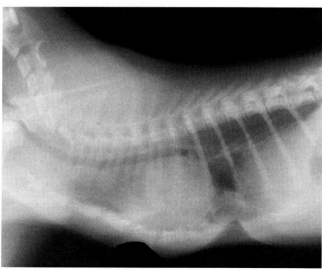

A

B

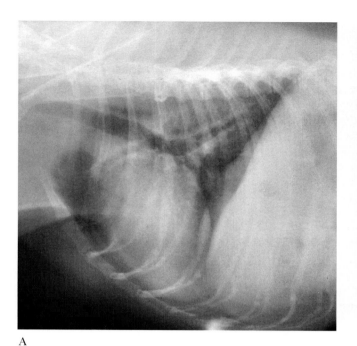
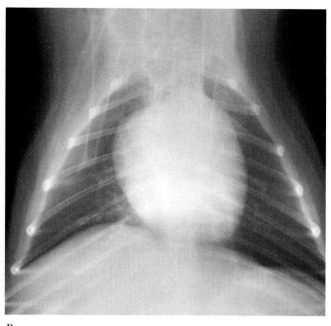

A   B

Figure 2–44. (A&B) A 5-year-old female mixed breed dog presented with a 4-month history of chronic cough, which had not responded to antibiotics and bronchial dilators. The thoracic cavity is markedly widened at its caudal aspect in both (A) the lateral and (B) the ventrodorsal radiographs. The sternum diverges at an acute angle from the thoracic spine. This thoracic conformation is referred to as pigeon chest. **Diagnosis:** Normal thorax.

DIAPHRAGMATIC ABNORMALITIES

The variation in appearance of the normal diaphragm due to variations in breed, species, position, x-ray beam geometry, phase of respiration, and abdominal content make recognition of diaphragmatic abnormalities difficult. Although the basic shape of the diaphragm is fairly constant, contour alterations occur frequently.

Diaphragmatic abnormalities that may be recognized radiographically include changes in shape, width, outline, and position. The diaphragmatic outline may be deformed from masses arising from the diaphragm, from the pleural space, or from abdominal masses that protrude through the diaphragm. The diaphragm's outline and position may change with diaphragmatic hernia or diaphragmatic paralysis.

MASSES

Masses may arise from or involve the diaphragm; pleural or mediastinal tumors may metastasize to or involve the diaphragm. Solitary or multiple masses may protrude from the diaphragm altering its normal shape. Diaphragmatic granulomas or adhesions may occur in association with chronic pleural disease; focal or multifocal diaphragmatic irregularities may be produced. The patient's history or analysis of fluid obtained from thoracocentesis is necessary for differentiation of these lesions, because the radiographic appearance will be similar.

Sonographic evaluation from the abdominal side of the diaphragm may reveal an abnormal shape to the diaphragm. However, this can be difficult to appreciate unless there is fluid between the diaphragm and liver. Discriminating between diaphragmatic, pleural, or mediastinal masses, diaphragmatic hernias with herniation of a liver lobe and caudal or accessory lung lobe masses can be challenging. The manner in which the mass moves (whether with the lung or the diaphragm) may be a useful feature in determining the origin of a mass in the region of the diaphragm.

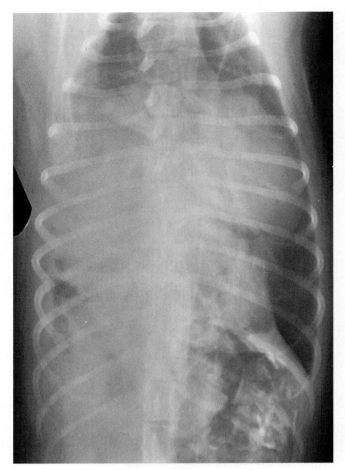

A

Figure 2–45. (A&B) A 2-year-old male mixed breed dog presented following thoracic trauma. The dog had mild respiratory distress. There are multiple gas-filled loops of intestine noted within the right ventral hemithorax. There are many bone fragments noted within the stomach, which has been displaced into the ventral thorax. The cardiac silhouette is displaced into the left hemithorax. **Diagnosis:** Diaphragmatic hernia.

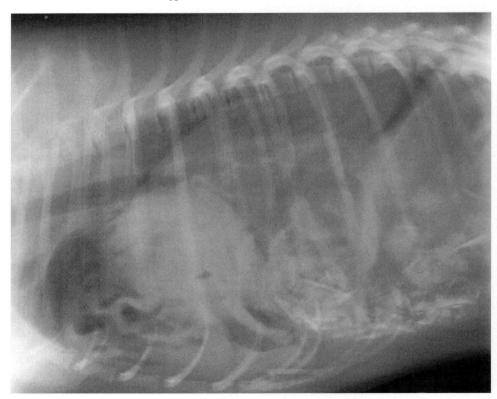

B

HERNIAS

Diaphragmatic hernias allow protrusion of abdominal viscera through the diaphragm. These protrusions alter the shape of the diaphragm.

Diaphragmatic Hernia

Several different acquired and congenital diaphragmatic hernias may occur.[47-49] These include traumatic or congenital diaphragmatic hernia, hiatal hernia, and pericardial diaphragmatic hernia. Although congenital diaphragmatic hernias occur, most diaphragmatic hernias are traumatic. Many congenital diaphragmatic hernias are associated with sternal anomalies. In most cases, the diagnosis of traumatic diaphragmatic hernia can be easily confirmed radiographically. When large amounts of pleural fluid are present and only a portion of the liver is herniated, the diagnosis may be difficult. The presence of gas-, food-, or fluid-filled portions of the gastrointestinal tract within the pleural space is the most reliable radiographic evidence of diaphragmatic hernia (Fig. 2–45). The bowel should be recognized because of its typical size, shape, and density. Obstruction of the bowel may occur and result in bowel distention, which could turn a chronic diaphragmatic hernia into an acute condition. Loss of the diaphragmatic outline is a sign of diaphragmatic hernia; however, this may occur with any type of pleural fluid and with pulmonary, pleural, or caudal mediastinal masses that arise from or contact the diaphragm. Diaphragmatic hernias usually result in displacement of the thoracic viscera (Fig. 2–46). The degree and direction of the displacement will vary with the hernia site and amount of abdominal viscera within the pleural space. On occasion, only the stomach will herniate into the pleural space and become distended with gas. This will appear as a homogeneous gas density that has no pulmonary vessels and which displaces the cardiac silhouette and pulmonary parenchyma. It is critical that gastric involvement in diaphragmatic hernias be recognized, because these can become acute, life-threatening emergencies if the stomach dilates and significantly interferes with respiration.

In addition to the thoracic radiographic changes, the abdominal radiograph will also be useful. The stomach may be positioned closer to the diaphragmatic outline when the liver herniates into the thorax. In many obese cats and in several dogs, the falciform ligament contains enough fat to outline the ventral abdominal margin of the diaphragm. Loss of this shadow in an obese animal with pleural fluid, but without peritoneal fluid, indicates a diagnosis of diaphragmatic hernia. In some animals with diaphragmatic hernia, the absence of normal viscera from the abdomen will permit the diagnosis of diaphragmatic hernia. Rib fractures, especially those involving the caudal ribs, may also be detected. Diaphragmatic tears may occur without herniation and may not be radiographically detectable.

Barium contrast examinations of the stomach and small intestine may be helpful when the diagnosis is not obvious on the survey film. Positioning of the stomach close to the diaphragm or identification of bowel within the thorax confirms the diagnosis of diaphragmatic hernia.

Positive and negative contrast peritoneography have been used to evaluate the diaphragm.[50] Injection of 1 to 2 ml per kilogram body weight of water-soluble positive-contrast into the peritoneal cavity followed by right and left lateral, sternal, and dorsal recumbent radiographs allows complete evaluation of the diaphragm. Identification of contrast within the pleural space confirms the diagnosis of diaphragmatic rupture (Fig. 2–47). Air, carbon dioxide, or nitrous oxide may also be used. The gas is injected into the peritoneal cavity, and its identification in the pleural cavity confirms the diagnosis (Fig. 2–48). Positional maneuvers including horizontal beam radiography can be used to float the gas between the liver and the diaphragm thereby outlining the abdominal surface of the diaphragm. In chronic diaphragmatic hernias, adhesions of the viscera to the diaphragm can interfere with contrast flow into the pleural space and result in a false-negative study.

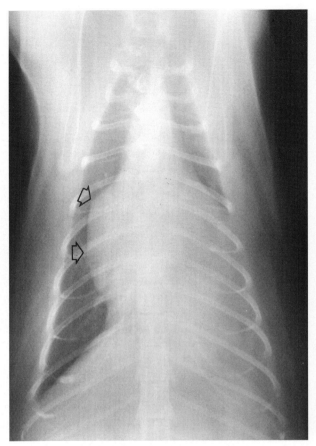

A

Figure 2–46. (A&B). A 10-year-old male cat presented with a 12-day history of hematuria and stranguria. Abdominal radiographs were obtained and, because of the appearance of the thorax on the abdominal radiographs, thoracic radiographs were obtained. There is a loss of the normal diaphragmatic shadow on the left side. There is a soft tissue and fat density located within the caudal ventral left hemithorax. The cardiac silhouette is displaced to the right and dorsally (*arrows*). **Diagnosis:** Diaphragmatic hernia.

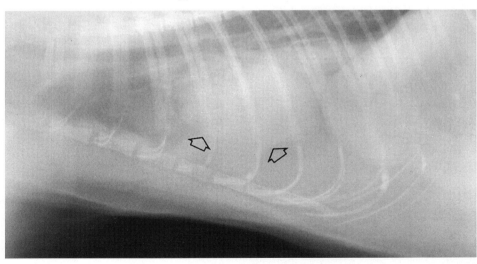

B

Positional radiographs may also be used to evaluate the diaphragm when pleural fluid is present. Right, left, sternal, and dorsal recumbent radiographs using both horizontally and vertically directed x-ray beams will shift the pleural fluid and outline different portions of the diaphragm. These positional maneuvers also permit complete evaluation of the stomach when it contains both gas and fluid. Positioning of the pylorus or body close to the diaphragm will indicate that the liver is small or herniated.

Congenital diaphragmatic hernias are seen infrequently. It is difficult to clinically distinguish them from traumatic hernias, because the radiographic signs are the

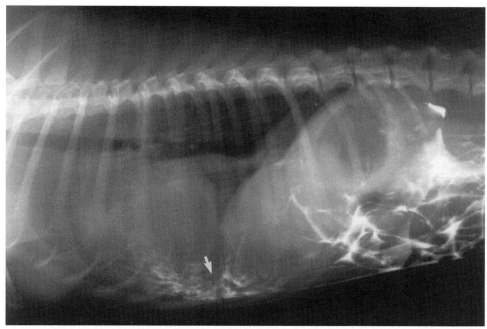

Figure 2–47. A 2-year-old male Cairn terrier presented with mild exercise intolerance. The dog had run away a week prior to being found and presented. Examination of survey radiographs revealed an increased density in the caudal and ventral portion of the thorax. A positive contrast celiogram reveals extravasation of the contrast media across the diaphragm and into the thoracic cavity (*arrow*). **Diagnosis:** Diaphragmatic hernia.

same. Congenital defects are most often on the ventral midline and the xiphoid is frequently involved. Malformation of the sternum including absence or splitting of the xiphoid or alteration in the shape and number of the sternebrae may be identified.

Sonographic changes associated with diaphragmatic hernias are usually restricted to the identification of hydrothorax and abdominal structures in abnormal locations (Fig. 2–49).[21] The most commonly involved organ is the liver. It is important to carefully identify a structure as liver because atelectatic lung, lung lobe torsion, and pulmonary or pleural neoplasms can closely mimic the sonographic appearance of liver.

It is usually very difficult to specifically identify a diaphragmatic rent, because the diaphragm itself is rarely seen. The hyperechoic line that is normally seen between the liver and lung is really the interface between the diaphragm (tissue) and lung (air). If there is a diaphragmatic defect, the interface between liver and lung will also appear as a thin, hyperechoic line.

Esophageal Hiatal Hernia

Although hernias may potentially occur around the caval or aortic hiatus, only those around the esophageal hiatus have been reported.[51–55] Esophageal hiatal hernias have been subdivided into three types (axial hiatal hernia, paraesophageal hernia, and combined hernia). An oval or semicircular soft tissue density may be visible protruding from the diaphragm in the lateral radiograph at the level of the esophageal hiatus. The soft tissue density will extend on the ventrodorsal view into the caudal mediastinum on or slightly to the left of the midline. Secondary esophageal dilation with food, fluid, or gas may be identified. Gas within the stomach will outline the rugal fold pattern and allow recognition of the stomach's position cranial to the diaphragm. In some instances, the rugal folds may be traced caudally through the diaphragmatic opening into the abdominal portion of the stomach (Fig. 2–50). Many hiatal hernias are termed "sliding" (i.e., the stomach may move into and out of the caudal mediastinum on sequential radiographs). An esophageal contrast

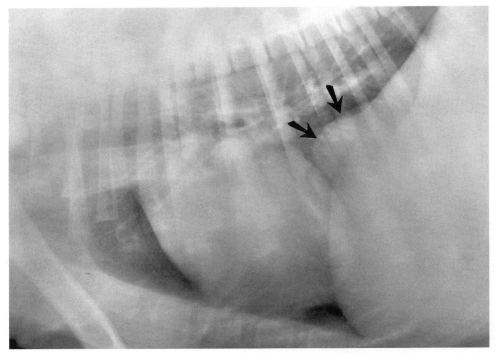

A

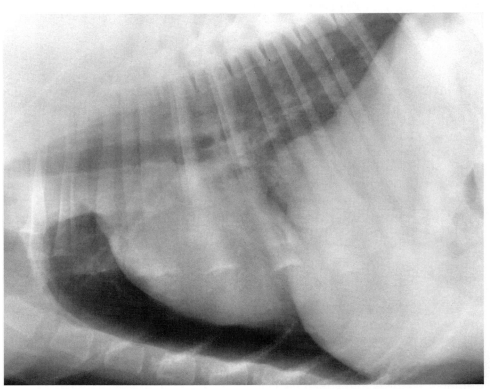

B

Figure 2–48. (A&B) A 6-month-old male mixed breed dog presented after thoracic trauma. The animal was mildly dyspneic. (A) On the lateral thoracic radiograph the diaphragm appeared to be irregular (*arrows*). No other abnormalities are noted. Carbon dioxide was introduced into the peritoneal cavity through a plastic catheter, and (B) a second lateral thoracic radiograph was obtained. Air is present within the pleural space separating the heart from the sternum. This is indicative of communication between the peritoneal and pleural cavities due to a diaphragmatic hernia. The diaphragmatic tear was at the level of the diaphragmatic irregularity. **Diagnosis:** Diaphragmatic hernia with herniation of a small portion of the liver.

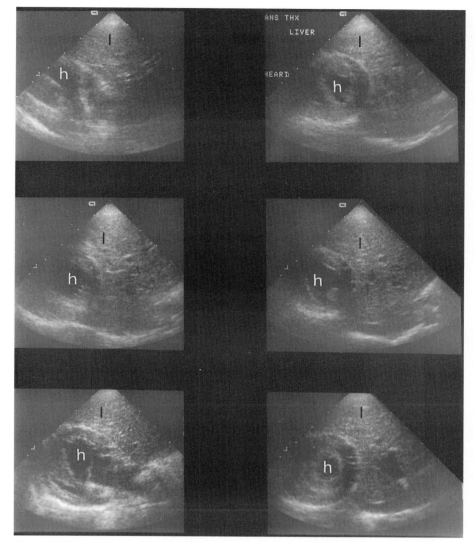

Figure 2–49. A 5-year-old male Yorkshire terrier presented due to an acute onset of dyspnea. Right parasternal short-axis views reveal the presence of liver (*l*) adjacent to the heart (*h*). The diaphragm is not visible. **Diagnosis:** Diaphragmatic hernia.

study is necessary in most instances to distinguish between axial hiatal hernia, in which the stomach protrudes through the esophageal hiatus, and paraesophageal hernia, in which the stomach protrudes through a diaphragmatic opening lateral to the hiatus. Sonographically, the stomach may be seen protruding cranially beyond the rest of the abdominal viscera with a hiatal hernia.

Pericardial Diaphragmatic Hernia

Pericardial diaphragmatic hernia (PDH) usually causes a pumpkin-shaped cardiac silhouette and is, therefore, one of the differential diagnostic considerations in dogs with generalized cardiac enlargement.[46,56,57] If gas-filled gastrointestinal structures are within the pericardial sac, the diagnosis may be radiographically evident (Fig. 2–51). The diaphragmatic defect in these animals is often small and not radiographically detectable. In cats with congenital PDH, the presence of a dorsal peritoneopericardial mesothelial remnant (a distinct curvilinear soft tissue opacity between the cardiac silhouette and diaphragm) is highly indicative of the diagnosis (Fig. 2–52).[56] Sonographicaly, PDH is recognized by the presence of abdominal viscera within the pericardial sac. This condition is discussed more completely in the section on cardiac abnormalities.

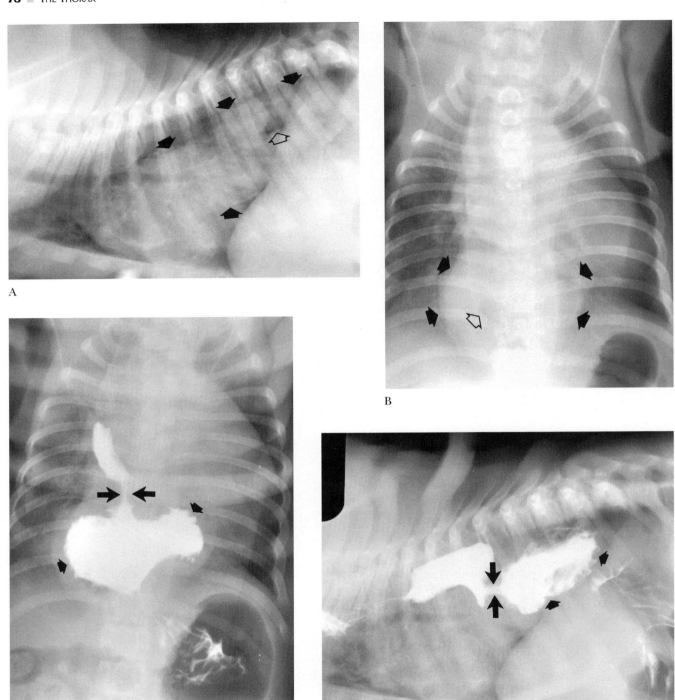

A

B

C

D

Figure 2–50. (A,B,C,D) A 3-month-old, male Shar-Pei presented with a history of labored breathing over a period of several weeks. (A) Lateral and (B) ventrodorsal thoracic radiographs revealed a soft tissue-dense mass located in the caudal mediastinum. This density obliterates a portion of the caudal dorsal cardiac silhouette (*closed arrows*) and is visible on the midline in (B). There is a gas bubble within this soft tissue density (*open arrows*). An esophagram was performed with (C) ventrodorsal and (D) lateral radiographs. The caudal thoracic esophagus is dilated. There is a constriction in the esophagus at the level of T–8 (*large arrows*). Caudal to this constriction, the contrast column widens into a large hollow viscus. There are irregularities in the margins of this structure, which represent rugal folds (*small arrows*). An additional constriction is noted caudal to this area of dilation. Contrast can be traced from that point into the intra-abdominal portion of the stomach. The radiographic findings are indicative of hiatal hernia. The size of the barium containing bowel and the presence of rugal folds identify the intrathoracic portion of the stomach. **Diagnosis:** Esophageal hiatal hernia.

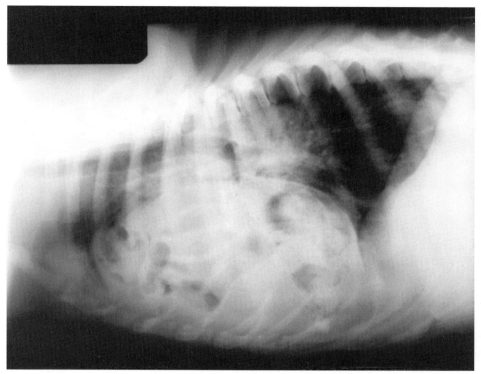

Figure 2–51. A 1-year-old male old English sheepdog presented with exercise intolerance. On physical examination the heart sounds were muffled. The lateral radiograph reveals a severely enlarged cardiac silhouette with multiple air-filled tubular structures within it. **Diagnosis:** Pericardial diaphragmatic hernia with loops of bowel trapped within the pericardial sac.

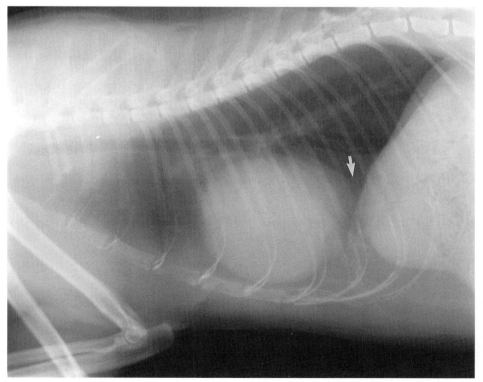

Figure 2–52. An 8-year-old female domestic long-haired cat was examined for abdominal distension. The lateral view of the thorax revealed an enlarged cardiac silhouette. The liver appears to be slightly smaller than normal. The dorsal peritoneopericardial mesothelial remnant (*arrow*) can be seen. **Diagnosis:** Congenital pericardial diaphragmatic hernia.

HYPERTROPHIC MUSCULAR DYSTROPHY

Thickening and irregularity of the diaphragmatic contour, megaesophagus, and cardiomegaly have been described in dogs and cats with hypertrophic muscular dystrophy.[58] Decreased liver echogenicity, peritoneal fluid, hepatic, splenic and renal enlargement, increased renal cortical echogenicity, and adrenal mineralization may be demonstrated on ultrasound examination. Concentric left ventricular hypertrophy, increased left ventricular systolic and diastolic dimensions, and increased endocardial echogenicity have also been reported.

ABNORMAL FUNCTION

The position of the diaphragm varies with respiratory phase, recumbency, and pressure from abdominal contents. In lateral recumbency, the dependent crus is usually cranial to the opposite crus. Asymmetry between diaphragmatic crura may be a normal variation; however, if one crus is consistently located cranial to the opposite crus despite positional changes, the possibility of a functional diaphragmatic abnormality should be considered. Displacement of one or both diaphragmatic crura may result from adhesions or diaphragmatic paralysis. It may also result from pulmonary, pleural, or abdominal diseases. Functional evaluation of the diaphragm usually requires fluoroscopy.

PLEURAL ABNORMALITIES

Pleural abnormalities that can be detected include intra- and extra-pleural masses and air or fluid accumulation in the pleural space. Specific radiographic and sonographic changes are described for evaluating these conditions.

PLEURAL AND EXTRAPLEURAL MASSES

Masses that involve the thoracic wall may extend into the thorax, although they may not penetrate the pleura. These chest wall masses are often referred to as extrapleural masses. The intact pleural covering produces a smooth distinct margin over the inner surface of these masses. A convex interface with the adjacent lung and concave edges at the point of attachment to the chest wall (referred to as a shoulder) may be seen (Fig. 2–53). These masses are usually widest at their point of attachment. Rib destruction, bony proliferation, soft tissue mineralization and distortion of intercostal spaces may be seen. Although the presence of a bony lesion identifies the mass as extrapleural, the absence of bone lesions does not exclude that possibility. The often smaller, external portion of the mass may also be identified. Pleural fluid, more often observed with pleural than extrapleural or pulmonary masses, is usually minimal, occurring after the mass becomes rather large. Most extrapleural masses are neoplastic, often arising from the rib or costal cartilage, although some inflammatory lesions may be encountered. When an intrapulmonary lesion is located at the edge of a lung lobe and contacts the parietal pleura, it can appear similar to a pleural or extrapleural mass. The shape of the soft tissue density and evaluation of the point of junction between chest wall and lung lesion may distinguish between pulmonary and extrapleural masses.[59] Pulmonary masses are usually round and lack the "shoulder" observed with extrapleural masses. Obtaining opposite lateral views will be helpful in distinguishing between pulmonary and pleural or extrapleural masses. In some instances, biopsy, needle aspirate, or surgery is the only way to make a definitive diagnosis. Fluoroscopic examination, computed tomography, ultrasonography, and/or pleurography have been recommended; however, they are rarely required.

Herniation of abdominal viscera through a diaphragmatic tear may mimic the appearance of a pleural or extrapleural mass. Positional radiographs, evaluation of the abdomen, and careful evaluation of the diaphragm will usually identify the hernia.

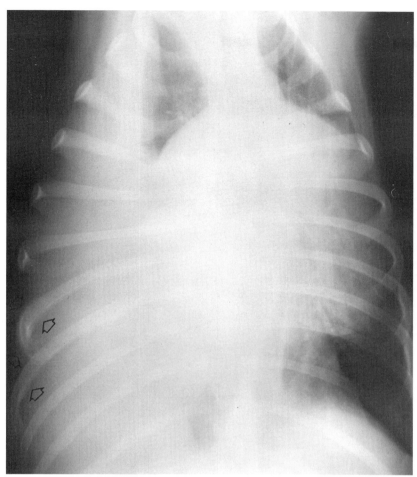

A

Figure 2–53. (A&B) A 2-year-old male mixed breed dog presented with a history of having been kicked by a horse 2 weeks previously. Soft tissue swelling was present on the right thoracic wall. The dog had evidence of mild respiratory distress. There is a soft tissue density in the right hemithorax. The cardiac silhouette and trachea are displaced to the left. The diaphragmatic outline is obliterated. There is bony proliferation on the cortical margins of the 8th and 9th ribs. There is destruction involving the ventral aspect of the 8th rib at the costochondral junction (*arrows*). There is irregular soft tissue mineralization noted in this area. The radiographic changes are indicative of a pleural mass that has displaced the cardiac silhouette. Although other causes of pleural fluid and mass should also be considered in a differential diagnosis, the bony lesion indicates that the mass is extrapleural and arising from the ribs. **Diagnosis:** Fibrosarcoma.

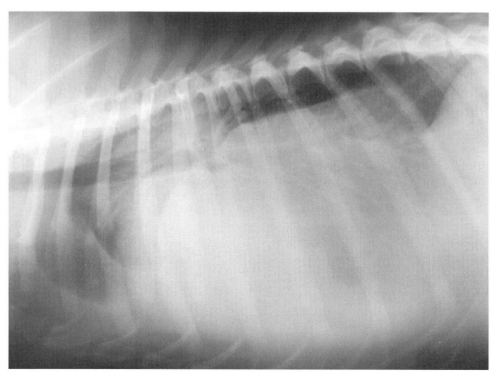

B

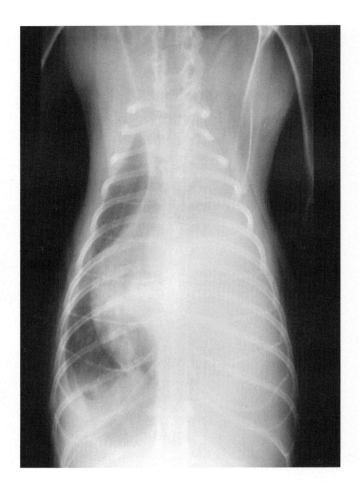

Figure 2–54. A 5-year-old male cat presented with dyspnea and pale mucous membranes. A diaphragmatic hernia had been repaired 4 months earlier. In the ventrodorsal radiograph there is a soft tissue density that obliterates the entire left thoracic cavity. The cardiac silhouette and trachea are displaced to the right. There is a small amount of fluid present in the pleural space on the right side. This fluid outlines the lung lobes and separates them from the lateral thoracic wall. The radiographic changes are indicative of a soft tissue density within the left hemithorax. This could be a mass or trapped pleural fluid. A thoracocentesis was performed and purulent material was removed. **Diagnosis:** Loculated pyothorax.

Encapsulated or loculated pleural fluid, granulomatous masses, or pleural neoplasms may produce radiographic evidence of pleural masses (Fig. 2–54). Primary and metastatic pleural neoplasms are rare. They are often hidden by the presence of pleural fluid and are not identified until the fluid is removed.[60] A fluid collection that does not conform to the normal linear or triangular shape of the pleural space as defined by the lung lobes, or a fluid density that maintains its position and shape despite alteration in the animal's position during radiography, is indicative of a pleural mass. Rib involvement is unusual. Uneven lung compression or displacement of the heart or other mediastinal structures can also be observed.

As a screening technique for pleural lesions, ultrasound is usually impractical because of the large area that must be evaluated. The transducer must be placed immediately over the lesion to be identified. However, once an area of interest is identified radiographically, the area may be readily evaluated to determine the tissues involved and the character (cystic or solid) of the lesion. Observing movement of the mass with respiration, which identifies the mass as intrapulmonary, and identifying the position of the lung lobes when the mass is pleural are useful in discriminating among diaphragmatic hernias and pleural and pulmonary masses. Once a lesion is imaged, the sonogram can be used to guide a needle for biopsy or aspiration.[21]

PLEURAL FLUID (HYDROTHORAX)

The radiographic appearance of pleural fluid depends upon the nature and amount of the fluid and the presence or absence of co-existing thoracic disease. Pleural fluid will obliterate normal fluid-dense structures and will highlight air-containing structures (Fig. 2–55). In the lateral radiograph, the cardiac apex and diaphragmatic outline may be obliterated. Because of their elastic nature, the lung lobes will retain

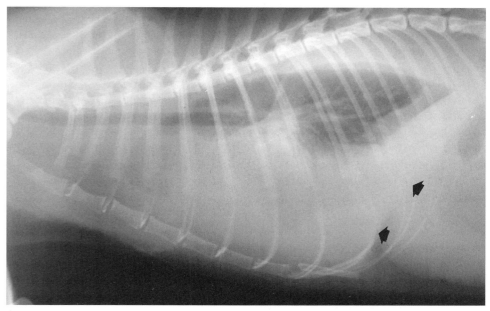

A

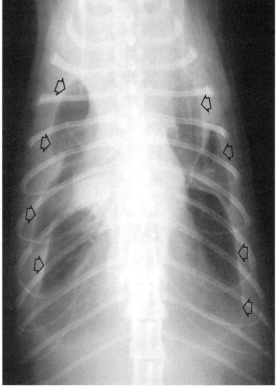

B

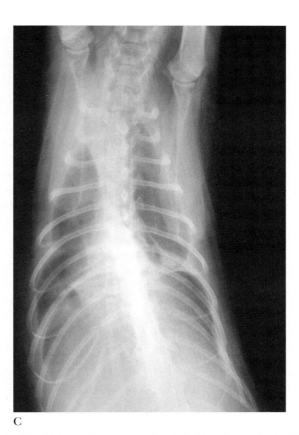

C

Figure 2–55. (A,B,C) A 2-year-old female cat was presented with a history of dyspnea and muffled heart sounds. (A) Lateral, (B) ventrodorsal, and (C) erect ventrodorsal thoracic radiographs were obtained. In the (B) ventrodorsal radiograph, the margins of the lung lobes are visible (*open arrows*) outlined by a fluid density that separates them from the lateral thoracic wall and outlines the interlobar fissures. The cardiac silhouette is obscured. In the (A) lateral radiograph, the diaphragmatic margins are obscured on the thoracic side—the fat in the abdomen identifies the abdominal side of the diaphragm (*closed arrows*). The radiographic changes are indicative of pleural fluid. Because the cranial mediastinum could not be evaluated on the ventrodorsal radiograph an (C) erect ventrodorsal radiograph was obtained using a horizontally directed x-ray beam. The lung lobes moved into the cranial thorax with gravitation of the pleural fluid caudally. This radiographic finding indicates that an anterior mediastinal mass was not present. **Diagnosis:** Pleural fluid. A thoracocentesis was performed and pyothorax was diagnosed.

their normal shape and fluid will accumulate in the interlobar fissures dorsal and ventral to the lung lobes. This outlines the lung lobes, accentuating their margins, and produces a "scalloping" or "leafing" of the lobes. Fluid collecting between lung lobes produces linear- or triangular-shaped densities at the anatomic sites of the interlobar fissures. If fluid has been present for a significant length of time (weeks to months), fibrin deposition or inflammation of the visceral pleura may result in rounding of the lung lobe margins. The volume of fluid that is present will determine the extent to which the heart and diaphragm are obliterated, the width of the interlobar fissures, and the amount of separation between the lung and the dorsal and ventral thoracic wall. In animals with freely moveable pleural fluid, right and left lateral recumbent radiographs differ, because the mediastinum will not prevent fluid movement from one side to the other and the dependent lung lobes will collapse to a greater extent than the nondependent lobes. Failure of the fluid to shift position in opposite lateral recumbent radiographs indicates that the fluid is trapped, the mediastinum is abnormally thickened, the fluid is fibrinous, or a pleural mass is present.[60]

The dorsoventral and ventrodorsal radiographs appear different when free pleural fluid is present due to gravity's effect on the heart, lung, and fluid.[61] In the ventrodorsal view, the pleural fluid accumulates dorsally on either side of the vertebral column. The cardiac silhouette will usually be visible, surrounded by aerated lung. The costodiaphragmatic recesses or costophrenic angles will become rounded or blunted. If only a small amount of fluid is present it may be localized to the "paraspinal gutters" and may be only minimally apparent on the ventrodorsal view. More often, fluid will be evident (i.e., separating the lungs from the lateral thoracic wall, separating individual lung lobes) on both views. This is dependent on the amount of fluid and is usually more obvious in the ventrodorsal when compared to the dorsoventral view. Pleural fissure lines will be evident outlining the lung lobes in both views. The pattern and distribution of these lines will change with the view. Part of the diaphragmatic outline will be obliterated in either view; however, the cupula or dome will be less obvious in the dorsoventral view and the crura will be obscured in the ventrodorsal view. In the dorsoventral radiograph, the pleural fluid will gravitate to the sternum, the cardiac silhouette will be obliterated, and the mediastinum will appear widened. The differences between ventrodorsal and dorsoventral views may be used to determine the nature of the pleural fluid and to detect masses or other lesions that might be masked by the fluid. A change in the fluid distribution with changes in the animal's position indicates that adhesions and large amounts of fibrin are not present. Areas of the thorax masked by fluid in one view may be evaluated in another view.

Horizontal beam radiographs are also useful in detecting and evaluating pleural fluid. Because the fluid should move with gravity, the region of interest should be up and the fluid should move to the dependent side, unless it is fibrinous in nature, trapped by adhesions, or a fluid-dense mass is present.

Inflation of the lung lobes should displace the pleural fluid evenly. If fluid accumulates in the area of a lung lobe and does not move away with normal respiration, an abnormality or disease within that lung lobe should be suspected. Positional maneuvers can be performed to evaluate the lung lobe, although the lesion often will not be apparent until the pleural fluid is removed (Fig. 2–56).

The role that pleural fluid accumulation plays in the misdiagnosis of pulmonary disease should not be minimized. A fibrinous pleural fluid that "traps" over a lung lobe may give the appearance of pulmonary lobar disease. The presence of internal pulmonary structure within the density (air bronchogram signs, bronchial thickening, etc.) indicates the presence of pulmonary disease; however, the absence of a pulmonary pattern suggests pleural disease but does not exclude pulmonary involvement. Confirmation may require ultrasound or computed tomography.

Fat accumulates in the mediastinum, dorsal to the sternum, adjacent to the pericardium, and beneath the parietal pleura in obese dogs and cats. This may be mistaken for pleural fluid; however, this fat density does not completely obliterate the diaphragm or cardiac silhouette and, therefore, it can be recognized as a fat density.

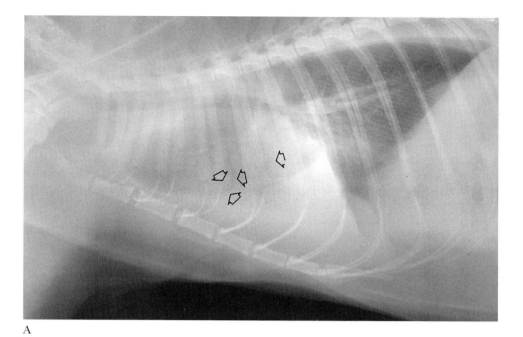

A

B

C

Figure 2–56. (A,B,C) A 10-year-old male castrated cat presented with a 1-day history of an acute onset of dyspnea. There was no history of thoracic trauma. (A) Lateral, (B) ventrodorsal, and (C) erect ventrodorsal radiographs were obtained. There is pleural fluid noted especially in the right cranial thorax. The cardiac silhouette is obscured. There are bronchial structures present in the area of the right cranial lung lobe anterior to the cardiac silhouette in (A) (*arrows*). In (C) the erect ventrodorsal radiograph, the soft tissue density remains in the right cranial thorax indicating that it is a solid mass or trapped fluid. Most of the pleural fluid drains into the caudal thorax. The radiographic findings are indicative of pleural fluid with disease in the right cranial lung lobe. This could be the result of bacterial pneumonia or other infiltrate in the lung lobe. **Diagnosis:** Lung lobe torsion. An exploratory thoracotomy was performed and a right cranial lung lobe torsion was identified. The pleural fluid was chylous.

Despite a large amount of density in the ventral thorax, the pleural fissure lines will not be observed when fat rather than fluid accumulates in the pleural space. Changes in the animal's position will not change the position of this fat density.

Pleural thickening and outlining of pleural interlobar fissures due to pleural fibrosis and/or calcification may be observed in older animals. This will be similar to the changes that occur with small amounts of pleural fluid; however, thickened pleural fissures are linear while pleural fluid accumulations are triangular with the peripheral portion of the density usually wider than the central portion. A change in the animal's position without an appropriate change in the appearance of these lines will identify the fibrotic or calcific nature of these densities.

Pleural fluid will only displace thoracic viscera because of gravitational effects. In the presence of large amounts of fluid, the heart will move toward the most dependent portion of the thoracic cavity. This displacement causes the trachea to appear elevated on the lateral view, which may create the false impression of cardiomegaly.[62] Displacement of the cardiac silhouette in a direction against the effect of gravity, compression of the tracheal lumen, displacement of the carina caudally, or a localized elevation of the trachea indicate that a mass is present within the fluid. Loculated or encapsulated fluid may mimic this effect.

Sonography will reliably demonstrate even small amounts of pleural fluid if the transducer is placed on the most dependent portion of the chest or over an area of trapped fluid.[21] The presence of fibrin tags on pleural surfaces indicates chronicity of the fluid accumulation. If the fluid contains a lot of floating debris, pyothorax may be present. A pleural mass that was not identified radiographically due to the lack of density difference between the fluid and the mass may be identified (Fig. 2–57). Lung masses, atelectasis, or pneumonia may also be identified.

The causes of hydrothorax are numerous and include right heart failure, neoplasia, hypoproteinemia, infection, traumatic rupture of vascular or lymphatic structures, and inflammation.[21,47,56,59,63–68] The nature of the fluid cannot be determined

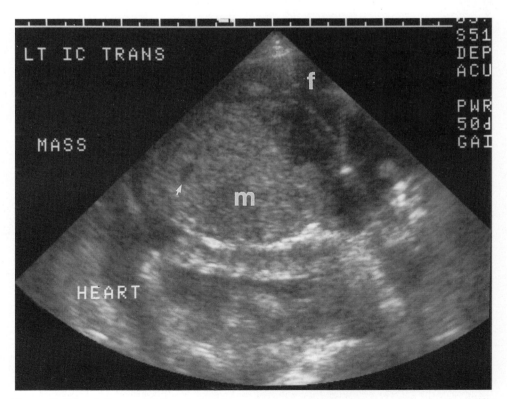

Figure 2–57. A 5-year-old female keeshound presented with dyspnea and anemia. Radiographs revealed a hydrothorax. A right parasternal long-axis view revealed the presence of pleural fluid (*f*) and a heteroechoic mass (*m*) with a small cystic area (*arrow*) arising from the visceral pleura and lying adjacent to the heart. **Diagnosis:** Hemangiosarcoma.

using ultrasound; however, identification of intrathoracic abnormalities such as an enlarged right heart, pericardial fluid or mass, pleural mass, diaphragmatic hernia, or lung lobe torsion will provide important clues to the diagnosis.

PLEURAL AIR (PNEUMOTHORAX)

Air within the pleural space is referred to as pneumothorax. Some minor differences can be observed when comparing right with left lateral recumbent radiographs and dorsoventral with ventrodorsal radiographs of animals with pneumothorax; however, the major features are the same (Fig. 2–58).[69] In the lateral radiograph, these

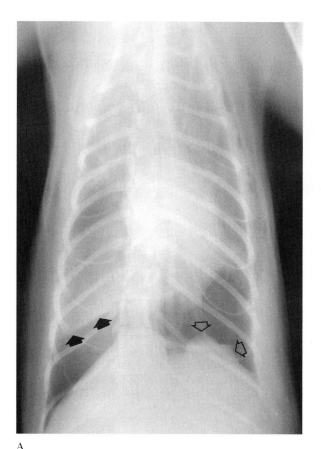

Figure 2–58. (A&B) A 1-year-old female cat showed evidence of respiratory distress after surgery for the repair of a diaphragmatic hernia. There is air within the pleural space separating the lungs from the lateral thoracic wall. (A) In the ventrodorsal radiograph and (B) lateral radiograph there is atelectasis of the right caudal lung lobe (*closed arrows*). There is irregularity of the diaphragm at the site of diaphragmatic hernia repair (*open arrows*). (B) In the lateral radiograph there is air within the peritoneal cavity due to surgery (*large arrows*). The radiographic findings are indicative of pneumothorax subsequent to diaphragmatic hernia repair. The marked increase in pulmonary density in the right caudal lung lobe indicates that there is pathology within this lung lobe. This is most likely residual atelectasis or pulmonary contusion. **Diagnosis:** Pneumothorax. Atelectasis of the right caudal lung lobe. The pneumothorax and lung lobe atelectasis resolved after chest tube placement and continued aspiration of the pleural space.

A

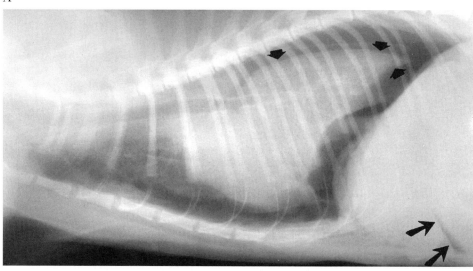

B

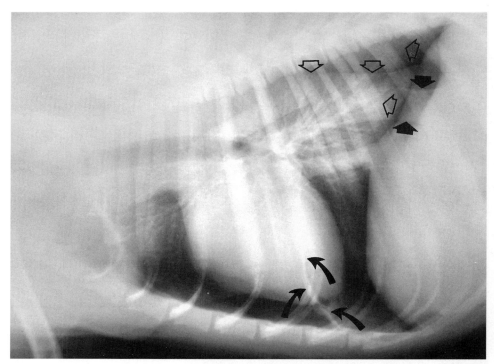

Figure 2–59. A 1-year-old male mixed breed dog was presented after thoracic trauma. The dog had evidence of mild respiratory distress. In this lateral radiograph, the collapsed caudal lung lobes are outlined by air within the pleural space (*open arrows*). The cardiac silhouette is separated from the sternum. The esophagus can be seen in the caudal thorax (*solid straight arrow*). There is a thin soft tissue-dense linear structure present in the caudal ventral thorax (*curved arrows*). This represents a portion of the caudal mediastinum, which is outlined by the pleural air. **Diagnosis:** Pneumothorax.

features include separation of the lung lobes from the ventral and dorsal thoracic wall, separation of the heart from the sternum, separation of the lung lobes from the diaphragm, and an overall increase in pulmonary density due to lung lobe atelectasis. Air may become trapped within the mediastinum as the animal is rotated (Fig. 2–59). This will produce soft tissue-dense well-defined lines (mediastinal folds), usually in the caudal (post cardiac) mediastinum extending from the cardiac apex to the sternum or diaphragm.[70]

In the ventrodorsal and dorsoventral radiograph, the lungs will be separated from the lateral thoracic wall by air density. This is identified by the lack of pulmonary vasculature and airways traversing the air density beyond the border of the lung. The density of the lung lobes will increase due to atelectasis. Air may be identified between the lungs and the diaphragm. On occasion, air may accumulate between the heart and lung lobes and may become trapped within the mediastinum outlining the mediastinal folds but not the individual mediastinal structures.

A lateral radiograph obtained using a horizontal x-ray beam is helpful for detecting small amounts of pleural air. Furthermore, small amounts of pleural air may be accentuated by obtaining radiographs at expiration rather than at inspiration.

As with pleural fluid, air should move freely within the pleural space and distribute evenly rising to the highest point within the thorax. The lungs should collapse uniformly. If this does not occur and one lung lobe or a portion of a lung lobe is denser than the others, lung lobe disease should be suspected. Additional radiographs or repeat evaluation after removal of the pleural air may be helpful in these instances. Unilateral pneumothorax is rare; however, if previous or co-existing pleural or mediastinal disease has produced adhesions or pleural thickening, a unilateral pneumothorax can occur.

Pneumothorax is most often secondary to trauma and can occur with or without rib fractures. Spontaneous pneumothorax refers to those that occur in the absence

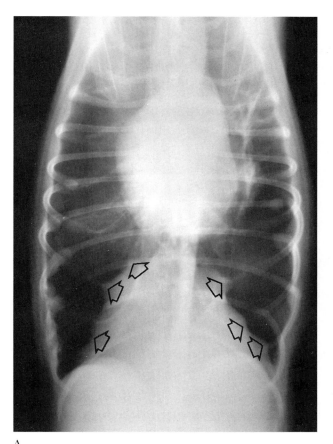

Figure 2–60. (A&B) An 8-year-old male mixed breed dog presented with an acute onset of respiratory distress associated with thoracic trauma. There is air present in the pleural space separating the lungs from the thoracic wall and diaphragm. The caudal lung lobes are collapsed and the cardiac silhouette is separated from the sternum. The diaphragm is displaced caudally. The diaphragmatic attachments to the sternebra and dorsal diaphragmatic attachments to the lumbar vertebral bodies are evident (*arrows*). The marked caudal diaphragmatic displacement and lung lobe collapse is indicative of a tension pneumothorax. There are incidental findings of old, healing fractures involving the ribs on both the right and left caudal thoracic wall. **Diagnosis:** Tension pneumothorax. This resulted from a tear in the left caudal lung lobe.

A

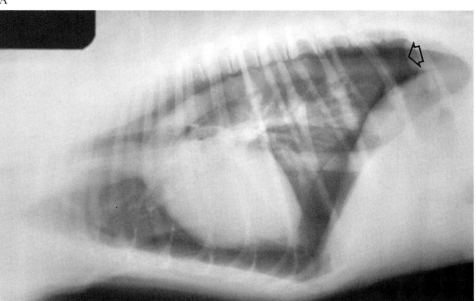

B

of trauma resulting from rupture of a lung tumor, abscess, or bulla, or from pleural tears.[71–73]

Tension pneumothorax occurs when a tear in the visceral pleura functions as a one-way valve and air continues to accumulate within the pleural space. Under these circumstances, intrapleural pressure may exceed atmospheric pressure (Fig. 2–60). Severe lung lobe collapse, flattening, or caudal displacement of the diaphragm into the abdomen and "tenting" of the diaphragm at its costal attachments may be evident. The thorax may be widened (barrel-chested) and the mediastinum may shift away from the side in which the air has accumulated (if the mediastinum is intact). This emergency condition should be recognized and treated immediately.

Pneumothorax may be mimicked by overexposure of the radiograph, overlying skin folds, over-inflation of the lung, or hypovolemia. If this is suspected, a high intensity ("hot") light should be used to determine if the pulmonary vessels and airways extend to the thoracic wall. Lung lobe margins remain almost parallel to the thoracic wall when the lungs collapse due to pneumothorax. Any apparent margins that are not parallel are probably artifacts. Skin folds can often be traced beyond the thoracic wall. Separation of the heart from the sternum is a sign of mediastinal shift and is not pathognomonic for pneumothorax. Full inflation of the right middle lung lobe in a deep-chested breed or over-inflation of the lung can produce this same separation. Any time radiographic changes suggest the presence of pleural air on one radiograph but the diagnosis cannot be supported by another view, the diagnosis is suspect.

MEDIASTINAL ABNORMALITIES

Abnormalities of the mediastinum that may be radiographically detected include changes in size, shape, and position and alteration in density. The mediastinum is divided into cranial (pre-cardiac), middle, and caudal (post cardiac) portions. The trachea is the only structure in the cranial mediastinum that can be consistently identified on thoracic radiographs. It therefore serves as a landmark or reference point for evaluation of cranial mediastinal lesions, especially masses.

The size of the mediastinum varies among different individuals due to the accumulation of fat and the presence of the thymus in young animals. This normal variation must be considered before an abnormality is diagnosed. In a fat animal, a widened mediastinum that has a smooth margin and does not displace or compress the trachea is normal.

MASSES

Cranial mediastinal masses produce an increased thoracic density, because they displace the air-filled lung (Figs. 2–61 and 2–62). Usually located in the ventral thorax, they may also obscure the cardiac silhouette. Although esophageal or periesophageal masses will usually displace the trachea ventrally, most mediastinal masses, if large enough, will displace the trachea dorsally and away from the midline (usually to the right). The tracheal lumen may be compressed and the cardiac silhouette and tracheal bifurcation (normally located at the 5th or 6th intercostal space in the dog and almost always in the 6th intercostal space in the cat) will often be displaced caudally and dorsally. The mass, if large enough, may interfere with esophageal peristalsis and a gas-, fluid-, or food-filled esophagus will be evident at the thoracic inlet. Sternal lymphadenopathy or masses in the area of the sternal lymph nodes will produce a soft tissue density in the ventral cranial mediastinum. These masses typically have a convex dorsal margin and are located over the 2nd to 4th sternebrae. This aids in distinguishing them from fat accumulation, which often occurs in the same area. Mediastinal margin irregularity or a change in contour are much more specific signs of a mediastinal mass than is widening alone. In the ventrodorsal radiograph, the widened mediastinum may extend on both sides of the vertebral column blending with the margins of the cardiac silhouette. The trachea may be displaced to the right or left depending on the origin of the mass. The cranial margins of the cranial lung lobes will be displaced laterally, and the entire lobes may be displaced caudally. Masses in the tip of either cranial lung lobe may contact the mediastinum and mimic a mediastinal mass. Distinction between these may be impossible without the use of computed tomography. Irregularity of the mediastinal margin is most often the result of a mediastinal mass rather than fat or fluid accumulation. There are several causes of mediastinal masses including neoplasia, cyst, trapped fluid, abscess, or granuloma.[68,74–79]

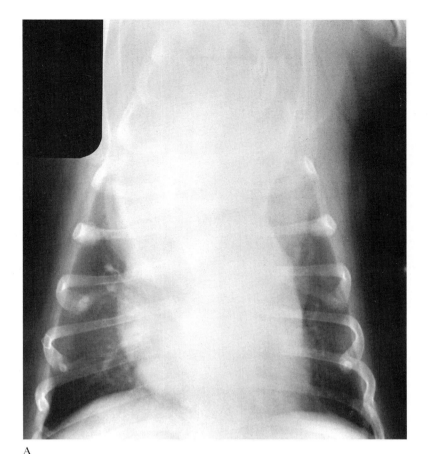

A

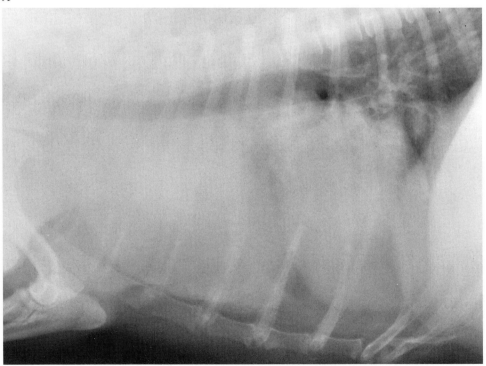

B

Figure 2–61. (A&B) A 10-year-old spayed dachshund presented with mammary gland masses. There is a large, soft tissue-dense mass in the cranial thorax. There are areas of calcification associated with this mass, especially ventrally and cranially. (A) On the ventrodorsal and (B) lateral radiographs the cranial mediastinum is widened, the trachea is displaced to the right and dorsally, and the cardiac silhouette is displaced caudally. There is no evidence of pleural fluid. The radiographic findings are indicative of a cranial mediastinal mass. **Diagnosis:** Thymoma. This mass was unrelated to the mammary gland neoplasms.

Sonography will reveal most cranial mediastinal masses. Very large masses are readily imaged from anywhere on the cranial thoracic wall. Smaller masses may require using the heart as a sonographic window. Sternal lymph node enlargement (which may not contact the heart) may require the use of a parasternal window. Regardless of the imaging portal, evaluation will reveal the presence of mass and allow

91

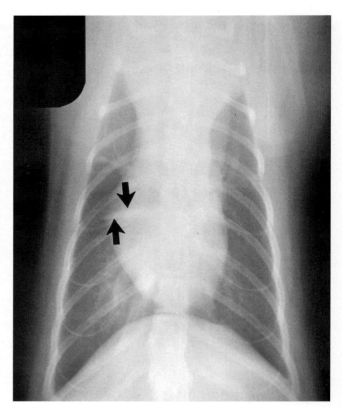

A

Figure 2–62. (A&B) An 8-month-old male cat presented a 2-week history of intermittent dyspneic episodes and vomiting. There is a soft tissue density in the cranial mediastinum. The trachea is elevated and compressed. The cranial lung lobes tips are displaced laterally and the lobes are displaced caudally. There is a small amount of pleural fluid present in the fissure between the right middle and caudal lung lobes (*arrows*). The radiographic findings are indicative of a cranial mediastinal mass. **Diagnosis:** Lymphoma.

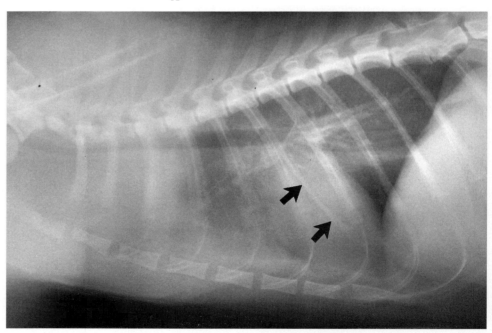

B

for the determination of whether it is cystic, solid, or predominately solid with some cystic elements. The relationship of the mass to various vascular structures may be apparent (Fig. 2–63). Exact identification of the tissue of origin of the mass cannot usually be made with ultrasound. However, sonography can be used to guide a needle for aspiration or biopsy.

Other than esophageal masses (cardiac, aortic, or pericardial masses will be discussed separately), masses in the mid-portion of the mediastinum usually involve

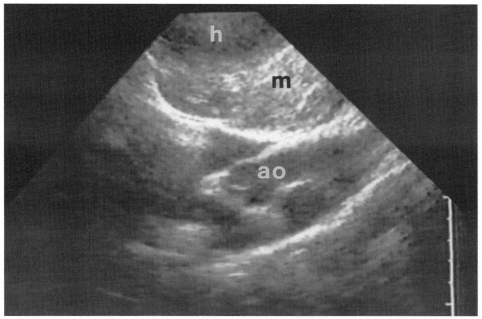

Figure 2–63. A 7-year-old German shepherd dog presented with anorexia, weight loss, and hypercalcemia. Radiographs revealed a moderate to severe hydrothorax. A right parasternal long-axis view revealed a mass (*m*) immediately cranial to the heart base [aorta (*ao*)]. Hydrothorax (*h*) is also present. **Diagnosis:** Lymphoma.

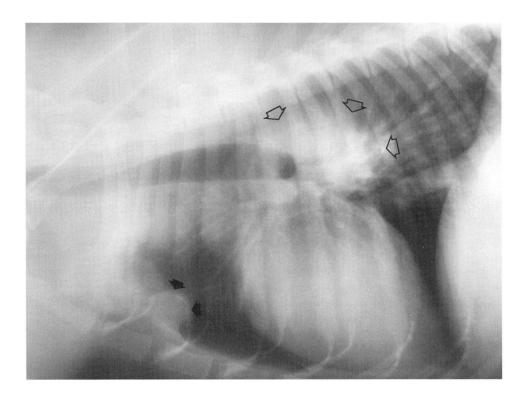

Figure 2–64. A 4-year-old female German shorthair pointer presented with generalized peripheral lymphadenopathy. There is a soft tissue density in the cranial ventral thorax, which represents sternal lymphadenopathy (*closed arrows*). There is an additional soft tissue density that surrounds the tracheal bifurcation (*open arrows*). The caudal main stem bronchi are displaced ventrally. The radiographic findings are indicative of sternal and tracheobronchial lymphadenopathy. **Diagnosis:** Lymphoma.

the mediastinal and/or tracheobronchial lymph nodes (Fig. 2–64). Tracheal or bronchial compression or deviation may be the only visible radiographic change because the lymph node borders are often obscured by concurrent increased pulmonary density or by contact with the heart. The trachea may be elevated cranially to its bifurcation, and the main caudal lobe bronchi depressed ventrally caudal to this point. Narrowing of the tracheal and bronchial lumina may also be evident. These changes help distinguish tracheobronchial masses from hilar pulmonary infiltrates (which do not displace or compress the airways), left atrial enlargement (which may elevate the left main caudal lobe bronchus), and esophageal masses (which may depress the entire trachea, both bronchi and the cardiac silhouette).

Sonography can occasionally be used to evaluate masses in the mid-portion of the mediastinum. Tracheobronchial lymphadenopathy can sometimes be imaged as masses adjacent to the cardiac base using the heart as a sonographic window. Fine needle aspiration can rarely be performed using sonographic guidance.

Caudal mediastinal masses most often arise from or involve the esophagus and will be discussed in that section. A contrast esophagram is helpful in distinguishing caudal mediastinal abscesses and tumors from esophageal masses or foreign bodies. Diaphragmatic masses and hernias may occupy the caudal mediastinum and should be considered whenever a soft tissue density is present in this area.

MEDIASTINAL FLUID

Fluid (blood, edema fluid, exudate) may accumulate in the cranial, middle, and/or caudal mediastinum with or without the presence of pleural fluid.[80] Detection is very difficult in obese animals; however, this diagnosis should be considered in a thin animal with a widened cranial, middle, or caudal mediastinum. Sonography can provide confirmation of this diagnosis.

Mediastinal density does not increase markedly as the mediastinum becomes filled with fluid or replaced by a mass. The increased density can be detected only when the mediastinum displaces the air-filled lung.

MEDIASTINAL AIR (PNEUMOMEDIASTINUM)

Air may accumulate within the mediastinum itself (pneumomediastinum) or within the esophagus. This may occur as a result of tracheal, bronchial, or esophageal perforation, perforating wounds at the thoracic inlet, or dissection of subcutaneous emphysema (Fig. 2–65). Pneumomediastinum with accompanying pulmonary interstitial infiltrate has been reported secondary to paraquat toxicity. Pneumomediastinum may progress to pneumothorax, however the opposite very rarely occurs. Mediastinal air may dissect retroperitoneally or beyond the thoracic inlet into the cervical fascia and subcutaneously.

Air within the mediastinum will delineate the normally unidentifiable mediastinal structures (Fig. 2–66).[70,81] The cranial mediastinum may have a granular pattern that results from a mixture of air and fluid densities. The external tracheal margin will become sharply defined. The cranial vena cava, azygous vein, esophagus, and sometimes the aortic arch and left subclavian and brachycephalic arteries may become visible. The air may dissect caudally and outline the descending aorta and main pulmonary artery. Continued caudal migration may produce a pneumoretroperitoneum, which outlines the abdominal aorta, its main branches, and both kidneys. Pneumomediastinum may extend into the pericardial sac creating a pneumopericardium. The thin tissue-dense pericardium will become distinctly separate from the cardiac silhouette and the surface irregularities of the heart will become visible.

The cause of pneumomediastinum is rarely evident on the survey radiograph. Contrast studies of the trachea or esophagus may be helpful in unusual cases in delineating perforation with mediastinal extension and pneumomediastinum (see Fig. 2–65). Since pneumomediastinum is usually self-limiting, contrast injections into external wounds to demonstrate communication with the mediastinum are usually unnecessary.

A mild degree of pneumomediastinum can be easily overlooked. In animals with over-inflated lungs or pneumothorax, an erroneous impression of pneumomediastinum may be created, especially if delineation or definition of the descending aorta is used as the sole criterion for the diagnosis. Additional radiographic changes

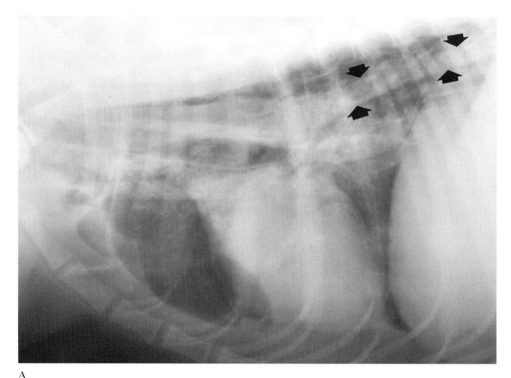

A

B

Figure 2–65. (A&B) A 4-year-old spayed collie presented 2 weeks after having been poisoned. The oral and lingual mucosa were necrotic. The dog was having difficulty breathing. The dog had responded to initial treatment but developed an acute depression and vomited blood 24 hours prior to admission. (A) A lateral thoracic radiograph revealed a marked accumulation of air within the cranial mediastinum. The cranial mediastinal structures are outlined. The aorta can be traced beyond the diaphragm into the abdomen (*arrows*). The radiographic findings are indicative of pneumomediastinum. (B) An esophagram was performed. Contrast material can be seen outside the esophageal lumen in the cranial thorax (*arrows*). This is indicative of esophageal perforation. **Diagnosis:** Pneumomediastinum secondary to esophageal perforation. This dog was euthanized due to the severity of the esophageal injury.

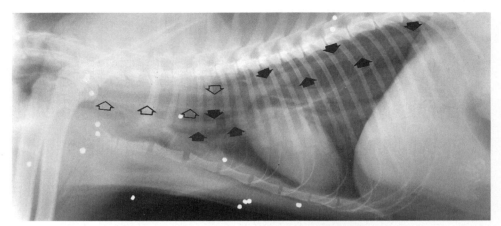

Figure 2–66. A 2-year-old female cat presented with a unknown history of multiple external wounds and subcutaneous emphysema. On the lateral radiograph, gas is noted in the soft tissues at the thoracic inlet. The air dissects into the cranial mediastinum. The outer tracheal wall is distinctly outlined (*open arrows*). The cranial vena cava and the aortic arch are also outlined distinctly (*closed arrows*). The azygous vein is clearly delineated. There are multiple shotgun pellets in the soft tissues over the thorax. **Diagnosis:** Pneumomediastinum. This resulted from extension of the subcutaneous emphysema from the external wounds in the cervical soft tissues. There was no evidence of tracheal or esophageal perforation. The mediastinal air resolved without treatment.

should be present before a diagnosis of pneumomediastinum is made. Ultrasound is of no value in detecting or determining the cause of pneumomediastinum.

TRACHEAL ABNORMALITIES

Tracheal abnormalities include those affecting the tracheal size, shape, density, and position as well as those affecting tracheal function. Most tracheal abnormalities can be adequately evaluated on non-contrast radiographs.[82] Evaluation and comparison of radiographs obtained at inspiration and expiration are required for detection of functional abnormalities. The ventrodorsal or dorsoventral radiograph is less valuable than the lateral radiograph because superimposition of the vertebral column occurs; however, this view should not be ignored.

TRACHEAL HYPOPLASIA

Tracheal hypoplasia is obvious in severely affected dogs.[25,83] The uniformly small tracheal diameter will be evident in both lateral and ventrodorsal radiographs. The entire trachea from the larynx to the main stem bronchi is usually involved, although congenital hypoplasia of shorter segments of the trachea has been described.[25] The tracheal diameter is often 50% or less than the laryngeal diameter. The hypoplastic trachea retains its normal ovoid shape in contrast to the more elliptical shape observed in tracheal collapse. The normal trachea should be wider than the cranial-caudal dimension of the proximal third of the 3rd rib.[25] Tracheal hypoplasia occurs most frequently in brachycephalic dogs (e.g., English bulldogs, pugs, etc.); however, other breeds have been affected (Fig. 2–67).

Narrowing of the entire trachea may also result from mucosal inflammation or exudate accumulation. The inflammation must be severe for radiographic detection and, although cases have been described, the radiographic diagnosis is difficult and rare (Fig. 2–68).[84]

Localized or segmental tracheal stenosis may be congenital, secondary to local inflammation and fibrosis, or secondary to trauma (Figs. 2–69 and 2–70). The stenosis is usually circumferential and involves one or more tracheal rings. The mucosal surface is usually smooth, although the tracheal rings may be deformed. Distinction between acquired and congenital localized tracheal stenosis is not radiographically possible; however, congenital localized stenosis is extremely uncommon. The major

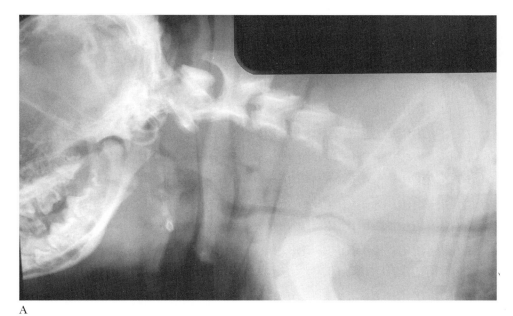

A

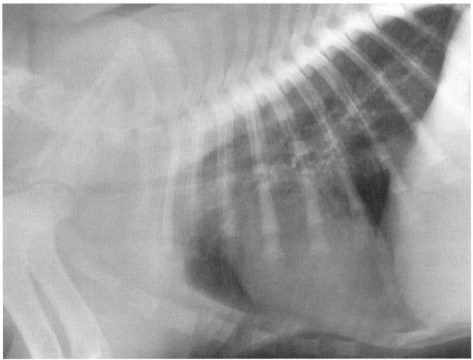

B

Figure 2–67. A 4-month-old male English bulldog presented with a 3-week history of difficulty breathing. (A) A lateral radiograph of the cervical soft tissues and (B) a lateral thoracic radiograph revealed that the entire trachea was small in diameter. The laryngeal area was indistinct due to overlying soft tissue density. **Diagnosis:** Hypoplastic trachea.

distinction must be made between localized stenosis and intramural or intraluminal masses.

TRACHEAL AVULSION OR PERFORATION

Tracheal avulsion or rupture is usually traumatic. An interruption in the tracheal wall may be visible. The avulsed ends may be widely separated or a thin, soft tissue-dense band or line may separate the avulsed portions. Pneumomediastinum is frequently, but not always, present.

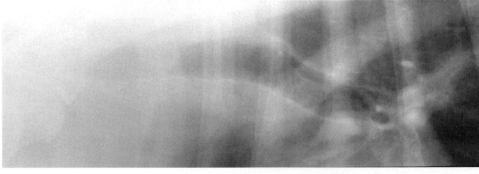

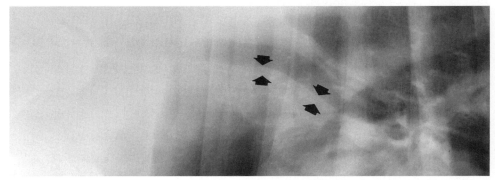

A

Figure 2–68. (A&B) A 6-year-old male Doberman pinscher presented with a 2-week history of epistaxis. (A) Thoracic radiographs were obtained before the dog was anesthetized for aspiration and flushing of the nasal passages. (B) The second radiograph was obtained after anesthesia. Marked thickening of the tracheal wall is evident (*arrows*) when (B) is compared with (A). This is due to accumulation of exudate in the trachea. This resulted from the nasal cavity and frontal sinus irrigation. **Diagnosis:** Tracheitis.

B

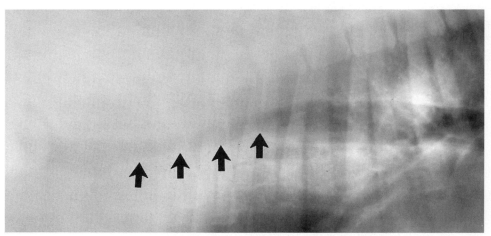

Figure 2–69. A 6-month-old male German shepherd dog presented with a 1-week history of inspiratory and expiratory stridor. On the lateral thoracic radiograph the trachea is narrowed and irregular in the area of the thoracic inlet (*arrows*). The mucosal surface is irregular, and the tracheal wall appears thickened. The radiographic changes are indicative of tracheal stenosis. This was thought to be caused by trauma. The affected area of the trachea was resected. Pathologic examination revealed congenital tracheal deformity. **Diagnosis:** Congenital tracheal stenosis.

Tracheal perforation is rarely recognized radiographically. Pneumomediastinum is often present, but the site of the perforation can rarely be identified even when contrast studies are performed.

TRACHEAL MASSES

Extraluminal masses may displace or deform the trachea. These usually arise from mediastinal structures and are described in that section (see *Mediastinal Structures* elsewhere in this chapter). Because the trachea is somewhat rigid, extraluminal

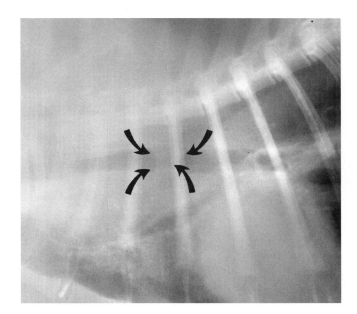

Figure 2–70. A 4-year-old male cat presented with acute respiratory distress, which occurred 1.5 weeks after a fractured mandible had been repaired. On the lateral thoracic radiograph, there is marked narrowing of the tracheal lumen at the level of the 4th intercostal space (*arrows*). This is indicative of a localized tracheal stenosis. **Diagnosis:** Tracheal stenosis. This portion of the trachea was resected. The etiology of the tracheal stenosis was not determined.

masses produce a gradually curving displacement of the trachea. Although displacement is the most common finding with an extraluminal mass, the tracheal lumen can become narrowed if the mass surrounds the trachea or compresses it against a solid structure such as the heart, aorta, spine, or cervical muscles.[85]

Intramural lesions cause thickening of the tracheal wall with luminal deformities. The curvature of the mass will be more abrupt than the gradual curve of the trachea, which accompanies extraluminal masses. The degree of tracheal displacement depends upon the amount of the mass that extends outside the tracheal wall and the compressibility of the adjacent tissues. The mucosal surface of the trachea is usually smooth (Figs. 2–71 and 2–72).

Intraluminal lesions are more common than intramural lesions. Granulomas, neoplasms, polyps, and foreign objects may be encountered. Masses may be solitary or multiple and are often eccentric. They produce rounded or cauliflower shaped densities within the tracheal lumen. The attachment site of the mass blends with the normal tracheal mucosa. Most benign and malignant neoplasms produce solitary masses that may occur anywhere within the tracheal lumen.[85] Tracheal granulomas due to *Oslerus osleri* are often multiple and occur in the distal third of the trachea and in the main stem bronchi.[86] Tracheal wall thickening may also be present.

Although other soft tissue densities may overlap the tracheal lumen and mimic intraluminal masses, careful inspection of the lesions will reveal their true nature. Intratracheal masses will usually have distinct margins that are surrounded by air and at least one indistinct or poorly defined margin at the point of tracheal attachment. Superimposed soft tissue masses will have less distinct margins if surrounded by fat and will have all sides visible if surrounded by air (i.e., on the outside of the animal). If an intraluminal lesion is not identified on both lateral and ventrodorsal radiographs, the radiograph that showed the lesion should be repeated and should be centered on the region of interest to confirm the location of the mass. Ultrasound has little value in evaluation of tracheal abnormalities.

TRACHEAL FOREIGN BODIES

Dense tracheal foreign objects are easily detected; small tissue-dense objects are more easily overlooked. Larger tracheal foreign bodies may lodge at the tracheal bifurcation.[87] Smaller foreign bodies usually pass into and obstruct an individual bronchus (the right caudal being the most commonly involved).[88] This may lead to local inflammation and bronchial thickening. Ideally, the foreign object should be identified on at least two radiographs, preferably at right angles to each other. When

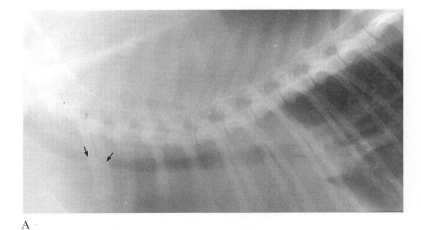

A

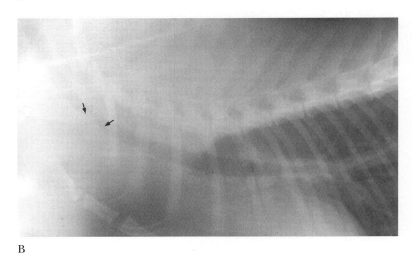

B

Figure 2–71. (A&B) A 9-year-old female cat presented with an acute onset of respiratory distress. On the two lateral thoracic radiographs that were obtained there is a soft tissue density in the trachea at the level of the 1st rib (*arrows*). The tracheal lumen is narrowed. The margins of the mass are distinct. The radiographic findings indicate an intraluminal tracheal mass. **Diagnosis:** Metastatic neoplasm within the trachea.

Figure 2–72. A 7-year-old neutered male domestic shorthair cat presented with dyspnea of 3 days' duration. The lateral radiograph reveals the presence of a sharply marginated mass within the lumen of the trachea (*arrows*). The mass could not be seen on the ventrodorsal view due to the superimposed spine and sternum. **Diagnosis:** Tracheal chondroma. The mass was successfully removed at surgery.

this is not possible, two similarly positioned radiographs, with one centered on the lesion, are preferred. The sharp distinct margins resulting from the air surrounding the tracheal foreign body may not always be observed.

Radiographic studies using barium or water-soluble iodine-containing contrast agents may be used for tracheal evaluation.[89,90] However, these are rarely necessary if the patient is well positioned and properly exposed survey radiographs are obtained.

TRACHEAL DISPLACEMENT

The trachea is an easily identified landmark when evaluating intrathoracic masses. When displaced, the tracheal position indicates the origin of the mass. Ventral displacement of the cranial thoracic trachea may occur secondary to esophageal enlargement, periesophageal masses, or other dorsal mediastinal masses. Dorsal tracheal displacement occurs in association with masses arising within the mediastinum ventral to the trachea, from right atrial enlargement or tumors, or from heart base masses. Dorsal displacement of the trachea immediately cranial to the bifurcation may be due to right atrial, heart base, or tracheobronchial lymph node masses. Dorsal displacement of the trachea caudal to the tracheal bifurcation occurs with left atrial enlargement. Ventral displacement may be due to esophageal enlargement, periesophageal caudal mediastinal masses, or tracheobronchial lymph node enlargement. The degree of ventral main stem bronchial displacement is more severe with lymph node enlargement than with esophageal lesions. Many esophageal lesions displace both the heart and trachea, while lymph node enlargement affects mostly the trachea and main stem bronchi. Left ventricular enlargement will elevate the trachea at the bifurcation.

Mediastinal shifts away from the midline may be easily detected by identifying the trachea's position. Whether the shift is due to a mass pushing in the direction of the shift or to the collapse of the lung lobe with shifting toward the collapsed side cannot be determined solely from tracheal position.

Dorsal displacement of the cranial thoracic trachea may be observed on the recumbent lateral view when pleural fluid is present. This may mimic the displacement that accompanies a cranial mediastinal mass, but it is due to a shift in the position of the lungs. Compression of the tracheal lumen indicates that a mass is present within the pleural fluid; in the absence of tracheal compression, a mass may or may not be present.

Tracheal displacement to the left is prevented by the aorta; it can occur when a right aortic arch is present. Mediastinal shifts that include the heart will permit leftward tracheal displacement. Right-sided displacement of the trachea between the thoracic inlet and bifurcation is seen in many normal dogs and is more pronounced in brachycephalic breeds. Right-sided displacement of the trachea may also occur with heart base masses and esophageal enlargement. Most ventral mediastinal masses displace the trachea dorsally and do not move it to either the right or left.

The tracheal bifurcation may be displaced caudally. In the cat, the tracheal bifurcation is almost always visualized at the 6th intercostal space and any deviation caudal to this strongly suggests the presence of a cranial mediastinal mass. In dogs, the tracheal bifurcation occurs at the 5th or 6th intercostal space. The possibility of a cranial mediastinal mass should be considered if there is displacement caudal to the 6th intercostal space.

Tracheobronchial lymphadenopathy, especially when associated with chronic disease, may cause narrowing as well as displacement of the trachea and/or main stem bronchi. These are reliable signs of lymphadenopathy, which can be seen despite obliteration of the lymph node margins by a pulmonary infiltrate.

TRACHEAL COLLAPSE

The tracheal diameter may change very slightly with respiration and coughing in normal animals.[91] When marked luminal narrowing occurs during normal or forced respiration, tracheal collapse is present. Although dorsoventral narrowing is most

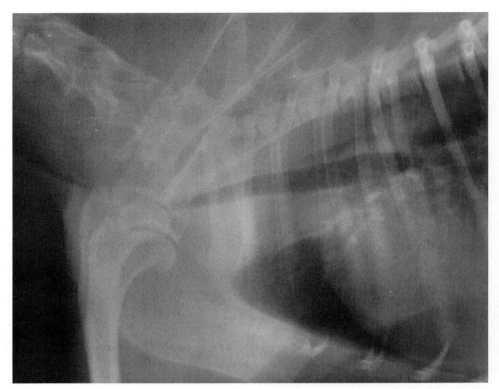

Figure 2–73. An 8-year-old male Yorkshire terrier presented with a 5-year history of a honking cough. On this lateral radiograph there is marked narrowing of the trachea cranial to the thoracic inlet. This is evident in the radiograph obtained at inspiration. **Diagnosis:** Extrathoracic tracheal collapse.

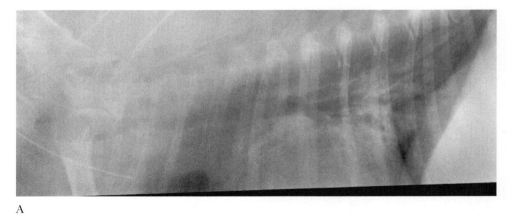

A

B

Figure 2–74. (A&B) A 12-year-old male poodle presented with harsh lung sounds and respiratory distress, especially when excited. (A) Inspiratory and (B) expiratory lateral thoracic radiographs were obtained. The trachea appears normal on (A). On (B) the entire intrathoracic trachea narrows markedly. There is extensive calcification of the tracheal rings. The left atrium is enlarged. **Diagnosis:** Intrathoracic tracheal collapse.

common, congenital side-to-side (lateral) narrowing may occur. The extent and location of the narrowing will vary. Narrowing of the caudal cervical trachea is more common at inspiration; at expiration intrathoracic tracheal narrowing is usually seen (Figs. 2–73 and 2–74). The narrowing may extend through the thoracic inlet, which probably accounts for some variation. Left atrial enlargement may cause narrowing or collapse the tracheal bifurcation or main stem bronchi (Fig. 2–75).

Both inspiratory and expiratory lateral radiographs that include the entire trachea should be obtained if tracheal collapse is suspected. Inducing a cough will accentuate the collapse; however, obtaining a radiograph at the time of the cough may be difficult.

Fluoroscopic examination is useful in evaluating and documenting tracheal collapse. Contrast studies using intratrachealy administered barium or water-soluble iodinated contrast agents have been described; however, these rarely provide additional useful information beyond that obtained from carefully positioned, properly exposed, survey radiographs.[89,90]

A lateral radiograph obtained while the animal's head and neck are dorsiflexed is recommended for evaluation of tracheal collapse.[91] This view accentuates the tracheal narrowing and may be useful, especially relative to the tracheal diameter at the thoracic inlet. A tangential cross-sectional projection of the trachea has also been described for evaluation of tracheal collapse. The animal is positioned in sternal recumbency and the head and neck are dorsiflexed. The x-ray beam is directed caudally and ventrally to strike the trachea tangentially at the thoracic inlet. Although this view is difficult to obtain because of patient resistance, it may provide additional information (Fig. 2–76).

The amount of tracheal collapse that occurs during coughing in normal dogs has not been defined. A clear-cut distinction between normal narrowing and tracheal

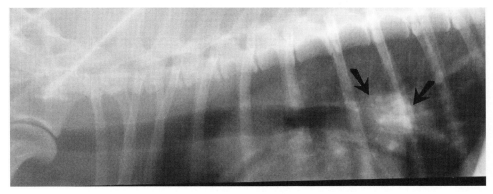

A

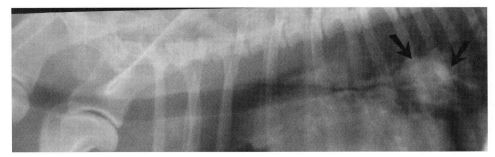

B

Figure 2–75. (A&B) A 14-year-old male cocker spaniel presented with a several month history of chronic cough. (A) On the lateral radiographs taken on inspiration the trachea appears normal size. (B) On the lateral radiograph taken at expiration the trachea narrows markedly at the tracheal bifurcation. This is indicative of collapse of the tracheal bifurcation and mainstream bronchi. Enlargement of the left ventricle and left atrium is present. The left atrium is seen extending caudal and dorsal to the tracheal bifurcation (*arrows*). **Diagnosis:** Collapse of the tracheal bifurcation and mainstem bronchi. Left heart enlargement consistent with mitral valve insufficiency.

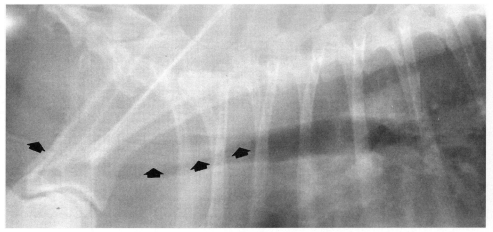

A

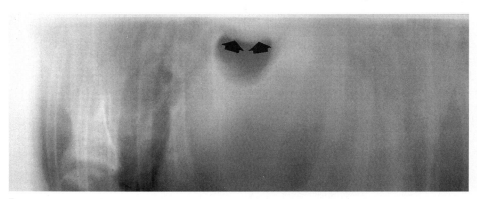

B

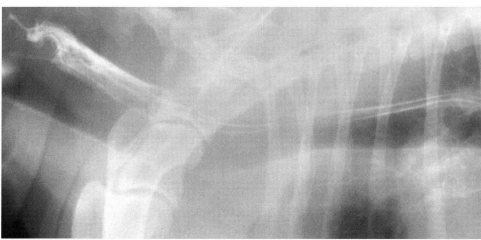

C

Figure 2–76. (A,B,C) A 13-year-old male poodle presented with a 6-month history of chronic non-productive cough. (A) On the lateral thoracic view, there is a soft tissue density super-imposed on the tracheal shadow in the caudal cervical region extending into the thoracic inlet (*arrows*). This creates an impression of tracheal collapse. (B) On a skyline projection of the trachea the lumen appears normal. There is slight indentation of the dorsal trachea (*arrows*). An esophagram was performed (C). The position of the esophagus can be seen overlying the trachea. **Diagnosis:** Normal trachea with no evidence of tracheal collapse.

collapse cannot be made. If the tracheal diameter narrows more than 50% with nor-mal respiration or coughing, a diagnosis of tracheal collapse should be considered.

An overlap of the trachea by the esophagus at the thoracic inlet may be seen. Care-ful examination of the radiograph will reveal the tracheal lucency with the superimposed esophagus. This is probably due to a flaccid dorsal trachealis muscle with esophageal indentation (see Fig. 2-76). The trachea may also rotate slightly causing the trachealis muscle to become dorso-lateral instead of dorsal. Indentation of the trachea by the esophagus due to laxity of the trachealis muscle may represent a type of collapsing trachea.

Animals with tracheal collapse may also have cardiac, pulmonary, or bronchial disease; therefore, the radiographic evaluation should include the entire respiratory tract. Tracheal collapse occurs most frequently in old, obese, small breed dogs. It rarely occurs in cats.[92]

ESOPHAGEAL ABNORMALITIES

Radiography is an important part of the clinical evaluation of animals with esophageal abnormalities. Survey radiographs provide useful information. Additional information can be obtained with esophageal contrast studies. A static (radiographic) contrast exam provides some functional information; however, a complete functional evaluation requires a dynamic (fluoroscopic) contrast exam. Cineradiographic or videotape with slow motion and reverse capabilities are necessary to record and completely evaluate the separate, rapidly occurring phases of swallowing.

Ultrasound is rarely useful in the evaluation of the intrathoracic esophagus. The cervical esophagus may be identified dorsal to, or left and lateral to, the trachea. The hyperechoic gas and mucous within the lumen helps identify the esophagus.

ESOPHAGEAL DILATION (MEGAESOPHAGUS)

Generalized Dilation

The esophagus may become distended with air, fluid, or food material (Fig. 2–77). It will be evident in the lateral radiograph as a tubular structure dorsal, lateral, and sometimes ventral to the trachea, dorsal to the heart base, and between the aorta and caudal vena cava caudal to the heart. The fluid- or food-filled esophagus may be recognized because of the increased density or granular pattern of gas, bone, and tissue density located in the region through which the esophagus passes. The air-filled esophagus will decrease the thoracic density and a pair of thin, linear fluid densities corresponding to the dorsal and ventral esophageal walls may be detected. The ventral wall may drape ventral to the trachea in the cranial mediastinum, pass dorsal to the heart base, drape ventral to the caudal vena cava, and then rise to the level of esophageal hiatus. The dorsal esophageal wall may be obliterated by contact with the longus coli muscles and may be evident only from the midthoracic area passing obliquely to the diaphragm at the esophageal hiatus. In the dorsoventral radiograph, the esophageal wall may be visible on the right side as a thin, tissue-dense line progressing caudally or caudolaterally to the tracheal bifurcation and then angling to intersect the midline at the esophageal hiatus. The left side of the esophagus may be evident in the cranial thorax angling toward the midline at the heart base. The wall is not visible as it passes to the right of the aortic arch but usually becomes visible caudal to the tracheal bifurcation; it curves slightly lateral before tapering toward the midline at the esophageal hiatus. Caudal to the heart, the converging esophageal walls have been described as a cone- or funnel-shaped with the apex at the esophageal hiatus. The dilated food, fluid, or air-filled esophagus may produce indirect radiographic evidence of its presence such as ventral or rightward tracheal displacement and ventral displacement of the heart.

Generalized esophageal enlargement may be due to many different conditions. In young animals, idiopathic megaesophagus is the most common cause. In adults, the list of possible causes is lengthy and includes various central nervous system or neuromuscular disorders (e.g., myasthenia gravis, lead poisoning, polyneuritis,

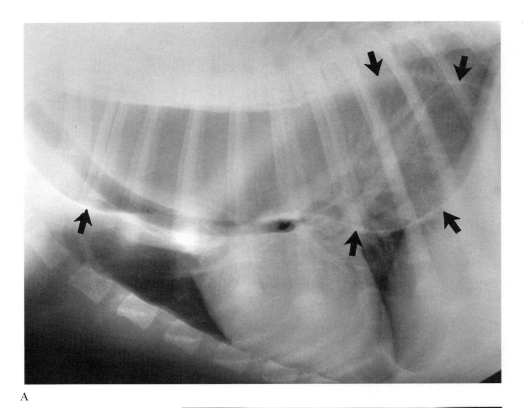

A

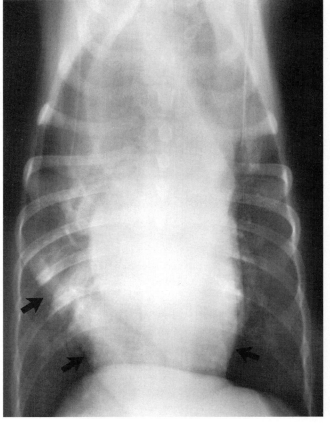

B

Figure 2–77. (A&B) A 6-month-old female Great Dane presented with 3-month history of chronic regurgitation. The thoracic esophagus is dilated and filled with air. The esophageal walls are visible (*arrows*). The trachea is displaced ventrally and to the right. The cardiac silhouette is displaced ventrally. **Diagnosis:** Megaesophagus.

polymyositis); endocrinopathies (e.g., hypothyroidism, hypoadrenocorticism); and other conditions such as chronic esophagitis, tumor, foreign body, stricture, hiatal hernia, gastric volvulus, and anesthesia.[93,94]

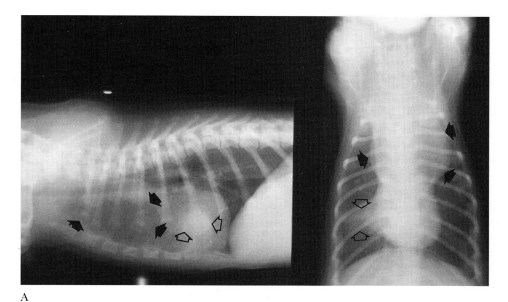

A

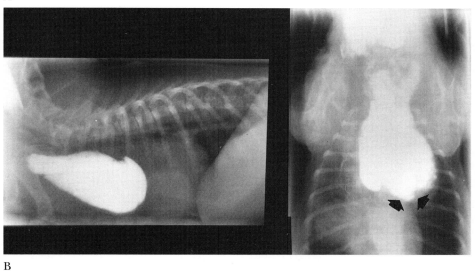

B

Figure 2–78. (A&B) A 3-month-old female dachshund presented with a history of regurgitation after the owner started feeding the dog solid food. The regurgitation occurred shortly after ingestion. (A) Ventrodorsal and lateral thoracic radiographs were obtained. The cranial mediastinum is widened. There is an air-filled density in the cranial mediastinum (*solid arrows*). This is indicative of a dilated cranial thoracic esophagus. There is a localized alveolar pattern infiltrate in the right middle lung lobe (*open arrows*). This is due to aspiration pneumonia. (B) An esophagram was performed. The esophageal dilatation cranial to the cardiac silhouette is identified. The esophagus caudal to the cardiac silhouette is normal. The area of stenosis is evident on the lateral and ventrodorsal radiographs (*arrows*). **Diagnosis:** Vascular ring anomaly. Persistent right aortic arch.

Localized Dilation

Localized esophageal dilation in a young dog is most often due to a vascular ring anomaly (Fig. 2–78).[95–97] The most common of these is a persistent right aortic arch; however, other vascular ring anomalies, such as the double aortic arch and aberrant left and right subclavian arteries, may occur. These abnormalities produce esophageal dilation cranial to the heart base. This dilation may displace the trachea ventrally on the lateral radiograph. In the ventrodorsal view, the esophageal dilation may be identified in the cranial mediastinum on the left side. The right aortic arch prevents tracheal displacement and, therefore, the rightward tracheal displacement, usually observed with idiopathic megaesophagus, does not occur. The aortic shadow, normally observed slightly to the left of the vertebral column, may be superimposed on the vertebral column and not evident on the ventrodorsal radiograph. In some animals with vascular ring anomalies, the caudal thoracic esophagus will also dilate. In these animals, a constriction at the heart base, which is not present in idiopathic megaesophagus, may be identified even on the non-contrast radiograph. If necessary, this constriction can be confirmed by a contrast esophagram. This caudal esophageal dilation is secondary to the ring's interference with normal esophageal peristalsis.

The specific vascular ring anomaly cannot be defined without an angiographic study, and even then it is frequently not identifiable. Angiography is rarely performed because of this difficulty and because persistent right aortic arches are the most common vascular ring anomalies.

Localized esophageal dilation may be seen with acquired and congenital diverticulae, localized esophagitis, foreign bodies, or proximal to esophageal strictures. Motility disturbances may lead to pulsion diverticulae while periesophageal inflammation, fibrosis, and adhesions may produce traction diverticulae. These may occur at any point within the esophagus (Fig. 2–79). A slight local dilation may be observed at the thoracic inlet especially in normal brachycephalic dogs. A small amount of air may be seen within the esophagus at this point on a non-contrast study; however, a contrast esophagram is usually required to demonstrate this local dilation. It lacks clinical significance.

Esophageal strictures may occur at any site, with the more common being at the thoracic inlet, over the base of the heart, or near the gastroesophageal junction. The

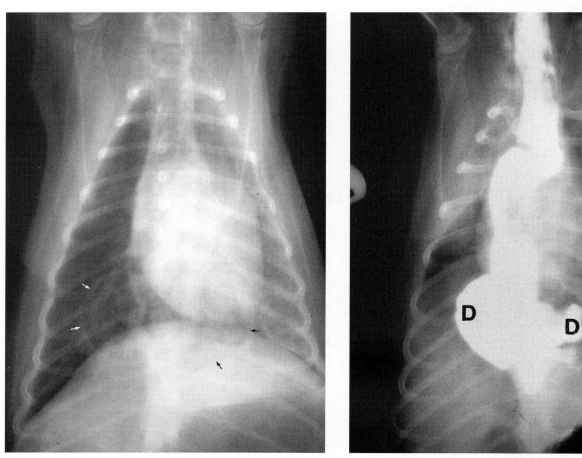

A B

Figure 2–79. (A&B) A 4-year-old pug presented with regurgitation of 2 weeks' duration. (A) A ventrodorsal radiograph revealed two thin-walled, air-filled structures (*arrows*) on the midline nearly adjacent to the diaphragm. (B) An esophagram performed 2 days later revealed mild dilation of the entire esophagus as well as focal dilations (D) immediately cranial to the diaphragm. **Diagnosis:** Esophageal diverticulae.

esophagus proximal to the lesion may be dilated. Diagnosis of a stricture requires a contrast esophagram (Fig. 2–80). It may be necessary to mix the barium with food because liquid barium may pass through without interference if the stricture is mild. Treatment may be performed by balloon catheter dilation with positioning of the balloon under fluoroscopic guidance.[98,99]

Many patients swallow air during radiography, and a localized air accumulation within the esophagus must be identified on at least two radiographs and must be consistent in size, shape, and location to be considered significant. Local accumulations of food or bony material are more significant. Unless the density can be identified as a foreign object, an esophageal contrast study is needed to evaluate the cause of the food accumulation. With time, a local esophageal dilation may become generalized.

Esophageal Masses

The shape of the esophagus may be altered by extraluminal, intramural, and intraluminal masses, as well as by generalized and localized esophageal dilation.[100] Masses are usually inflammatory or neoplastic in origin and may arise from the esophagus or the adjacent mediastinum. A soft tissue density may be identified in the mediastinum on non-contrast radiographs. This mass may produce a localized or generalized esophageal dilation with air or food accumulating proximal to the soft tissue density. In most instances, an esophageal contrast study is required to determine the nature of the soft tissue density; however, the air pattern within or around the density may provide a clue to its nature.

EXTRALUMINAL MASSES

A smooth gradual displacement of the esophagus with an uninterrupted mucosal surface is indicative of an extraluminal mass. The air or contrast column may be merely displaced or thinned as it passes through or around the lesion. Contrast or air will not accumulate within the lesion unless there is esophageal perforation and a periesophageal mediastinal abscess. Either neoplastic or inflammatory mediastinal masses or hernias may produce this lesion.

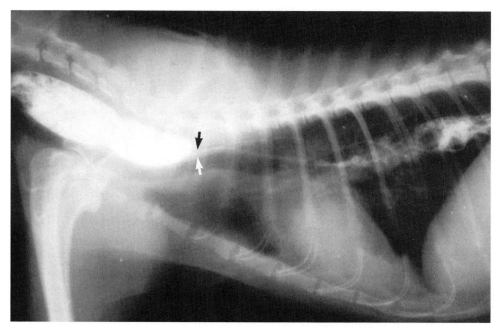

Figure 2–80. A 1-year-old neutered female cat presented for regurgitation of 1-week duration. The cat had been neutered 2 weeks prior to the onset of signs. An esophagram reveals dilation of the cranial esophagus, which terminates into an abruptly narrowed area (*arrows*). The distal esophagus is normal in size. **Diagnosis:** Esophageal stricture.

INTRAMURAL MASSES

Intramural masses may be circumferential (annular) or eccentric. Esophageal displacement will be minimal depending on the lesion's size. Contrast or air may accumulate proximal to these lesions if they are circumferential or obstructive. The mucosal surface is usually smooth and intact. A thin column of contrast may be observed within the center or at the edge of the lesion. Tumors and granulomas may produce this type of lesion (Fig. 2–81).[101–103]

INTRALUMINAL MASSES

Intraluminal masses, including foreign bodies, allow contrast or air passage around their edges as well as within them. This often breaks up the bolus of contrast and causes some of it to remain within and/or around the mass. The mucosal surface will be rough and uneven. Pedunculated tumors, granulomas, and foreign bodies will produce this type of lesion.

In some instances, a lack of normal esophageal peristalsis will prevent the contrast media from reaching the lesion. In these cases, an erect lateral or ventrodorsal radiograph using a horizontal x-ray beam may be valuable in demonstrating the margins of the lesion (Fig. 2–82).

ESOPHAGEAL DENSITY

The density of the esophagus will vary depending on its content. Gas, fluid, food, or a mixture of these may be normally observed within the esophagus. A small amount of air or food present within the esophagus on a single radiograph is not abnormal; however, if this is identified on multiple radiographs, an esophageal contrast study is recommended. Any food material that is retained within the esophagus is abnormal.

ESOPHAGEAL DISPLACEMENT

The esophagus may be displaced by mediastinal, heart base, or hilar masses. The direction of the displacement will indicate the origin of the mass. An esophagram is usually required to identify the position of the esophagus.

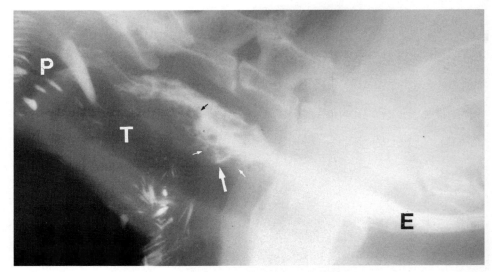

Figure 2–81. A 3-year-old mixed breed dog presented with dysphagia and weight loss. Attempts at swallowing were labored. An esophagram revealed multiple mural masses in the proximal cervical esophagus (*arrows*). The caudal cervical esophagus appeared normal (*E*). Also identified are the trachea (*T*) and pharynx (*P*). Endoscopic examination revealed multiple mural masses in the area, which were biopsied. **Diagnosis:** Granulomatous esophagitis (Histoplasmosis).

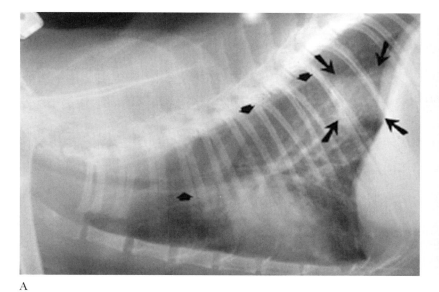

A

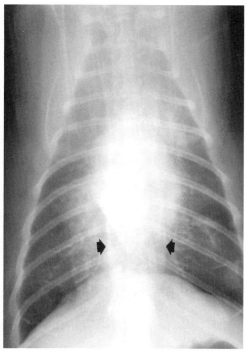

B

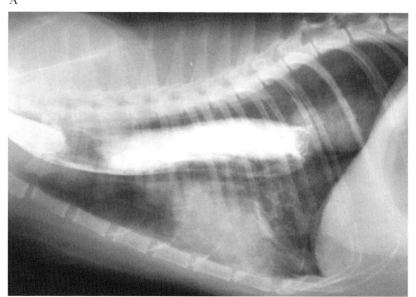

C

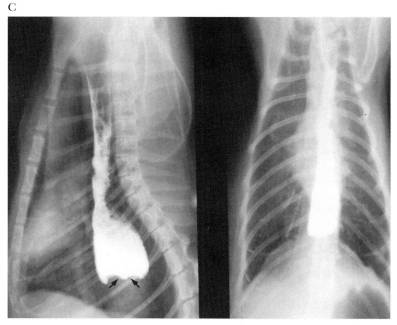

D

Figure 2–82. (A,B,C,D) A 13-year-old spayed cat presented with a 1-month history of chronic vomiting. There is dilation of the thoracic esophagus. The esophageal walls are visible in both the (A) lateral and (B) ventrodorsal radiographs (*short arrows*). The trachea and cardiac silhouette are ventrally displaced. There is a soft tissue density identified in the caudal mediastinum at the level of the esophageal hiatus (*long arrows*). There is an increase in pulmonary interstitial density. The radiographic findings are indicative of esophageal dilation with a mass or foreign body in the caudal thoracic esophagus. (C) An esophagram revealed the contrast material outlined the dilated thoracic esophagus and did not extend beyond the level of the soft tissue density. (D) Erect lateral and erect ventrodorsal radiographs were obtained using a horizontal x-ray beam. The contrast material has moved into the caudal thoracic esophagus and outlines the soft tissue-dense mass. There is indentation of the contrast column with a central outpouching indicating constriction of the esophageal lumen (*arrows*). The radiographic findings are indicative of a soft tissue mass in the caudal thoracic esophagus. The erect radiographs with the horizontal x-ray beam are useful in demonstrating the mass more completely. **Diagnosis:** Squamous cell carcinoma of the caudal thoracic esophagus.

Masses around the esophageal hiatus, caudal mediastinal abscesses or tumors, esophageal granulomas or tumors, hiatal or paraesophageal hernias, gastroesophageal intussusception, or diaphragmatic masses may be differentiated by an esophageal contrast study. Caudal mediastinal or diaphragmatic masses are extraluminal and may displace the esophagus but will not involve the esophageal mucosa.

ESOPHAGEAL FOREIGN BODIES

Esophageal foreign bodies may be radiopaque and easily identified or tissue-dense and less readily detected.[104] Foreign bodies usually lodge at the thoracic inlet, cranial to the heart base, or cranial to the esophageal hiatus (Figs. 2–83, 2–84 and 2–85).[105,106] Identification of these foreign objects on the ventrodorsal radiograph is often difficult because of the overlying vertebral column. Esophageal dilation cranial to the foreign object may provide a clue to its presence, but an esophageal contrast study may be necessary to outline it. If an esophageal foreign body is identified or suspected, the thoracic radiograph must be carefully evaluated for evidence of mediastinal or pleural fluid and/or air, which indicate esophageal perforation. Aspiration pneumonia may be present if the animal has been vomiting. If esophageal perforation is suspected, an esophageal contrast study may be performed using a water-soluble iodine-containing contrast material.[107] The contrast study may not demonstrate contrast leakage despite non-contrast radiographic evidence of esophageal perforation because of adhesions or fibrosis, which may partially seal the perforation.[108] Esophagoscopy is the preferred method to delineate an esophageal perforation.

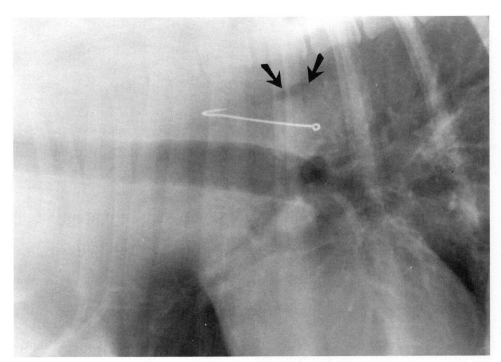

Figure 2–83. A 7-year-old female springer spaniel presented with a history of having swallowed a fish hook 2 days earlier. On this lateral thoracic radiograph the fish hook is readily identified dorsal to the heart base. There is a soft tissue density surrounding the fish hook, and there is gas in the soft tissues dorsal to this density (*arrows*). The radiographic findings indicate perforation of the esophagus by the fish hook with air within the mediastinum. The soft tissue density that surrounds the fish hook may represent bait that was on the fish hook at the time it was swallowed. **Diagnosis:** Fish hook in the thoracic esophagus with penetration of the mucosa. The fish hook was removed by endoscopy. Additional air was present in the mediastinum after removal of the fish hook. A contrast esophagram was performed 3 days after foreign body removal and there was no evidence of leakage of contrast material at the site of foreign body perforation. No complications were encountered.

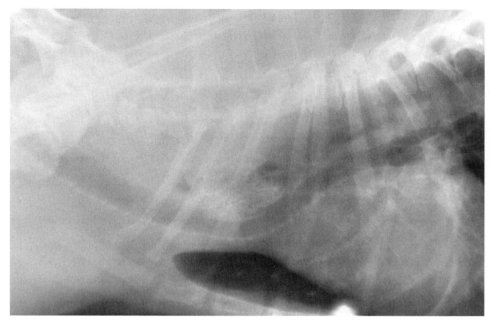

Figure 2–84. A 5-year-old spayed Boston terrier was presented with a history of regurgitating immediately after eating. On the lateral thoracic radiograph the trachea is ventrally displaced at the level of the thoracic inlet. There is a radiopaque object dorsal to the trachea. This object has a bone density and trabecular pattern. It represents a portion of a vertebral body that is lodged within the esophagus. There is gas noted in the esophagus surrounding this foreign object. The portion of the esophagus distal to this foreign body also contains a small amount of fluid and gas. **Diagnosis:** Esophageal foreign body. There is no evidence of esophageal perforation. The esophageal foreign body was removed by endoscopy. No complications were encountered.

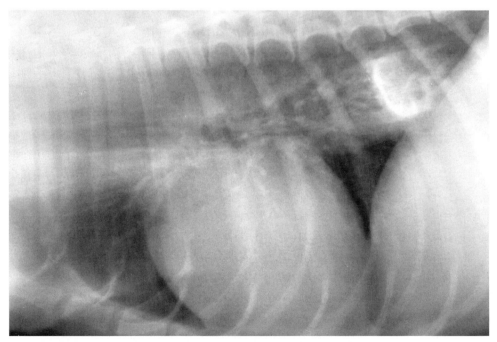

Figure 2–85. A 5-year-old female Lhasa apso presented with an acute onset of vomiting and diarrhea with abdominal distention. The dog was anorectic. On the lateral thoracic radiograph there is a radiodense foreign body in the esophagus anterior to the diaphragm. The bone density and trabecular pattern identify this object as a bone. There is a small amount of gas within the cranial thoracic esophagus dorsal to the trachea. **Diagnosis:** Esophageal foreign body. No complications were noted. The foreign body was displaced into the stomach with a fiberoptic endoscope.

ESOPHAGEAL FISTULAE

Tracheoesophageal and bronchoesophageal fistulae are rare in dogs and cats.[109-111] Mediastinal or pleural fluid or a localized pulmonary infiltrate may be observed in association with these fistulae. The diagnosis requires demonstration of a communication between the esophagus and the trachea or bronchus during an esophageal contrast study (Fig. 2–86). Aspirated contrast media must not be confused with a fistula. When a fistula is present, a larger amount of contrast will be present within the distal as compared to the proximal airway.

ESOPHAGEAL FUNCTION

Evaluation of esophageal function usually requires fluoroscopy; however, some indirect information can be obtained from both survey and contrast static images.[112] Generalized or localized esophageal dilation is a nonspecific finding that indicates reduced peristaltic activity and muscle tone. Megaesophagus is a general term used to describe a generalized esophageal dilation. It has been used synonymously with congenital idiopathic megaesophagus; however, there are many causes of esophageal dilation and the term megaesophagus does not indicate a specific etiology or disease entity.

The degree and extent of the esophageal dilation can best be radiographically determined by using contrast media. Those anatomic or structural alterations that could cause secondary esophageal dilation can be identified. In some instances, the contrast material will not reach the caudal thoracic esophagus due to esophageal hypomotility or a complete absence of peristalsis. Supporting the patient in an erect position and using a horizontal x-ray beam will frequently outline the caudal thoracic esophagus when peristaltic activity is insufficient to propel the contrast to that level. The weight of the contrast-filled esophagus may close the lower esophageal sphincter and block contrast passage when the animal is positioned in an erect posture. This can create the illusion of lower esophageal sphincter spasm or stenosis.

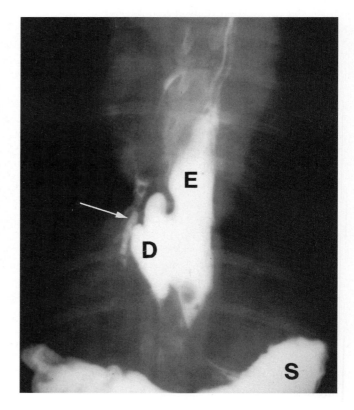

Figure 2–86. A 5-year-old male keeshound presented with chronic regurgitation and a recent onset of cough and inappetence. Survey radiographs suggested the presence of a mass in the area of the caudal esophagus. A contrast study of the esophagus (*E*) revealed the presence of a diverticulum (*D*) immediately cranial to the stomach (*S*) with a fistula into the bronchus (*arrow*). The bronchus is seen to taper distally and the amount of contrast diminishes in the more cranial portion of the bronchus. **Diagnosis:** Bronchoesophageal fistula.

Gastroesophageal Reflux

Reflux of gastric contents into the thoracic esophagus may be observed during esophageal and gastric contrast studies, especially in cats. If the contrast is immediately returned to the stomach by esophageal peristalsis, the reflux is not significant. Persistence of the contrast in the thoracic esophagus or esophageal dilation and/or mucosal irregularity are indicative of esophageal inflammatory disease.[54] However, it may be difficult to determine whether this is secondary to chronic reflux or a primary esophageal or lower esophageal sphincter disorder.

CARDIAC ABNORMALITIES

In animals with cardiac disease, both the size and shape of the heart can be evaluated radiographically. Variation of the heart's size and shape among different breeds and individuals makes the radiographic evaluation challenging. Several important factors that must be remembered when radiographically evaluating the heart include:

1. The cardiac silhouette is a summation shadow of all four cardiac chambers and the major vessels smoothed out by the pericardium.
2. The cardiac size and shape vary with the stage of the cardiac cycle.
3. The apparent cardiac size will vary with the respiratory phase.
4. The "normal" cardiac size and shape varies with thoracic conformation.

Many animals with cardiac disease have normal cardiac silhouettes. This occurs because there is a wide range of shapes and sizes among normal animals, some cardiac diseases do not cause cardiomegaly, and many cardiac diseases must be present for a period of time before cardiac size alterations develop.

Echocardiography provides a great deal more information about the heart than does survey radiography. Echocardiography allows for the determination of the thickness of various portions of the myocardium, the diameters of various chambers and great vessels, the motion of valves, septum, and other structures, and even determination of the direction and velocity of blood flow through various parts of the heart and great vessels. It is very important that proper care be taken in the performance of the echocardiogram. Measurements must be made at precisely the proper site and the beam angle. Doppler evaluations must be performed with equal attention to procedure to ensure that artifacts, such as aliasing, are not mistaken for valid measurements.

CARDIOMEGALY

Cardiomegaly is a non-specific term that indicates that the cardiac silhouette exceeds the expected dimension for an animal of a specific breed, age, and physique. Moderate and severe degrees of cardiomegaly are readily detected, but a mild degree may be overlooked or diagnosed incorrectly. The radiograph cannot differentiate among cardiomegaly due to muscular hypertrophy, chamber dilation, or small amounts of pericardial fluid. The radiographic diagnosis in those animals with a mild degree of cardiomegaly should be ignored if it is not supported by clinical, electrocardiographic, echocardiographic, or other (non-cardiac) radiographic findings.

Because the radiograph depicts the cardiac silhouette and not just the heart, the cardiac silhouette may appear enlarged although the heart size is normal. This can be due to age, obesity, physique, thoracic conformation, phase of respiration, phase of cardiac cycle, or geometry of the x-ray image. The cardiac silhouette may appear slightly larger (relative to the thoracic dimensions) in young dogs. This characteristic usually disappears around 4 to 6 months of age. Older dogs seem to have a larger cardiac silhouette than do young mature dogs. This characteristic may be largely due to asymptomatic compensated cardiac disease. Fat can accumulate around the heart, both inside and outside the pericardial sac, in obese animals. This will result in an enlarged cardiac silhouette. Animals that are in good physical shape and are bred or used for athletic activities such as racing seem to have a larger heart than non-racing animals with similar thoracic conformation.

Cardiomegaly may result from cardiac and extracardiac diseases. Fluid overload, myocardial disease, valvular insufficiency, anemia, or cardiovascular shunts may produce cardiac dilation.[113] Hypertrophy results from increased resistance to cardiac output, elevated systemic pressure, or idiopathic causes. When evaluating cardiac size, both a lateral and dorsoventral or ventrodorsal radiograph should be examined. If the cardiac silhouette appears enlarged on only one view, the enlargement is probably artifactual.

In the lateral radiograph, the heart may enlarge cranially, caudally, and/or dorsally. Cranial and caudal enlargement increase the cardiac size relative to the intercostal spaces. This must always be evaluated relative to the dog's thoracic conformation. Cranial cardiac enlargement is mostly right ventricular with cranial dorsal enlargement associated with the right auricular appendage, pulmonary artery, and aortic arch. The cranial cardiac border bulges anteriorly, accentuating its normal curvature. The cardiac-sternal contact increases. The cranial border may appear straight and become more vertical when the cardiac enlargement becomes marked.

Caudal enlargement is mainly left ventricular with caudodorsal enlargement associated with the left atrium. The cranially directed curve of the normal caudal cardiac border gradually becomes straighter and more vertically directed. The slight indentation that is sometimes observed between the left atrium and ventricle becomes flattened. The caudal vena cava becomes dorsally displaced at the point where it contacts the heart. Overlap between the heart and the diaphragm increases; however, the reliability of this change depends on consistently obtaining an inspiratory radiograph.

Dorsal enlargement of the cardiac silhouette will increase the apico-basilar cardiac dimension and decrease the normal caudoventral angulation of the trachea. This must always be interpreted with consideration of the animal's thoracic conformation. Generally, right heart enlargement elevates the trachea cranial to the tracheal bifurcation, left ventricular enlargement causes elevation at the bifurcation, and left atrial enlargement causes elevation caudal to the bifurcation. These changes rarely occur as isolated events and a considerable amount of overlap is observed.

In the dorsoventral or ventrodorsal radiograph, cardiac enlargement may be cranial, caudal, or to either side. The cranial cardiac margin blends with the cranial mediastinum and evaluation of this dimension is difficult. Cranial right enlargement, usually associated with the right atrium, accentuates the curvature of this cardiac margin. Cranial left enlargement, usually associated with the aortic arch and main pulmonary artery (rarely the right atrial appendage), produces bulges (knobs) on this part of the cardiac margin. Caudal left enlargement is usually associated with the left ventricle and results in a rounder silhouette. Caudal cardiac silhouette enlargement also causes rounding of the cardiac apex, which results in a flattened or blunted tip. This is best documented in a ventrodorsal rather than a dorsoventral radiograph. Enlargement of the cardiac silhouette in a cranio-caudal dimension, resulting in an increased apico-basilar dimension and elongation of the cardiac silhouette, is mainly associated with left ventricular enlargement.

Enlargement of the cardiac silhouette on the right side is mostly due to right ventricular enlargement. The location of the cardiac apex relative to the midline is critical. An apex shift to the left will decrease the appearance of right-sided cardiomegaly, while a shift toward the right will increase the apparent enlargement. Enlargement of the right cardiac margin accentuates its normal convexity. The cardiac apex shifts to the left and the distance from the cardiac margin to the right thoracic wall decreases. Enlargement of the cardiac margin on the left side is mostly due to left ventricular enlargement. The normal, relatively straight, left cardiac margin becomes more convex and the distance to the left thoracic wall decreases. Apex shift to the right is an uncommon occurrence. Left atrial appendage enlargement produces a convex bulge at the three- to five o'clock position. This occurs with moderate to marked enlargement and is rarely seen without left ventricular enlargement.

Because the shape of the normal heart differs in the comparison of ventrodorsal and dorsoventral radiographs, re-evaluation of a patient should include use of the same view each time—consistent and accurate positioning are more important than the specific position used.

Cardiomegaly in cats differs in appearance from that observed in dogs. On the lateral radiograph, this produces a bulging cardiac contour, because enlargement is most apparent in the cranial-dorsal and caudo-dorsal portion of the silhouette. The cardiac silhouette may be elongated and tracheal elevation may be observed. On the dorsoventral radiograph, cardiac enlargement usually produces changes in the right and left cranial margins. This increases the dimension cranially while maintaining a relatively normal caudal dimension producing a somewhat triangular or valentine-shaped cardiac silhouette.

The nature of the cardiac enlargement depends on the specific cardiac disease that is present, as well as the duration and severity of the disease. Once a diagnosis of cardiomegaly is made, the cardiac silhouette should be evaluated critically for evidence of a specific chamber or major vascular enlargement. Previous radiographs are invaluable in detecting cardiomegaly and specific chamber enlargement.

Usually, a diagnosis of cardiomegaly is not made from an echocardiographic examination. The information obtained is more cardiac chamber specific than simply a general assessment of overall cardiac size. M-mode and two-dimensional measurements are usually made from leading edge (acoustic interface closest to the transducer) to leading edge. Diastolic dimensions are measured at the Q or R wave of the ECG. Systolic measurements are obtained at the point of peak downward septal movement.

Right Atrial Enlargement

Right atrial enlargement is not radiographically identified unless the atrium becomes severely enlarged. When present, it is usually associated with evidence of generalized right heart disease (Fig. 2–87). The exception to this is when a right atrial thrombus or neoplasm is present.

On the lateral radiograph, an enlarged right auricular appendage will produce a convex bulge on the cranial dorsal margin of the cardiac silhouette. That portion of the trachea cranial to the bifurcation may be mildly displaced dorsally over the heart base.

On the ventrodorsal or dorsoventral radiograph, the enlarged right atrium will produce a bulge on the right cranial cardiac margin at approximately the nine- to eleven o'clock position. Severe enlargement may protrude across the midline to the left cranial cardiac margin.

An echocardiogram can identify right atrial enlargement prior to it being radiographically evident. Although normal diameters have not been well defined, the right atrium should not appear larger than the left atrium on the right parasternal long axis view or the left parasternal 4-chamber view.

Right Ventricular Enlargement

Right ventricular enlargement causes accentuation of the cranial convexity of the cardiac silhouette on the lateral radiograph; it eventually causes a vertically oriented cardiac border (Fig. 2–88). Contact between the cardiac silhouette and the sternum increases, the cardiac apex becomes elevated or separated from the sternum, and the trachea may become elevated cranial to or at the bifurcation as a result of right ventricular enlargement. If a line is drawn from the tracheal bifurcation to the cardiac apex, the amount of the cardiac silhouette cranial to this line will be greater than the normal two-thirds of the total cardiac area.

In the ventrodorsal or dorsoventral radiograph, right ventricular enlargement will make the right cardiac margin become more convex and the distance to the right

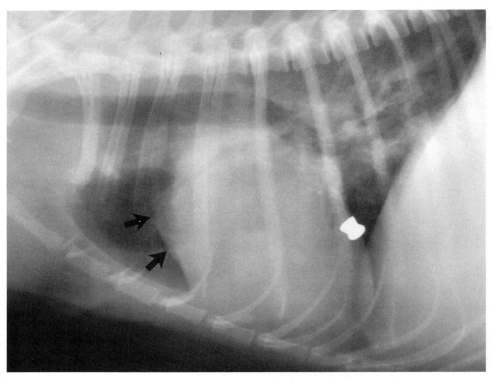

A

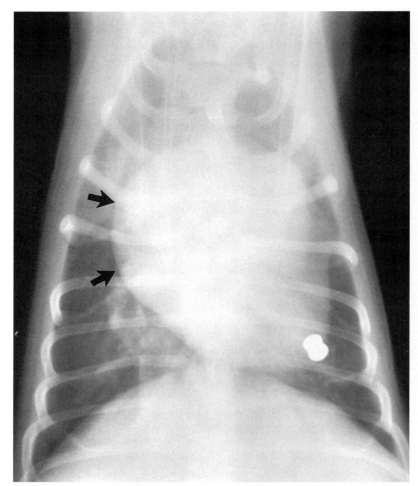

Figure 2–87. (A&B) A 7-year-old male mixed breed dog presented with a 5-day history of anorexia and lethargy. The abdomen was distended. (A) On the lateral thoracic radiographs there is a bulge present on the cranial aspect of the cardiac silhouette (*arrows*). The trachea is mildly elevated cranial to the tracheal bifurcation and there is sternal contact as well as elevation of the cardiac apex from the sternum. (B) On the ventrodorsal radiograph a bulge is present on the right cranial aspect of the cardiac silhouette (*arrows*), as is rounding of the right side of the cardiac silhouette and shifting of the cardiac apex into the left hemithorax. The radiographic changes are indicative of right atrial enlargement. The right ventricle is also enlarged. There is an incidental finding of a radiopaque air rifle pellet within the soft tissues. **Diagnosis:** Enlarged right ventricle and atrium. This was due to tricuspid insufficiency.

B

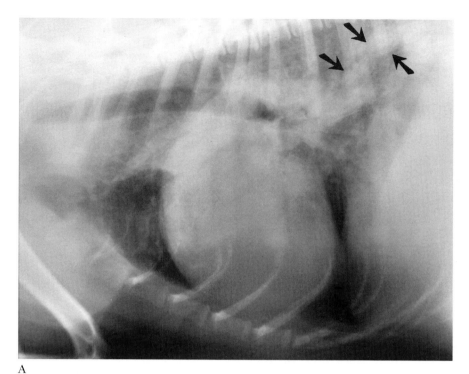

A

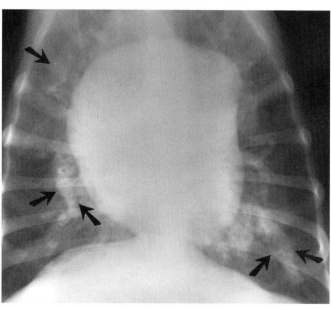

B

Figure 2–88. (A&B) A 6-year-old female mixed breed dog presented with a history of poor exercise tolerance, lethargy, and abdominal distention. The cardiac silhouette is enlarged. (A) On the lateral radiograph the cranial aspect of the cardiac silhouette is rounded and the cardiac apex is elevated from the sternum. (B) On the ventrodorsal radiograph the right side of the cardiac silhouette is rounded. There is a bulge on the left side of the cardiac silhouette in the area of the main pulmonary artery segment. The pulmonary arteries are enlarged and tortuous (*arrows*) on both radiographs. There is an increase in pulmonary interstitial density, especially in the caudal dorsal lung lobes. **Diagnosis:** Dirofilariasis.

thoracic wall will decrease. The cardiac apex will shift to the left. As the cardiac apex becomes elevated from the sternum, the right ventricle may bulge caudally beyond the interventricular septum producing two bulges on the caudal cardiac margin (an apparent double apex). If a line is drawn from the cardiac apex to the point where the cranial mediastinum merges with the right cranial cardiac border, more than half of the heart area will be to the right of this line.

Radiographic evidence of right ventricular enlargement can be due to either dilation of the right ventricular cavity or hypertrophy of the right ventricular myocardium. An echocardiogram can determine if either or both of these lesions are present. The normal diameter of the right ventricular cavity (at end-diastole) is not well defined in the dog, but it should not exceed 33% to 50% of the diameter of the left ventricle as measured on the right parasternal long axis view. The diameter in the cat (at end-diastole) should not exceed 7 mm.[18] Likewise, the normal thickness of the right ventricular free wall is poorly defined but should be approximately 33% to 50% of the thickness of the interventricular septum or left ventricular free wall.[31]

Main Pulmonary Artery Enlargement

On the lateral radiograph, a markedly enlarged main pulmonary artery may bulge cranial to the cranial dorsal cardiac border (Fig. 2–89). In most cases, the enlarged pulmonary artery does not extend beyond the cardiac margin or is lost within the soft tissue density of the cranial mediastinum.

On the ventrodorsal or dorsoventral radiograph, the enlarged main pulmonary artery bulges beyond the left cranial cardiac margin at the one- to two o'clock position. The cranial border of the bulge may blend with the shadow of the cranial mediastinum. In a slightly overexposed radiograph, the caudal border may be traced back to the origin of the right and left main pulmonary arteries.

Slight bulging in the area of the main pulmonary artery may be observed in normal dogs. This may be due to rotation of the heart within the thorax, exposure of the radiograph during systole, or malpositioning of the animal.

The main pulmonary artery is best seen on the right parasternal short axis view high on the base through the pulmonic valve region. The pulmonary artery is normally the same diameter as the valvular orifice. The right and left pulmonary arteries normally have a smaller diameter than the main pulmonary artery.

Left Atrial Enlargement

On the lateral radiograph, the silhouette of the enlarged left atrium produces a "wing-shaped" shadow caudal to the tracheal bifurcation and dorsal to the caudal vena cava (Fig. 2–90). The caudal cardiac margin becomes straight and forms a sharp angle with the dorsal cardiac margin. Caudal to the tracheal bifurcation, the main stem bronchi are elevated, and the left bronchus is more markedly affected.

On the ventrodorsal or dorsoventral radiograph, the enlarged left auricular appendage may bulge beyond the left cardiac margin producing a convex bulge at about two- to five o'clock. The atrium may be evident as an increased density between the caudal main stem bronchi. An overexposed radiograph will demonstrate the widened angle between the main stem bronchi, which results from the displacement by the enlarged atrium.

Echocardiographically, the normal diameter of the left atrium has been defined for both the dog and cat using the right parasternal long axis left ventricular outflow view. In general, the left atrial diameter should be approximately the same as the aorta (at the level of the aortic valve) as imaged on the right parasternal long axis view. The left atrium may also be viewed using the left parasternal 4-chamber view and the right parasternal short axis view.

Left Ventricular Enlargement

On the lateral radiograph, the normal convexity of the caudal cardiac margin may become accentuated in mild left ventricular enlargement (Fig. 2–91). This will progress until the caudal cardiac margin becomes straightened and more upright; it will eventually become perpendicular to the sternum. The caudal vena cava becomes elevated, sloping upward from the diaphragm to the heart. The tracheal bifurcation is also elevated and the thoracic trachea may be parallel to the thoracic vertebral bodies or slope dorsally from the thoracic inlet to its bifurcation.

On the ventrodorsal or dorsoventral radiograph, the normally straight left cardiac margin becomes more convex and the distance from its margin to the left thoracic wall decreases. The cardiac apex becomes rounded and blunt. It moves toward the midline and rarely shifts into the right hemithorax. The cranio-caudal dimension of the cardiac silhouette increases. A line drawn from the junction of the right cardiac

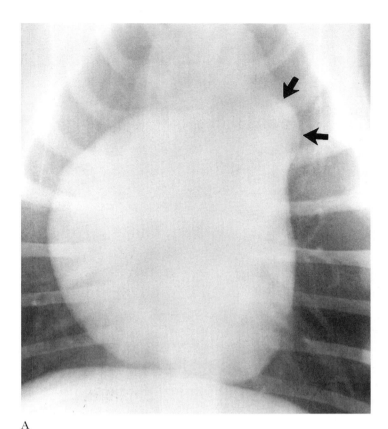

A

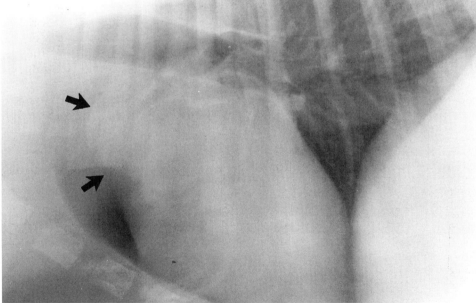

B

Figure 2–89. (A&B) A 5-month-old female Airedale presented for evaluation of a Grade 5/6 holosystolic murmur. The cardiac silhouette is enlarged. (A) On the ventrodorsal radiograph the right margin of the cardiac silhouette is rounded. A bulge is present in the area of the pulmonary artery segment (*arrows*). (B) On the lateral radiograph there is increased sternal contact and cranial bulging of the cardiac margin. The pulmonary artery enlargement is also evident cranial to the cardiac silhouette (*arrows*). The pulmonary vessels appear small. The radiographic findings are indicative of right heart and main pulmonary artery segment enlargement. **Diagnosis:** Pulmonic stenosis.

border with the cranial mediastinum to the cardiac apex will divide the heart unequally with a larger area on the left side.

Radiographic evidence of left ventricular enlargement can be due to either dilation of the left ventricular cavity and/or hypertrophy of the ventricular myocardium. The echocardiogram can determine if either or both of these processes are present. The normal diameter of the left ventricle and thickness of the interventricular septum and left ventricular free wall have been defined.[18] In cats, the left ventricular diameter ranges from 1.1 to 1.5 cm in diastole, and from 0.6 to 0.9 cm in systole. The

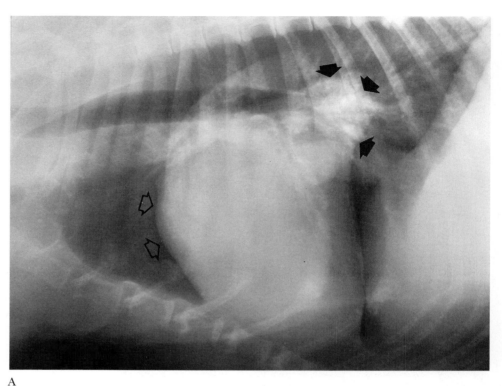

A

Figure 2–90. (A&B) A 13-year-old male miniature poodle presented with a chronic moist cough. The cardiac silhouette is markedly enlarged. The left atrium is enlarged on both (A) the lateral and (B) ventrodorsal radiographs. The caudal cardiac border is straightened, and the main stem bronchi are both elevated and compressed. On (B) a bulge is noted on the cardiac silhouette in the three to five o'clock position, and on (A) a wing-shaped density is present on the caudal dorsal cardiac margin (*closed arrows*). These findings indicate left atrial enlargement. The cardiac apex is rounded and the caudal cardiac margin is straight. The tracheal elevation on (A) indicates left ventricular enlargement. The right side of the cardiac silhouette is also rounded and there is a bulge on the cranial aspect of the cardiac silhouette indicating right atrial enlargement (*open arrows*). The radiographic changes are indicative of generalized cardiomegaly. **Diagnosis:** Mitral and tricuspid insufficiency with bi-atrial and bi-ventricular enlargement.

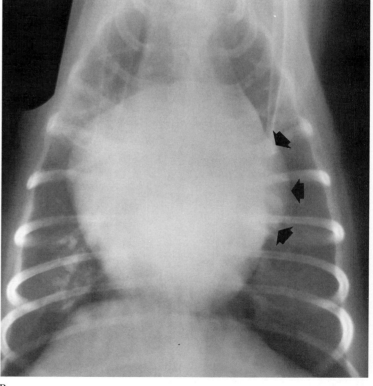

B

thickness of the intraventricular septum ranges from 0.25 to 0.5 cm in diastole and from 0.5 to 0.8 cm in systole. The left ventricular free wall thickness ranges from 0.25 to 0.5 cm in diastole and from 0.4 to 0.8 cm in systole.

In dogs, the cardiac measurements vary in a relationship that is not linear but has been indexed to body weight.[31] In a 12 kg dog, the left ventricular diameter in dias-

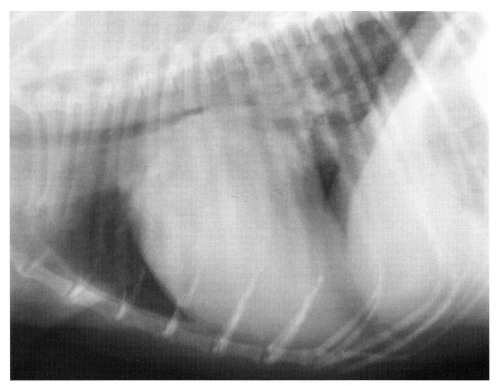

A

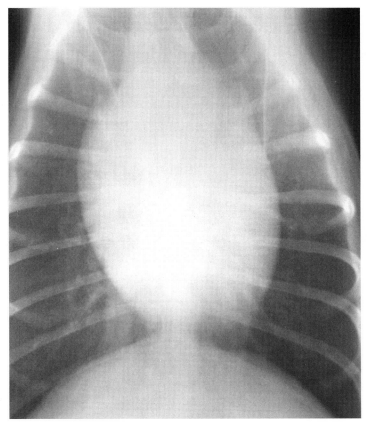

B

Figure 2–91. (A&B) A 10-year-old female miniature poodle presented with a 4-day history of coughing. On the lateral and ventrodorsal thoracic radiographs the cardiac silhouette is enlarged and elongated. The left cardiac margin is rounded, and there is elevation of the tracheal bifurcation. The caudal cardiac margin is straight and upright. The radiographic changes are indicative of left ventricular enlargement. **Diagnosis:** Left ventricular and atrial enlargement. This was due to mitral insufficiency.

tole is 3.4 cm, while in a 24 kg dog it is 4.3 cm. The left ventricular diameter in systole is 2.1 cm for a 12 kg dog, while for a 24 kg dog the systolic diameter is 2.9 cm. The diastolic width of the intraventricular septum for a 12 kg dog is 0.72 cm, while in a 24 kg dog the width is 0.84 cm. The systolic dimension of the interventricular septum is 1.09 cm for a 12 kg dog and 1.2 cm for a 24 kg dog. The diastolic left ventricular free wall measurement is 0.62 cm for a 12 kg dog and 0.75 cm for a 24 kg dog. During systole, the left ventricular free wall measures 0.95 cm for the 12 kg and 0.11 cm for the 24 kg dog.

Aortic Arch Enlargement

On the lateral radiograph, the enlarged aortic arch may be evident as a bulge on the cranial dorsal cardiac margin (Fig. 2–92). This enlargement is not often seen be-

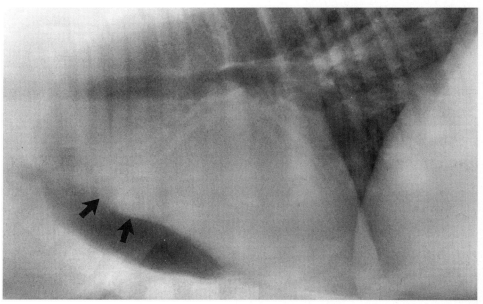

A

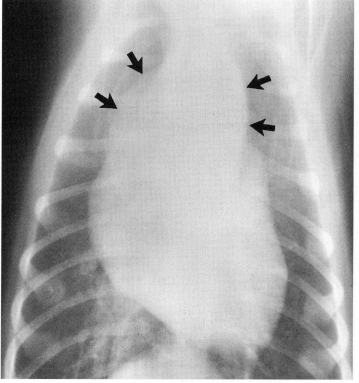

Figure 2–92. (A&B) A 3-month-old, female collie was presented for evaluation of a Grade 5/6 holosystolic murmur. The cardiac silhouette is normal size. (A) On the lateral radiograph the caudal margin of the cardiac silhouette appears straight and there is a bulge on the cranial dorsal margin (*arrows*) of the cardiac silhouette. (B) On the ventrodorsal radiograph a bulge is present in the cranial mediastinum cranial to the cardiac silhouette (*arrows*). The radiographic findings are indicative of aortic arch enlargement. **Diagnosis:** Aortic stenosis.

B

cause the aortic arch is within the cranial mediastinum and is in contact with the rest of the heart. In normal older cats and some normal chondrodystrophic dogs, a small aortic bulge may be identified.

On the ventrodorsal or dorsoventral radiograph, the cranial bulging of the aorta may be hidden within the mediastinum or produce a widened mediastinum. If the enlargement involves the descending aorta (as in patent ductus arteriosus), the bulge will be observed along the left margin of the descending aorta. If the enlargement involves the ascending aortic arch (as in aortic stenosis), the bulge will be observed cranial to the cardiac silhouette.

The proximal ascending aorta is easily visualized by echocardiography. As seen on the right parasternal, long axis, left ventricular outflow tract view, the aorta begins with the aortic valves, then is followed by a slight dilation (sinus of Valsalva) and then continues cranial and then dorsal. In some patients, part of the aortic arch can be visualized. Dilation of this segment is readily recognized, and the diameter can be compared with published normals (1.9 cm–12 kg; 2.4 cm–24 kg).[31] Dilation of the aorta distal to this region usually is not exhibited on the echocardiogram, because the air-filled lung blocks transmission of sound to these regions (e.g., at the level of ductus arteriosus).

MICROCARDIA

Microcardia is a non-specific term that is used to denote a smaller than normal cardiac silhouette (Fig. 2–93). It generally reflects a decrease in circulating blood volume. This may occur from hypovolemic shock, dehydration, or emaciation and has been reported with Addison's disease.[114] The hypovolemia and hypoperfusion also cause the caudal vena cava and pulmonary arteries to appear small. Microcardia may be diagnosed incorrectly when the heart appears small in comparison to the lungs as a result of over-inflation of the lungs or tension pneumothorax.

On the lateral radiograph, an abnormally small heart may not contact the sternum. It will measure 2½ intercostal spaces, or less, in width and its height will be less than 50% of the lateral thoracic dimension. The apex often appears more sharply pointed than normal. The heart will be almost perpendicular to the sternum.

On the ventrodorsal or dorsoventral radiograph, the cardiac silhouette will occupy less than 50% of the thoracic diameter and will be separated from the diaphragm by lucent lung. The heart may be oval in shape due to its upright position within the thorax.

Echocardiographically, hypovolemia is recognized by a decrease in the diameter of all chambers and great vessels. Cardiac wall thicknesses will remain normal or be slightly increased, and fractional shortening may be normal or increased.

HEART DISEASE AND CONGESTIVE HEART FAILURE

Heart disease (a structural or functional heart abnormality) may be present for a long time before an animal develops congestive heart failure—circulatory inadequacy resulting in congestive changes in other organs. The presence of an enlarged cardiac silhouette is not an indicator of heart failure. Rather, changes in extracardiac structures are used to define congestive heart failure. These changes may be divided into those associated with left heart failure and those associated with right heart failure.

Congestive left heart failure develops in stages. Pulmonary venous congestion may be recognized radiographically when the size of the pulmonary vein exceeds the size of the adjacent pulmonary artery. This is followed by interstitial pulmonary edema, which produces a blurring of vascular margins beginning in the perihilar area and radiating peripherally in a nearly symmetrical fashion. This, then, progresses to a more diffuse, poorly-defined alveolar infiltrate. In some dogs with cardiomyopathy (especially those with chronic left heart failure), a nodular pattern may be present.

Figure 2–93. (A&B) A 10-year-old female Doberman pinscher was presented with a history of collapse. The cardiac silhouette is small. The pulmonary vessels and caudal vena cava also appear small. The radiographic findings are indicative of microcardia and hypovolemia. **Diagnosis:** Hypoadrenocorticism (Addison's disease).

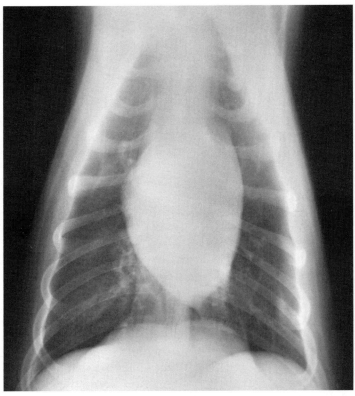

A

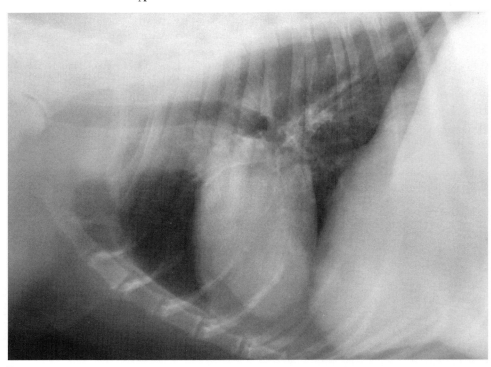

B

Pleural fluid may follow the pulmonary edema. Although decreased cardiac output may reduce the size of the aorta, this is not generally recognized radiographically. Congestive left heart failure usually occurs after left heart enlargement; however, the left heart size may be normal with acute left heart failure secondary to conditions such as ruptured chordae tendineae or myocarditis.

While echocardiography is generally superior to conventional radiography for evaluating cardiac morphology, motion, myocardial function, and blood flow patterns, it cannot evaluate the pulmonary parenchyma or pulmonic vessels. Therefore, echocardiography alone cannot make a diagnosis of congestive left heart failure. Radiographic evidence is required.

Congestive right heart failure results in systemic venous congestion. Enlargement of the caudal vena cava usually occurs. This cannot always be identified radiographically, because the normal caudal vena cava size varies with cardiac cycle and respiration. Hepatomegaly, splenomegaly, ascites, and pleural and/or pericardial effusions may be observed radiographically in patients with congestive right heart failure.

The sonographic diagnosis of congestive right heart failure requires evaluation of the heart as well as the size of the post cava and hepatic veins. The size of the caudal vena cava and hepatic veins is evaluated subjectively. The enlargement that occurs with right heart failure is marked and easily recognized after a few normal livers have been examined. The presence of ascites is helpful in confirming the diagnosis of right heart failure. Right heart enlargement or pericardial fluid along with dilation of the hepatic veins and post cava is indicative of congestive right heart failure.

SPECIFIC CARDIAC DISEASES

When evaluating either the thoracic radiograph or echocardiogram, it is useful to categorize cardiac disease as either acquired or congenital. The radiograph, only one part of the cardiac evaluation, should not be used as the sole basis for a definite diagnosis. The echocardiogram may allow a definite diagnosis. If there is a disparity between clinical, electrocardiographic, echocardiographic, and radiographic findings, an angiocardiogram is recommended to establish a definitive diagnosis.[115]

CONGENITAL CARDIAC DISEASES

There are specific radiographic and echocardiographic features described for most congenital cardiac diseases.[115–117] Because some variation exists, one or more of the expected features in any specific case may be absent. Unless specified, the features described apply to both dogs and cats.

PATENT DUCTUS ARTERIOSUS

Patent ductus arteriosus (PDA) is the failure of the fetal patent ductus arteriosus to close at birth. This situation usually results in a left to right shunting of blood, which causes increased blood flow through the lungs and the left side of the heart (Fig. 2–94). As a result, the left ventricle, left atrium, pulmonary arteries, and pulmonary veins are all enlarged and/or increased in number.[118,119] An aneurysmal dilation occurs in the descending aorta and in the main pulmonary artery. The aortic aneurysm produces a bulge usually seen on the ventrodorsal radiograph along the left side of the aorta at the level of the 4th or 5th intercostal space. Additionally, a pulmonary arterial aneurysmal dilation (knob) will be visible at the same level or slightly caudal to the aortic aneurysm, and a third bulge (enlarged left atrial appendage) may be visible caudal to the pulmonary aneurysm.

The echocardiogram in dogs with patent ductus arteriosus will reveal left atrial and left ventricular dilation. The E-point septal separation (point of maximal mitral valve opening to left ventricular septal echo) is greater than normal (Fig. 2–95). Fractional shortening will be either normal or diminished (subsequent to the ventricular dilation). In some cases, the aneurysmal dilation of the aorta will be identified but the dilation of the pulmonary artery is rarely seen. In some cases with long-standing disease, there may be right ventricular dilation. Direct visualization of the

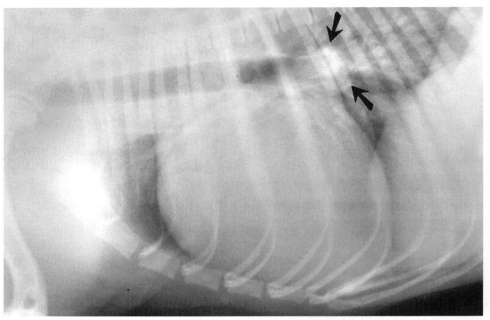

A

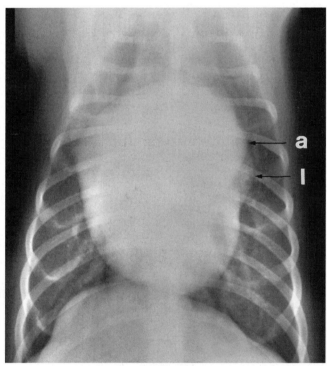

B

Figure 2–94. A 9-month-old female cocker spaniel was presented for evaluation of a continuous murmur. The cardiac silhouette is markedly enlarged. (A) On the lateral radiograph the cranial and caudal cardiac margins appear rounded and a soft tissue density is present in the area of the left atrium (*arrows*). (B) On the ventrodorsal radiograph there are bulges on the left cardiac margin at the site of aorta (*a*) and left atrium (*l*). The cardiac apex is rounded. The pulmonary vessels appear increased in size. The radiographic findings indicate left-sided cardiomegaly with pulmonary arterial and aortic aneurysmal dilatations. The increased size of pulmonary vessels indicate the presence of a left to right shunt. **Diagnosis:** Patent ductus arteriosus.

ductus is uncommon but may be accomplished by using a parasternal short-axis view at the heart base.[120] Doppler studies may reveal a continuous flow disturbance and a high velocity retrograde flow toward the pulmonic valve in the proximal pulmonary artery.[121] Mitral regurgitation is often identified as well.

Most dogs with PDA have typical radiographic and echocardiographic findings; however, all changes are not present in every case. The severity and duration of the shunt will influence the appearance. Cats with PDA have similar changes; however, as with dogs, it is unusual for all radiographic changes to be present.

After ligation of the ductus, the pulmonary vessels return quickly to normal size. The left heart also decreases (returns to the normal) in size, although this may take longer and left heart enlargement often persists when mitral regurgitation is present preoperatively.

A PDA with right to left shunting produces a different spectrum of echocardiographic and radiographic changes.[121] The right ventricle is enlarged due to elevated right ventricular pressure. The aortic aneurysm will not be observed; however, a pulmonary knob will be present and the main pulmonary arteries are often enlarged, tortuous, and blunted. The size of the pulmonary veins will be normal. A contrast echocardiogram may reveal the presence of bubbles in the aortic root after intravenous injection.[120]

AORTICOPULMONARY SEPTAL DEFECT (WINDOW)

Aorticopulmonary septal defect (a window of communication between the aorta and pulmonary artery near their origin at the base of the heart) produces hemodynamic effects similar to those seen with a PDA.[122,123] The radiographic and echocardiographic changes are similar, except that the aorta and pulmonary artery lack the degree of aneurysmal dilation seen in PDA.

AORTIC STENOSIS

Aortic stenosis, whether valvular, subvalvular, or supravalvular, has consistent radiographic features (see Fig. 2–92).[124,125] An enlarged aortic arch will be visible extending cranially into the cranial mediastinum; although, in many affected animals this is masked by the cranial mediastinum. The cardiac silhouette may appear elongated with a broad apex due to the left ventricular enlargement. The remainder of the heart and thoracic structures usually are normal.

Echocardiographic findings may be specific for the site of anomaly. Subvalvular aortic stenosis (SAS) may be seen either as a discrete membrane or focal ridge just below the aortic valve, or as a more elongated ("tunnel-type") narrowing of the left ventricular outflow tract (Fig. 2–96). Usually, this is most noticeable on the septal side. Other findings associated with SAS may include hypertrophy of the left ventricle, normal to increased fractional shortening, coarse systolic fluttering of the aortic valve, partial premature closure of the aortic valve, and systolic anterior motion (SAM) of the septal leaflet toward the interventricular septum in early systole (Fig.

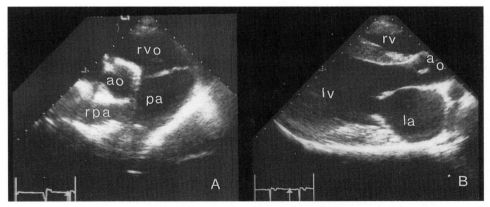

Figure 2–95. (A&B) A 2-year-old male neapolitan mastiff presented with failure to gain weight and labored breathing after exercise. Auscultation revealed a continuous (machinery) murmur. Radiographs revealed generalized cardiomegaly and prominent pulmonary arteries. (A) A right parasternal short-axis view reveals marked dilation of the right ventricular outflow tract (*rvo*), as well as the main (*pa*) and right (*rpa*) pulmonary arteries. (B) The right parasternal long-axis aortic outflow view reveals dilation of the left atrium (*la*) and left ventricle (*lv*). Also identified are the right ventricle (*rv*) and aorta (*ao*). **Diagnosis:** Patent ductus arteriosus.

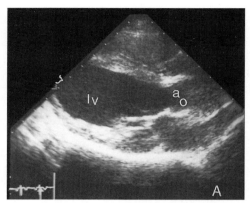
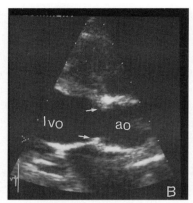

Figure 2–96. A 6-month-old male rottweiler presented with a Grade 4/6 systolic ejection type murmur that was best heard at the left heart base. (A) A right parasternal long-axis aortic outflow view revealed the left ventricle (*lv*) and aorta (*ao*). (B) A close-up view of the aortic outflow tract revealed a focal hyperechoic band (*arrows*) narrowing the left ventricular outflow tract (*lvo*) immediately beneath the aortic valve leaflets. **Diagnosis:** Aortic stenosis.

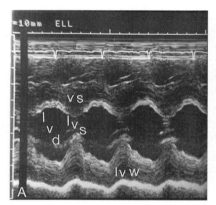
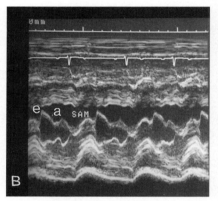

Figure 2–97. (A&B) (A) An M-mode view at the level of the left ventricle reveals the normal structures: *vs*–interventricular septum, *lvd*–left ventricular cavity in diastole, *lvs*–left ventricular cavity in systole, and *lvw*–left ventricular free wall. The fractional shortening (LVED-LVS/LVED) is increased (approximately 55%). (B) An M-mode view at the level of the mitral valve reveals abnormal valve motion with systolic anterior motion of the septal leaflet (*sam*). Also defined are the E-point (*e*) and A-point (*a*). **Diagnosis:** Systolic anterior motion of the mitral valve and increased fractional shortening consistent with aortic stenosis.

2–97). SAM can be so severe (prolonged) that the septal leaflet of the mitral valve closes in mid-systole and acts as an aortic outflow obstruction. Although the post stenotic aneurysmal dilation of the aorta can be seen, the degree of aneurysmal dilation is variable and may not be readily noted. Valvular stenosis is difficult to identify. In this condition, the valve leaflets may appear thickened with a decreased range of motion. Supravalvular lesions are very rare but would show an obvious constriction distal to the aortic valve.

Doppler studies are useful in the diagnosis of aortic stenosis. Turbulent flow beyond the stenosis and a delayed peak in aortic velocity may be seen.[121] Aortic regurgitation (insufficiency) can often be demonstrated. Estimation of the pressure gradient across the stenosis can be made but this may not be accurate in all cases because of decreased cardiac output and the subsequent drop in velocity across the valve, as well as angular changes in the relationship between the left ventricle and aortic outflow tract.[38] In some cases, the degree of stenosis is so mild that obvious changes in cardiac morphology and function are not apparent on two-dimensional or M-mode studies. Doppler studies are helpful in these cases.

VENTRICULAR SEPTAL DEFECT

The size and location of the septal defect and the amount of blood and direction of blood flow through the shunt determine the radiographic changes that are observed (Fig. 2–98). In many septal defects, the cardiac silhouette and pulmonary vessels are

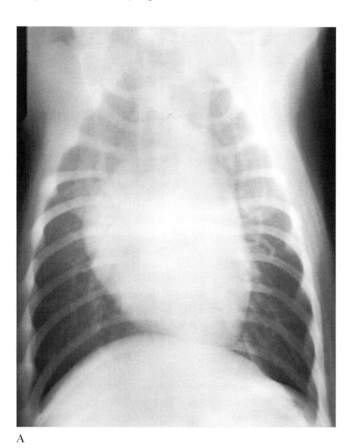

Figure 2–98. (A&B) A 5-month-old, male golden retriever presented for evaluation of a Grade 5/6 systolic murmur. The dog was asymptomatic. (A) On the ventrodorsal radiograph the cardiac silhouette is mildly enlarged and appears elongated. (B) On the lateral radiograph there is slight elevation of the trachea. The right and left cardiac margins appear rounded in (A). The radiographic findings indicate mild cardiomegaly. **Diagnosis:** Ventricular septal defect.

A

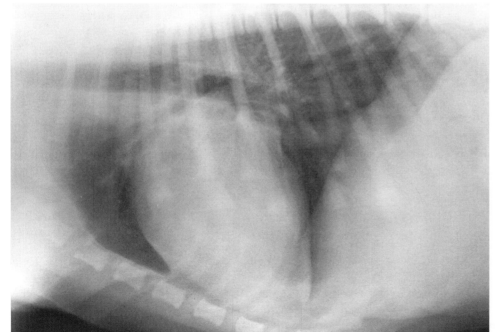

B

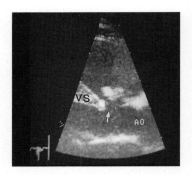

Figure 2–99. A 6-month-old male rottweiler presented with a Grade 4/6 systolic ejection-type murmur that was best heard at the heart base. The right parasternal long-axis aortic (*ao*) outflow view reveals a focal defect (*arrow*) high upon the interventricular septum (*vs*). Doppler studies confirmed the defect. **Diagnosis:** Ventricular septal defect.

radiographically normal. When radiographic changes are present, enlargement of the right ventricle is usually more obvious than left ventricular enlargement, although both occur. Pulmonary arterial and venous enlargement may be evident; however, the size and number of vessels depend on the volume of blood shunting from left to right. The vessels appear normal or only slightly overperfused in most cases.

The echocardiographic changes are likewise dependent upon the size of the defect and the amount of blood that is shunted. Typically, septal defects are located close to the aortic root ("high") (Fig. 2–99). They vary in size from pin-points to those involving the majority of the interventricular septum. Defects less than 1 cm in size may be difficult or impossible to image. The majority of VSD's occur in the membranous (thin) part of the septum. An apparent defect may be seen in normal individuals in this area due to dropout of echoes because the tissue is so thin. It is important to be able to define the septal defect in multiple (repeatable) imaging planes to ensure that it is not an artifact. In most instances, an increase in image intensity (bright echo at the junction of the defect—T sign) is noted at the edge of the defect adding support to the diagnosis.[120] Associated findings can include dilation of the left atrium, left and right ventricle, and increased fractional shortening. Contrast sonography (bubble studies) can be used to help identify ventricular septal defects. In those that have right-to-left shunting of blood, the bubbles may be seen in the left ventricle before they appear in the left atrium. In those that shunt from left-to-right, there may be an area of apparent diminished bubble numbers in the right ventricle due the shunting of non-contrast laden blood across the septum into the area. Doppler studies (particularly color flow) are more sensitive and may detect both left-to-right and right-to-left shunts. Turbulent flow usually will be apparent at the site of the defect.

PULMONIC STENOSIS

Similar radiographic findings will be present regardless of whether a pulmonic stenosis is subvalvular, valvular, or supravalvular (Figs. 2–89 and 2–100). Enlargement of the right ventricle and a post-stenotic dilation of the main pulmonary artery are present in most cases.[126] The size of the pulmonary vessels may be small or normal.

Echocardiographic findings in pulmonic stenosis are consistent with the radiographic changes. Aneurysmal dilation of the main pulmonary artery is usually apparent (Fig. 2–101). Thickened, domed pulmonic valves may also be seen. The results of the stenosis (right ventricular hypertension) may lead to thickening of the right ventricular free wall and interventricular septum, which can be identified by echocardiography. The right ventricular diameter may be increased. If severe, the increased right ventricular pressures may cause paradoxical septal motion—a situation in which the interventricular septal motion parallels that of the left ventricular free wall, nearly obliterating any fractional shortening and severely reducing stroke

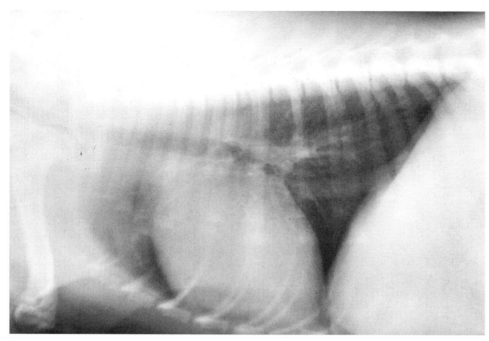

A

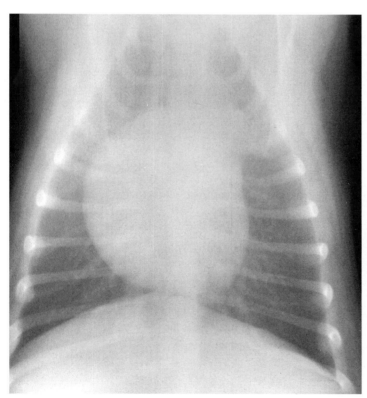

B

Figure 2–100. (A&B) A 5-month-old female West Highland white terrier presented for evaluation of a Grade 5/6 holosystolic murmur. There were no clinical signs associated with this murmur. The cardiac silhouette shows increased sternal contact and rounding of the cranial border on the lateral view. The ventrodorsal view reveals an enlargement of the main pulmonary artery segment is identified. The pulmonary vessels appear small. **Diagnosis:** Pulmonic stenosis.

volume. Doppler studies are used to estimate the pressure gradient across the valve, which aids in choosing between medical and surgical treatments. Patients with gradients exceeding 80 mm Hg are candidates for immediate treatment, while those with gradients from 40 to 80 mm Hg are not usually treated and are re-evaluated periodically. Treatment planning for balloon valvuloplasty frequently utilizes echocardiography to determine the size of the outflow tract and annulus.[127,128]

TETRALOGY OF FALLOT

Tetralogy of Fallot is the combination of a pulmonic stenosis, ventricular septal defect, overriding (rightward displaced) aorta, and right ventricular hypertrophy (Fig. 2–102). The cardiac silhouette size is usually normal or only slightly enlarged. The right ventricular margin may be slightly more round and the left ventricular margin straighter than normal. Both changes result in a somewhat rectangular-shaped heart. The post-stenotic pulmonary artery dilation is usually small and not radiographically visible. A striking radiographic feature is the decreased pulmonary vascular size and hyperlucent lung. The aorta may be small, but radiographic recognition is difficult.

The echocardiographic findings are consistent with the intrinsic pathology. The interventricular septal defect is usually "high" in the membranous portion of the septum. The aortic root is seen "straddling" the septal defect (Fig. 2–103). The main pulmonary artery usually shows a mild aneurysmal dilation. The right ventricular free wall is thickened. The left atrium may be small. The shunting of blood may be confirmed with contrast ("bubble") or Doppler studies.

EISENMENGER'S COMPLEX

This is a rare defect with a right-to-left shunt and is similar to Tetralogy of Fallot except that there is no pulmonic stenosis present.[129] Mild or moderate right-sided cardiomegaly is present. The pulmonary vessels may be enlarged, tortuous, and blunted. Angiocardiography may be required to establish the diagnosis.

COR TRIATRIATUM DEXTER

Cor triatriatum dexter is a rare anomaly in which there is a septum at the orifice of the vena cava into the right atrium. Radiographic abnormalities are limited to enlargement of the caudal vena cava, hepatomegaly, and ascites.[130,131] Echocardiography reveals separation of the right atrium into two segments with the caudal vena cava entering the smaller segment. Hepatic venous distension is often observed. The diagnosis may be confirmed by angiocardiography.

Figure 2–101. A 3-year-old spayed female English bulldog presented with ascites and a Grade 5/6 systolic heart murmur that was best heard over the left heart base. A right parasternal short-axis view reveals narrowing of the valvular orifice (*). There is a dilation (*D*) of the main pulmonary artery (*pa*) distal to the narrowing. Other structures noted are the aorta (*ao*), right ventricular outflow tract (*rvo*), pulmonary artery (*pa*), right pulmonary artery (*rpa*), and left pulmonary artery (*lpa*). **Diagnosis:** Pulmonic stenosis.

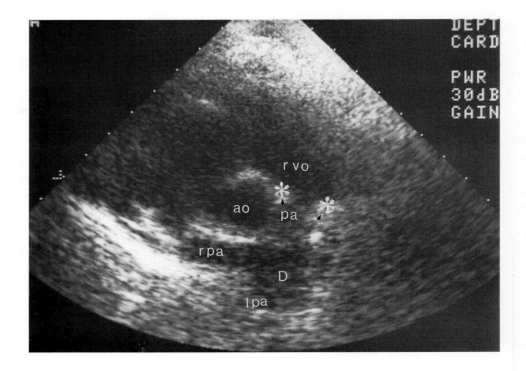

ATRIOVENTRICULAR VALVE MALFORMATIONS

Atrioventricular valve malformation may affect the mitral valve, the tricuspid valve, or both. The pathology may include an enlarged valve annulus, short and thick valve leaflets, short and stout chordae tendineae, and upward malposition of papillary muscles.[132] These changes result in valvular insufficiency.

Mitral valve insufficiency results in mitral regurgitation and subsequent left heart

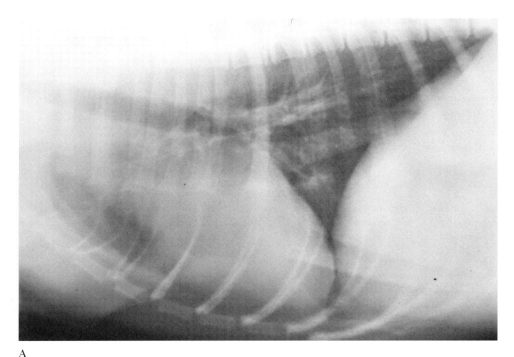

A

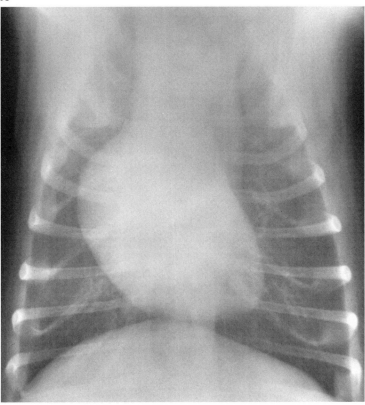

B

Figure 2–102. (A&B) A 6-month-old male Scottish terrier was presented with a Grade 5/6 systolic murmur. The dog had exercise intolerance and was cyanotic. The cardiac silhouette shows slight right-sided enlargement. The pulmonary vessels appear smaller than normal. No other abnormalities are noted. The radiographic findings are indicative of congenital heart disease, most likely Tetralogy of Fallot. **Diagnosis:** Tetralogy of Fallot.

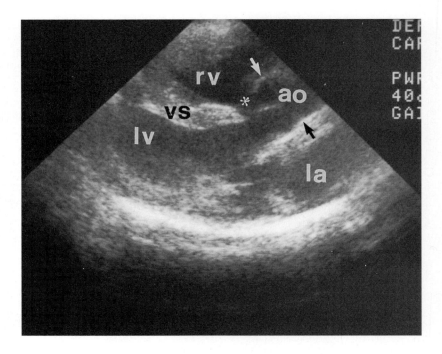

Figure 2–103. A 1-year-old male mixed-breed dog was presented for exercise intolerance. A Grade 5/6 systolic heart murmur was present. A right parasternal long-axis aortic outflow view reveals the presence of a defect (*) in the interventricular septum (*vs*). The origin (*arrows*) of the aorta (*ao*) is positioned astride the interventricular septum. Also seen are the right ventricle (*rv*), left ventricle (*lv*), and left atrium (*la*). **Diagnosis:** Tetralogy of Fallot (the pulmonic stenosis and right ventricular hypertrophy were seen on other views).

failure. Radiographic findings of congenital mitral valve insufficiency (like acquired mitral valve insufficiency) usually include massive left atrial dilation and moderate to severe left ventricular enlargement.[133] Pulmonary edema may be present if the dog is in left heart failure. Tricuspid insufficiency results in tricuspid regurgitation, and subsequently leads to right heart failure. Radiographic findings include right atrial dilation (this is only radiographically apparent if massive) and right ventricular enlargement (see Fig. 2–87). Pleural or abdominal effusion may be present if right heart failure occurs. Combinations of the above findings may be noted if both conditions coexist (Fig. 2–104).

Echocardiographic findings of mitral insufficiency include marked left atrial dilation, left ventricular dilation, and mild left ventricular hypertrophy. Malformations may include displaced papillary muscles, abnormal chordae tendineae, and shortened and/or thickened valve leaflets. Prolapse of the valve leaflets (displacement of one or more valve leaflets into the atrium) may be seen. Fractional shortening is typically normal or increased but may be decreased late in the course of disease.[134,135] Carefully performed Doppler studies will confirm a diagnosis of mitral regurgitation. Because the regurgitant flow may be narrow or directed angularly into the left atrium, the study requires Doppler mapping (i.e., sampling at multiple locations throughout the atrium), which is time consuming but usually effective. The use of color Doppler readily confirms the diagnosis and requires a great deal less time to perform.[136]

Echocardiographic findings of tricuspid insufficiency include severe right atrial dilation and right ventricular enlargement. Abnormal papillary muscles, chordae tendineae, and valvular prolapse may be seen (Fig. 2–105). Positioning of the valves low in the ventricle away from the annulus may be seen in Ebstein's anomaly. Doppler findings will be similar to those seen with mitral regurgitation.

ATRIAL SEPTAL DEFECTS

Atrial septal defects are uncommon and rarely cause changes that are radiographically apparent. Large defects with significant shunting of blood flow may cause right heart enlargement and dilation of pulmonary arteries and veins.

Echocardiography is more sensitive in determining the presence of atrial septal defects. Shunting of blood may be detected with a contrast ("bubble") study, because there frequently is bi-directional flow through the defect. Doppler echocardiogra-

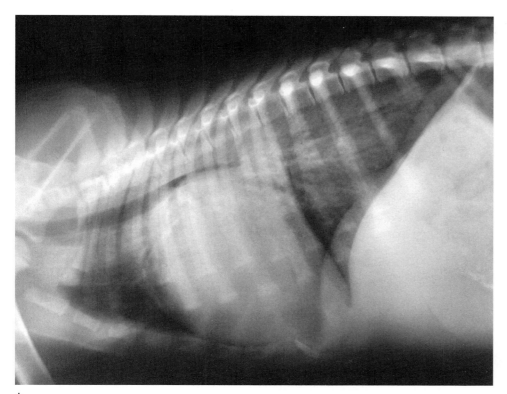

A

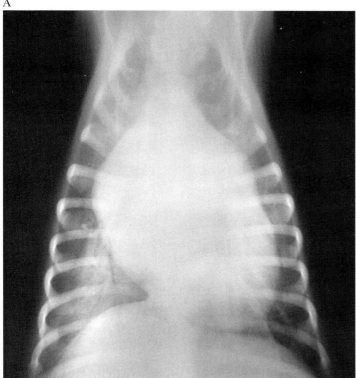

B

Figure 2–104. (A&B) A 3-month-old female mixed breed dog presented with an acute onset of respiratory distress. A Grade 4/6 systolic murmur was detected on physical examination. The cardiac silhouette is markedly enlarged. (A) On the lateral radiograph the caudal cardiac margin is straightened. The trachea is elevated. There is increased sternal contact and bulging of the cranial margin of the cardiac silhouette. (B) On the ventrodorsal radiograph the cardiac silhouette is enlarged and the apex is rounded. The cardiac silhouette appears elongated. There is an alveolar pulmonary infiltrate in the right caudal lung lobe. The radiographic findings are indicative of congenital heart disease with left heart failure. **Diagnosis:** Congenital mitral and tricuspid insufficiency.

phy has the highest degree of sensitivity and specificity in the detection and quantification of atrial septal defects.

PRIMARY ENDOCARDIAL FIBROELASTOSIS

Endocardial fibroelastosis has been reported in dogs, has also been reported in Siamese cats, and has been documented as a congenital anomaly in Burmese cats.[137]

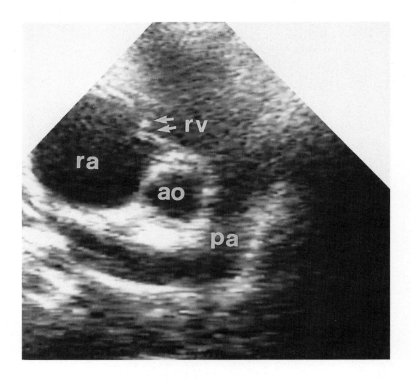

Figure 2–105. A 2-year-old male German shepherd dog was presented with exercise intolerance. A Grade 2/6 systolic murmur was present and the jugular veins were distended. A right parasternal shot-axis view of the heart base revealed dilation of the right atrium (*ra*) and right ventricle (*rv*) as well as prolapse of the tricuspid valve leaflets (*arrows*). Also identified are the aorta (*ao*) and pulmonary artery (*pa*). **Diagnosis:** Tricuspid valve dysplasia with prolapse.

Radiographically, left heart enlargement or generalized cardiomegaly may be seen. Expected echocardiographic findings would include hyperechoic endocardium and dilation of the left atrium and ventricle.

COMBINED CONGENITAL DEFECTS

There have been several reports of animals with multiple congenital cardiac anomalies.[138–140] Their radiographic and echocardiographic appearance will reflect both the anatomic defects as well as their alterations in hemodynamics.

ACQUIRED CARDIAC DISEASES

ACQUIRED ATRIOVENTRICULAR (MITRAL/TRICUSPID) VALVULAR INSUFFICIENCY

Insufficiency of the mitral and/or the tricuspid valve is seen frequently in older, mostly small breed dogs and is usually the result of endocardiosis. Endocardiosis (also sometimes termed mucoid valvular degeneration and myxomatous transformation of the AV valves) is a degenerative process that results in thickened, shortened, nodular, and/or distorted valve leaflets.[141] While it may affect any heart valve, the mitral and tricuspid valves are most commonly involved. A less common cause of valvular insufficiency is trauma to the heart resulting in disruption of part or all of the valve.[142] The radiographic signs depend upon the site and severity of the lesion and are a result of valvular insufficiency. Left ventricular and left atrial enlargement are observed with mitral valve insufficiency (see Fig. 2–75). The degree of chamber enlargement and the change with time is useful in determining the severity and in monitoring progression of the mitral insufficiency. The observed radiographic changes include normal cardiac size and shape, cardiomegaly, cardiomegaly and pulmonary venous congestion, or cardiomegaly and pulmonary edema. Animals with mitral endocardiosis also frequently have tricuspid valve endocardiosis. They may have tricuspid insufficiency and radiographic evidence of right ventricular and right atrial enlargement.

There is a poor correlation between the cardiac size and shape and the likelihood

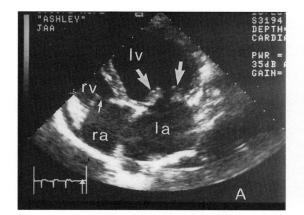

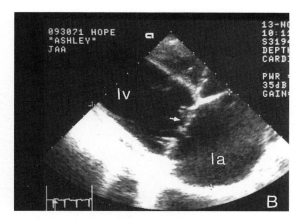

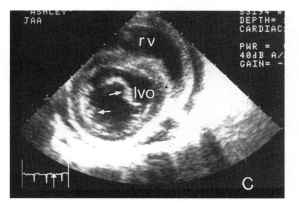

Figure 2–106. A 14-year-old neutered male Cairn terrier was presented for coughing. A Grade 5/6 systolic murmur was present. (A) A left parasternal 4-chamber view reveals dilation of the left atrium (*la*) and left ventricle (*lv*). The right ventricle (*rv*) and right atrium (*ra*) are normal. The leaflets of the tricuspid valve (*small arrow*) are normal. The leaflets of the mitral valve (*large arrows*) are shortened and grossly thickened. The apparent discontinuity of the interatrial septum is due to artifact. (B) A right parasternal long-axis 4-chamber view reveals left atrial (*la*) and left ventricular (*lv*) dilation. There is mild prolapse of the thickened, irregular septal leaflet of the mitral valve (*arrow*) into the left atrium. (C) A right parasternal short-axis view at the level of the mitral valve reveals the thickening and irregularity of the mitral valve leaflets (*arrows*). The left ventricular outflow tract (*lvo*) and right ventricle (*rv*) are also identified. **Diagnosis:** Mitral valve insufficiency secondary to endocardiosis.

that the dog will develop right- and/or left-sided failure. Animals with mild degrees of cardiomegaly may develop congestive heart failure as readily as those with more obvious cardiomegaly.

The echocardiographic findings are similar to those seen with congenital valvular insufficiency. Specifically, there usually is dilation of the left atrium and left ventricle (Fig. 2–106). The M-mode study of the left ventricle will usually reveal increased fractional shortening as the ventricle attempts to compensate for the loss of ventricular output due to the mitral insufficiency. Careful study of the mitral valve leaflets frequently will reveal that they are shortened, thickened, and irregular. Nodular changes may be observed. If severe, prolapse of the mitral valve leaflet into the left atrium may also be seen.

CARDIOMYOPATHY

Canine dilated cardiomyopathy most commonly occurs in 2- to 7-year-old male large and giant breed dogs.[143] Varying degrees of right and left side cardiomegaly will be observed (Fig. 2–107). In many instances, an alteration in the cardiac shape will be much more noticeable than the total cardiomegaly. Bulging in the atrial areas may be observed. Pulmonary edema or effusions into the pleural and/or peritoneal cavities may also be seen.

Cats with dilated cardiomyopathy usually show generalized cardiomegaly. They may also have prominence of the atria resulting in a "valentine" shape (Fig. 2–108). Pleural or peritoneal effusion, pulmonary edema, and arterial thromboembolism may also be present. Feline dilated cardiomyopathy is uncommon now that commercial diets have been adequately supplemented with taurine.

The echocardiographic findings of both canine and feline dilated cardiomyopathy include dilation of the left ventricle and atrium, thinning of the myocardium, and decreased fractional shortening (Figs. 2–109 and 2–110).[144,145]

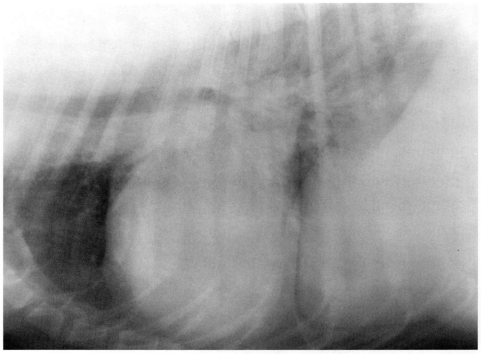

A

Figure 2–107. (A&B) A 9-year-old male Doberman pinscher presented with a 2-week history of tachycardia and coughing. The cardiac silhouette is markedly enlarged. (A) On the lateral radiograph, the caudal cardiac margin appears straight. There is elevation of the trachea. (B) On the ventrodorsal radiograph, the left cardiac margin is rounded, and the cardiac apex is round. There is an alveolar pattern infiltrate in the left caudal lobe and interstitial pattern infiltrates throughout all lobes. There are several pleural fissure lines identified (*arrows*). The radiographic findings are indicative of generalized cardiomegaly with evidence of pulmonary edema. **Diagnosis:** Dilated cardiomyopathy with left heart failure.

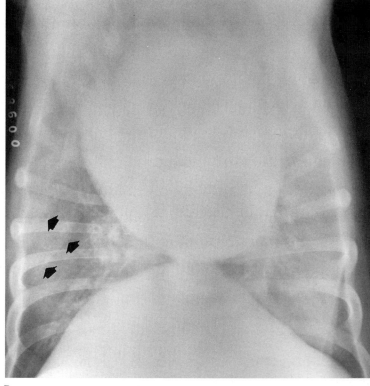

B

Hypertrophic cardiomyopathy occurs more frequently in cats than in dogs. There are no survey radiographic findings that can be used to differentiate dilated and hypertrophic cardiomyopathy (Fig. 2–111). The cardiac silhouette alterations are similar in all types of feline cardiomyopathy. The cardiac silhouette may be appear to be normal. More commonly, the cardiac silhouette will enlarge, particularly in moderate or severe cases.[146–148]

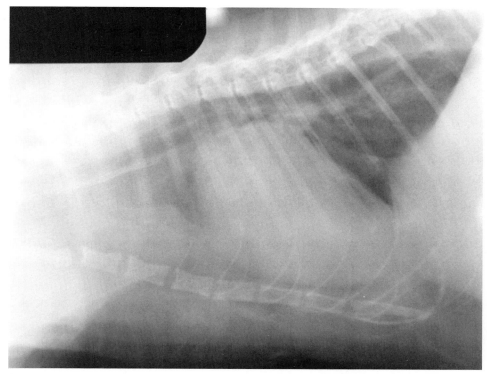

A

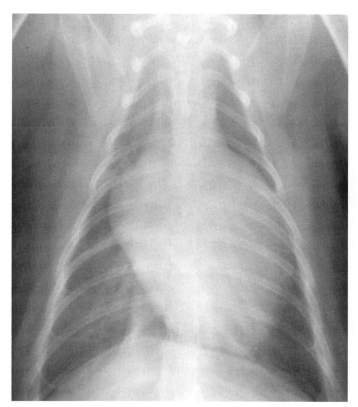

B

Figure 2–108. (A&B) A 2-year-old female cat presented with a 3-day history of progressive lethargy, anorexia, and weakness. There is marked cardiomegaly especially in the area of the atria, and the trachea is markedly elevated. The radiographic findings are indicative of generalized cardiomegaly and free pleural fluid. **Diagnosis:** Dilated cardiomyopathy.

Echocardiographic changes include hypertrophy of the left ventricular myocardium (including free wall, septum, or both), dilation of the left atrium, decreased ventricular lumenal diameter, and normal to increased fractional shortening (Fig. 2–112). Occasionally, the ventricle will be dilated and hypertrophied. This situation

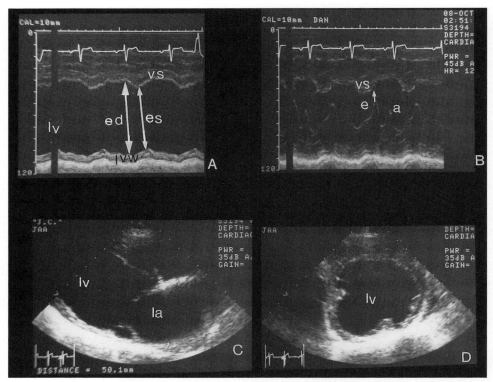

Figure 2–109. (A,B,C,&D) A 5-year-old male Doberman pinscher was presented with exercise intolerance. Auscultation revealed a Grade 4/6 murmur and irregular rhythm. An ECG revealed occasional ventricular premature beats. (A) An M-mode view of the left ventricle (*lv*) distal to the mitral valves reveals diminished fractional shortening. The end-diastolic diameter (*ed*) was 66 mm, and the end-systolic diameter (*es*) was 56 mm, giving a 15% fractional shortening value. Also identified are the interventricular septum (*vs*) and left ventricular wall (*lvw*). (B) An M-mode view at the level of the mitral valve reveals a marked E-point septal separation (*arrow*) of 10 mm. Identified are the E- and A-points as well as the interventricular septum (*vs*). (C) A right parasternal long-axis 4-chamber view demonstrated dilation of the left ventricle (*lv*) and left atrium (*la*). (D) A right parasternal short-axis view of the left ventricle (*lv*) demonstrated ventricular dilation and mild thinning of the myocardium. **Diagnosis:** Dilated cardiomyopathy.

Figure 2–110. (A&B) An 11-year-old neutered male domestic shorthair cat presented with anorexia and lethargy. A Grade 3/6 murmur was ausculted. (A) A right parasternal short-axis view of the left ventricle reveals both left (*lv*) and right ventricular (*rv*) dilation. (B) An M-mode view through the left ventricle reveals marked right (*rv*) and left (*lv*) ventricular dilation. Minimal change in the ventricular diameter is present between systole and diastole. **Diagnosis:** Dilated cardiomyopathy.

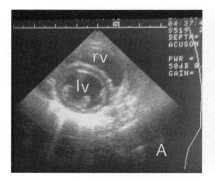

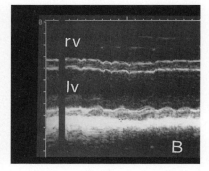

is frequently associated with feline hyperthyroidism. On rare occasions, a thrombus may form in the left atrium or ventricle (Fig. 2–113).

Restrictive (also termed intermediate or unclassified) cardiomyopathy has been described.[149,150] The major factor in restrictive cardiomyopathy is diastolic dysfunction. The lesions are usually related to endocardial, subendocardial, or myocardial fibrosis. Radiographic changes are indistinguishable from those seen with hypertrophic cardiomyopathy. Echocardiographic findings are variable. The most common feature is severe left atrial dilation. Other changes may include normal to thickened myocardium, and normal to slightly decreased fractional shortening and

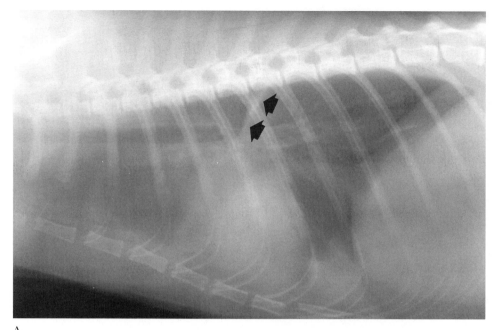

A

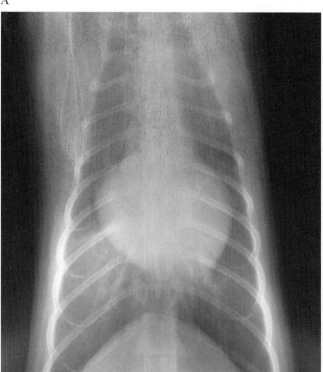

B

Figure 2–111. (A&B) A 1-year-old male cat presented with a 2-week history of lethargy and anorexia. The cat had a Grade 4/6 holosystolic murmur. The cardiac silhouette is markedly enlarged. The ventrodorsal view reveals marked bi-atrial prominence. There is a small amount of pleural fluid in the caudal mediastinum. A pleural fissure line is present dorsal to the cardiac silhouette (*arrows*). The caudal vena cava appears enlarged. The radiographic findings are indicative of generalized cardiomegaly with pleural fluid. **Diagnosis:** Hypertrophic cardiomyopathy.

ventricular diameter. Distortion of the left ventricular chamber and an irregular and highly echogenic endocardium may be seen. Mitral valve regurgitation may be demonstrated with Doppler studies in these cases.

ENDOCARDITIS AND MYOCARDITIS

The size and shape of the cardiac silhouette usually are normal with either acute endocarditis or myocarditis.[151] Radiographic evidence of heart failure may be present despite the heart's normal size and shape.

Echocardiography may reveal hyperechoic vegetative masses on either the aortic

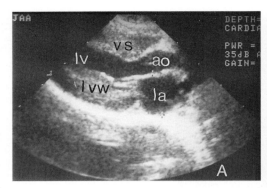
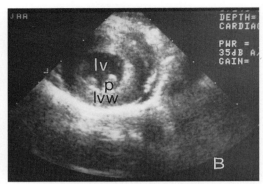

Figure 2–112. (A&B) A 9-year-old neutered male domestic shorthair cat was presented with dyspnea. A gallop rhythm was auscultated. Radiographs revealed mild cardiomegaly, pulmonary edema, and a minimal pleural effusion. (A) A right parasternal long-axis aortic outflow view reveals dilation of the left atrium (*la*). The left ventricular free wall (*lvw*) and interventricular septum (*vs*) are thickened. The left ventricular cavity (*lv*) is diminished. The aorta (*ao*) is normal. These findings were confirmed on an M-mode study which was utilized for mensuration. (B) A right parasternal short axis view of the left ventricle shows the thickened left ventricular free wall (*lvw*) and narrowed left ventricular cavity (*lv*). The papillary muscles (*p*) are clearly defined. **Diagnosis:** Hypertrophic cardiomyopathy.

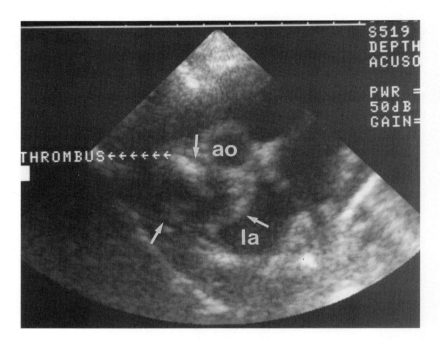

Figure 2–113. A 12-year-old neutered male domestic shorthair cat was presented with dyspnea, tachycardia, and a Grade 4/6 heart murmur. A right parasternal short-axis view at the level of the aorta (*ao*) reveals a large thrombus (*arrows*) in the left atrium (*la*). **Diagnosis:** Hypertrophic cardiomyopathy and left atrial thrombus.

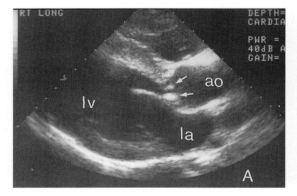
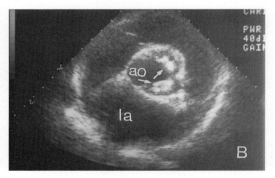

Figure 2–114. (A&B) A 4-year-old male Great Dane presented with a history of hematuria of 4 months' duration. Urinalysis revealed pyuria (with pus casts) and an *Escherichia coli* was cultured. A Grade 3/6 systolic ejection type murmur had developed a week prior to examination. (A) A right parasternal long-axis aortic outflow view revealed echogenic masses (*arrows*) on the aortic valve cusps. Identified are the left atrium (*la*), left ventricle (*lv*), and aorta (*ao*). (B) A right parasternal short-axis view at the aortic level reveled the echogenic masses (*arrows*) on the left and right cusps of the aortic valve. Identified are the aorta (*ao*) and left atrium (*la*). **Diagnosis:** Bacterial endocarditis of the aortic valve secondary to pyelonephritis.

or mitral valves with endocarditis (Fig. 2–114). These may even calcify. Diastolic flutter of the anterior mitral valve leaflet may occur due to aortic insufficiency.

COR PULMONALE

Cor pulmonale indicates right heart enlargement secondary to pulmonary disease. Any disease that inhibits normal pulmonary blood flow and causes pulmonary hy-

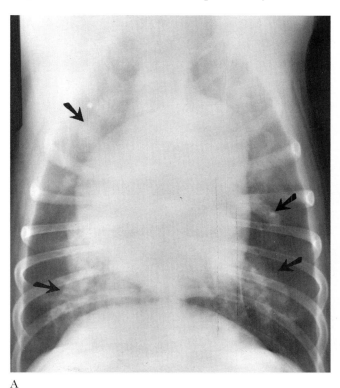

A

Figure 2–115. (A&B) A 6-year-old female boxer presented with a 1-month history of coughing and syncopal attacks. There is marked right-sided cardiomegaly with rounding of the right side of the cardiac silhouette on (A) the ventrodorsal radiograph, and cranial bulging of the cardiac silhouette on (B) the lateral radiograph. The cardiac apex is elevated from the sternum. The pulmonary arteries are enlarged and tortuous (*arrows*). There is an interstitial pattern infiltrate, which most severely involves the caudal dorsal lung lobes. The radiographic findings are indicative of heartworm disease. **Diagnosis:** Dirofilariasis.

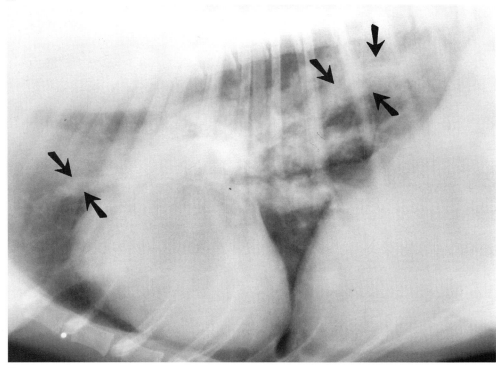

B

pertension may produce cor pulmonale. Right ventricular enlargement, enlargement of the main pulmonary artery, and enlargement and/or tortuosity of the pulmonary arterial branches are the major radiographic features. Dirofilariasis is likely the most common cause of cor pulmonale.[152–154] The nature and extent of the underlying lung pathology varies (Fig. 2–115).

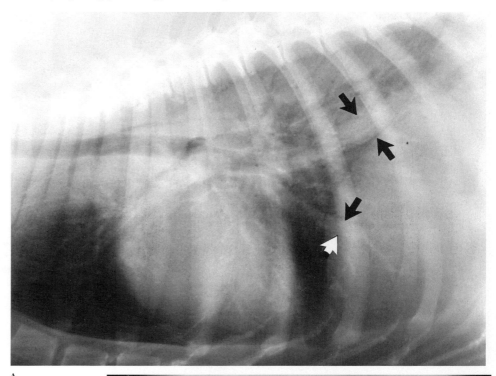

A

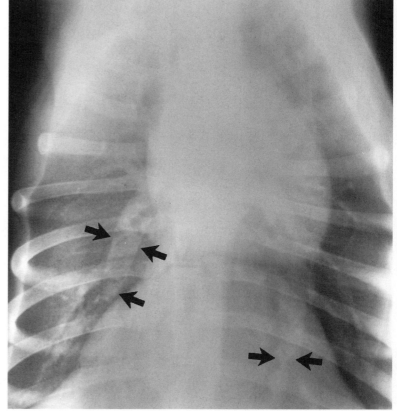

B

Figure 2–116. (A&B) A 6-year-old female bullmastiff presented with a 1-day history of respiratory distress and harsh lung sounds. There is a generalized interstitial pattern infiltrate, and the pulmonary arteries are enlarged and tortuous (*arrows*). There is mild right heart enlargement with bulging on the cranial aspect of the cardiac silhouette on (A) the lateral radiograph. The radiographic findings are indicative of pulmonary infiltrate with eosinophilia secondary to heartworm disease. **Diagnosis:** Eosinophilic pneumonitis secondary to heartworm disease. Microfilaria were not detected in this dog's blood; however, the heartworm antigen test was positive.

The echocardiographic findings reflect the pulmonary hypertension. Dilation of the main pulmonary artery and right ventricle as well as hypertrophy of the right ventricle can be seen. In severe cases, there may be dilation of the right atrium and signs of right heart failure.

DIROFILARIASIS

Thoracic radiographs may be normal in mild or early dirofilariasis.[155] Enlargement of the right heart and caudal lung lobe arteries may be observed as early as 6 months after infection.[154] Pulmonary artery enlargement (larger than the adjacent vein), irregular saccular peripheral arterial dilations (tortuosity), loss of normal arterial arborization (pruning), and sudden termination of a large artery (blunting) may be observed (see Figs. 2–2 and 2–115).[156] Other pulmonary parenchymal abnormalities that may be observed range from a mild increase in pulmonary density to severe, focal alveolar pattern infiltrates associated with pulmonary embolism or lung lobe infarction. In cases of occult dirofilariasis (absence of demonstrable microfilaria), a diffuse, patchy interstitial infiltrate may be present throughout the lung. This infiltrate may partially obscure margins of the peripheral pulmonary vessels (Fig. 2–116).

Thromboembolism, infarction, or secondary bacterial pneumonia may produce large areas of interstitial and alveolar pattern infiltrates. This may be observed in animals with active infection but is more frequent after treatment for adult heartworms. Granulomas have been reported infrequently in both microfilaremic and occult heartworm cases. These pulmonary masses have no specific characteristics—only the presence of the typical arterial changes suggests their origin.

It is difficult to radiographically detect reinfection in dogs that have been previously treated for heartworms. Some regression of the cardiac and pulmonary abnormalities occurs after treatment; however, in many cases the cardiomegaly and pulmonary arterial changes persist despite the absence of parasites.

The most common echocardiographic findings reflect pulmonary hypertension. Hypertrophy of the right ventricle and dilation of the main pulmonary artery may be present. In severe cases, there may be dilation of the right atrium and signs of right heart failure. Identification of individual worms is difficult because of their small diameter. Large numbers of worms may be identified as linear echogenic structures in the right heart and main pulmonary arteries (Fig. 2–117).[157]

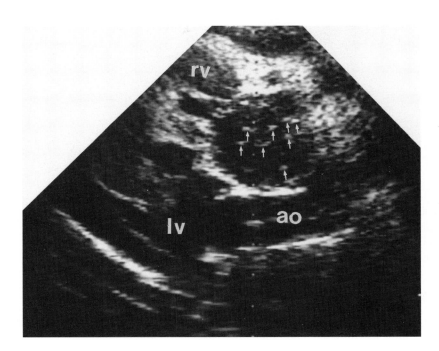

Figure 2–117. A 5-year-old male mixed breed dog was presented for exercise intolerance. A right parasternal long-axis aortic outflow view revealed multiple, highly echogenic, small foci (*arrows*) in the right atrium. The foci were composed of short, parallel line pairs. The right atrium and right ventricle (*rv*) were dilated. The aorta (*ao*) and left ventricle (*lv*) are identified. **Diagnosis:** Dirofilariasis.

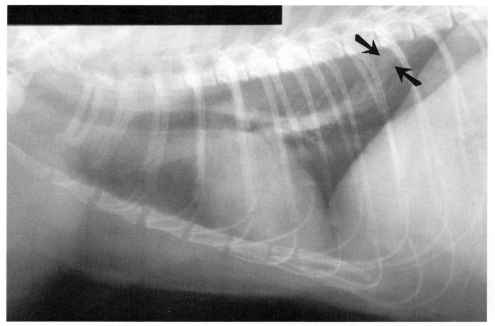

A

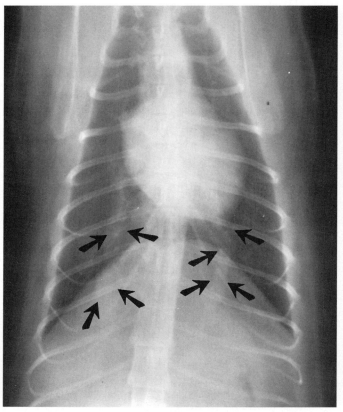

B

Figure 2–118. (A&B) A 4-year-old female cat presented with a history of chronic cystitis. A Grade 3/6 systolic murmur and gallop rhythm were picked up on routine physical examination. There is mild cardiomegaly. The caudal lobar pulmonary arteries are enlarged and tortuous (*arrows*). The remainder of the lung is normal. The radiographic findings are indicative of heartworm infestation. **Diagnosis:** Dirofilariasis.

Dirofilariasis in cats produces changes similar to those in dogs with mild to moderate infections.[151] Right ventricular enlargement is less frequent. Enlarged, irregular pulmonary arteries and a mild increase in interstitial pulmonary density may be present (Fig. 2–118).

CARDIAC MASSES

Various primary tumors and granulomas have been described.[158–163] The radiographic appearance of these depends upon the location of the mass and its hemo-

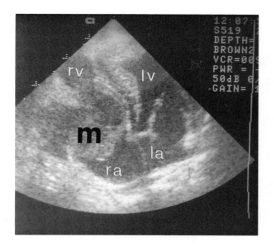

Figure 2–119. A 9-year-old spayed female Labrador retriever presented with abdominal distension and lethargy of 2-weeks' duration. A left parasternal long-axis 4-chamber view revealed a large heteroechoic mass (*m*) within the right atrium (*ra*). Also identified are the right ventricle (*rv*), left atrium (*la*), and left ventricle (*lv*). **Diagnosis:** Right atrial fibrosarcoma.

dynamic effects upon various cardiac structures. The majority of the masses described have been noted on echocardiography. These may present as focal thickenings of cardiac muscle or masses that project into the lumen of various cardiac chambers (Fig. 2–119).

PERICARDIAL DISEASE

PERICARDIAL EFFUSION

Generalized enlargement of the cardiac silhouette may be observed with concurrent left and right heart disease or with pericardial disease (Figs. 2–120 and 2–121).[164,165] With concurrent left and right heart disease, the cardiac silhouette retains some of its normal contour with greater curvature of the right and cranial cardiac margins and prominence of the left atrium. If a significant amount of pericardial effusion surrounds the heart, it will smooth the outline of the cardiac silhouette. The heart base retains its normal shape. This results in a pumpkin- or soccer ball-shaped cardiac silhouette. The nature of an effusion cannot be radiographically determined, nor can small amounts of pericardial fluid be radiographically recognized.

Pericardial effusion may result in cardiac tamponade. In this situation, the pulmonary vessels are often small and the caudal vena cava may be enlarged. This finding is sometimes helpful when distinguishing between generalized cardiomegaly and pericardial disease.

Introduction of a significant volume of air into the pericardial sac after an equal amount of fluid has been removed by pericardiocentesis allows for further evaluation of the possible causes of pericardial effusion.[164,165] It is important to use both left and right lateral as well as ventrodorsal and dorsoventral views when performing this study, because there usually is some residual fluid left in the pericardial sac, which obscures visualization of the dependent portion of the pericardial sac and heart. The heart and pericardium should then be evaluated for the presence of masses. While echocardiography has replaced pneumopericardiography in many cases, there are some instances in which the echocardiogram fails to demonstrate a mass that is diagnosed by the radiographic study.

Echocardiography is very sensitive at detecting even small amounts of pericardial fluid. It may be difficult to distinguish pericardial from pleural fluid; however, careful examination of the heart will demonstrate the fact that the pericardial fluid outlines or conforms to the contour of the heart and does not cause retraction or outlining of the lung lobes. The nature of the fluid is indicated in part by its echogenicity. Fluid containing numerous echogenic foci suggests it contains particulate matter (e.g., pus). The presence of long bands of echogenic material suggests the presence of fibrin tags and suggests the idea that the condition is chronic.

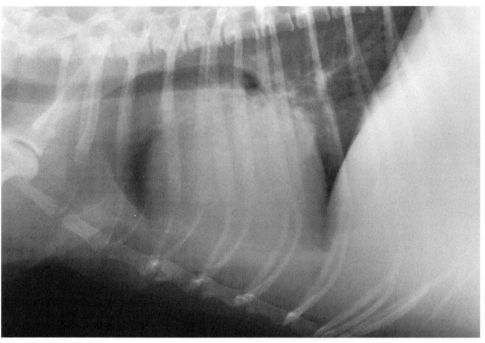

A

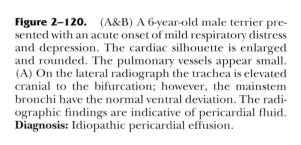

Figure 2–120. (A&B) A 6-year-old male terrier presented with an acute onset of mild respiratory distress and depression. The cardiac silhouette is enlarged and rounded. The pulmonary vessels appear small. (A) On the lateral radiograph the trachea is elevated cranial to the bifurcation; however, the mainstem bronchi have the normal ventral deviation. The radiographic findings are indicative of pericardial fluid. **Diagnosis:** Idiopathic pericardial effusion.

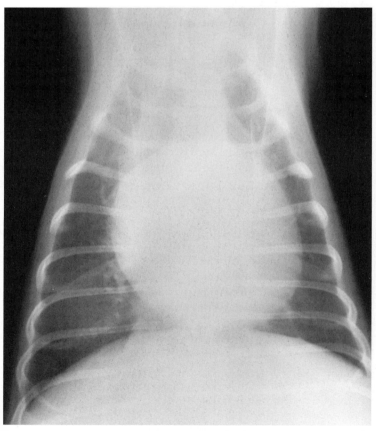

B

Cardiac tamponade occurs when the internal pericardial pressure rises to a level at which it interferes with right heart function. The increased pericardial pressure is transmitted through the right ventricular free wall and results in elevated right ventricular pressure, limited diastolic filling, and, eventually, in paradoxical septal motion (PSM) resulting in reduced stroke volume. It also interferes with right atrial fill-

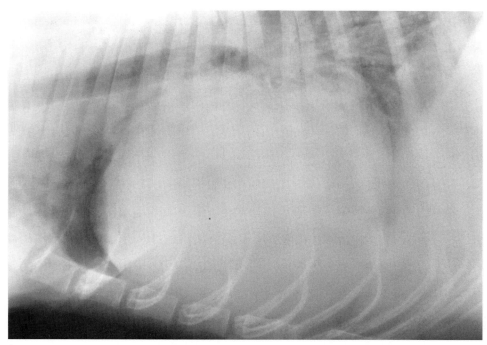

A

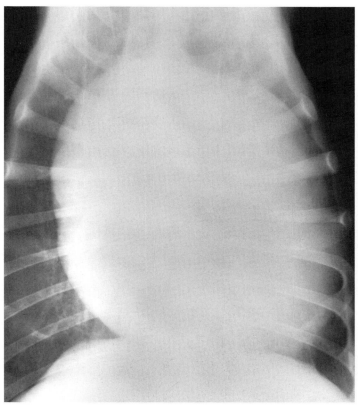

B

Figure 2–121. (A&B) A 4-year-old male German shepherd dog presented with a 2-week history of lethargy and weight loss. The owners noted labored respiration and abdominal distention 24 hours prior to presentation. The cardiac silhouette is markedly enlarged and rounded. (A) On the lateral radiograph the trachea is mildly elevated cranial to the tracheal bifurcation; the main stem bronchi deflect ventrally beyond the tracheal bifurcation. The radiographic findings are indicative of pericardial fluid. **Diagnosis:** Hemopericardium secondary to right atrial hemangiosarcoma. The diagnosis was determined by pericardiocentesis and necropsy examination.

ing and causes diastolic collapse of the right atrium (Fig. 2–122). This leads to congestive right heart failure and decreased left heart output. The effects on the right ventricle may be seen as a bowing of the interventricular septum or the presence of paradoxical septal motion. In this situation (PSM), the movement of the left ventricular free wall and the interventricular septum are identical to each other and they remain parallel and roughly equidistant from each other throughout the entire cardiac cycle resulting in minimal ventricular contraction (Fig. 2–123).[166] The free margin of the right auricular appendage can be observed to move inward during diastole, and the heart can be observed to move within the pericardial sac. The pericardium itself may be identified as a thin curvilinear echogenic structure.

The cause of pericardial fluid accumulation is not determined in many cases. Diseases that must be considered when pericardial fluid is present include bacterial, protozoal, or mycotic infection, heart base or right atrial neoplasms, pericardial

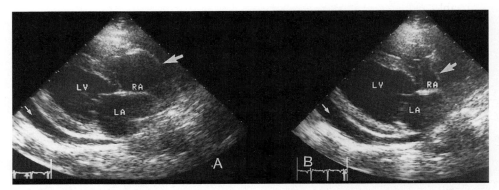

Figure 2–122. An 8-year-old male Labrador retriever presented with exercise intolerance and ascites of 3 months' duration. (A) A right parasternal long-axis 4-chamber view in early diastole reveals a moderate pericardial effusion (*small arrow*). Identified are the left atrium (*LA*), left ventricle (*LV*), and right atrium (*RA*). The right atrial free wall is apparent (*large arrow*). (B) A right parasternal long-axis 4-chamber view in late diastole reveals collapse of the right atrium (*large arrow*). The pericardial effusion is still evident (*small arrow*). The cause of the effusion was not determined. **Diagnosis:** Idiopathic pericardial effusion and cardiac tamponade.

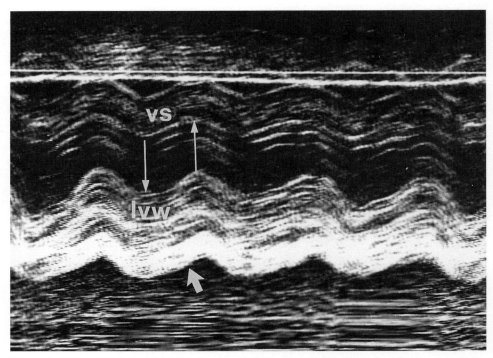

Figure 2–123. A 9-year-old female keeshound presented with ascites and exercise intolerance of several weeks' duration. An M-mode echocardiogram of the ventricles reveals paradoxical septal motion—left ventricular free wall (*lvw*) and interventricular septum (*vs*) move in parallel (*long, thin arrows*). Pericardial effusion and pericardial thickening (fibrin deposition?) are apparent (*large arrow*). **Diagnosis:** Pericardial effusion and tamponade with paradoxical septal motion.

diaphragmatic hernia, hypoalbuminemia, uremia, right heart failure, immune pericarditis, atrial rupture, pericardial cysts, visceral leishmaniasis, feline infectious peritonitis, and idiopathic causes.[135,163,167–172] Masses involving the right atrium or heart base can frequently be detected (Fig. 2–124). In a few cases, the mass may not be visualized and a positive or negative contrast pericardiogram may confirm the diagnosis. The silhouette should be evaluated carefully to identify fluid- or gas-filled bowel or omental fat when a peritoneopericardial diaphragmatic hernia is present. The term *idiopathic benign pericardial effusion* is used when a specific etiology cannot be established.

PERICARDIAL MASSES

Pericardial masses usually produce pericardial fluid and rarely alter the smooth curvature of the cardiac silhouette. Echocardiography frequently allows identification of the masses.[158] Masses may be solid or cystic and may represent tumors, granulomas, or cysts (Fig. 2–125).

RESTRICTIVE PERICARDIAL DISEASE

Chronic infection or inflammation may result in pericardial fibrosis and a restrictive pericardial disease. Recognition of this condition is difficult; however, the presence of an irregularly shaped cardiac silhouette in a patient with right heart failure without right-sided cardiomegaly suggests the diagnosis of restrictive pericardial disease. No specific echocardiographic findings have been reported, but a thickened or irregular pericardium may be identified (Fig. 2–126).

PERICARDIAL DIAPHRAGMATIC HERNIA

Pericardial diaphragmatic hernia will result in a pumpkin-shaped or soccer ball-shaped cardiac silhouette. The condition is easily recognized when intestines or fat

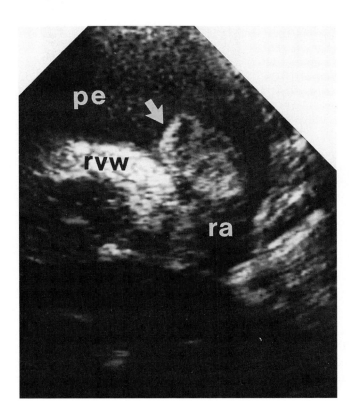

Figure 2–124. A 9-year-old spayed female golden retriever was presented with ascites. Auscultation revealed muffled heart sounds. An electrocardiogram revealed dampened complexes with electrical alternans. A right parasternal long-axis 4-chamber view revealed severe pericardial effusion (*pe*). A large, complex mass (*arrow*) with cystic areas is present on the right atrium (*ra*). Also identified is the right ventricular free wall (*rvw*). **Diagnosis:** Right atrial hemangiosarcoma.

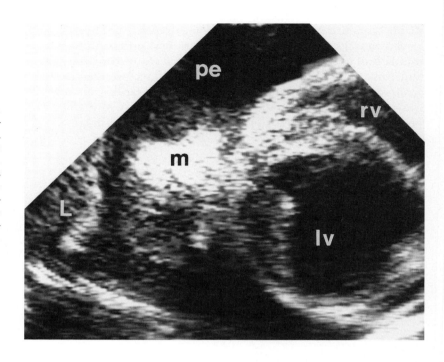

Figure 2–125. A 1-year-old male German shepherd dog was presented with ascites. Auscultation revealed muffled heart sounds. A right parasternal short-axis view through the ventricles revealed severe pericardial effusion (*pe*) and a complex mass (*m*) with cystic areas caudal to the heart. The mass did not move with the heart beat. No diaphragmatic discontinuity could be visualized. Also identified are the liver (*L*), left ventricle (*lv*), and right ventricle (*rv*). A pericardiectomy was performed. **Diagnosis:** Pericardial cyst.

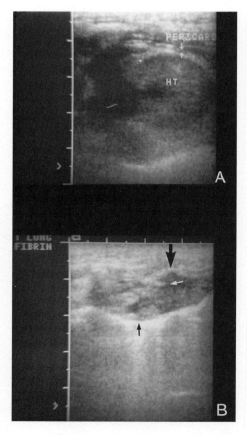

Figure 2–126. (A&B) A 3-year-old neutered male domestic shorthair cat presented with respiratory distress of 2 months' duration. (A) A right parasternal short-axis view of the heart revealed mild pleural effusion and thickening of the pericardium. (B) A longitudinal view of the pleural space revealed the parietal pleura (*large black arrow*) and visceral pleura (*small black arrow*) were displaced by a fluid that contained numerous echogenic, filamentous fibrin tags (*small white arrow*). **Diagnosis:** Pleuritis and pericarditis—a causative agent was not identified.

are present within the pericardial sac. It is more difficult to distinguish this condition from other pericardial diseases when the liver and/or spleen are herniated or when there is fluid as well as the liver or spleen within the pericardial sac. A sternal deformity, absent, split, or malformed xiphoid, or absence of sternebrae is often seen with this condition. A dorsal mesothelial remnant has been described in cats.[56]

This is evident as a curvilinear soft tissue structure in the caudal ventral mediastinum ventral to the caudal vena cava. Affected animals usually are asymptomatic; however, liver abnormalities such as cirrhosis or tumor may result from the presence of the liver within the pericardial sac for a long time period. The condition is congenital and is the result of incomplete separation of the pleural and peritoneal cavities.

Ultrasound will readily distinguish between pericardial fluid and liver or spleen within the pericardial sac.

ABNORMALITIES OF THE AORTA

ANEURYSM

Aortic abnormalities, other than those associated with congenital cardiac disease (e.g., patent ductus arteriosus, aortic stenosis) or vascular ring anomalies, are uncommon. Aneurysmal dilation in the descending aorta (patent ductus) or aortic arch (aortic stenosis) may be observed in those cases. Aneurysmal dilations of the descending aorta may occur secondary to *Spirocerca lupi* infestation in dogs and have been observed as an incidental finding in other asymptomatic dogs.[173] In these cases, an enlarged aortic shadow will be visible, especially on the lateral radiograph.

COARCTATION OF THE AORTA

Coarctation of the aorta (narrowing, usually severe, of the aortic lumen) has rarely been reported in dogs.[84,174,175] The lesion will be evident radiographically as a post-stenotic aneurysmal dilation. An angiographic study may be required to establish the diagnosis. Echocardiography will rarely be helpful because the lesion is likely to be located away from the heart and lack a sonographic window.

TUMOR

Aortic body tumors originate from the baroreceptor tissue within the aortic arch. A localized dorsal deviation of the trachea cranial to the bifurcation may be evident when the mass becomes large (Fig. 2–127). This usually is an abrupt deviation, initially dorsally and then ventrally, near the ascending aorta. On the dorsoventral or ventrodorsal view, the trachea may be displaced abruptly to the right as it passes the aortic arch. Aortic body tumors may extend dorsal to the trachea. Invasion of the cranial thoracic vertebral bodies may occur. Pericardial effusion may accompany aortic body tumors. Flexion of the head and neck will produce dorsal deviation of the trachea in the cranial mediastinum cranial to the heart base, and this has been mistaken for evidence of an aortic body or heart base tumor. Deviation of the trachea to the right on ventrodorsal or dorsoventral radiographs is also observed in both normal and obese brachycephalic dogs. The abrupt nature of the tracheal displacement observed with heart base tumors is an important feature in differentiating a tumor from this normal variation.

Echocardiography will frequently reveal the presence of an aortic body tumor. They are most common between the aorta and pulmonary artery. The right parasternal short axis view of the cardiac base is the most common view used to identify these masses (Fig. 2–128).

CALCIFICATION

Calcification of the aorta is rare. It has been observed in association with lymphosarcoma, renal secondary hyperparathyroidism, atherosclerosis, and Cushing's disease.[176] Thin, linear calcification will be seen extending along the margins of the aorta (Fig. 2–129). The aortic valves may be involved.

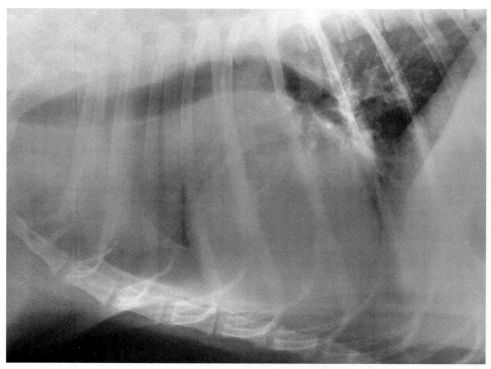

A

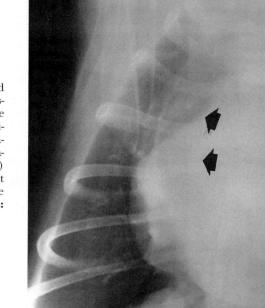

Figure 2–127. A 7-year-old male mixed breed dog presented with respiratory distress, which had been gradual in onset. There is a soft tissue density in the cranial mediastinum extending to the heart base. The trachea is displaced dorsally in (A) the lateral radiograph and markedly to the right in (B) the ventrodorsal view (*arrows*). The abrupt nature of the tracheal deviation indicates the presence of a heart base mass. **Diagnosis:** Aortic body tumor.

B

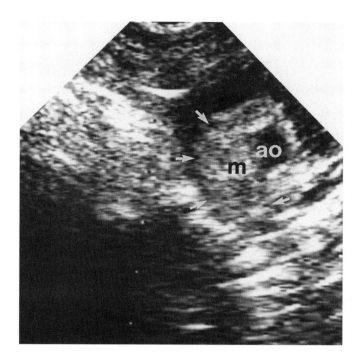

Figure 2–128. A 7-year-old male Samoyed presented with exercise intolerance. A right parasternal short-axis view at the level of the aorta revealed the presence of a mass (*m–arrows*) between the aorta (*ao*) and pulmonary artery. **Diagnosis:** Aortic body tumor.

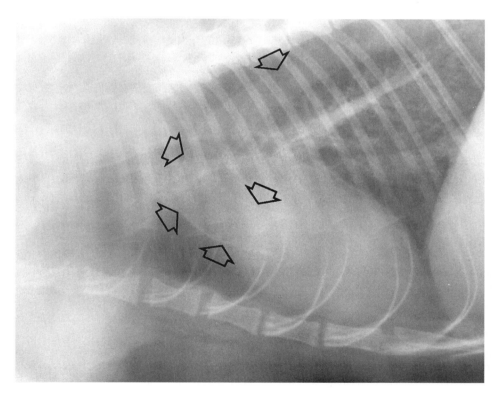

Figure 2–129. A 4-year-old male cat presented with a history of anemia and a heart murmur. On the lateral thoracic radiograph the cardiac silhouette is mildly enlarged and irregularly shaped. There is calcification of the margins of the aorta (*arrows*). The calcification extends into the ascending and descending aorta. **Diagnosis:** Aortic calcification. The etiology was not determined. The cat's clinical signs were due to lymphocytic leukemia.

ABNORMALITIES OF THE CAUDAL VENA CAVA

Isolated abnormalities of the caudal vena cava are extremely rare.[177,178] Although most right heart diseases will eventually cause the caudal vena cava to dilate, its size varies normally with cardiac cycle and phase of respiration. Invasion of the caudal vena cava by masses extending from the right atrium, liver, kidney, or adrenal glands or masses of dirofilaria may alter the shape of the vena cava. Diaphragmatic abnormalities also may alter the shape of the caudal vena cava. The size of the caval foramen may be altered after repair of a diaphragmatic hernia.

PULMONARY ABNORMALITIES

The first step in evaluating the lung on a thoracic radiograph is to be certain that the technical quality of the radiograph is adequate. Next, evaluate the overall pulmonary density by comparing the right lung to the left. Similar densities and patterns should be present in comparable areas. If available, previous radiographs should be compared directly. If areas of abnormally increased or decreased density are observed, they should be evaluated according to the portion (i.e., ventral, dorsal, peripheral, middle, hilar) or number of lung lobes involved. The symmetry or asymmetry of the suspect lesion and distribution of the abnormality should be noted. It should be determined if a lesion centers on the pulmonary hilus and extends outward, seems more severe in the middle or peripheral lung, or is uniformly dispersed throughout the lung.[179] Next, the pattern of pulmonary density should be determined. The defined patterns include the alveolar, interstitial, bronchial, or vascular pattern.[180] Many infiltrates will have features of more than one type of pattern. The predominant pattern is used to develop the list of differential diagnoses.

PULMONARY PATTERNS

ALVEOLAR PATTERN

Alveolar patterns result from flooding of pulmonary acini with fluid. An acinus consists of that portion of lung that is distal to a terminal bronchiole (i.e., the respiratory bronchioles, alveolar ducts, alveolar sacs, and alveoli). Each acinus has multiple communications with the adjacent acini via multiple interalveolar pores (pores of Cohn). An acinus, which represents the basic unit of the end-air spaces, is the smallest pulmonary unit that is individually visible on a radiograph.

An alveolar pattern is due to flooding of the end-air spaces (acini) with some type of fluid (pus, blood, edema) or, rarely, with cellular material. As individual acini become filled, the fluid then spreads to adjacent acini through the interalveolar pores. This results in the typical radiographic pattern of a poorly marginated ("fluffy") density. The areas of density may spread and their poorly-defined borders will coalesce. This process may spread until all acini within a lung lobe are filled. If this happens, there may be a sharply marginated border seen at the edge of a lung lobe due to the dense connective tissue or pleura blocking further spread of the fluid into the adjacent lung lobe. As the number of fluid-filled adjacent acini increases, the air-filled, large, and medium sized bronchial structures may become evident as linear radiolucent branching structures (Fig. 2–130). This is referred to as the air bronchogram sign. The air-filled bronchi are surrounded by a tissue/fluid density, and the bronchial wall and adjacent vessel are not seen as individual structures. When a bronchus branches perpendicular to the x-ray beam it will be seen as a round, radiolucent dot.

Recognition of an alveolar pattern is important, because it identifies the abnormal density as being within the end-air spaces rather than within the interstitial space, pleural space, mediastinum, or outside the thoracic cavity. It also strongly suggests a fluid nature of the infiltrate. Finally, it suggests that an attempt to aspirate material via the airways (e.g., a transtracheal wash or bronchoscopic lavage) will likely yield diagnostic material.

INTERSTITIAL PATTERN

Interstitial pattern infiltrates have been described as a fine linear, reticular, or nodular pattern of density.[180] This pattern produces either a fluid-dense haze, which obscures or obliterates vascular outlines, or distinct linear densities or distinct nodules. Interstitial pattern infiltrates do not produce air bronchogram signs.

The fine linear pattern of infiltrate may be due to the presence of fluid or cells (including neoplastic) or fibrosis within the supporting tissues of the lung. Many lin-

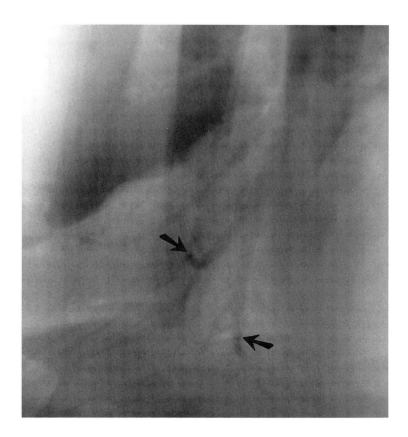

Figure 2–130. A 6-month-old female Great Dane presented with a 2-week history of a cough. A soft tissue density was present in the right cranial lung lobe. A close-up of the lung lobe infiltrate is illustrated, and the radiolucent branching structure indicative of an air bronchogram sign is visible. Several air-filled end-on bronchi are visible as radiolucent dots (*arrows*). These findings indicate the presence of air-filled bronchi and fluid-filled acini. Discrete margins are absent except at the lobar border. This is an alveolar pattern. The infiltrate may consist of pus, edema, or hemorrhage. **Diagnosis:** Bacterial pneumonia.

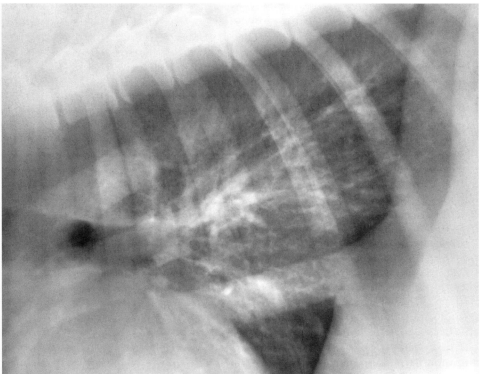

Figure 2–131. A 7-year-old male German shepherd dog presented with a mass in the caudal abdomen. Thoracic radiographs were obtained to evaluate the dog for the presence of pulmonary metastases. A photographic enlargement of the caudal lung lobes is illustrated. The pulmonary vessels are obscured by a pattern of linear soft tissue densities. This represents pulmonary interstitial fibrosis and is a common finding among the normal features of the lungs of an aged dog that have no clinical signs. **Diagnosis:** Pulmonary fibrosis.

ear and branching densities may be evident. Viewed in summation, these can produce a net-like or reticular pattern (Fig. 2–131). At the points where these linear densities converge, small tissue-dense dots may become evident producing a fine nodular interstitial pattern.

The nodular pattern is caused by aggregations of cells (e.g., seen with metastatic neoplasia) within the supporting tissues of the lung. A separate subcategory is the nodule that is caused by focal infiltration of viscous or predominately cellular material into a single acinus or a few acini, but which does not have the typical spread of fluid through the interalveolar pores. This type of nodular pattern (acinonodular pattern) is typical of granulomatous pneumonia.

Interstitial patterns may be classified as chronic or active according to their radiographic appearance. An active interstitial infiltrate is characterized by poorly defined, wide linear interstitial densities with extensive blurring of vascular margins. As the condition becomes chronic, or resolves with fibrosis, the interstitial densities become thinner and better defined and the vascular borders become more clearly visible.

Recognition of an interstitial pattern is important, because it identifies the abnormal density as being within the supporting tissues of the lung rather than within the end-air spaces, pleural space, mediastinum, or outside the thoracic cavity. It also strongly suggests a cellular nature of the infiltrate. Finally, it suggests that an attempt to aspirate material via the airways will not likely yield diagnostic material. Rather, direct sampling (e.g., fine needle aspirate, biopsy) is more likely to be successful.

BRONCHIAL PATTERN

The bronchial pattern results from fluid or cellular infiltrate within the bronchial wall and peribronchial and perivascular connective tissue of the lung. It results in bronchial wall thickening and outlining of many bronchial structures not normally identified (Fig. 2–132). These bronchial structures may be seen as paired somewhat parallel lines that converge slightly and branch in pairs. These paired lines are thinner and do not taper, as do pulmonary vessels, maintaining a fairly uniform width throughout their course. They have been described as "railroad" or "tram tracks" because they converge slightly as they extend toward the lung periphery in a fashion similar to the way railroad tracks appear to converge as they get further away from an observer. When these structures branch perpendicular to the x-ray beam they produce a tissue-dense circle or "doughnut" with a radiolucent center. This pattern suggests that an attempt to aspirate material via the airways will be rewarding.

Another form of the bronchial pattern is seen with bronchiectasis. Two forms of bronchiectasis have been described: tubular and saccular. Tubular bronchiectasis consists of bronchial dilation and loss of the normal taper of the bronchial lumen as it progresses distally into the lung.[181] Saccular bronchiectasis consists of focal bronchial dilations. Both forms are frequently associated with bronchial thickening due to chronic inflammation.

VASCULAR PATTERNS

Vascular patterns are produced by an increase or decrease in the size, shape, and/or number of pulmonary arteries and veins. Evaluation of pulmonary vascular size is subjective, based on a recollection of other similar sized patients. Vessels radiographically appear as linear, tapering, branching, soft tissue-dense structures. When vessels branch perpendicular to the x-ray beam, they are seen as distinct round, solid densities that have the same or slightly smaller diameter than the parent vessel. The margins of the pulmonary vessels should be smooth and well defined. Vascular patterns without other pulmonary patterns are rarely observed in pulmonary diseases but may be observed in animals with cardiovascular disease.

DIFFERENTIAL DIAGNOSES USING PULMONARY PATTERNS

In addition to the symmetry, distribution, and pattern of a pulmonary lesion, changes in other thoracic structures should also be noted and used to narrow the

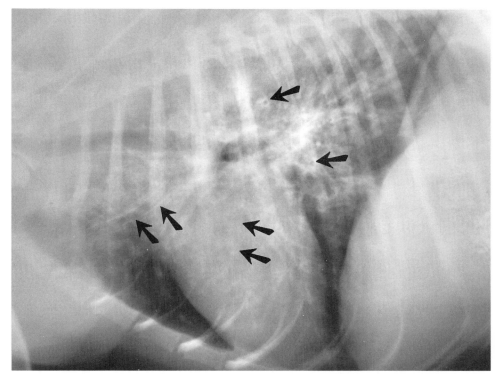

Figure 2–132. A 2-year-old male mixed breed dog was presented with a 3-week history of a cough. On the lateral thoracic radiograph, the pulmonary vessels are obscured by a diffuse increase in pulmonary densities. Several end-on bronchi and thickened bronchial walls are evident (*arrows*). The radiographic findings indicate a diffuse bronchial pattern and a mild interstitial pattern. **Diagnosis:** Eosinophilic bronchitis and pneumonitis. A transtracheal wash was performed and eosinophils were identified in the specimen. The dog was treated with corticosteroids and the pulmonary disease resolved.

differential diagnosis. The presence or absence of cardiac, lymph node, tracheal, esophageal, diaphragm, rib, or chest wall lesions will influence the probability of a specific diagnosis. However, in many cases only a ranking of differential diagnoses is possible. Pattern recognition provides useful clues in differentiating pulmonary diseases. In many cases, a mixture of patterns is observed. In those cases, the predominant pattern should be used to classify the density observed.[179] A classic example of this is the pathogenesis of left heart failure. In the early stages of congestive heart failure, an increased vascular pattern is present. This is followed by an interstitial pattern with loss of vascular outlines. Finally, this may progress to an alveolar pattern of infiltrates with loss of both vascular and bronchial wall shadows, coalescing "fluffy" densities, and, possibly, air bronchograms. Although many different pulmonary diseases can demonstrate various patterns during the course of disease, most diseases have typical infiltrate patterns at the time they present for radiography. For example, bacterial pneumonia usually presents with a focal alveolar pattern when first seen, although interstitial patterns will be visible very early in the disease and when the infiltrate has nearly resolved. Recognition of the pattern and its distribution may suggest certain diagnoses, eliminate others, and generally narrow the list of probable diagnoses (Table 2–2).

The infiltrate pattern provides a strong clue to the next logical diagnostic test. Diseases that have their infiltrates in the bronchi or end-air spaces may be amenable to diagnosis by transtracheal aspiration or bronchoscopy. Diseases with infiltrates confined to the pulmonary interstitium usually will require either open biopsy or fine needle aspiration.

Table 2-2. Radiographic Patterns of Pulmonary Abnormalities

A. Alveolar Pattern
  1. Focal or Multifocal
    a. Bacterial pneumonia
    b. Aspiration pneumonia
    c. Pulmonary edema
    d. Pulmonary hemorrhage (trauma, coagulopathy)
    e. Embolus
    f. Lung lobe torsion
    g. Atelectasis
    h. Parasitic pneumonia (Capillaria, Aleurostrongylus, larval migrans, Toxoplasma)
    i. Immune (pulmonary infiltrates with eosinophilia, allergic)
    j. Neoplasia
  2. Disseminated or Diffuse
    a. Cardiogenic (left heart failure) pulmonary edema
    b. Non-cardiogenic pulmonary edema
      1) Allergic
      2) Central nervous system
      3) Post ictal
      4) Electric shock
      5) Toxic (ANTU)
      6) Post expansion (shock lung, adult respiratory distress syndrome)
      7) Uremic
      8) Upper airway obstruction
B. Interstitial Pattern
  1. Nodular Patterns
    a. Parasitic pneumonia
    b. Mycotic pneumonia
    c. Feline infectious peritonitis
    d. Eosinophilic granulomatosis
    e. Lymphomatoid granulomatosis
    f. Congestive left heart failure
    g. Neoplasia
    h. Abscess
  2. Linear or Reticular Patterns
    a. Age
    b. Inhalation (smoke, dust)
    c. Immune (PIE, allergic)
    d. Left heart failure
    e. Mycotic pneumonia
    f. Hemorrhage (coagulopathy)
    g. Metastatic or primary neoplasia
    g. Lymphoma
    h. Dirofilariasis
    i. Viral pneumonia
    k. Mineralization
C. Bronchial Patterns
  1. Bronchitis (Allergic, viral, bacterial)
  2. Chronic Bronchitis
  3. Bronchiectasis
D. Vascular Pattern
  1. Increased
    a. Left to right cardiac or vascular shunts (PDA, VSD, ASD)
    b. Pulmonary venous congestion (left heart failure)
    c. Arteriovenous fistula (peripheral)
    d. Pulmonary hypertension
    e. Dirofilariasis
  2. Decreased
    a. Right to left cardiac shunts (Tetralogy of Fallot, Reverse PDA)
    b. Pulmonic stenosis
    c. Hypovolemia (shock, dehydration, Addison's disease)
    d. Emphysema
    e. Thromboembolism
    f. Right heart failure
    g. Pericardial disease (tamponade, effusion, restrictive pericarditis)
  3. Abnormal Branching
    a. Dirofilariasis
    b. Hypertension

DISEASES ASSOCIATED WITH ALVEOLAR PATTERNS

BACTERIAL PNEUMONIA

Bacterial pneumonia is characteristically seen with an alveolar pattern infiltrate.[180] Bacterial pneumonia may involve any lung lobe, or portion thereof, and may be focal

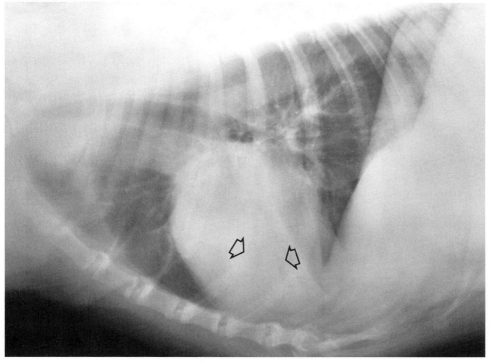

A

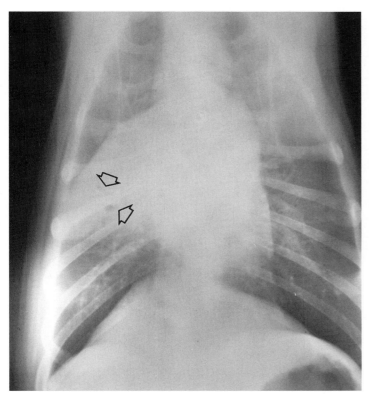

B

Figure 2–133. (A&B) A 12-year-old female Irish setter presented with a 24-hour history of labored respiration and coughing. There is an infiltrate, which is homogeneous within the right middle lung lobe. The margins of the infiltrate are sharply defined by the lobar borders. Air bronchograms are present (*arrows*). The radiographic findings are consistent with bacterial pneumonia. **Diagnosis:** Bacterial pneumonia.

or multifocal (Figs. 2–133, 2–134 and 2–135). Bronchial pneumonia (that which has pathogen spread through the airways) tends to be lobar in distribution. Hematogenous pneumonia (that which has pathogen spread via the vascular system) tends to have a patchy, multifocal distribution.[180] Tracheobronchial or sternal lymphadenopathy and pleural fluid are rarely present with either type of bacterial pneumonia. Spontaneous pneumothorax and/or pyothorax may result from chronic bacterial pneumonia secondary to lung abscessation.[71]

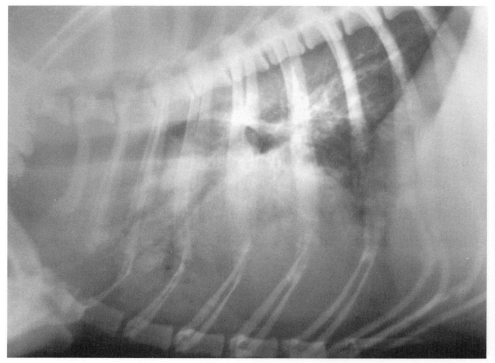

A

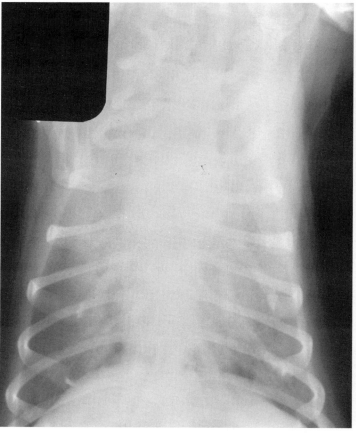

B

Figure 2–134. (A&B) A 10-year-old male dachshund presented with a 6-month history of chronic nasal discharge. The dog also had harsh lung sounds and a Grade 2/6 systolic murmur. There is a fluid-dense infiltrate in the cranial lung lobes bilaterally. The infiltrate is coalescent and poorly marginated. There are air bronchograms noted within these lung lobes, especially in the cranial ventral lung. This is consistent with a bacterial or aspiration pneumonia. **Diagnosis:** Bacterial pneumonia.

ASPIRATION PNEUMONIA

Aspiration pneumonia produces similar focal or multifocal alveolar patterns (Fig. 2–136). The pattern depends upon the amount and nature of the material aspirated and the severity of the lung's reaction. A large volume of material or a material that

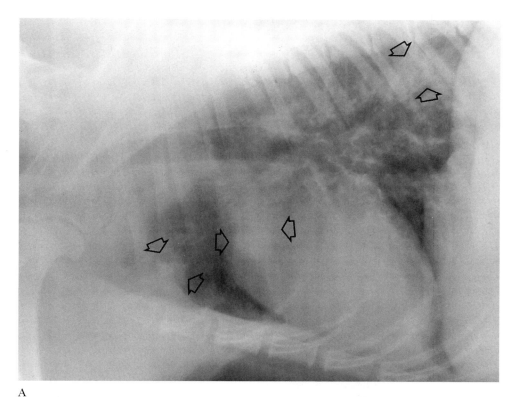

A

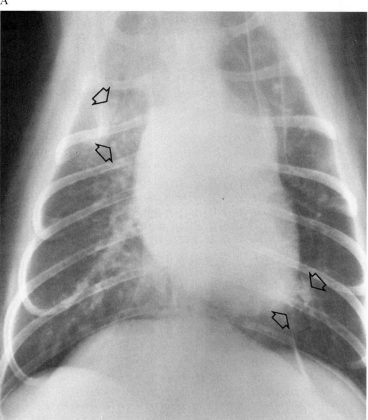

B

Figure 2–135. (A&B) A 7-year-old female mixed breed dog presented for evaluation of a productive cough that had persisted for 7 months following exposure to smoke. There are focal areas of pulmonary density in the left caudal and right cranial lung lobes (*arrows*). There is a diffuse increase in pulmonary bronchial and interstitial densities. The diffuse pulmonary density is secondary to the previous smoke inhalation and represents interstitial fibrosis. The focal areas of density (patchy alveolar pattern infiltrates) are most likely due to secondary bacterial infection. **Diagnosis:** Bacterial pneumonia secondary to chronic interstitial and bronchial fibrosis due to smoke inhalation.

is very irritating is more likely to cause a severe alveolar pattern. The distribution of the infiltrates may depend on the animal's position when the material is aspirated. Passively aspirated (e.g., during sedation or anesthesia) material is most likely to go to the most dependent or first accessible lung lobe (frequently the right cranial

Figure 2–136. (A&B) An 8-year-old male Doberman pinscher presented with a 4-month history of regurgitation, which had been occurring spontaneously and sporadically. The esophagus is dilated throughout the thorax. In both (A) and (B) the esophageal walls are evident as thin, soft tissue densities (*closed arrows*). The trachea and cardiac silhouette are displaced ventrally. There are areas of focal alveolar pattern infiltrates within the right cranial, left cranial, and left caudal lung lobes (*open arrows*). These are typified by their coalescence and poorly-defined borders. Air bronchogram signs are not present. The radiographic findings are indicative of aspiration pneumonia. **Diagnosis:** Megaesophagus with aspiration pneumonia. The dog was hypothyroid and this was assumed to be the cause of the megaesophagus.

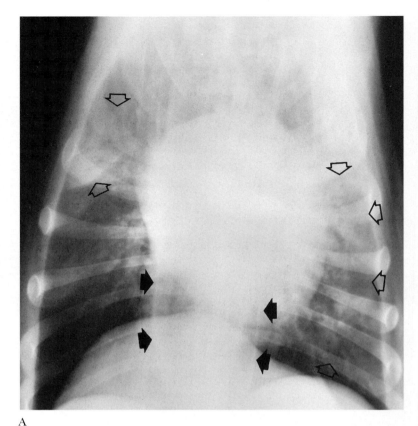

A

B

lobe). The right caudal lung lobe is more likely to be the lobe involved if the aspiration is forceful or the aspirated material is solid (e.g., foxtails, other plant material, etc.), because the bronchus to this lobe is the straightest in relation to the trachea. Dilation of the esophagus in conjunction with this type of a pulmonary pattern suggests that the aspiration pneumonia may be coincidental to megaesophagus.

PARASITIC PNEUMONIA

Toxoplasmosis may produce multifocal alveolar pattern infiltrates in the lungs. This is an unusual presentation.[182] Capillaria and Aleurostrongylus may also produce multifocal alveolar infiltrates.

VIRAL PNEUMONIA

Viral pneumonia rarely produces alveolar pattern infiltrates without secondary infection with bacteria. An exception to this is the pneumonia that is associated with Calicivirus in cats. This has been reported to be a rapidly progressive pneumonia that reveals a severe, diffuse alveolar pattern infiltrate.[183]

PULMONARY INFILTRATES WITH EOSINOPHILIA

A syndrome has been described in which dogs develop medium to large areas of alveolar pattern infiltrates (Fig. 2–137).[184,185] In some cases, associated findings may include lymphadenopathy and a bronchial/fine linear interstitial pattern. Less frequently seen are pleural effusions and nodular masses. The affected dogs usually have an associated eosinophilia. The exact cause of the eosinophilia frequently is not determined.

PULMONARY EDEMA (CARDIOGENIC AND NONCARDIOGENIC)

Pulmonary edema is the flooding of the end-air spaces with fluid. Pulmonary edema can be subdivided into that caused by left heart failure (cardiogenic pulmonary edema) and that due to other causes (noncardiogenic pulmonary edema).

Cardiogenic pulmonary edema is the most frequently seen type of pulmonary edema. It is typified by alveolar pattern infiltrates that are located in the hilar and perihilar areas, but atypical distributions can occasionally be seen (Fig. 2–138). If particularly severe, the infiltrates may involve all portions of the lung (Fig. 2–139) and free pleural fluid may be observed. If radiographed early in the pathogenesis of

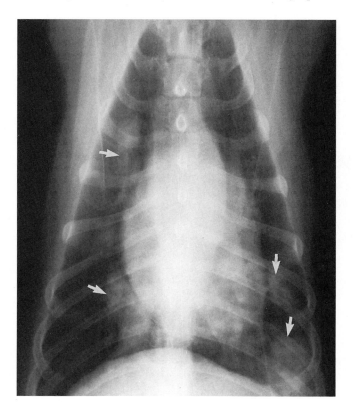

Figure 2–137. A 6-year-old male whippet presented for cough. An absolute eosinophilia was present. The dog was negative for dirofilariasis. The ventrodorsal radiograph revealed patchy areas of alveolar pattern infiltrate (*arrows*) in multiple lung lobes. **Diagnosis:** Pulmonary infiltrates with eosinophilia. (Reproduced with permission from Burk RL: Radiographic examination of the cardiopulmonary system. VCNA 1983; 13:241.)

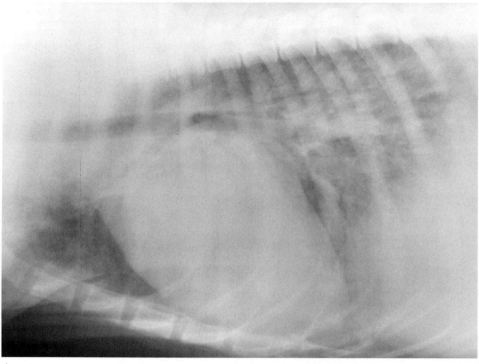

A

Figure 2–138. (A&B) A 4-year-old female Saint Bernard presented with acute respiratory distress. There is marked cardiomegaly, and the caudal cardiac margin is straightened. The tracheal bifurcation and mainstem bronchi are elevated. There is diffuse alveolar pattern infiltrate, which is most severe in the hilar area. Air bronchogram signs are present in the caudal lung lobes. The radiographic findings are indicative of left heart failure. **Diagnosis:** Left heart failure secondary to dilated cardiomyopathy.

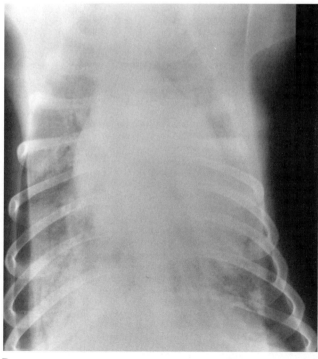

B

left heart failure or after successful treatment, the lesion may be predominately an interstitial pattern infiltrate. The lesions usually resolve from the periphery toward the hilus.

There are many causes of noncardiogenic pulmonary edema including neurological problems such as head trauma or seizures, electric shock, severe allergic disease, advanced uremia, pancreatitis, irritating inhalants (smoke/heat), near drowning, radiation damage, and acute respiratory distress syndrome.[186–192] The more

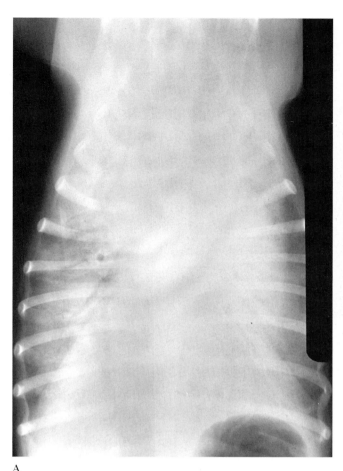

A

Figure 2–139. (A&B) A 6-year-old female Doberman pinscher presented with a 3-day history of an acute onset of dyspnea. The dog's heart rate was rapid. There is a diffuse alveolar pattern infiltrate typified by poorly-defined and coalescent densities involving all lung lobes. A few air bronchogram signs are present. The density is most severe in the hilar area and radiates outward from that point. (B) On the lateral radiograph the trachea and tracheal bifurcation are elevated. The mainstem bronchi are split (*arrows*). Although the entire outline of the cardiac silhouette cannot be seen, the tracheal alterations indicate left-sided cardiomegaly. The radiographic changes suggest congestive left heart failure. **Diagnosis:** Cardiomyopathy with congestive left heart failure.

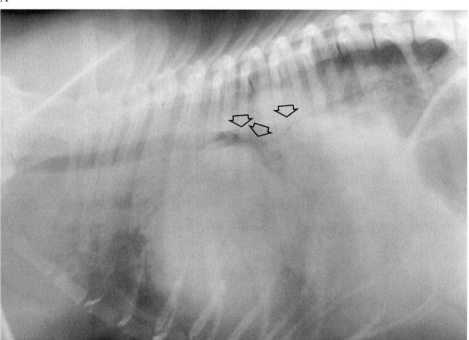

B

commonly seen lesions are typically in the dorsal and caudal portions of the caudal lung lobes and are most frequently associated with electric shock or seizures (Figs. 2–140 and 2–141). Other types of noncardiogenic edema may be more diffusely distributed.

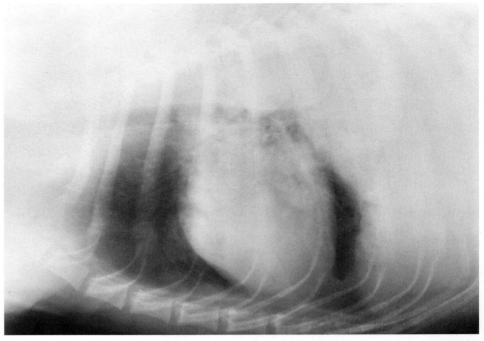

A

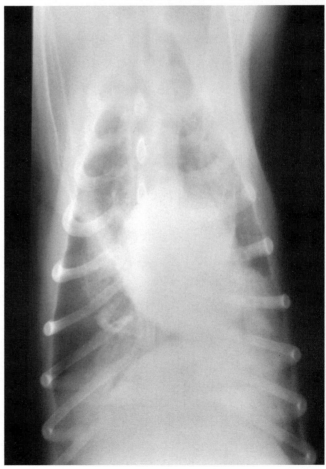

Figure 2–140. (A&B) A 4-year-old female German shepherd dog presented with a history of acute onset of respiratory distress associated with three seizure episodes. There is an alveolar pattern infiltrate typified by coalescent and poorly-defined densities in the dorsal portions of the caudal lung lobes. Air bronchogram signs are not present. The hilar region is less involved. The radiographic findings are consistent with a noncardiogenic pulmonary edema. **Diagnosis:** Post ictal pulmonary edema.

B

NEOPLASIA

The vast majority of primary and metastatic pulmonary tumors present as interstitial pattern infiltrates. However, there are several uncommon exceptions. These include squamous cell carcinoma of the bronchus, which usually results in partial or complete atelectasis of the affected lung lobe(s).[193] Alveolar cell carcinoma usually ap-

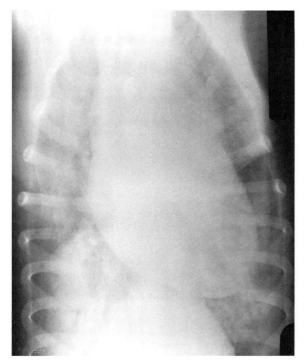

A

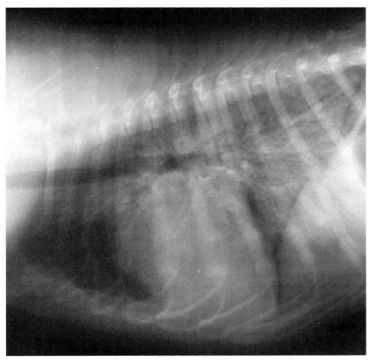

B

Figure 2–141. (A&B) A 6-month-old male German shepherd dog presented with a history of respiratory distress. An alveolar pattern infiltrate typified by poorly-defined and coalescent densities is present in the dorsal portions of the caudal lung lobes. A few air bronchogram signs are present. The hilar region is less severely involved. The radiographic findings are suggestive of a non-cardiogenic pulmonary edema. **Diagnosis:** Non-cardiogenic pulmonary edema secondary to electric shock. The owners discovered that the dog had been chewing on an electric lamp cord.

pears as multiple, poorly-defined foci of alveolar pattern infiltrates in one or more lung lobes. This may also be associated with a fine linear interstitial infiltrate. Bronchoalveolar carcinoma frequently presents as a large, focal area(s) of alveolar pattern infiltrate with multiple smaller areas of infiltrate or nodule formation in other lobes. Lymphosarcoma may rarely produce a focal or multifocal alveolar infiltrate.

PULMONARY HEMORRHAGE (CONTUSION)

Pulmonary hemorrhage or contusion may result from chest trauma or a coagulopathy. Rib fractures may or may not be present, however the presence of recent rib fractures or a history of recent trauma strongly suggests that the density is a contusion.

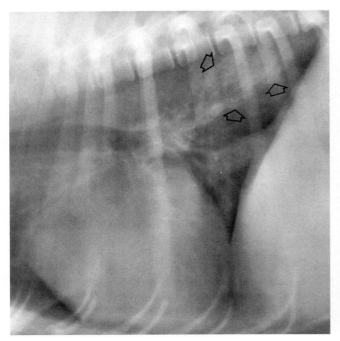
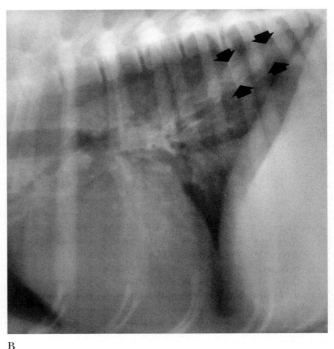

A   B

Figure 2–142.   A 4-year-old male mixed breed dog presented with a history of respiratory distress and fever occurring 1 week following treatment for heartworm disease. (A) In the initial thoracic radiograph there is a local area of interstitial density in the caudal dorsal lung (*open arrows*). This is indicative of pulmonary thrombosis or embolization secondary to heartworm treatment. (B) On the follow-up radiograph, repeated 10 days after presentation, an enlarged irregular pulmonary artery is evident in the caudal dorsal lung lobe (*closed arrows*). This most likely represents thrombosis of the pulmonary artery. **Diagnosis:** Pulmonary thrombosis/embolization secondary to treatment for dirofilariasis.

Any lung lobe or portion of a lobe may be involved. Pneumothorax, pneumomediastinum, hydrothorax, and diaphragmatic hernia can be concomitantly seen with lung contusion. Uneven lung lobe density in conjunction with bilateral pneumothorax and/or hydrothorax suggests that a pulmonary infiltrate is present in the lobe that is most dense, and, in the presence of trauma, this is likely to be a pulmonary contusion.

PULMONARY EMBOLIC DISEASE

Pulmonary embolic disease may occur in conjunction with dirofilariasis (Fig. 2–142), hyperadrenocorticism, glomerulonephritis, coagulopathies, and other clinical syndromes.[65,194–196] Survey radiography is relatively insensitive in the detection of this problem. Pulmonary scintigraphy or angiography is more likely to confirm the diagnosis.[39] Radiographically, pulmonary emboli may occasionally produce a decreased pulmonary density due to oligemia distal to the arterial thrombosis. More commonly, an alveolar pattern infiltrate due to the hemorrhage, necrosis, and inflammation is present. These patterns are seen only if major pulmonary arteries are occluded. Obstruction of minor arteries will not lead to radiographic changes because the collateral circulation present at that level prevents significant oligemia to the tissues. If a thrombosis is caused by dirofilariasis, enlarged, tortuous, or irregularly shaped pulmonary vessels usually are visible.

LUNG LOBE TORSION

Lung lobe torsion usually presents with hydrothorax. A solitary lung lobe that has a severe alveolar pattern infiltrate and also has an abnormal shape may be seen.[197,198] The involved lung lobe will become dense, and air bronchograms may be evident

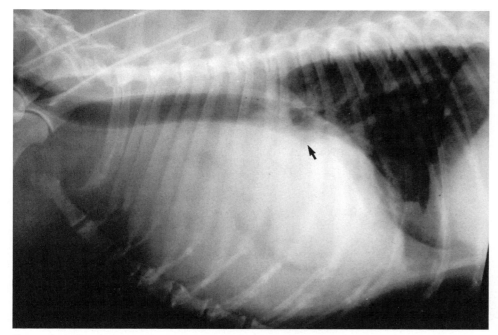

Figure 2–143. A 4-year-old male Afghan hound presented for a sudden onset of dyspnea. Auscultation revealed dull lung sounds in the left cranial thorax. Examination of the lateral radiograph reveals a homogeneous density in the cranial lung lobe area. Close examination reveals an abrupt obstruction of the left cranial lung lobe bronchus (*arrow*). **Diagnosis:** Torsion of the left cranial lung lobe.

early in the disease. Later, the lung will fill completely with fluid and the air bronchograms will disappear (Figs. 2–56 and 2–143). The main lobar bronchus may remain aerated and visible for a short distance. Abrupt termination of the bronchus after it branches from the trachea may be seen. The right middle lung lobe is most frequently affected, with the right and left cranial lung lobes the next most frequent.[67] Lung lobe torsion is more common in deep-chested breeds of dogs but may be seen in other breeds as well as in cats.[67,197]

ATELECTASIS

Atelectasis is collapse of a lung lobe. This occurs when the end-air spaces are no longer filled with air, and it results in the affected lobe being homogeneously tissue-dense with a loss of normal volume.[199] Mediastinal shifts and compensatory hyperinflation of other lung lobes may be noted in association with atelectasis. Complete atelectasis will not have any air-filled structures and no air bronchograms will be present. There seems to be a predilection for atelectasis of the right middle lung lobe in cats. The cause of this is unknown. The general causes of atelectasis include airway obstruction (due to tumor, hypertrophy of luminal epithelium, or foreign matter), compression (as seen with tumor, hydrothorax, or hypostatic congestion), or pneumothorax (loss of negative pleural pressure resulting in collapse of a lobe or lobes) (Figs. 2–58 and 2–144).

DISEASES ASSOCIATED WITH INTERSTITIAL PATTERNS

These diseases may present as a primarily linear/reticular or nodular pattern. While overlap frequently exists between these disease, and even some overlap exists between alveolar and interstitial patterns, the feature that is demonstrated most frequently on the radiograph is the one that should be utilized in developing a list of possible diagnoses.

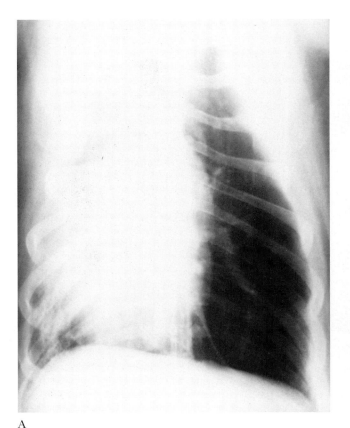
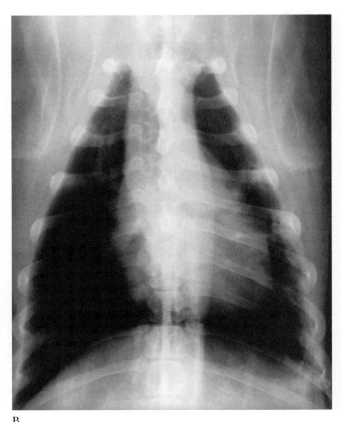

A   B

Figure 2–144. (A&B) A 9-year-old male rottweiler presented with an oral mass. Radiographs of the thorax were taken immediately after completing radiographs of the skull. (A) Examination reveals a dense alveolar pattern infiltrate in the right lungs. The cardiac silhouette is shifted to the right. (B) Repeat radiograph taken immediately after several positive pressure ventilations were made reveals normal lung morphology. **Diagnosis:** Iatrogenic atelectasis and hypostatic congestion of the right lung.

Disseminated or diffuse interstitial pulmonary patterns may be subdivided into chronic or active infiltrates. In chronic interstitial patterns, the linear and circular densities will be thin and fairly well defined, and the pulmonary vessel margins will be minimally blurred. Well-defined nodular densities of various sizes, many of which can be calcified, may be present. In contrast, more active infiltrates are wider, less well defined and vessel margins may be more blurred.

LINEAR/RETICULAR INTERSTITIAL PATTERNS

PARASITIC PNEUMONIA

Parasitic pneumonia may be seen with *Capillaria aerophilia, Filaroides milksi,* and *Aleurostrongylus abstrusus* infections.[200–204] These are uncommon, but in severe cases they may produce focal or multifocal alveolar or interstitial pulmonary patterns. Peribronchial densities may be present throughout the lung and multifocal nodular densities are seen (Fig. 2–145). The most obvious changes reportedly involve the caudal lung lobes. Visceral larval migrans may produce multifocal interstitial densities in the caudal dorsal lung lobes. This is very rare even in severe Toxocara infestation. Leishmaniasis has also been reported to cause an interstitial pattern.[205]

VIRAL PNEUMONIA

Viral pneumonia rarely produces radiographic changes. A fine linear/reticular pattern may occasionally be seen (Fig. 2–146). Many times if infiltrates are present they

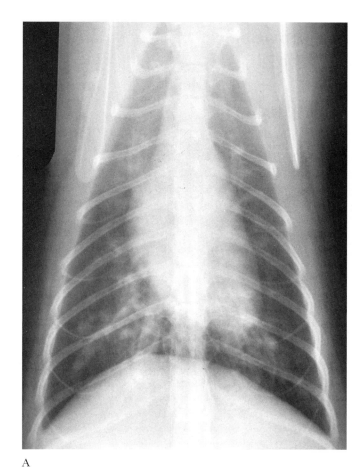

Figure 2–145. (A&B) A 2-year-old female cat presented with a 1.5-month history of coughing and dyspnea. There is an increase in pulmonary interstitial and peribronchiolar densities noted throughout the lungs. The vascular structures are obscured. The bronchial walls are thickened. The radiographic findings are indicative of allergic or parasitic pneumonia. **Diagnosis:** Aleurostrongylus pneumonia. The parasite was recovered on a tracheal wash.

A

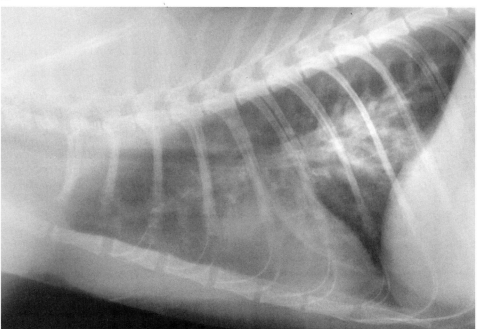

B

are due to secondary bacterial infection. Calicivirus pneumonia in cats has been reported to progress to an alveolar pattern infiltrate.[181]

IMMUNE (ALLERGIC) PULMONARY DISEASE

A combination of a fine linear or reticular pattern that may be superimposed onto an equally prominent bronchial pattern may be seen with pulmonary disease caused

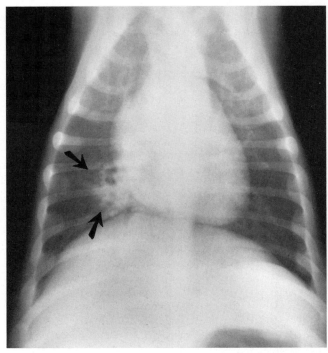

Figure 2–146. (A&B) A 3-month-old female Doberman pinscher presented with a 1-week history of cough. There is a focal area of interstitial density in the right caudal lung lobe (*arrows*). There is a generalized increase in pulmonary interstitial densities. These findings suggest viral pneumonia complicated by secondary bacterial infection. **Diagnosis:** Canine distemper.

A

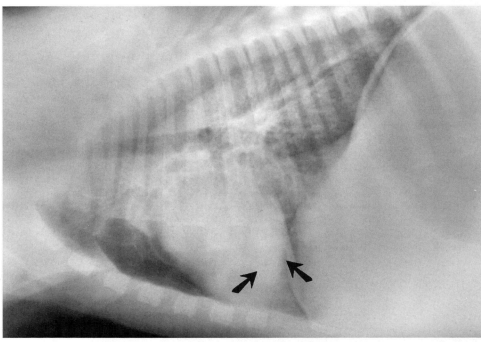

B

by allergic reaction to locally present (e.g., parasites) or inhaled antigens (Figs. 2–147 and 2–148). These changes reflect the infiltration of eosinophils and round cells into bronchial, peribronchial, and interstitial tissues. Small nodules may be present if large accumulations of infiltrate occur in a single area. This condition has also been termed allergic pneumonia or allergic pneumonitis. A relatively frequent example of this disseminated or diffuse fine linear or reticular interstitial infiltrate occurs with occult dirofilariasis. However, this specific etiology usually can be recognized because of the cardiovascular changes.

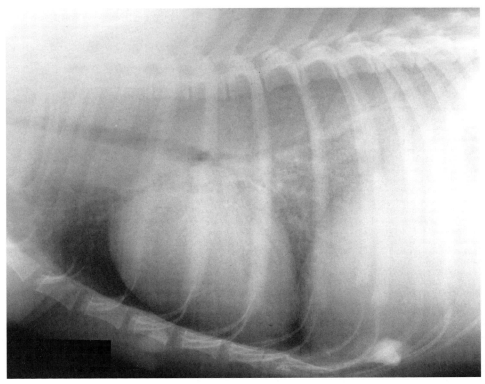

A

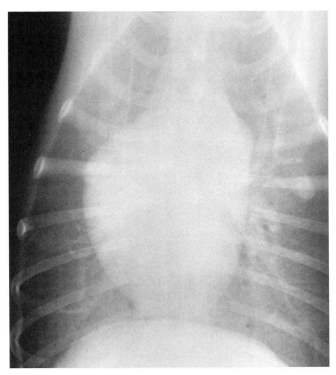

B

Figure 2–147. (A&B) A 3-year-old male pit bull presented with a 3-month history of a dry, non-productive cough. There is a diffuse increase in pulmonary interstitial densities with loss of normal vascular structures. There is a mild right-sided cardiomegaly. The radiographic findings indicate a severe interstitial pulmonary infiltrate. **Diagnosis:** Eosinophilic pneumonitis.

CONGESTIVE LEFT HEART FAILURE

An early stage of left heart failure will produce interstitial edema, which starts in the hilar region and progresses peripherally. With interstitial edema, the enlarged pulmonary veins may still be partially visible. Left-side cardiac enlargement with a large

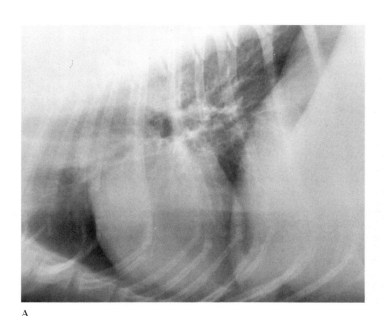

A

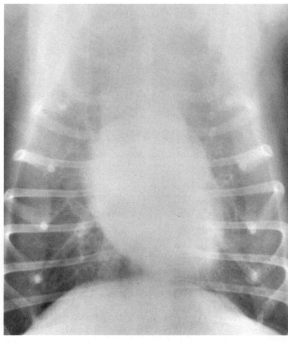

B

Figure 2–148. (A&B) A 9-year-old male dachshund presented with an 8-month history of a non-productive cough. There is a generalized increase in bronchial and interstitial densities. This is indicative of allergic pulmonary disease. **Diagnosis:** Eosinophilic pneumonitis.

left atrium is most often observed. On occasion, the pulmonary density is more severe in one lung lobe. When this occurs, a superimposed bacterial infection or other process should also be suspected.

LYMPHOMA

Lymphoma involving the pulmonary parenchyma is less common than other presentations of this disease. When present, it will typically produce a disseminated interstitial infiltrate, which is often more severe in the perihilar area (Figs. 2–149 and 2–150). Multifocal nodular densities, alveolar infiltrates, and pleural fluid have been observed. Tracheobronchial, sternal, and/or extrathoracic lymphadenopathy may be present and provide important information leading to the diagnosis.

METASTATIC NEOPLASIA

A poorly defined, diffuse interstitial pattern and, rarely, an alveolar pattern may occasionally be present (Fig. 2–151). This has been described as lymphangitic metastases or pulmonary carcinomatosis, although neoplasms other than metastatic carcinoma may produce this pattern. Coalescence of the densities produces more solid appearing masses or nodules without air bronchograms. Bronchial compression, distortion, or displacement may be visible. Lymphadenopathy is infrequent and air bronchograms rarely occur.

PULMONARY HEMORRHAGE

Diffuse pulmonary hemorrhage may occur in animals with disseminated intravascular coagulation or other coagulopathies such as warfarin poisoning or von Willebrand's disease. A disseminated or diffuse interstitial or alveolar pattern may be present if the disorder is not severe. An alveolar pattern is the more common finding. Pleural fluid (hemorrhage) may also be present.

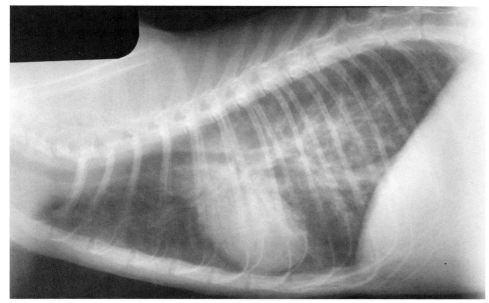

A

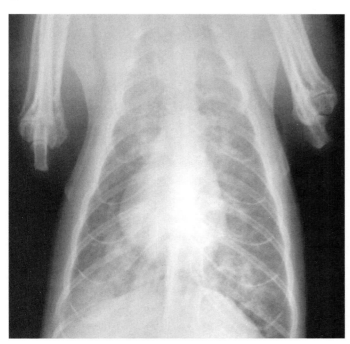

B

Figure 2–149. (A&B) A 3-year-old spayed cat presented with a several month history of weight loss and anorexia. The cat had developed respiratory distress. There is a marked increase in pulmonary interstitial densities distributed throughout the lung. The infiltrate is more severe in the right caudal lung lobe. The pulmonary vascular structures are obscured. Many end-on bronchi are identified. **Diagnosis:** Lymphoma. The pulmonary infiltrate was thought to represent an allergic or parasitic pneumonia. The diagnosis of lymphoma was made at necropsy. A similar pulmonary pattern may be observed with feline infectious peritonitis.

AZOTEMIA

Azotemia can very rarely provoke an interstitial or alveolar inflammatory response. Hemorrhage or bacterial infection may produce a focal or multifocal alveolar or interstitial infiltrate in conjunction with uremia.[192] Pleural and pericardial effusions have been observed. Pulmonary and/or pleural calcification may be present with chronic renal failure (Fig. 2–152).

OLD AGE—INTERSTITIAL FIBROSIS

Chronic disseminated or diffuse interstitial pulmonary patterns, including fine linear and reticular patterns as well as calcified, discrete nodules, may be observed in thoracic radiographs of old dogs and cats.[206] The calcified nodules may be either old

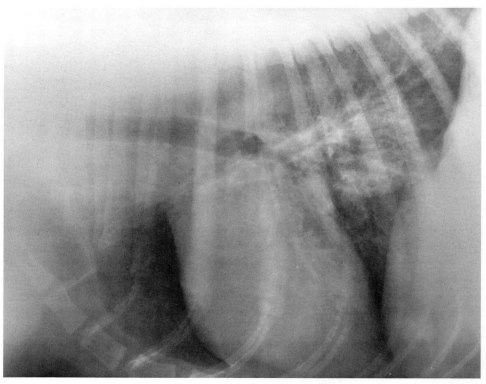

A

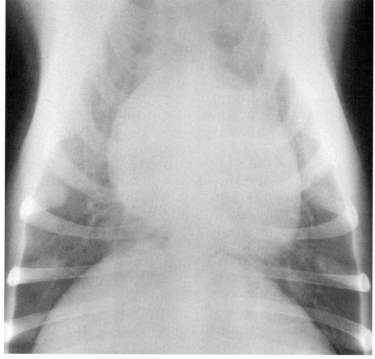

B

Figure 2–150. (A&B) A 5-year-old male Doberman pinscher presented with generalized lymphadenopathy. There is a diffuse increase in pulmonary interstitial densities. The vascular structures are obscured. **Diagnosis:** Lymphoma. The diagnosis was confirmed by lymph node biopsy.

granulomas that dystrophically calcified or pulmonary osteomata—islands of bone within the lung whose cause is unknown. The general causes of these changes may include long-term inhalation of irritating smoke or dust particles or prior pulmonary disease, which has healed leaving scarring within the lung.

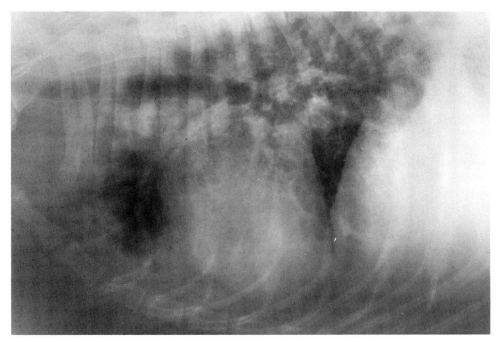

A

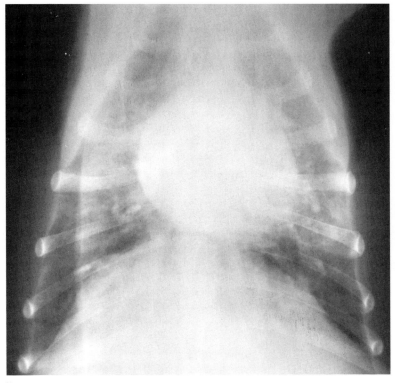

B

Figure 2–151. (A&B) A 14-year-old female Doberman pinscher presented with a 3-month history of weight loss. The dog was depressed and dehydrated. There is a diffuse increase in pulmonary interstitial densities throughout the lung. These densities are poorly defined. Well-defined nodular densities are not identified. The radiographic findings may be due to disseminated neoplasia, granulomatous disease, or chronic infection. **Diagnosis:** Diffuse metastatic neoplasia. A lung aspirate was performed and metastatic carcinoma was detected.

PNEUMOCONIOSIS

Inhalation of irritating substances such as smoke or dust particles can produce pulmonary fibrosis without inducing a severe inflammatory response. This may occur acutely but more commonly develops over a long period without apparent clinical signs. The diffuse or disseminated pulmonary interstitial density will often be mild and is frequently seen with advanced age.[207]

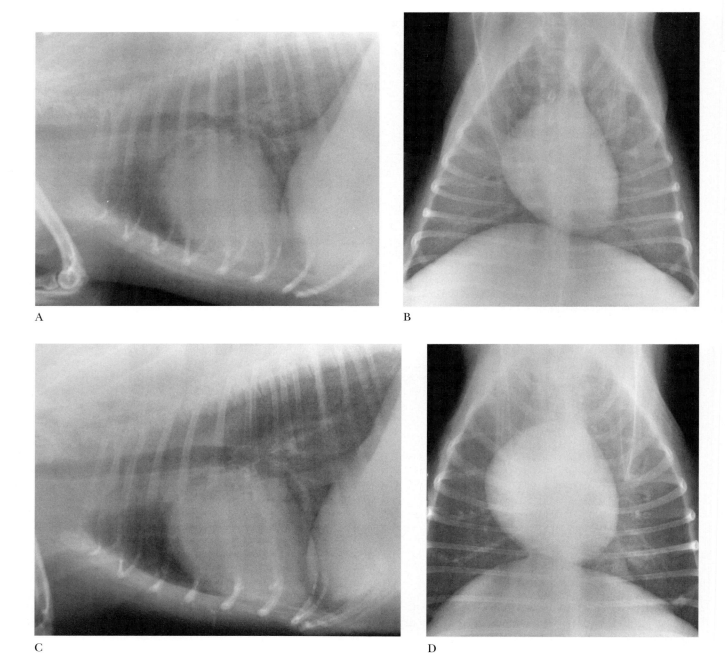

A

B

C

D

Figure 2–152. (A,B,C,D) A 6-year-old female schnauzer presented with a 2-week history of anorexia, depression, and vomiting. (A&B) Thoracic radiographs were obtained at the time of admission. (C&D) Follow-up radiographs were obtained 2 weeks later following treatment of the dog for chronic renal failure. In (A&B) there is a diffuse increase in pulmonary interstitial densities. The vascular structures are poorly defined. In (C&D) the pulmonary interstitial densities have increased in severity. The densities are sharply defined and appear mineralized. **Diagnosis:** Pulmonary interstitial mineralization associated with chronic renal failure.

NODULAR PULMONARY PATTERN

The term *nodular pulmonary pattern* is used to describe solid spherical or oval soft tissue densities that are distinctly outlined within the lung. Most nodules originate within the interstitial tissue, enlarge and compress the surrounding pulmonary parenchyma, and may grow to distort or compress the bronchi. They may represent

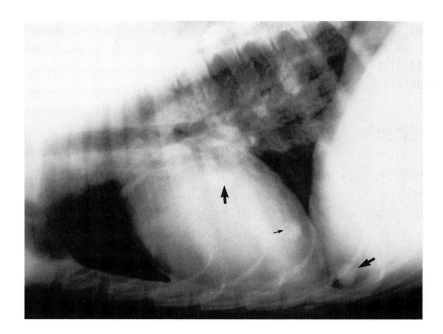

Figure 2–153. A 5-year-old female beagle was presented with exercise intolerance and hemoptysis. A lateral radiograph reveals multiple nodular densities (*arrows*) throughout all lung lobes. Close examination revealed one (*small arrow*) to be cavitated. **Diagnosis:** Paragonimiasis.

solid masses or fluid-filled, cyst-like structures. Nodular lung lesions may be well- or poorly circumscribed, solitary or multiple, and may become very large.

PARASITIC PNEUMONIA

Parasitic pneumonia may be seen with *Capillaria aerophilia* and *Aleurostrongylus abstrusus* infestations. These infestations are uncommon but in severe cases may produce focal or multifocal interstitial or alveolar pulmonary patterns. Peribronchial densities may be present throughout the lung and multifocal nodular densities are common.[200–204] The most obvious change reportedly involves the caudal lung lobes. Larval migrans may produce multifocal interstitial densities in the caudal dorsal lung lobes. This is very rare even in severe toxocara infestation.

Another form of parasitic pneumonia is infestation with *Paragonimus kellicotti*. Infestation is typified by the presence of clearly defined interstitial nodular densities throughout the lungs (Fig. 2–153). Classic lesions will have a radiolucency in the periphery of the lesion (as the flukes inhabit the interstitium immediately adjacent to a bronchus). Lesions are most common in the right caudal lung lobe. Pneumocysts (which may be septated) may also be seen. Pneumothorax has also been noted, on occasion.[208–210]

FELINE INFECTIOUS PERITONITIS

Feline infectious peritonitis occasionally produces disseminated interstitial or nodular densities.[211] Pleural and peritoneal fluid are more commonly observed.

MYCOTIC PNEUMONIA

Mycotic pneumonia usually will produce disseminated interstitial nodular pulmonary infiltrates (Fig. 2–154).[212–215] While the infiltrate does not often progress to a diffuse alveolar pattern, focal alveolar or interstitial infiltrates may occur. Multiple small (miliary) and various size nodular densities may be present. Tracheobronchial lymphadenopathy is frequently seen (Fig. 2–155). Occasionally, this may be masked by extensive pulmonary infiltrate. Coalescence of the pulmonary densities usually produces granulomatous masses rather than alveolar patterns. Cavitation rarely occurs within the pulmonary granulomas. Blastomycosis, coccidioidomycosis, and

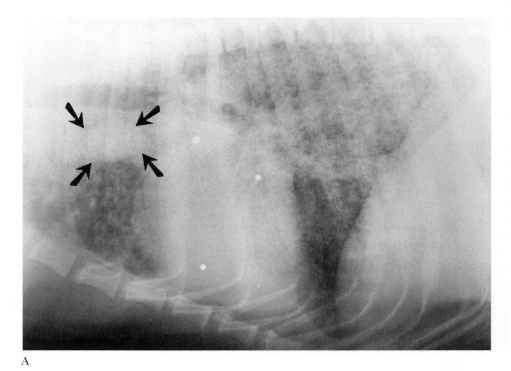

A

B

C

Figure 2–154. (A,B,C) A 6-year-old male mixed breed dog that had a 2-week history of decreased exercise tolerance. There is a generalized increase in pulmonary interstitial densities. There is a soft tissue density in the mediastinum cranial to the cardiac silhouette (*arrows*). The radiographic findings are indicative of a generalized interstitial pulmonary infiltrate with cranial mediastinal lymphadenopathy. The differential diagnosis should include neoplasia and mycotic disease. **Diagnosis:** Blastomycosis.

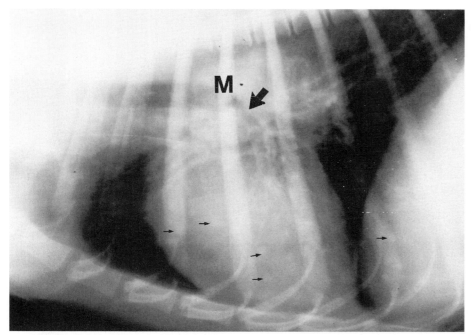

Figure 2–155. A 3-year-old springer spaniel presented with inappetence, dyspnea, and fever. The lateral radiograph revealed multiple pulmonary nodules (*small arrows*) and a mass (*M*) at the base of the heart. The caudal mainstem bronchi are ventrally displaced (*arrow*) by the mass. **Diagnosis:** Histoplasmosis with pulmonary nodules and tracheobronchial lymph node enlargement.

histoplasmosis all produce similar radiographic changes. Tracheobronchial lymphadenopathy is somewhat less frequent in blastomycosis, and lymph node calcification is observed more often in histoplasmosis. Calcification of pulmonary nodules may be observed as a sequelae to the active disease (Fig. 2–156). Cryptococcosis, aspergillosis, and nocardiosis rarely produce pulmonary lesions. When present, they are more likely to be focal or multifocal interstitial densities or granulomas.

EOSINOPHILIC GRANULOMATOSIS

Eosinophilic granulomatosis has been described in conjunction with dirofilariasis.[185] It is typified by the presence of large nodular masses and some degree of fine linear/reticular pulmonary markings (Fig. 2–157).

LYMPHOMATOID GRANULOMATOSIS

Lymphomatoid granulomatosis has been described with large, nodular pulmonary masses.[216] Other findings that have been frequently noted include lobar consolidation and tracheobronchial lymphadenopathy. Less common findings have included mild hydrothorax, sternal and mediastinal lymphadenopathy, and a diffuse interstitial lung pattern.

CONGESTIVE LEFT HEART FAILURE

On rare occasion, congestive left heart failure will present as an acinonodular pattern (Fig. 2–158). This pattern of fine nodular densities tends to coalesce toward the pulmonary hilus. The pattern is seen more often with chronic heart failure due to dilated cardiomyopathy.

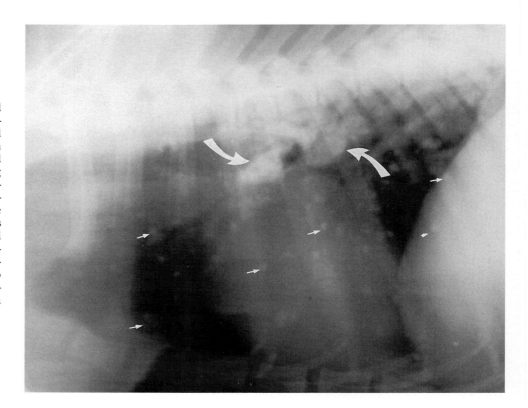

Figure 2–156. A 9-year-old female Brittany spaniel presented with mammary gland masses. The lateral radiograph revealed multiple calcified nodules throughout all lung lobes (*small arrows*). No evidence of tissue density was present in any of the nodules. The tracheobronchial lymph nodes were enlarged and calcified (*curved arrows*). **Diagnosis:** Calcified nodules and tracheobronchial lymph nodes due to prior Histoplasmosis. No evidence of metastatic neoplasia was found.

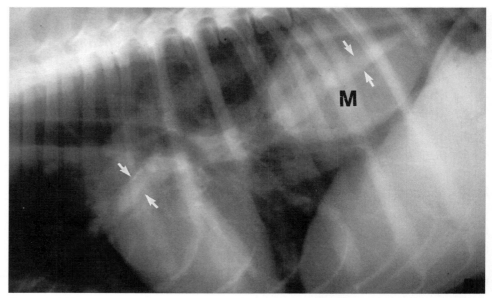

Figure 2–157. A 6-year-old male German shepherd dog presented with exercise intolerance, anorexia, and weakness. The lateral radiograph revealed markedly dilated pulmonary arteries (*arrows*) and a large mass (*M*) in the caudal lung. Microfilaria were present on a direct blood smear. **Diagnosis:** Eosinophilic granuloma. At necropsy fragments of a dead adult *D. immitis* were present in the mass.

GRANULOMA OF FOREIGN MATERIAL

Granulomatous lesions may form around any foreign material that is inhaled and stays within the lung. Such material could include plant matter (plant awns) or iatrogenic substances (Fig. 2–159).

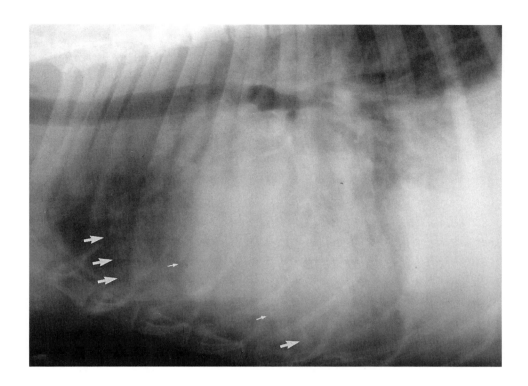

Figure 2–158. An 8-year-old male Doberman pinscher presented with an acute onset of dyspnea. A murmur and arrhythmia were ausculted. The lateral radiograph revealed multiple nodular densities (acinonodular pattern) throughout all lung lobes (*arrows*). The cardiac silhouette was enlarged. **Diagnosis:** Dilated cardiomyopathy with pulmonary edema. The infiltrate cleared over night with treatment of the heart condition.

PRIMARY PULMONARY NEOPLASIA

Differentiating primary from metastatic neoplasia (or other forms of nodular pulmonary disease) is difficult. Although solitary nodules are more likely to be primary neoplasms, the possibility of a solitary metastasis or granuloma cannot be excluded.

Bronchogenic carcinoma is the most common tumor type. Bronchogenic carcinomas usually arise in the periphery of the lung and usually are solitary (Fig. 2–160).[193,217,218] Necrosis within the center of the mass combined with communication with an airway may result in air accumulation within the soft tissue-dense mass. Cavitation may be evident radiographically as a decreased (air) density within the tissue-dense mass. Cavitation is reportedly more frequent in bronchogenic carcinoma and squamous cell carcinoma. It may also occur within pulmonary abscesses, traumatic cysts, or hematomas.

Occasionally, calcification is identified radiographically within primary or metastatic lung tumors. Small, amorphous calcification may be present within large neoplastic tissue-dense masses (Fig. 2–161).

Bronchoalveolar carcinoma may appear as a solitary nodule in the middle or peripheral lung areas. However, a more common appearance is that of a poorly-defined mass.

Radiographically apparent tracheobronchial lymphadenopathy is an uncommon finding with primary or secondary lung tumors. It occurs most often in association with multicentric lymphosarcoma or granulomatous disease.

METASTATIC PULMONARY NEOPLASIA

Metastatic pulmonary neoplasia occurs more frequently than primary lung tumors. Multiple, well-defined, variable size nodular densities located in the middle or peripheral portions of the lung that are not cavitated and do not displace or obstruct bronchi are observed most often (Figs. 2–162 and 2–163).[4,193,218-220] Concomitant tracheobronchial lymphadenopathy is uncommon. A poorly defined diffuse interstitial

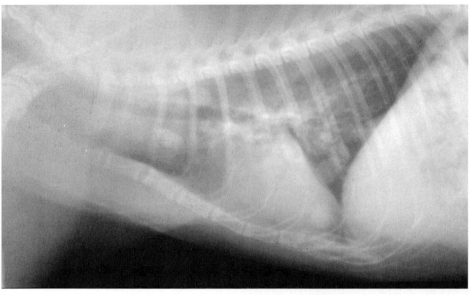

A

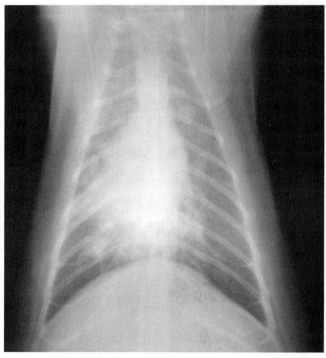

B

Figure 2–159. (A&B) An 11-year-old spayed female Siamese cat presented with a 2-year history of chronic coughing. The cough responded slightly to treatment with antibiotics and cortisone. Multiple nodules of varying sizes are present throughout all lung lobes. The right middle lobe is atelectatic. The radiographic findings are indicative of multiple soft tissue masses, which may be neoplastic or granulomatous. Aspiration of one of these nodules revealed a granulomatous reaction secondary to lipid material. **Diagnosis:** Granulomas secondary to aspiration of mineral oil.

pattern and, rarely, an alveolar pattern may occasionally be present. The wide variety of radiographic lesions reported with pulmonary metastasis results partly from the characteristics of the primary neoplasm. It also results from concomitant pulmonary hemorrhage, edema, inflammation, infection, or necrosis.

PULMONARY ABSCESS

Focal, walled-off accumulations of septic matter may occasionally occur within the lung. If chronic, there may be a discrete mass with no other associated changes (Fig. 2–164). If more acute, associated inflammation may surround the mass yielding less distinct borders.

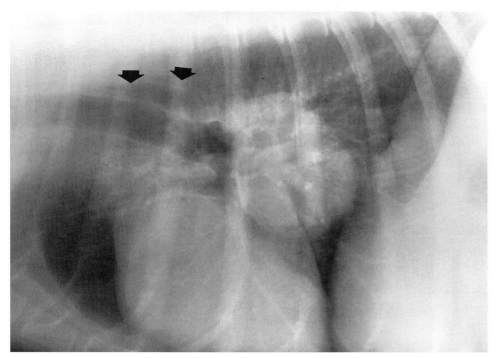

A

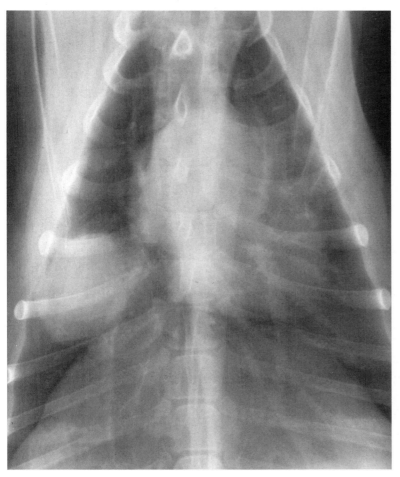

B

Figure 2–160. (A&B) A 10-year-old female mixed breed dog presented with multiple mammary tumors. There is a large soft tissue-dense mass present in the right caudal lung lobe. The margins of the mass are well defined. No other masses are noted. There is a small amount of gas present in the cranial thoracic esophagus (*arrows*). This is a normal finding. **Diagnosis:** Primary lung tumor. Although a solitary large metastatic neoplasm may be encountered, it is much less likely than a primary lung tumor.

Figure 2–161. (A&B) An 8-year-old male German shepherd dog presented with a history of lethargy and collapse. A large soft tissue-dense mass is present in the right cranial lung lobe. There are several areas of calcification noted within this soft tissue-dense mass. There is an increase in density in the right middle lung lobe overlying the cardiac silhouette (*arrows*). This represents atelectasis secondary to bronchial compression by the mass. **Diagnosis:** Primary lung tumor.

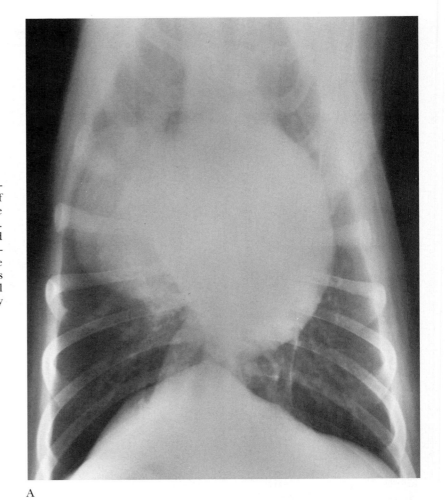

A

B

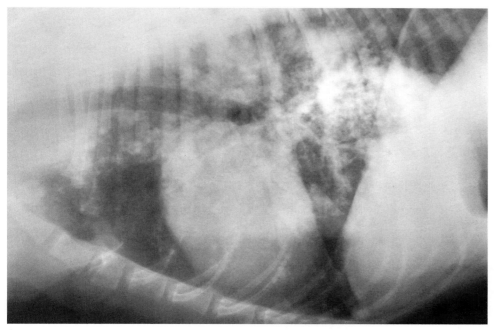

A

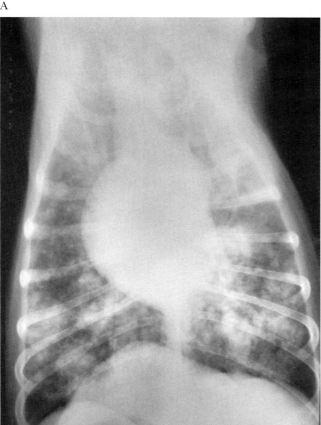

B

Figure 2–162. (A&B) A 12-year-old female mixed breed dog presented with an acute onset of dyspnea, depression, and ataxia. There was a mass present in the area of the left thyroid gland. There is a diffuse increase in pulmonary interstitial density. Discrete nodular soft tissue densities of varying size are scattered throughout the lung. The presence of nodular masses in conjunction with the diffuse interstitial density indicates a diagnosis of metastatic tumor. **Diagnosis:** Metastatic thyroid adenocarcinoma.

DISEASES ASSOCIATED WITH BRONCHIAL PATTERNS

ALLERGIC AND VIRAL BRONCHITIS

A marked peribronchial infiltrate occurs in cats with allergic pulmonary disease (Fig. 2–165).[221,222] This is due to an accumulation of eosinophils and mononuclear inflammatory cells in the bronchial walls and both the peribronchial and interstitial

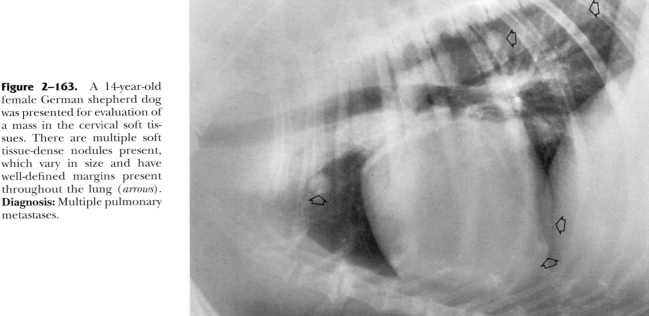

Figure 2–163. A 14-year-old female German shepherd dog was presented for evaluation of a mass in the cervical soft tissues. There are multiple soft tissue-dense nodules present, which vary in size and have well-defined margins present throughout the lung (*arrows*). **Diagnosis:** Multiple pulmonary metastases.

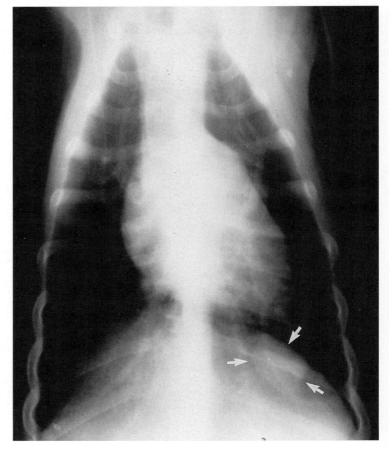

Figure 2–164. A 7-year-old male mixed breed dog presented with a cough of 1 month's duration. The ventrodorsal radiograph revealed a solitary mass in the left caudal lung lobe (*arrows*). Differential considerations included neoplasia, granuloma, or abscess. **Diagnosis:** Pulmonary abscess.

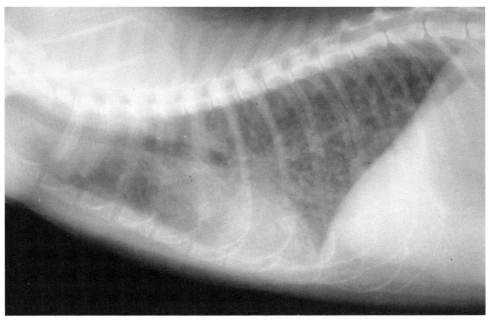

A

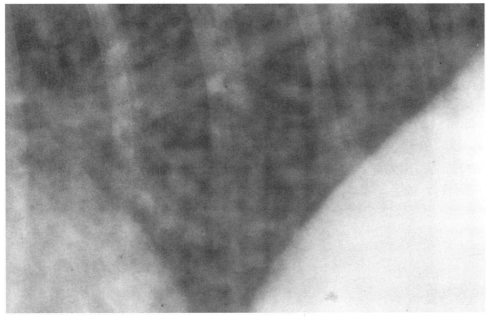

B

Figure 2–165. (A&B) A 4-year-old spayed female domestic shorthair cat presented with acute dyspnea and cyanosis. (A) The lateral radiograph reveals a severe bronchial pattern throughout all lung lobes. (B) The close up view reveals multiple pairs of poorly-defined parallel lines ("tram lines") and circular structures ("doughnuts") indicative of the bronchial and peribronchial infiltrate. **Diagnosis:** Feline "bronchitis/asthma" syndrome.

tissues. If severe, allergic bronchial disease can produce an interstitial edematous infiltrate. If the disease becomes chronic, pulmonary interstitial (peribronchial) fibrosis may result. Viral tracheobronchitis in dogs and most upper respiratory viruses in cats do not produce radiographic changes unless they are complicated by secondary bacterial infection.

Figure 2–166. (A&B) A 5-year-old female cocker spaniel presented with a 6-month history of a cough. There is marked thickening of the bronchial walls with dilation and irregularity of the bronchi (*arrows*). This produces an increased pulmonary interstitial density that obscures the normal pulmonary vascular structures. This is indicative of severe bronchiectasis. **Diagnosis:** Bronchiectasis.

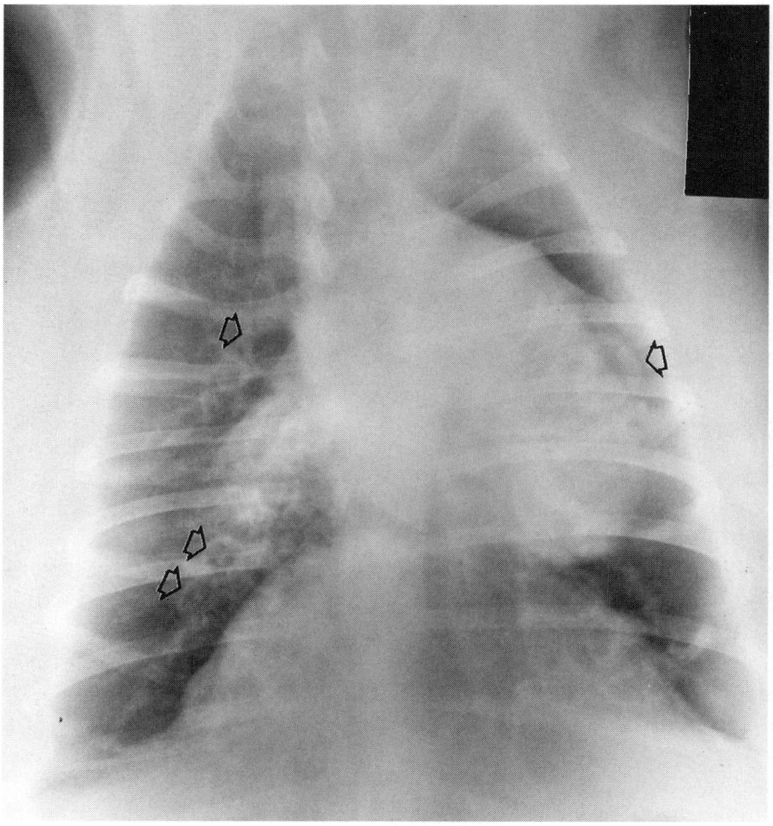

A

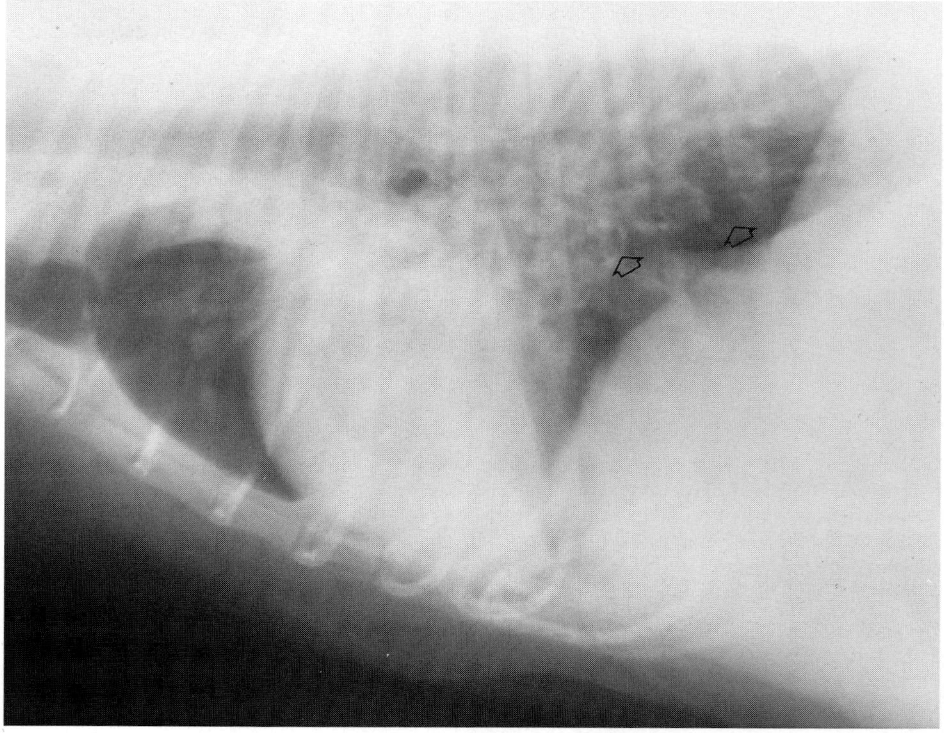

B

BRONCHIAL DYSGENESIS

Bronchial dysgenesis and associated lobar emphysema have been reported. The major radiographic findings have been areas of hyperlucent lung due to emphysema. On necropsy, there were marked bronchial changes including lack of normal cartilage, haphazard arrangements of cartilage, and bronchial torsion.[223,224] Bronchography might be helpful in these cases.

CHRONIC BRONCHITIS

Chronic bronchitis in the dog and cat is typified by the presence of thickened bronchial walls which, when viewed in cross section, appear as circles or tiny nodules with a radiolucent lumen ("doughnuts") or nearly parallel fine radiopaque lines ("tram lines").[225] These findings are common in older individuals but should not be considered "normal aging." Rather, this indicates the frequency of the underlying pathology.

BRONCHIECTASIS

Bronchiectasis represents an unusual bronchial pattern—it is the loss of the normal pattern of bronchial tapering.[181,226–229] Associated with this is a change in bronchial epithelium and mucous characteristics, loss of ciliary function, and bronchial wall thickening (Fig. 2–166). These changes predispose toward chronic bacterial infection with focal or multifocal alveolar or interstitial patterns and both chronic and active interstitial infiltrates.

Both tubular and saccular bronchiectasis have been described. In tubular bronchiectasis, the bronchi are dilated centrally and fail to taper until they do so abruptly in the periphery of the lung (Fig. 2–167).[181] In saccular bronchiectasis, there are focal dilations that are present along the bronchi. Air will be trapped within the focal dilations, and they will appear as round or oval hyperlucent areas (Fig. 2–168). Exudate may also accumulate and produce a mixture of dense and lucent foci within the lung.

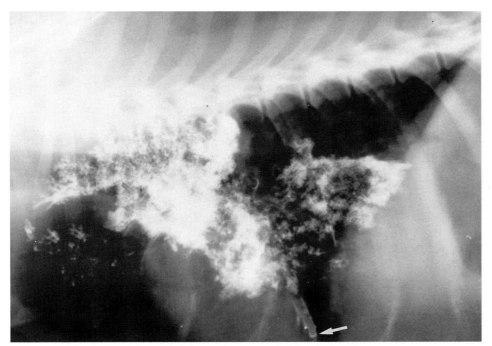

Figure 2–167. A 5-year-old Cairn terrier presented with a chronic cough. Survey radiographs revealed bronchial thickening and a loss of normal tapering. A late-phase view of a bronchogram revealed the dilated bronchus with minimal tapering and acute blunting (*arrow*). This bronchus is too large to be this far in the periphery. The blunting is due to an endobronchial mucus plug. **Diagnosis:** Tubular bronchiectasis.

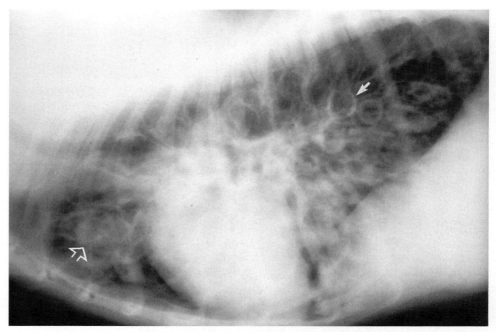

Figure 2–168. A 1-year-old male mixed breed dog presented with a history of chronic respiratory problems. The lateral radiograph revealed multiple, round, thick-walled air-filled structures (*solid arrow*). Some structures were filled with a fluid density (*open arrow*). **Diagnosis:** Saccular bronchiectasis.

Kartagener's syndrome consists of a triad of problems including sinusitis, situs inversus, and bronchiectasis.[226,227,229]

DISEASES ASSOCIATED WITH DECREASED PULMONARY DENSITY

Although abnormal increases in pulmonary density are much more commonly observed and more easily recognized, both focal and diffuse decreases in pulmonary density may be encountered. Usually, a large degree of pathology must be present before the condition can be detected radiographically. Focal areas of decreased pulmonary density may be detected more easily due to the contrast within the surrounding normal lung. Recognizing a generalized decrease in lung density is more difficult. An expiratory radiograph will often accentuate the difference between the normal lung density and the area of lucency.

Intrapulmonary or subpleural bullae or blebs are the most frequently observed focal lucencies, although other cavitary lesions occur. Emphysema is a lesion that is characterized by an abnormal increase in the size of the air spaces distal to the terminal bronchioles—either from dilation of the alveoli or destruction of their walls. It may be focal or diffuse. Decreased blood flow (oligemia) may be focal or diffuse and may result in an apparent decreased pulmonary density, which may be recognized radiographically.

PULMONARY BULLAE AND BLEBS

Pulmonary bullae and blebs produce oval, round, or spherical radiolucent areas with a thin, smooth tissue-dense margin (Fig. 2–169). They may be congenital or secondary to previous trauma or infection.[230] Their smooth, thin wall distinguishes them from other cavitary lesions. Although the term *bulla* usually indicates a lesion within the lung and the term *bleb* usually indicates a subpleural lesion, the terms are often used interchangeably. Pneumomediastinum or pneumothorax may occur as

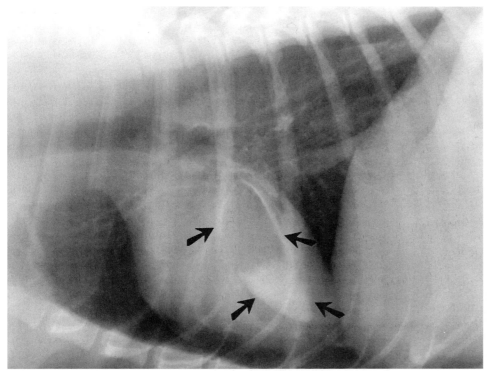

Figure 2–169. A 2-year-old female mixed breed dog was radiographed after thoracic trauma. The dog showed evidence of mild respiratory distress. On the lateral thoracic radiograph there is a fluid- and air-filled structure evident and superimposed on the cardiac silhouette (*arrows*). The structure has thin, soft tissue-dense walls. The cardiac silhouette is separated from the sternum. The left caudal lung lobe is separated from the thoracic vertebral bodies by an air density. **Diagnosis:** Traumatic bulla and pneumothorax.

sequelae to rupture of bullae or blebs. Many traumatic bullae contain both air and fluid. A radiograph obtained using a horizontal x-ray beam may demonstrate the air-fluid interface. Computed tomography has been used to demonstrate bullae that were not apparent on survey radiography.[41]

CAVITARY LESIONS

A tissue-dense mass within the lung may become necrotic and communicate with an airway allowing air accumulation within the mass and producing a cavitary lesion.[231] Cavitation may occur with primary and secondary neoplasms, granulomas, and intrapulmonary abscesses (Figs. 2–170 and 2–171). Cavitary lesions generally have thicker, more irregular walls than bullae or blebs. It is nearly impossible to differentiate the cause of the cavitary lesion based solely on its radiographic features.

EMPHYSEMA

Focal areas of emphysema are uncommon and are usually accompanied by chronic bronchial and interstitial disease (Fig. 2–172). They are often masked by the increased pulmonary density, which results from the bronchial or interstitial infiltrate. Chronic bronchitis and bronchiectasis may result in focal emphysematous areas.

Generalized emphysema, deep inspiration, and over-inflation result in similar radiographic changes. The diaphragm appears flattened and the dome is positioned caudally to approximately the level of T–13 or L–1. The cardiac silhouette often appears small. The lungs appear hyperlucent with well-defined and small pulmonary vessels. Bronchial structures may appear normal, reduced, or increased in number, size, or wall thickness. Radiographs should be obtained at both full inspiration and

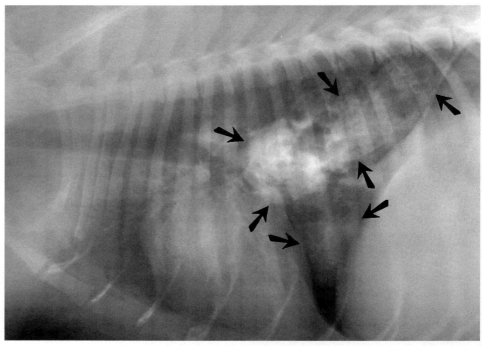

A

Figure 2–170. (A&B) A 2-year-old male cocker spaniel presented with a 6-month history of chronic, productive cough. There are soft tissue densities in the left caudal and accessory lung lobes (*arrows*). There are irregular air-dense cavities within the soft tissue density. The radiographic findings indicate chronic infection with cavitation. This may indicate a foreign body pneumonia. **Diagnosis:** Chronic bacterial pneumonia with a cavitated mass. The left caudal lung lobe was surgically removed because the dog did not respond to antibiotic therapy.

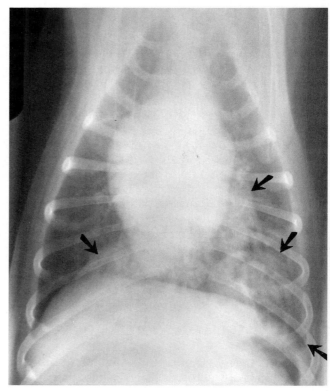

B

expiration when generalized emphysema is suspected. There are many possible underlying causes, which include bronchial dysgenesis.[224,225]

OLIGEMIA

Assessment of lung perfusion is subjective and difficult. Technical errors, variation in thoracic conformation, and alterations resulting from different respiratory phases

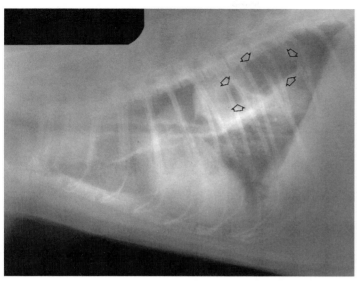
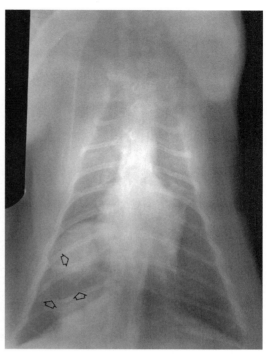

A   B

Figure 2–171. (A&B) A 6-year-old male cat that was presented with a 4-month history of intermittent pyrexia and cough. On the (A) lateral and (b) ventrodorsal radiographs there is a soft tissue density in the right caudal lung lobe. There are multiple air-containing cavities within this soft tissue density (*arrows*). The margins of the soft tissue density are well-defined. The radiographic findings indicate a large cavitated mass. This may represent a pulmonary abscess or a neoplasm. **Diagnosis:** Abscessed right caudal lung lobe.

complicate the evaluation. A decrease in lung perfusion may be focal or diffuse. A diffuse reduction in lung perfusion is most often associated with right-to-left cardiac shunts (Eisenmenger's complex), decreased pulmonary blood flow (pulmonic stenosis), or decreased circulating blood volume (hypovolemia).

Focal reduction in pulmonary perfusion usually is due to pulmonary thrombosis. Although associated radiographic changes are uncommon, radiographic signs may occasionally be present. These signs include uneven vascular diameters, unequal-sized pulmonary arteries (when right and left lung lobes are compared), a small pulmonary vein when compared to the adjacent pulmonary artery, absence of vascular shadows within a normal-sized lung lobe, and an enlarged central pulmonary artery with abrupt reduction in arterial diameter (Fig. 2–173).[196] Right-sided cardiomegaly with or without main pulmonary artery enlargement and pleural fluid may also be present.

DISEASES ASSOCIATED WITH PULMONARY CALCIFICATION

Calcification may occur within normal pulmonary structures as well as in intrapulmonary lesions. It may be associated with normal aging changes, pulmonary diseases, or systemic disorders.

Calcification of the main stem bronchi may be present in dogs of any age; however, the degree of calcification and the number of smaller bronchi that become calcified usually increases with age. Thin linear and circular calcified densities become apparent (Fig. 2–174). Small nodular calcifications may also be evident in thoracic radiographs of aged dogs. These may be pleural or intrapulmonary and are probably either osteomata or calcified granulomas resulting from previous inflammation.[41] They are without clinical significance but must be differentiated from other active granulomas and neoplasms. The density of the nodules combined with their

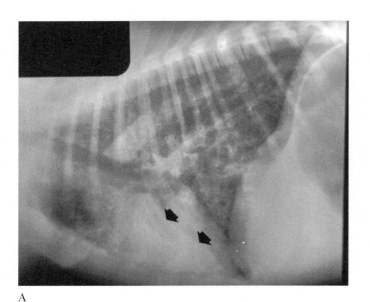

A

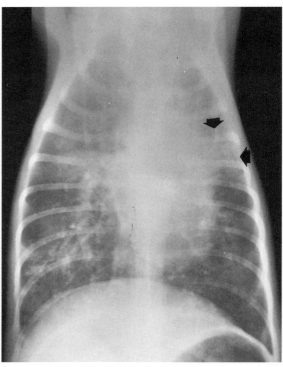

B

Figure 2–172. A 1-year-old male Shetland sheepdog presented with a 6-month history of cough. There is a severe bronchial pattern with bronchial thickening and calcification. Multiple peribronchial and interstitial densities are present throughout the lung lobes. The diaphragm is flattened and displaced caudally. There is a localized area of alveolar infiltrate evident in the caudal subsegment of the left cranial lung lobe (*arrows*). The radiographic findings are suggestive of bacterial pneumonia with interstitial fibrosis and hyperinflation due to chronic emphysema. **Diagnosis:** Chronic bacterial pneumonia and emphysema.

Figure 2–173. (A&B) A 5-year-old cat presented with acute respiratory distress. On two ventrodorsal thoracic radiographs there is a decrease in density within the right lung lobes. The pulmonary arteries and veins in the left lung lobes are evident (*arrows*); the right caudal lung lobe artery is small and the pulmonary vein is not identified. The radiographic findings are indicative of oligemia of the right lung lobes with hyperinflation. **Diagnosis:** Thrombosis of the pulmonary artery in the right caudal lung lobe. The diagnosis was confirmed by a selective arteriogram. The etiology was not determined.

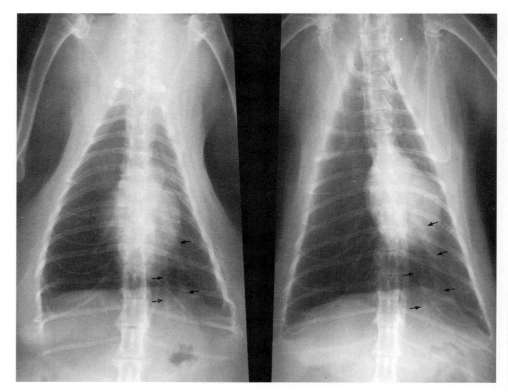

A   B

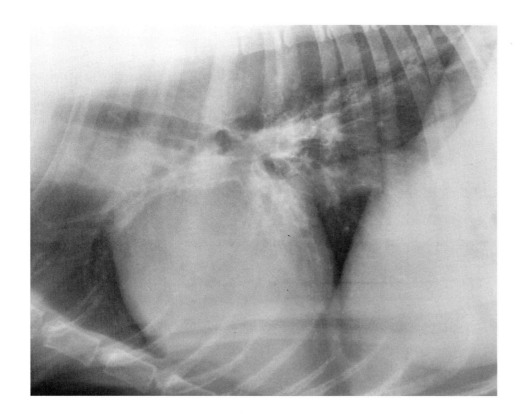

Figure 2–174. An 11-year-old male pit bull presented for weakness and muffled heart sounds. On a close-up photograph of the lateral thoracic radiograph there are areas of bronchial calcification evident. These are common findings in an older dog. There were no thoracic abnormalities. **Diagnosis:** Bronchial calcification.

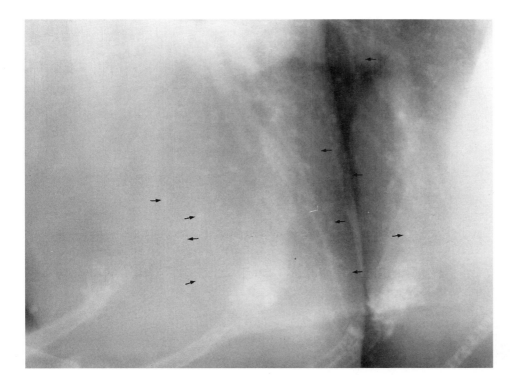

Figure 2–175. A 13-year-old female mixed breed dog presented with multiple mammary tumors. A close-up view of the lateral thoracic radiograph reveals multiple small mineralized densities superimposed over the cardiac silhouette (*arrows*). The small uniform size and calcified density of these nodules indicate that they are pulmonary or pleural osteomas. There is no evidence of pulmonary metastasis. **Diagnosis:** Pulmonary or pleural osteomas.

small, usually uniform size and distinct margins identifies them as pulmonary or pleural osteomas rather than neoplasms (Fig. 2–175).

Fungal granulomas, parasitic granulomas, primary and metastatic neoplasm, and abscesses may become partially or completely calcified.[214] Tracheobronchial lymph node calcification has also been observed (see Fig. 2–156).[214]

Systemic diseases, such as Cushing's disease, primary and secondary hyperparathyroidism, and hypervitaminosis D, can produce varying degrees of intrapulmonary calcification. These changes usually are distributed evenly throughout the lung and involve the bronchial walls and pulmonary interstitial tissue. Small nodular calcifications may be present.[232] Many of these animals have other soft tissue calcifications (e.g., vascular or subcutaneous). Some instances of rapidly progressive pulmonary calcification have been described in which the etiology was not established.

CERVICAL SOFT TISSUE ABNORMALITIES

PHARYNGEAL ABNORMALITIES

Abnormalities of the oral or nasal pharynx may produce clinical signs indicating either respiratory or swallowing disorders or a combination of both. Respiratory disorders may result from pharyngeal or retropharyngeal masses, swelling, foreign bodies, or trauma. Swallowing disorders rarely produce radiographic changes unless they are due to pharyngeal masses.

A carefully positioned lateral view with the animal's head and neck extended provides the most useful information. Ventrodorsal and dorsoventral views are rarely helpful. Slight rotation or flexion of the head and neck can produce artifactual increases in laryngeal density and create an illusion of a soft tissue mass. If the animal is swallowing at the time of radiographic exposure, the normal pharyngeal airway may be artifactually eliminated. Thus, all abnormalities identified should be confirmed with a well-positioned, properly exposed lateral radiograph (Fig. 2–176). Both pharyngeal and laryngeal abnormalities may occur without apparent radiographic changes. Endoscopy should be performed regardless of the radiographic findings if clinical signs indicate an abnormality in these areas.

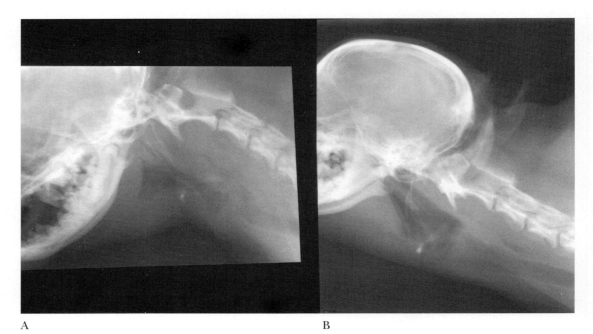

A   B

Figure 2–176. A 5-year-old female Chihuahua was presented with a respiratory stridor of 2 weeks' duration. Lateral radiographs of the larynx were obtained. (A) The initial lateral radiograph of the larynx was obtained with the animal's neck flexed. The oral pharynx appears to be compressed. The larynx is indistinct. A mass in the oral pharynx was suspected. (B) A second lateral radiograph was obtained with the head and neck extended. The laryngeal structures appear normal in this radiograph. **Diagnosis:** Normal larynx.

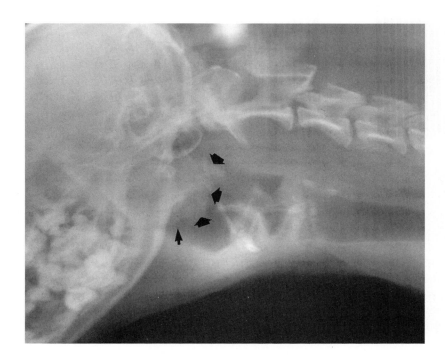

Figure 2–177. An 11-year-old female mixed breed dog presented with a history of respiratory distress, which had gradually increased over a 3-month period. There is a large soft tissue mass in the region of the caudal nasal and oral pharynx (*arrows*). This mass appears to be attached to the caudal aspect of the soft palate and is obliterating both the oral and nasal pharynx. No other abnormalities are noted. **Diagnosis:** Melanoma.

FOREIGN BODIES

Radiopaque foreign objects (e.g., bones or metallic objects) are readily identified. Their location should be confirmed on a ventrodorsal as well as a lateral radiograph. Subcutaneous or retropharyngeal air or soft tissue swelling may be visible if mucosal penetration has occurred. Detecting tissue-dense foreign material may be impossible if it is completely embedded into the pharyngeal soft tissues. However, the air normally present within the pharynx should outline these objects if they project into the pharyngeal lumen. Soft tissue swelling or retropharyngeal masses may result from trauma to the pharynx secondary to a foreign body.

MASSES

Intraluminal and retropharyngeal masses may narrow the pharyngeal lumen (Fig. 2–177). These may be associated with the tonsils, retropharyngeal lymph nodes, or salivary glands, or may arise from the pharyngeal mucosa or surrounding muscles. A decreased pharyngeal airway, displacement of the soft palate, larynx, or hyoid bones, or distortion of the pharyngeal shape may be observed radiographically (Fig. 2–178). If the mucosal surface of the pharynx is intact, the margins of the mass will be smooth. Irregularity of the margin and air within the mass indicates that the mucosal surface has been penetrated. The surrounding bony structures (i.e., skull, cervical vertebrae, hyoid bones) should be evaluated carefully for radiographic evidence of involvement.

SOFT PALATE

Elongation or swelling of the soft palate may be recognized radiographically. Careful positioning is mandatory when attempting to evaluate the position of the soft palate and larynx. In the normal dog, the rostral tip of the epiglottis should reach the caudal aspect of the soft palate. An elongated soft palate will extend beyond the epiglottis and into the laryngeal airway. The soft palate may also be thickened; however, this is an ambiguous radiographic change because the thickness of the soft

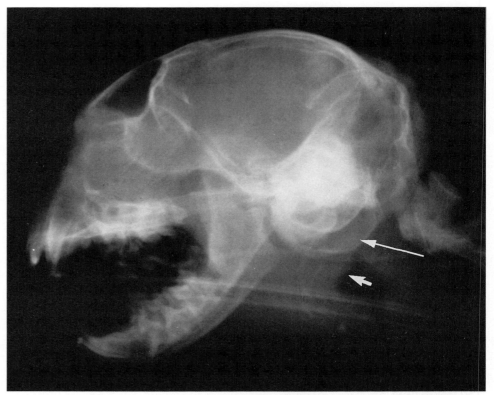

Figure 2–178. A 1-year-old neutered male domestic shorthair cat presented with a chronic nasal discharge. The lateral view reveals the presence of a tissue-dense mass in the nasopharynx (*short arrow*) and a tissue density within the osseous bulla (*long arrow*). **Diagnosis:** Auropharyngeal polyp.

palate can vary with the stage of normal respiration. A diagnosis of soft palate thickening requires persistent thickening on several sequential radiographs. Visual inspection of the palate is more reliable than radiography for evaluating soft palate thickness.

LARYNGEAL ABNORMALITIES

Laryngeal abnormalities may occur as a result of pharyngeal or retropharyngeal diseases as well as with intrinsic laryngeal disease. Therefore, the pharyngeal region should always be included and evaluated when the laryngeal area is radiographed. Laryngeal anatomy is complicated but most structures can be evaluated. The hyoid bones, laryngeal cartilages, and airway should be evaluated carefully. Artifacts induced by malpositioning and those resulting from swallowing motions during radiography frequently create an illusion of laryngeal disease. A suspicious area should be identified on at least two radiographs with the animal's head and neck extended. Visual inspection of the laryngeal airway and surrounding structures usually provides more information than radiography; however, lesions arising from the soft tissues around the larynx or from the bony structures can be best evaluated radiographically.

HYOID BONES

The hyoid bones can be readily evaluated. They are usually symmetrical and uniformly mineralized. Although hyoid bone abnormalities are rare, these bones may be fractured or dislocated in association with laryngeal trauma. This most often oc-

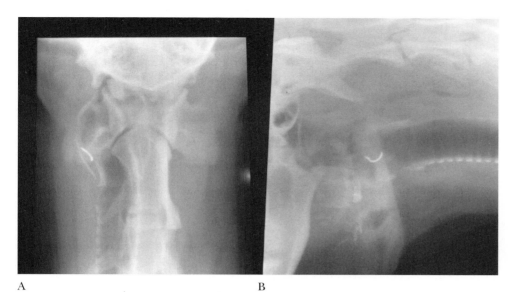

A   B

Figure 2–179. (A&B) A 4-year-old female mixed breed dog presented with a history of having swallowed a fish hook. (A) Ventrodorsal and (B) lateral radiographs of the laryngeal area revealed gas and mineralized densities within the soft tissues overlying the larynx. This was due to a previous surgical attempt at removal of the fish hook. The fish hook fragment can be seen in the larynx on the right side. It appears to be contained within the thyroid cartilage area. **Diagnosis:** Opaque foreign object in the larynx. This foreign object was identified and removed by endoscopy.

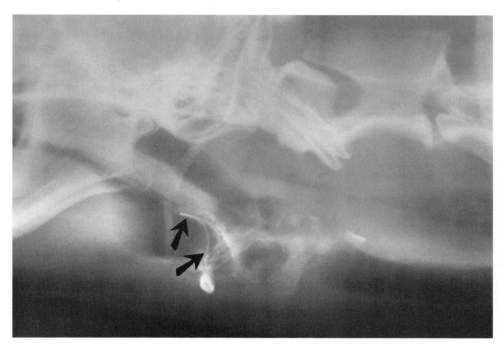

Figure 2–180. A 13-year-old male miniature schnauzer presented with a history of chronic cough. On the lateral radiograph of the larynx there is a radiopaque foreign object ventral to the epiglottis (*arrows*). This was identified as a fragment of a plastic catheter that was imbedded in the epiglottis. It was secondary to a previous transtracheal aspiration. **Diagnosis:** Laryngeal foreign body.

curs secondary to bite wounds or choke chain injuries. Avulsion of the hyoid bones from the larynx may be observed. Soft tissue tumors are rare; however, they may displace or destroy the hyoid bones. Infection rarely affects hyoid bones.

FOREIGN BODIES

Radiopaque foreign bodies are easily detected and should be identified on both lateral and ventrodorsal radiographs (Figs. 2–179 and 2–180). Tissue-dense foreign material may mimic laryngeal masses, inflammation, edema, or hemorrhage. Laryngoscopy is recommended if a foreign object is suspected.

LARYNGEAL MASSES

Laryngeal tumors and granulomas may arise from or involve the epiglottis, laryngeal cartilages, or vocal folds.[233] The soft tissue-dense mass will obliterate at least part of

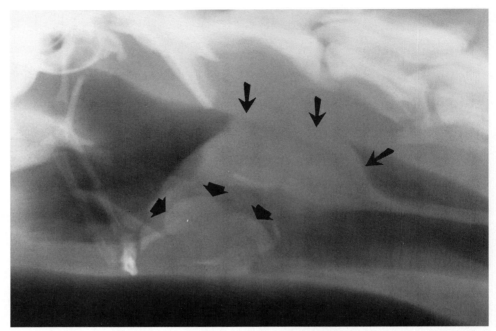

Figure 2–181. A 2-year-old male Labrador retriever was presented with a 1.5 year history of progressive respiratory disorder. There is a large soft tissue-dense mass in the region of the laryngeal cartilages (*wide arrows*). It appears to involve both the arytenoid and thyroid cartilages. A second soft tissue-dense mass is evident dorsal to the cricoid cartilage (*long arrows*). The esophagus caudal to this mass contains a small bolus of air. **Diagnosis:** Granuloma.

the laryngeal airway and may distort the normal architecture. Distinction between neoplasms and granulomata cannot be made based on radiographic changes (Fig. 2–181).

LARYNGEAL SWELLING

Edema, hemorrhage, or inflammation of the larynx may produce similar radiographic signs. The airway will become more dense and the laryngeal ventricles will be obliterated. The swelling must be severe before it can be detected radiographically. In most normal brachycephalic dogs, the larynx is indistinct and recognition of mucosal swelling or edema is difficult. Eversion of the laryngeal saccule is rarely identified but may produce obliteration of the normal air density and mimic laryngeal edema.

LARYNGEAL STENOSIS

Congenital or acquired laryngeal stenosis may deform the larynx and narrow or obliterate the airway. Acquired stenosis may occur following trauma or laryngeal surgery. The luminal deformity or irregular cartilaginous calcification may be recognized radiographically.

LARYNGEAL PARALYSIS

Laryngeal paralysis does not usually produce any radiographic abnormalities. The shape of the lateral ventricles may become more rounded instead of elliptical or may be obliterated. Obstruction of the laryngeal airway may result in distention of the pharynx as the animal attempts to inhale. The cervical trachea may narrow and the thoracic trachea may dilate if resistance to airflow is marked.

EXTRALUMINAL MASSES

Displacement of the larynx from its normal position may be associated with lesions arising from the pharynx or retropharyngeal area. Unfortunately, the position of the larynx varies greatly in normal animals depending on the head and neck position. When obvious displacement is present, the direction in which the larynx is displaced provides a clue to the origin of the mass.

THYROID AND PARATHYROID DISORDERS

Thyroid masses in dogs are usually large by the time of diagnosis. They may displace the trachea and be apparent on survey radiographs. Sonography can be useful in evaluating the thyroid. The normal thyroid gland appears normally shaped and fairly small (Fig. 2–182). Masses may be unilateral or bilateral (Figs. 2–183 and 2-184).

Feline hyperthyroidism is typified by diffuse enlargement (but not massive enlargement) of one or both thyroid glands. Sonography has been used to define size and determine if cystic areas are present within the glands (Fig. 2–185).[234]

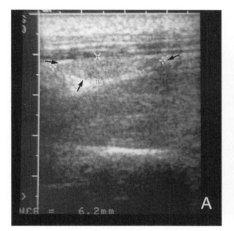
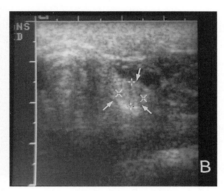

Figure 2–182. A 2-year-old male Chesapeake Bay retriever presented with polyuria, polydipsia, lethargy, weight loss, and hypercalcemia. Longitudinal (A) and transverse (B) sonograms of the left thyroid reveal a hyperechoic structure in the area of the thyroid. The size and architecture are normal. **Diagnosis:** Normal thyroid gland.

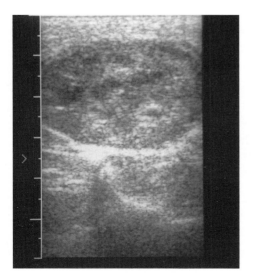

Figure 2–183. An 8-year-old spayed female chow chow presented with a cervical mass of 3-month duration. A transverse sonogram revealed an enlarged thyroid gland with complex architecture with multiple hypoechoic to anechoic areas. This may be due to hyperplasia or neoplasia with cystic areas. **Diagnosis:** Thyroid carcinoma.

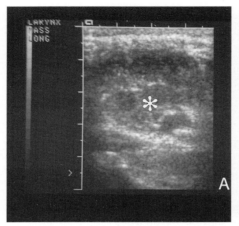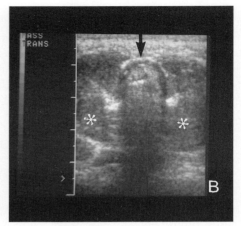

Figure 2–184. A 12-year-old spayed female mixed breed dog presented for panting and gagging. A palpable mass was present in the laryngeal region. Longitudinal (A) and transverse (B) sonograms revealed a mass (*) with complex architecture on both sides of the trachea (*arrow*). The area distal to the trachea on the transverse view is obscured by the presence of air in the trachea. **Diagnosis:** Thyroid carcinoma.

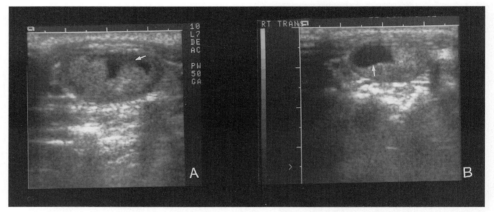

Figure 2–185. A 12-year-old spayed female domestic shorthair cat presented for a cervical swelling of 2-week duration. The longitudinal (A) and transverse (B) sonograms reveal an enlarged thyroid gland that contains an irregularly shaped anechoic structure (*arrow*). **Diagnosis:** Thyroid hyperplasia with cyst formation.

Sonography has also been used to identify enlarged parathyroid glands.[235] Abnormal glands were enlarged when compared to others in the opposite thyroid and were markedly hypoechoic.

SWALLOWING DISORDERS

Swallowing is a complex event that involves the pharynx, larynx, and esophagus. It cannot be evaluated without contrast administration and almost always requires a dynamic examination using cine or video fluoroscopy. The events must be examined slowly and repeatedly before a definite diagnosis can be reached. An esophagram with a single radiograph or series of radiographs may identify the site (i.e., oral, pharyngeal or esophageal) of the abnormality, but it rarely defines the functional problem. Therefore, patients with oral or pharyngeal dysphagia should be referred to hospitals that have fluoroscopic equipment.

Retention of food or barium in the oral pharynx suggests an oropharyngeal disorder. Contrast or food in the nasal pharynx may indicate the failure of the soft palate to close the nasal pharynx or it may indicate incoordination between pharyngeal muscle contraction and dorsal movement of the soft palate. Abnormal cricopharyngeal muscular activity may produce a cricopharyngeal achalasia (failure of the muscle to relax), chalazia (failure to contract with resulting sphincter incompetence), or incoordination between the pharyngeal muscle contraction and cricopharyngeal muscle relaxation. Aspiration of food or barium may indicate a lack of normal laryngeal movement, incoordination between the pharyngeal muscles and laryngeal muscles, or a sensory defect that does not allow the animal to detect the presence of food within the pharynx. Both liquid barium and barium-impregnated dog food should be used when studying animals with oropharyngeal disorders. Again, because of the complex nature of swallowing, static radiographs rarely produce a definite diagnosis.

REFERENCES

1. Spencer CP, Ackerman N, Burt JK. The canine lateral thoracic radiograph. Vet Radiol 1981;22:262.
2. Forrest LJ. Radiology corner—Advantages of the three view thoracic radiographic examination in instances other than metastasis. Vet Radiol 1992;33:340.
3. Biller DS, Myer CW. Case examples demonstrating the clinical utility of obtaining both right and left lateral thoracic radiographs in small animals. JAAHA 1987;23:381.
4. Lang L, Wortman JA, Glickman LT, et al. Sensitivity of radiographic detection of lung metastases in the dog. Vet Radiol 1986;27:74.
5. Barthez PY, Hornof WJ, Theon AP, et al. Receiver operating characteristic curve analysis of the performance of various radiographic protocols when screening dogs for pulmonary metastases. JAVMA 1994;204:237.
6. Grandage J. Posture, gravity, and radiologic interpretation. JAVRS 1979;22:80.
7. Ahlberg NE, Hoppe F, Kelter U, et al. A computed tomographic study of volume and x-ray attenuation of the lungs of beagles in various body positions. Vet Radiol 1985;26:43.
8. Pechman RD. Effect of dependency versus nondependency on lung lesion visualization. Vet Radiol 1987;28:185.
9. Steyn PF, Green RW. How patient positioning affects radiographic signs of canine lung disease. Vet Med 1990;85:796.
10. Grandage J. The radiology of the dog's diaphragm. JSAP 1974;15:1.
11. Suter PF. Radiographic examination. In: Ettinger SJ, Suter PF, eds. Canine cardiology. Philadelphia:WB Saunders Co, 1970;40.
12. Suter PF. Thoracic radiography: A text atlas of thoracic diseases in the dog and cat. Wettswil, Switzerland:Peter F Suter, 1984.
13. Carlisle CH, Thrall DE. A comparison of normal feline thoracic radiographs made in dorsal versus ventral recumbency. Vet Radiol 1982;23:3.
14. Ruehl WW, Thrall DE. The effect of dorsal versus ventral recumbency on the radiographic appearance of the canine thorax. Vet Radiol 1981;22:10.
15. Holmes RA, Smith FG, Lewis RE, et al. The effects of rotation on the radiographic appearance of the canine cardiac silhouette in dorsal recumbency. Vet Radiol 1985;26:98.
16. Silverman S, Suter PF. Influence of inspiration and expiration on canine thoracic radiographs. JAVMA 1975;166:502.
17. Fox PR, Bond BR, Peterson ME. Echocardiographic reference values in healthy cats sedated with ketamine hydrochloride. AJVR 1985;46:1479.
18. Moise NS. Echocardiography. In: Fox PR, ed. Canine and feline cardiology. New York:Churchill Livingstone Co, 1988;114.
19. Thomas WP. Two-dimensional, real-time echocardiography in the dog: Technique and anatomic validation. Vet Radiol 1984;25;50.
20. Thomas WP, Gaber CE, Jacobs GJ, et al. Recommendations for standards in transthoracic two-dimensional echocardiography in the dog and cat. JVIM 1993;7;247.
21. Stowater JL, Lamb CR. Ultrasonography of noncardiac thoracic diseases in small animals. JAVMA 1989;195:514.
22. Burk RL. Radiographic definition of the phrenicopericardiac ligament. JAVRS 1976;6:216.
23. Smallwood JE, George TF. Anatomic atlas for computed tomography in the mesaticephalic dog: Thorax and cranial abdomen. Vet Radiol Ultrasound 1993;34:65.
24. Feeney DA, Fletcher TF, Hardy, RM. Atlas of correlative imaging anatomy of the normal dog. Philadelphia: WB Saunders Co, 1991.
25. Suter PF, Colgrove DJ, Ewing GO. Congenital hypoplasia of the canine trachea. JAAHA 1972;20:773.
26. Burk RL, Corwin LA, Bahr RJ, et al. The right cranial lung lobe bronchus of the dog: Its identification in a lateral chest radiograph. JAVRS 1978;6:210.
27. Toal RL, Losonsky JM, Coulter DB, et al. Influence of cardiac cycle on the radiographic appearance of the feline heart. Vet Radiol 1985;26:63.
28. Ahlberg NE, Hansson K, Svensson L, et al. Radiographic heart-volume estimation in normal cats. Vet Radiol 1989;30:253.
29. Moon ML, Keene BW, Lessard P, et al. Age related changes in the feline cardiac silhouette. Vet Radiol Ultrasound 1993;34:315.

30. Buchanan JW, Bucheler H. Vertebral scale system to measure canine heart size in radiographs. JAVMA 1995;206:194.
31. Bonagura JD, O'Grady MR, Herring DS. Echocardiography: Principles of interpretation. VCNA 1985;15:1177.
32. Boon J, Wingfield WE, Miller CW. Echocardiographic indices in the normal dog. Vet Radiol 1983;24:214.
33. Piper FS, Reef V, Hamlin RL. Echocardiography in the domestic cat. AJVR 1979;40:882.
34. Jacobs G, Knight DV. M-mode echocardiographic measurements in nonanesthetized healthy cats: Effects of body weight, heart rate, and other variables. AJVR 1985;46:1705.
35. DeMadron E, Bonagura JD, Herring DS. Two-dimensional echocardiography in the normal cat. Vet Radiol 1985;26:149.
36. Morrison SA, Moise NS, Scarlett J, et al. Effect of breed and body weight on echocardiographic values in four breeds of dogs of differing somatype. JVIM 1992;6:220.
37. Kirberger RM, Bland-van den Berg P, Darazs B. Doppler echocardiography in the normal dog: Part I, velocity findings and flow patterns. Vet Radiol Ultrasound 1992;33:370.
38. Gaber C. Doppler echocardiography. Prob Vet Med 1991;3:479.
39. Koblik PD, Hornoff W, Harnagel SH, et al. A comparison of pulmonary angiography, digital subtraction angiography and 99M-Tc—DTPA/MAA ventilation-perfusion scintigraphy for detection of experimental pulmonary emboli in the dog. Vet Radiol 1989;30:159.
40. McKiernan BC, Johnson LR. Clinical pulmonary function testing in dogs and cats. VCNA 1992;22:1087.
41. Reif JS, Rhodes WH. The lungs of aged dogs: A radiographic-morphologic correlation. JAVRS 1966;7:5.
42. Burk RL. Computed tomography of thoracic diseases in dogs. JAVMA 1991;199:617.
43. O'Brien JA, Harvey CE, Tucker JA. The larynx of the dog: Its normal radiographic anatomy. JAVRS 1969;10:38.
44. Anderson M, Payne JT, Mann FA, et al. Flail chest: Pathophysiology, treatment and prognosis. Comp Cont Ed 1993;15:65.
45. Fossum TW, Boudrieau RJ, Hobson HP. Pectus excavatum in eight dogs and six cats. JAAHA 1989;25:595.
46. Evans SM, Biery DN. Congenital peritoneopericardial diaphragmatic hernia in the dog: A literature review and 17 additional case histories. Vet Radiol 1980;21:108.
47. Garson HL, Dodman HN, Baker OJ. Diaphragmatic hernia, analysis of 56 cases in dogs and cats. JSAP 1980;21:469.
48. Wilson GP, Newton CD, Burt JK. A review of 116 diaphragmatic hernias in dogs and cats. JAVMA 1971;159:1142.
49. Sullivan M, Lee R. Radiological features of 80 cases of diaphragmatic rupture. JSAP 1989;30:561.
50. Rendano VT. Positive contrast peritoneography: An aid in the radiographic diagnosis of diaphragmatic hernia. Vet Radiol 1979;20:67.
51. Ackerman N, Millman T. Esophageal hiatal hernia in a dog. Vet Radiol 1982;23:107.
52. Miles KG, Pope ER, Jergens AE. Paraesophageal hiatal hernia and pyloric obstruction in a dog. JAVMA 1988;193:1437.
53. Waldron DR, Moon M, Leib MS, et al. Oesophageal hiatal hernia in two cats. JSAP 1990;31:259.
54. Burnie AG, Simpson JW, Corcoran BM. Gastro-oesophageal reflux and hiatus hernia associated with laryngeal paralysis in a dog. JSAP 1989;30:414.
55. Callan MB, Washabau RJ, Saunders HM, et al. Congenital esophageal hiatal hernia in the Chinese shar-pei dog. JVIM 1993;7:210.
56. Berry CR, Koblik PD, Ticer JW. Dorsal peritoneopericardial mesothelial remnant as an aid to the diagnosis of feline congenital peritoneopericardial diaphragmatic hernia. Vet Radiol 1990;31:239.
57. Hay WH, Woodfield JA, Moon MA. Clinical, echocardiographic and radiographic findings of peritoneopericardial diaphragmatic hernia in two dogs and a cat. JAVMA 1989;195:1245.
58. Berry CR, Gaschan FP, Ackerman N. Radiographic and ultrasonographic features of hypertrophic feline muscular dystrophy in two cats. Vet Radiol Ultrasound 1992;33:357.
59. Lord PF, Suter PF, Chan KF, et al. Pleural, extrapleural and pulmonary lesions in small animals: A radiographic approach to differential diagnosis. JAVRS 1972;13:4.
60. Thrall DE, Goldschmidt MH. Mesothelioma in the dog: Six case reports. JAVRS 1978;19:107.
61. Groves TF, Ticer JW. Pleural fluid movement: Its effect on the appearance of ventrodorsal and dorsoventral radiographic projections. Vet Radiol 1983;24:99.
62. Snyder PS, Sato T, Atkins CE. The utility of thoracic radiographic measurement for the detection of cardiomegaly in cats with pleural effusion. Vet Radiol 1990;31:89.
63. Glaus TM, Rawlings CA, Mahaffey EA, et al. Acute thymic hemorrhage and hemothorax in a dog. JAAHA 1993;29:489.
64. Glaus TM, Jacobs GJ, Rawlings CA, et al. Surgical removal of heartworms from a cat with caval syndrome. JAVMA 1995;206:663.
65. Bunch SE, Metcalf MR, Crane SW, et al. Idiopathic pleural effusion and pulmonary thromboembolism in a dog with autoimmune hemolytic anemia. JAVMA 1989;195:1748.
66. Fossum TW. Severe bilateral fibrosing pleuritis associated with chronic chylothorax in five cats and two dogs. JAVMA 1992;201:317.
67. Lord PF, Greiner TP, Greene RW, et al. Lung lobe torsion in the dog. JAAHA 1973;9:473.
68. Stobie D, Carpenter JL. Lymphangiosarcoma of the mediastinum, mesentery, and omentum in a cat with chylothorax. JAAHA 1993;29:78.
69. Myer CW. Pneumothorax: A radiography review. JAVRS 1978;19:12.
70. Fagin BD. A radiographic approach to diagnosing pneumomediastinum. Vet Med 1988;83:571.
71. Forrester SD. Pneumothorax in a dog with a pulmonary abscess and suspected infective endocarditis. JAVMA 1992;200:351.

72. Dallman MJ, Martin RA, Roth L. Pneumothorax as the primary problem in two cases of bronchoalveolar carcinoma in the dog. JAAHA 1988;24:710.

73. Holtsinger RH, Beale BS, Bellah JS, et al. Spontaneous pneumothorax in the dog: A retrospective analysis of 21 cases. JAAHA 1993;29:195.

74. Salisbury SK, Forbes S, Blevins WE. Peritracheal abscess associated with tracheal collapse and bilateral laryngeal paralysis in a dog. JAVMA 1990;196:1273.

75. Postorino NC, Wheeler SL, Park RD, et al. A syndrome resembling lymphomatoid granulomatosis in the dog. JVIM 1989;3:15.

76. Liu SK, Patnaik AK, Burk RL. Thymic branchial cysts in the dog and cat. JAVMA 1983;182:1095.

77. O'Dair HA, Holt PE, Pearson GR, et al. Acquired immune mediated myasthenia gravis in a cat associated with a cystic thymus. JSAP 1991;32:202.

78. Scott-Moncrieff JC, Cook JR, Lantz GC. Acquired myasthenia gravis in a cat with a thymoma. JAVMA 1990;196:1291.

79. Shaiken LC, Evans SM, Goldschmidt MH. Radiographic findings in canine malignant histiocytosis. Vet Radiol 1991;32:237.

80. Mason GD, Lamb CR, Jakowski RM. Fatal mediastinal hemorrhage in a dog. Vet Radiol 1990;31:214.

81. van den Broek A. Pneumomediastinum in seventeen dogs: Etiology and radiographic signs. JSAP 1986;27:747.

82. Harvey CE. Inherited and congenital airway conditions. JSAP 1989;30;184.

83. Coyne BE, Fingland RB. Hypoplasia of the trachea in dogs: 103 cases. JAVMA 1992;201:768.

84. Okin R. Pseudomembranous tracheitis resembling collapsed trachea in a golden retriever. Canine Pract 1985;12:22.

85. Carlisle CH, Biery DN, Thrall DE. Tracheal and laryngeal tumors in the dog and cat: Literature review and 13 additional patients. Vet Radiol 1991;32:1991.

86. Lappin MR, Prestwood AK. *Oslerus osleri*: Clinical case, attempted transmission and epidemiology. JAAHA 1988;24:153.

87. Dimski DS. Tracheal obstruction caused by tree needles in a cat. JAVMA 1991;199:477.

88. Lotti U, Niebauer GW Tracheobronchial foreign bodies of plant origin in 153 hunting dogs. Comp Cont Ed 1992;14:900.

89. Cantwell HD. Metrizamide insufflation bronchography: A new diagnostic approach. Vet Radiol 1981;22:184.

90. Myer W, Burt JK, Davis GQ. A comparative study of propyliodone and barium bronchography in the dog. JAVRS 1974;15:44.

91. O'Brien JA, Buchanan JW, Kelly DF. Tracheal collapse in the dog. JAVRS 1966;7:12.

92. Hendricks JC, O'Brien JA. Tracheal collapse in two cats. JAVMA 1985;187:418.

93. Zawie DA. Medical diseases of the esophagus. Comp Cont Ed 1987;9:1146.

94. Bartges JW, Nielson DL. Reversible megaesophagus associated with atypical primary hypoadrenocorticism in a dog. JAVMA 1992;201:889.

95. Van Gundy T. Vascular ring anomalies. Comp Cont Ed 1989;11:36.

96. Hurley K, Miller MW, Willard MD, et al. Left aortic arch and right ligamentum arteriosum esophageal obstruction in a dog. JAVMA 1993;203:410.

97. Fingeroth JM, Fossum TW. Late-onset regurgitation associated with persistent right aortic arch in two dogs. JAVMA 1987;191:981.

98. Hardie EM, Greene RT, Ford RB. Balloon dilatation for treatment of esophageal stricture: A case report. JAAHA 1987;23:547.

99. Burk RL, Zawie DA, Garvey MS. Balloon catheter dilation of intramural esophageal strictures in the dog and cat: A description of the procedure and a report of six cases. Semin Vet Med Surg 1987;2:241.

100. Ridgeway RL, Suter PF. Clinical and radiographic signs in primary and metastatic esophageal neoplasms of the dog. JAVMA 1979;174:700.

101. Fernandes FH, Hawe RS, Loeb WF. Primary squamous cell carcinoma of the esophagus in a cat. Comp Anim Pract 1987;1:16.

102. Wilson RB, Holcher MA, Laney PS. Esophageal osteosarcoma in a dog. JAAHA 1991;27:361.

103. Johnson RC. Canine spirocercosis and associated esophageal sarcoma. Comp Cont Ed 1992;14:577.

104. Rendano VT, Zimmer JF, Wallach MS, et al. Impaction of the pharynx, larynx and esophagus by avian bones in the dog and cat. Vet Radiol 1988;29:213.

105. Squires RA. Esophageal obstruction by a hairball in a cat. JSAP 1989;30:311.

106. Houlton JEF, Herrtage ME, Taylor PM. Thoracic esophageal foreign bodies in the dog: A review of ninety cases. JSAP 1985;26:521.

107. Vessal K. Evaluation of barium and gastrograffin as a contrast media for esophageal perforation and rupture. Am J Roentgenol 1975;123:307.

108. Parker NR, Walter PA, Gay J. Diagnosis and surgical management of esophageal perforation. JAAHA 1989;25:587.

109. Basher AWP. Surgical treatment of congenital: Bronchoesophageal fistula in a dog. JAVMA 1991;199:479.

110. Van Ee RT, Dodd VM, Pope ER, et al. Bronchoesophageal fistula and transient megaesophagus in a dog. JAVMA 1986;188:874.

111. Freeman LM, Rush JE, Schelling SH, et al. Tracheoesophageal fistula in two cats. JAAHA 1993;29:531.

112. Stickle RS. Radiographic evaluation of esophageal function in Chinese shar-pei pups. JAVMA 1992;201:81.

113. Yaphe W, Giovengo S, Moise NS. Severe cardiomegaly secondary to anemia in a kitten. JAVMA 1993;202:961.

114. Rendano VT, Alexander JE. Heart size changes in experimentally-induced adrenal insufficiency in the dog: A radiographic study. JAVRS 1976;17:57.

115. Buchanan JW, Patterson DF. Selective angiography and angiocardiography in dogs with congenital cardiovascular disease. JAVRS 1965;6:21.
116. Kirberger RM, Bland-van den Berg P, Grimbeek RJ. Doppler echocardiography in the normal dog: Part II, factors influencing blood flow velocities and a comparison between left and right heart blood flow. Vet Radiol Ultrasound 1992;33:380.
117. Stickle RL, Anderson LK. Diagnosis of common congenital heart anomalies in the dog using survey and non-selective contrast radiography. Vet Radiol 1987;28:6.
118. Ackerman N, Burk RL, Hahn AW, et al. Patent ductus arteriosus in the dog: A retrospective study of radiographic, epidemiologic, and clinical findings. AJVR 1978;39:1805.
119. Goodwin JK, Lombard CW. Patent ductus arteriosus in adult dogs: Clinical features of 14 cases (1981–1990). JAAHA 1992;28:349.
120. Kaplan PM. Congenital heart disease. Prob Vet Med 1991;3:500.
121. Olivier NB. Congenital heart disease in dogs. In: Fox PF, ed. Canine and feline cardiology. New York:Churchill Livingstone Inc, 1988;357.
122. Nelson W. Aorticopulmonary window. JAVMA 1986;188:1055.
123. Eyster GE, Dalley SB, Chaffee A, et al. Aorticopulmonary septal defect in a dog. JAVMA 1975;167:1094.
124. Levitt L, Fowler JD, Schuh JCL. Aortic stenosis in the dog: A review of 12 cases. JAAHA 1989;25:357.
125. Stepien RL, Bonagura JD. Aortic stenosis: Clinical findings in six cats. JSAP 1991;32:341.
126. Fingland RB, Bonagura JD, Myer CW. Pulmonic stenosis in the dog: 29 cases (1975–1984). JAVMA 1986;189:281.
127. Brownlie SE, Cobb MA, Chambers J, et al. Percutaneous balloon valvuloplasty in four dogs with pulmonic stenosis. JSAP 1991;32:169.
128. Bright JM, Jennings J, Toal R, et al. Percutaneous balloon valvuloplasty for treatment of pulmonic stenosis in a dog. JAVMA 1987;191:995.
129. Ware WA, Bonagura JD. Multiple congenital cardiac anomalies and Eisenmenger's syndrome in a dog. Comp Cont Ed 1988;10:932.
130. Jevens DJ, Johnston SA, Jones CA, et al. Cor triatriatum dexter in two dogs. JAAHA 1993;29:289.
131. Otto CM, Mahaffey M, Jacobs G. Cor triatum dexter with Budd-Chiari syndrome and a review of ascites in young dogs. JSAP 1990;31:385.
132. Liu SK. Cardiovascular pathology. In: Fox PF, ed. Canine and feline cardiology. New York: Churchill Livingstone Inc, 1988;641.
133. Buchanan JW. Selective angiography and angiocardiography in dogs with acquired cardiovascular disease. JAVRS 1965;6:5.
134. Lombard CW, Spencer CP. Correlation of radiographic, echocardiographic and electrocardiographic signs of left heart enlargement in dogs with mitral regurgitation. Vet Radiol 1985;26:89.
135. Sadanga KK, MacDonald MJ, Buchanan JW. Echocardiography and surgery in a dog with left atrial rupture and hemopericardium. JVIM 1990;4:216.
136. Bond BR. Problems in veterinary ultrasonographic analysis of acquired heart disease. Prob Vet Med 1991;3:520.
137. Zook BC, Paasch LH. Endocardial fibroelastosis in Burmese cats. Am J Pathol 1982;106:435.
138. Sisson D, Luethy M, Thomas WP. Ventricular septal defect accompanied by aortic regurgitation in five dogs. JAAHA 1991;27:441.
139. Lombard CW, Ackerman N, Berry CR, et al. Pulmonic stenosis and right-to-left atrial shunt in three dogs. JAVMA 1989;164:71.
140. Brown DJ, Patterson DF. Pulmonary artery atresia with intact ventricular septum and agenesis of the ductus arteriosus in a pup. JAVMA 1989;195:229.
141. Keene BW. Chronic valvular disease in the dog. In: Fox PF, ed. Canine and feline cardiology. New York: Churchill Livingstone Inc, 1988;409.
142. Kaplan PM, Fox PR, Garvey MS, et al. Acute mitral regurgitation with papillary muscle rupture in a dog. JAVMA 1987;191:1436.
143. Lombard CW. Echocardiographic and clinical signs of canine dilated cardiomyopathy. JSAP 1984;25:59.
144. Sisson DD, Knight DH, Helinski C, et al. Plasma taurine concentrations and m-mode echocardiographic measures in healthy cats and cats with dilated cardiomyopathy. JVIM 1991;5:232.
145. Pion PD. Clinical findings in cats with dilated cardiomyopathy and the relationship of findings to taurine deficiency. JAVMA 1992;201:267.
146. Peterson EN, Moise NS, Brown CA, et al. Heterogeneity of hypertrophy in feline hypertrophic heart disease. JVIM 1993;7:183.
147. Bond BR, Fox PR, Peterson ME, et al. Echocardiographic findings in 103 cats with hyperthyroidism. JAVMA 1988;192:1546.
148. Medinger TL, Bruyette DS. Feline hypertrophic cardiomyopathy. Comp Cont Ed 1992;14:479.
149. Fox PF. Feline myocardial disease. In: Fox PF, ed. Canine and feline cardiology. New York: Churchill Livingstone Inc, 1988;435.
150. Kienle RD, Thomas WP. Echocardiography. In: Nyland TG, Mattoon JS, eds. Veterinary diagnostic ultrasound. Philadelphia: WB Saunders Co, 1995;244.
151. Calvert CA. Endocarditis and bacteremia. In: Fox PF, ed. Canine and feline cardiology. New York: Churchill Livingstone Inc, 1988;419.
152. Calvert CA, Mandell CP. Diagnosis and management of feline heartworm disease. JAVMA 1982;180:550.
153. Losonsky JM, Thrall DE, Lewis RE. Thoracic radiographic abnormalities in 200 dogs with spontaneous heartworm infestation. Vet Radiol 1983;24:120.
154. Thrall DE, Badertscher RR, Lewis RE, et al. Radiographic changes associated with developing dirofilariasis in experimentally infected dogs. AJVR 1980;41:81.
155. Wong MM, Suter PF, Rhode EA. Dirofilariasis without circulating microfilaria: A problem in diagnosis. JAVMA 1973;163:133.

156. Carlisle DH. Canine dirofilariasis: Its radiographic appearance. Vet Radiol 1980;21:123.
157. Badertscher RR, Losonsky JM, Paul AJ, et al. Two-dimensional echocardiography for diagnosis of dirofilariasis in nine dogs. JAVMA 1988;193:843.
158. Thomas WP, Sisson D, Bauer TG, et al. Detection of cardiac masses in dogs by two-dimensional echocardiography. Vet Radiol 1984;25:65.
159. Swartout MS, Ware WA, Bonagura JD. Intracardiac tumors in two dogs. JAAHA 1987;23:533.
160. Krotje LJ, Ware WA, Niyo Y. Intracardiac rhabdomyosarcoma in a dog. JAVMA 1990;197:368.
161. Keene BW, Rush JE, Cooley AJ, et al. Primary left ventricular hemangiosarcoma diagnosed by endomyocardial biopsy in a dog. JAVMA 1990;197:1501.
162. Vicini DS, Didier PJ, Ogilvie GK. Cardiac fibrosarcoma in a dog. JAVMA 1986;189:1486.
163. Aronsohn M. Cardiac hemangiosarcoma in the dog: A review of 38 cases. JAVMA 1985;187:922.
164. Reed JR, Thomas WP, Suter PF. Pneumopericardiography in the normal dog. Vet Radiol 1983;24:112.
165. Thomas WD, Reed JR, Gomez JA. Diagnostic pneumopericardiography in dogs with spontaneous pericardial effusion. Vet Radiol 1984;25:2.
166. Berry CR, Lombard CW, Hager DA, et al. Echocardiographic evaluation of cardiac tamponade in dogs before and after pericardiocentesis: Four cases (1984–1986). JAVMA 1988;192:1597.
167. Font A, Durall N, Domingo M, et al. Cardiac tamponade in a dog with visceral leishmaniasis. JAAHA 1193;29:95.
168. Rush JE, Keene BW, Fox PR. Pericardial disease in the cat: A retrospective evaluation of 66 cases. JAAHA 1990;26:39.
169. Berry CR, Hager DA. Pericardial effusion secondary to chronic endocardiosis and left atrial rupture in a dog. Comp Cont Ed 1988;10:800.
170. Font A, Durall N, Domingo M, et al. Cardiac tamponade in a dog with visceral leishmaniasis. JAAHA 1993;29:95.
171. Sisson D, Thomas WP, Reed J, et al. Intrapericardial cysts in the dog. JVIM 1993;7:364.
172. Reed JR. Pericardial diseases. In: Fox PF, ed. Canine and feline cardiology. New York: Churchill Livingstone Inc, 1988;495.
173. Fox SM, Burns J, Hawkins J. Spirocercosis in dogs. Comp Cont Ed 1988;10:807.
174. Jacobs G, Patterson D, Knight D. Complete interruption of the aortic arch in a dog. JAVMA 1987;191:1585.
175. Herrtage ME, Gorman NT, Jeffries AR. Coarctation of the aorta in a dog. Vet Radiol Ultrasound 1992;33:25.
176. Liu SK, Tilley LP, Tappe JP, et al. Clinical and pathological findings in dogs with atherosclerosis: 21 cases (1970–1983). JAVMA 1986;189:227.
177. Malik R, Hunt GB, Chard RB, et al. Congenital obstruction of the caudal vena cava in a dog. JAVMA 1990;197:880.
178. Cornelius L, Mahaffey M. Kinking of the intrathoracic caudal vena cava in five dogs. JSAP 1985;26:67.
179. Burk RL. Radiographic examination of the cardiopulmonary system. VCNA 1983;13:241.
180. Suter PF, Chan KF. Disseminated pulmonary disease in small animals: A radiographic approach to diagnosis. JAVRS 1968;9:67.
181. Myer CW, Burt JK. Bronchiectasis in the dog: Its radiographic appearance. Vet Radiol 1973;14:3.
182. Meier H, Holzworth J, Griffiths RC. Toxoplasmosis in the cat—Fourteen cases. JAVMA 1957;131:395.
183. Ford RB. Infectious disease of the respiratory tract. In: Sherding RG, ed. The cat: Diseases and clinical management. New York: Churchill Livingstone Inc, 1989;367.
184. Lord PF, Schaer M, Tilley L. Pulmonary infiltrates with eosinophilia in a dog. JAVRS 1975;16:115.
185. Calvert CA, Mahaffey MB, Lappin MR. Pulmonary and disseminated eosinophilic granulomatosis in dogs. JAAHA 1988;24:311.
186. McEntee MC, Page RL, Cline JM, et al. Radiation pneumonitis in three dogs. Vet Radiol Ultrasound 1992;33:199.
187. Kerr LY. Pulmonary edema secondary to upper airway obstruction in the dog: A review of nine cases. JAAHA 1989;25:207.
188. Farrow CS. Near drowning in the dog. JAVRS 1977;18:6.
189. Lord PF. Neurogenic pulmonary edema in the dog. JAAHA 1975;11:778.
190. Kolata RJ, Burrows CF. The clinical features of injury of chewing electrical cords in dogs and cats. JAAHA 1981;17:219.
191. Orsher AN, Kolata RJ. Acute respiratory distress syndrome: A case report and literature review. JAAHA 1982;18:41.
192. Moon ML, Greenlee PG, Burk RL. Uremic pneumonitis-like syndrome in ten dogs. JAAHA 1986;22:687.
193. Miles KG. A review of primary lung tumors in the dog and cat. Vet Radiol 1988;29:122.
194. Klein MK, Dow SW, Rosychuk RAW. Pulmonary thromboembolism associated with immune-mediated hemolytic anemia in dogs: Ten cases. JAVMA 1989;195:246.
195. Burns MG, Keely AB, Hornof WJ. Pulmonary artery thrombosis in three dogs with hyperadrenocorticism. JAVMA 1981;178:388.
196. Fluckiger MA, Gomez JA. Radiographic findings in dogs with spontaneous pulmonary thrombosis or embolism. Vet Radiol 1984;25:124.
197. Brown NO, Zontine WJ. Lung lobe torsion in the cat. JAVRS 1976;17:219.
198. Miller HG, Sherrill A. Lung lobe torsion: A difficult condition to diagnose. Vet Med 1987;82:797.
199. Lord PF, Gomez JA. Lung lobe collapse: Pathophysiologic and radiologic significance. Vet Radiol 1985;26:187.
200. Rendano VT, Georgi JR, Fahnestock GR, et al. *Filaroides hirthi* lungworm infection in dogs: Its radiographic appearance. JAVRS 1979;20:2.

201. Pinckney RD, Studer AD, Genta RM. *Filaroides hirthi* infection in two related dogs. JAVMA 1988;193:1287.
202. Williams JF. Parasitic diseases of the respiratory tract. In: Kirk RW, ed. Current veterinary therapy VII. Philadelphia: WB Saunders Co, 1980.
203. Losonsky JM, Smith FG, Lewis RE. Radiographic findings of *Aleurostrongylus abstrusus* infection in cats. JAAHA 1978;14:348.
204. Losonsky JM, Thrall DE, Prestwood AK. Radiographic evaluation of pulmonary abnormalities after *Aleurostrongylus abstrusus* inoculation in cats. AJVR 1983;44:478.
205. Swenson CL, Silverman J, Stromberg PC. Visceral leishmaniasis in an english foxhound from an Ohio research colony. JAVMA 1988;193:1089.
206. Ford RB. Chronic lung disease in old dogs and cats. Vet Rec 1990;126;399.
207. Padrid P, Amis TC. Chronic tracheobronchial disease in the dog. VCNA 1992;22:1203.
208. Pechman RD. The radiographic features of pulmonary paragonimiasis in the dog and cat. JAVRS 1976;17:182.
209. Rochat MC, Cowell RL, Tyler RD. Paragonimiasis in dogs and cats. Comp Cont Ed 1990;12:1093.
210. Pechman RD. Pulmonary paragonimiasis in dogs and cats: A review. JSAP 1980;21:87.
211. Trulove SG, McMahon HA, Nichols R, et al. Pyogranulomatous pneumonia associated with generalized noneffusive feline infectious peritonitis. Feline Pract 1992;20:25.
212. Schmidt M, Wolvekamp P. Radiographic findings in ten dogs with thoracic actinomycosis. Vet Radiol 1991;32:301.
213. Millman TM, O'Brien TR, Sutter PF, et al. Coccidioidomycosis in the dog: Its radiographic diagnosis. JAVRS 1979;20:50.
214. Burk RL, Corley EA, Corwin LA. The radiographic appearance of pulmonary histoplasmosis in the dog and cat: A review of 37 case histories. JAVRS 1978;19:2.
215. Walker MA. Thoracic blastomycosis: A review of its radiographic manifestations in 40 dogs. Vet Radiol 1981;22:22.
216. Berry CR, Moore PF, Thomas WP, et al. Pulmonary lymphomatoid granulomatosis in seven dogs. JVIM 1990;4:157.
217. Koblik PD. Radiographic appearance of primary lung tumors in cats: A review of 41 cases. Vet Radiol 1986;27:66.
218. Suter PF, Carrig CB, O'Brien TR, et al. Radiographic recognition of primary and metastatic pulmonary neoplasms of dogs and cat. JAVRS 1974;15:3.
219. Adams WM, Dubielzig R. Diffuse pulmonary alveolar septal metastases from mammary carcinoma in the dog. JAVRS 1978;19:161.
220. Tiemessen I. Thoracic metastases of canine mammary gland tumors—A radiographic study. Vet Radiol 1989;30:249.
221. Moise S, Wiedenkeller D, Yeager A, et al. Clinical, radiographic, and bronchial cytologic features of cats with bronchial disease: 65 cases (1980–1986). JAVMA 1989;194:1467.
222. Brownlie SE. A retrospective study of diagnosis in 109 cases of lower respiratory disease. JSAP 1990;31:371.
223. LaRue MJ, Garlick DS, Lamb CR, et al. Bronchial dysgenesis and lobar emphysema in an adult cat. JAVMA 1990;197:886.
224. Hoover JP. Bronchial cartilage dysplasia with multifocal lobar bullous emphysema and lung torsions in a pup. JAVMA 1992;201:599.
225. Padrid PA, Hornof WJ, Kurpershoek CJ. Canine chronic bronchitis—A pathophysiologic evaluation of 18 cases. JVIM 1990;4:172.
226. Stowater JL. Kartageners syndrome in a dog. JAVRS 1976;17:174.
227. Edwards DF, Kennedy JR, Toal RL, et al. Kartagener's syndrome in a chow chow dog with normal ciliary ultrastructure. Vet Pathol 1989;26:338.
228. Hoover JP, Howard-Martin MO, Bahr RJ. Chronic bronchitis, bronchiectasis, bronchiolitis, bronchiolitis obliterans, and bronchopneumonia in a rottweiler with primary ciliary dyskinesia. JAAHA 1989;25:297.
229. Foodman MS, Giger U, Stebbins K, et al. Kartagener's syndrome in an old miniature poodle. JSAP 1989;30:96.
230. Barber DL, Hill BL. Traumatically induced bullous lung lesions in the dog: A radiographic report of three cases. JAVMA 1976;169:1085.
231. Silverman S, Poulos PW, Suter PF. Cavitary pulmonary lesions in animals. JAVRS 1976;17:134.
232. Berry CR, Ackerman N, Monce K. Pulmonary mineralization in four dogs with Cushing's syndrome. Vet Radiol Ultrasound 1994;35:10.
233. Flanders JA, Castleman W, Carberry CA, et al. Laryngeal chondrosarcoma in a dog. JAVMA 1987;190:68.
234. Wisner ER, Matoon TJ, Nyland TG, et al. Normal ultrasound anatomy of the canine neck. Vet Radiol Ultrasound 1991;32:185.
235. Wisner ER, Nyland TG, Feldman EC, et al. Ultrasonographic evaluation of the parathyroid glands in hypercalcemic dogs. Vet Radiol Ultrasound 1993;34:108.

Chapter Three

THE ABDOMEN

RADIOLOGY AND ULTRASOUND OF THE ABDOMEN

Abdominal radiography is indicated whenever clinical signs or laboratory findings indicate the presence of abdominal disease, or whenever a condition is present in which involvement of, or extension to, the abdomen is possible. These characteristics include: (1) gastrointestinal signs such as vomiting, diarrhea, tenesmus, anorexia, and unexplained weight loss; (2) urogenital signs such as polyuria, oliguria, anuria, stranguria, pyuria, hematuria, polydipsia, and vaginal or prepucial discharge or bleeding; and (3) non-specific signs such as palpable abdominal masses or organomegaly, suspected hernias or abdominal wall masses, anemia, and fever of unknown origin. If there is evidence of direct trauma, it is advisable to radiograph the abdomen to ensure that there is no internal damage. In cases where the origin of the medical problem is obscure and other means do not yield a diagnosis, or when an animal resists or resents abdominal palpation, abdominal radiography may be indicated as a screening technique.

Abdominal ultrasound usually is performed in association with abdominal radiography. In some cases, such as the diagnosis of pregnancy or in the presence of abdominal fluid, only the ultrasound examination will be performed. This decision is often based on the experience and training of the ultrasonographer. A combined ultrasound and radiographic evaluation usually provides more information than either study by itself.

TECHNICAL CONSIDERATIONS

Radiography of the abdomen should be performed utilizing a consistent set of technical factors. A formal technique chart should be used to establish the kilovolt (peak) (kV[p]) and milliamp-seconds (mAs) settings for all exposures. If the animal measures greater than 10 cm at the thickest portion of the abdomen within the field of view, a grid should be used to reduce the effects of scatter radiation. The grid will prevent a haziness that may be misinterpreted as intra-abdominal loss of detail due to pathologic causes. The exposure time should be minimized to reduce motion artifact caused by bowel movement. Although in some animals exposure times as long as 0.1 seconds will produce satisfactory results, exposure times of 0.03 seconds or less are recommended. The radiographs should always be viewed on a view box with the films consistently oriented. It is customary practice to view all lateral films with the head facing to the left, and to view all ventrodorsal or dorsoventral films with the right side of the patient on the left side of the view box (as if facing the examiner) and the cranial abdomen in the uppermost (superior) position. Consistency in radiograph orientation facilitates recognition and general familiarity with normal structures and aids in the interpretation process.

Clipping the hair is essential to achieving a good abdominal ultrasound. Limited examination of the abdomen may be possible in some animals with a thin hair coat.

Wetting the hair coat with alcohol before applying the ultrasound gel improves the contact between the skin and transducer. The choice of ultrasound transducer and gain settings depends on the patient's size, organ of interest, and availability of equipment. Usually the highest frequency transducer that can penetrate to the depth of the structure of interest without high gain settings is preferred. Although there is ongoing controversy over linear versus sector transducers, they each offer advantages and disadvantages. Linear transducers offer a wider near field but are less useful for examining structures through an intercostal window or beneath the rib cage. Most sector transducers have a smaller footprint and therefore can be manipulated between or under the ribs. A consistent, systematic search pattern is recommended. Usually this means starting in the anterior abdomen and continuing along the left side to the posterior abdomen and returning on the right side. All organs should be evaluated in at least two planes. Longitudinal and transverse planes are customary although oblique planes are extremely useful. Because the organs may be moveable and not oriented along the transverse, or sagittal, plane of the animal, the planes used are related to the organ being examined and not the patient.

POSITIONING AND VIEW

The routine views of the abdomen are the lateral and ventrodorsal views (Figs. 3–1 and 3–2). It is our preference to take the lateral view with the animal's right side down. This usually causes the pylorus to be fluid-filled, and in some animals it will appear radiographically as a perfectly round tissue density suggestive of a mass or ball. The other commonly used positions are the left lateral and dorsoventral views (Figs. 3–3 and 3–4). On the left lateral position the pylorus usually will contain air and may appear as a radiolucent, round structure.[1] The choice between the right and left lateral as the routine view is a matter of personal preference. The ventrodorsal view is clearly preferable to the dorsoventral view when evaluating abdominal structures, because positioning for the ventrodorsal view causes the abdomen to be stretched to its fullest possible length and the abdominal viscera are distributed evenly throughout the abdomen. Positioning for the dorsoventral view results in the abdomen being somewhat bunched up, and the viscera are tightly crowded into a minimized space. This crowding makes identification of various structural and pathologic changes (loss of detail or masses) much more difficult.

Other views of the abdomen are occasionally useful. When a specific organ of interest (e.g., uterus, urinary bladder, or liver) has restricted mobility relative to other abdominal structures (e.g., intestine, spleen, stomach), the more mobile organs may be displaced away from the organ of interest by using focal abdominal compression.[2,3] This is done by compressing the abdomen directly over the organ of interest with a relatively radiolucent device, such as a wooden salad spoon. The exposure technique should be reduced (a 50% reduction in mAs is the norm) to compensate for the decrease in abdominal thickness caused by the compression. This technique will result in a radiograph with the structure of interest relatively isolated from other organs that might have been creating confusing shadows. Another method of isolating relatively immobile abdominal organs radiographically is to position the animal so that gravity pulls the relatively freely moveable organs away from the area of interest. In facilities that have a table which tilts, this is done by securing the patient to one end of the table and then tilting it up 20° to 30° from horizontal.

A view that may be useful in cases where free peritoneal air is suspected is the left lateral decubitus. For this view, the animal is positioned in left lateral recumbency, and a radiograph is taken with a horizontally directed beam centered on the cranial abdomen. Normally, in this view, there will be liver lobe or fat seen adjacent to the diaphragm. If free air is present in the abdominal cavity, it will be trapped above the liver immediately below the diaphragm and right lateral abdominal wall.

Ultrasound examinations may be performed with the animal in dorsal or lateral recumbency. The choice is usually determined by the experience and training of the ultrasonographer. Some patients are more comfortable in lateral recumbency and

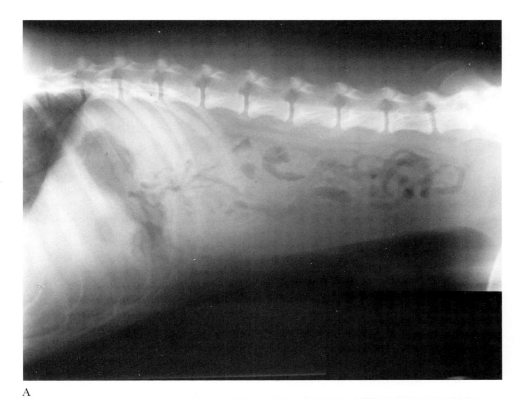

A

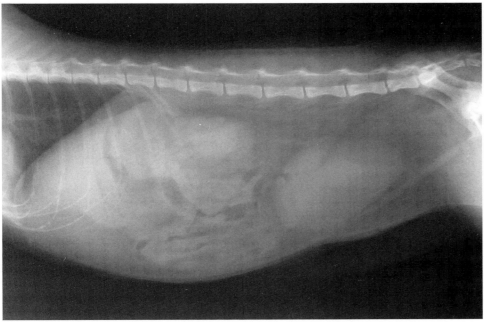

B

Figure 3–1. (A) A 4-year-old male cocker spaniel and (B) a 3-year-old male domestic short-haired cat. Both animals were clinically normal. The right lateral abdominal radiographs revealed normal anatomy. **Diagnosis:** Normal abdomen.

therefore that position can be used. For animals that resist both lateral and dorsal recumbency, the examination may be accomplished with the animal standing. Moving the animal and repeating the scan is helpful to document a change (or lack of change) in position of a lesion. This can help to distinguish bladder tumors (which remain fixed in location) from blood clots (which are moveable). Elevating the

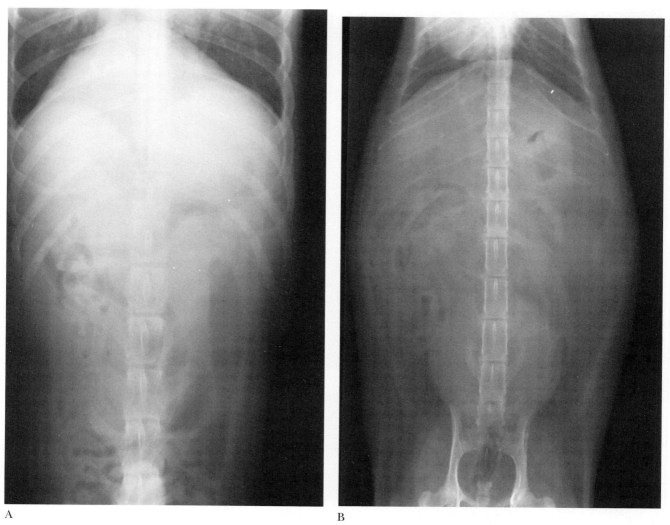

A   B

Figure 3–2.   The same animals as in Figure 3–1. The ventrodorsal view of (A) the dog and (B) the cat revealed normal anatomy. **Diagnosis:**Normal abdomen.

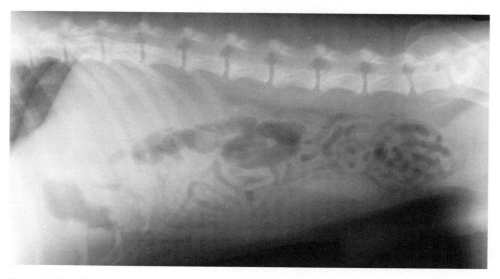

Figure 3–3.   The same dog as in Figure 3–1. The left lateral view of the abdomen demonstrated normal anatomy and gas in the pyloric region of the stomach. **Diagnosis:** Normal abdomen.

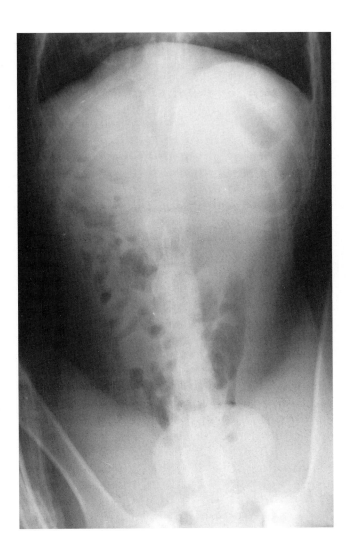

Figure 3–4. The same dog as in Figure 3–1. The dorsoventral view revealed a loss of diagnostic quality compared to the ventrodorsal view due to crowding of the viscera. **Diagnosis:** Normal abdomen.

head- or tail-end of the table may be useful for increasing access to the liver, in the former case, and to the bladder and prostate, in the latter instance. Rectal palpation may also be used to displace the prostate out of the pelvic canal making it more easily examined.

TECHNICAL EVALUATION OF THE RADIOGRAPH

Abdominal radiographs must first be evaluated for technical adequacy (positioning and exposure) before attempting to interpret the images for pathologic change. The radiographs should be exposed at the end (depth) of expiration to minimize the crowding and bunching of structures. Expiration can be evaluated by the position of the diaphragm on the lateral view. In full expiration, the diaphragmatic crura should cross the spinal column at approximately the 11th thoracic vertebra. The lateral view is assessed for rotation by determining if the lateral processes of the lumbar vertebrae and the ilia of the pelvis superimpose. The ventrodorsal view is evaluated by checking whether the dorsal spinous process bisects the vertebral body and whether the lateral vertebral processes are identical in appearance. Occasionally, when taking the ventrodorsal view the dog will twist or curl its body to one side. If this occurs, a repeat radiograph may be needed to eliminate this positioning artifact. Good radiographic technique will yield a radiograph that is neither too light nor too dark but one that readily differentiates the various radiographic densities. In some deep-chested dogs it may be necessary to use different radiographic techniques for the wider cranial as opposed to the narrower caudal abdomen. Presuming that these criteria are met, the radiographs may be evaluated. Both ventrodorsal and lateral views should be displayed simultaneously side-by-side so that any suspected change can be correlated on both projections.

RADIOGRAPHIC DETAIL

One can recognize various abdominal structures because of the differences between their radiographic densities. Whenever two structures of the same density touch, their margins will be obscured, and whenever two structures of different densities touch, a margin will be visible. The greater the difference in density (e.g., air against tissue versus fat against tissue) the more distinct the margin will be. The major contribution to abdominal detail is the difference in density between the mesenteric and omental fat and the tissue- (fluid-) dense viscera. Poor abdominal detail (a lack of contrast) may occur for several reasons. A cachectic animal will have poor abdominal detail and minimal soft tissue dorsal to the spine. The ventral midline will be displaced dorsal to its normal position (a "tucked up" appearance). Juvenile animals usually exhibit poor abdominal detail, presumably because of a lack of abdominal fat or the presence of a small amount of peritoneal fluid (Fig. 3–5).[4] The presence of fluid within the peritoneal cavity will obscure visceral detail and depending on the volume of fluid will produce abdominal distension (Fig. 3–6).

GENERAL TYPES OF RADIOGRAPHIC AND ULTRASOUND CHANGES

Analysis of a radiograph can reveal only the size, shape, density, position, and architecture of structures. Using this information, the veterinarian provides the necessary knowledge concerning anatomy, physiology, and pathology to develop an interpretation. Therefore, knowledge of the appearance of the normal structures and variations among individuals, breeds, and species is critical. If there is any doubt about a structure, it is helpful to refer to a radiograph of another animal of the same breed for comparison.

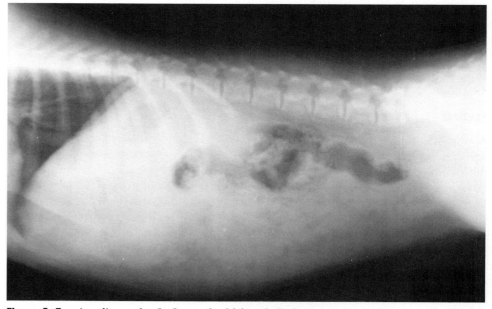

Figure 3–5. A radiograph of a 2-month-old female Doberman pinscher suspected of having eaten an earring. There is poor abdominal detail, which is normal for a juvenile animal. No foreign bodies are seen. **Diagnosis:** Normal juvenile abdomen.

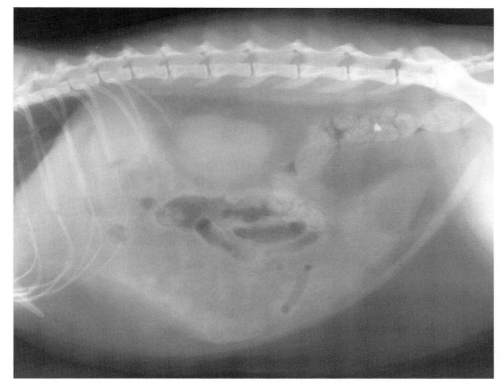

Figure 3–6. A 3-year-old female domestic short-haired cat with a 4-week history of anorexia and lethargy. There is a homogenous tissue density in the abdomen that prevents visualization of the normal abdominal structures. The ventral body wall is pendulous: this suggests the presence of intraabdominal contents. Differential diagnoses include peritoneal fluid accumulation, emaciation, or a juvenile abdomen. **Diagnosis:** Peritoneal effusion due to feline infectious peritonitis.

Ultrasound examination reveals the size, shape, echogenicity, position, and architecture of abdominal structures. It provides information about the internal structure of most tissue-dense abdominal organs that cannot be obtained from the radiograph. The ultrasound appearance of abdominal structures is influenced by the artifacts that occur during ultrasonography. These artifacts are discussed in Chapter 1 and should be reviewed and thoroughly understood before undertaking an abdominal ultrasound.

NORMAL RADIOGRAPHIC AND ULTRASOUND ANATOMY

ABDOMINAL BOUNDARY STRUCTURES

The abdomen is bordered dorsally by the spine, caudally by the pelvis, ventrally and laterally by the body wall, and cranially by the diaphragm. Immediately ventral to the spine is the sublumbar musculature (psoas muscles), which may be seen on both views. On the ventrodorsal view, the sublumbar muscles lie just lateral to the spine from the thoracolumbar junction to the pelvis. On the lateral view, they are fusiform tissue densities immediately ventral to the spine and extend from the thoracolumbar area to the pelvis. Immediately ventral to these muscles is the retroperitoneal space, a potential space that contains the kidneys, ureters, aorta, major blood vessels, sublumbar lymph nodes (external iliac, internal iliac, and coccygeal lymph nodes), and fat. Routinely, the ureters, major blood vessels, and lymph nodes are not seen. The aorta, a tubular structure running the length of the retroperitoneal space, and the deep circumflex iliac arteries (small, round tissue densities ventral to

L4 or L5), usually are seen. The retroperitoneal space continues around the caudal aspect of the abdomen at the pelvic canal and contains the prostate, bladder, uterus, and urethra. Laterally and ventrally, the body wall is composed of various muscles, fat, and skin. In particularly obese animals, these layers may be seen as individual sheets of tissue density separated from each other by fat. On the lateral view, the body wall is visibly thinner at the xiphoid, becomes thicker in the midabdomen, and continues at approximately the same thickness to its insertion at the pubis. On the ventrodorsal view, the lateral body walls are nearly the same thickness throughout their length. Cranially, the diaphragm separates the abdomen from the thorax. The diaphragm is composed of two crura and a central dome, which usually are seen readily. The differentiation of these parts is greater in deep-chested breeds and less in square-chested breeds. The peritoneal cavity is lined with the parietal peritoneum—a thin membrane which is not visible radiographically.

Ultrasound permits evaluation of the retroperitoneal space. The aorta and its branches, as well as the caudal vena cava, can be identified and traced from the diaphragm to the pelvic canal. Both longitudinal and transverse views should be obtained and the branches followed as far as possible. The vascular anatomy is helpful when examination of the adrenals is desired. In cooperative large dogs, normal lymph nodes may be identified at the root of the mesentery, at the ileocecocolic junction, and in the sublumbar retroperitoneal space. The psoas muscles and abdominal wall may be examined. The rectus abdominis muscles are usually visible as paired structures on either side of the ventral midline. They are uniformly echogenic, symmetrical in size and shape, and are thinner and less distinct cranially. The psoas muscles can be identified on either side of the aorta. They are heteroechoic and are symmetrical. The jejunal and medial iliac lymph nodes are most often seen during an ultrasound examination.[5] The iliac (sublumbar) lymph nodes can occasionally be seen but are not usually identified unless they are enlarged. The ureters cannot be traced through the retroperitoneal space, and even when markedly enlarged are often obscured by overlying intestines. The diaphragm can be seen as a bright echogenic line cranial to the liver. This actually represents the highly reflective interface between the diaphragm and the lung and not the diaphragm itself. When the diaphragm becomes thickened (such as in muscular dystrophy) it appears as a heteroechoic structure similar to other muscles.

SPECIFIC ABDOMINAL ORGANS

Liver

On the lateral abdominal radiograph of the dog, the liver, a homogeneously tissue-dense structure, is the most cranial organ extending caudally from the diaphragm to a line approximately parallel to the 13th rib, where it abuts the stomach (see Figs. 3–1 and 3–2). In breeds with shallow chests (Lhasa apso, etc.), the caudal ventral border of the liver may extend slightly caudal to the 13th rib and chondral cartilage; whereas, in deep-chested breeds (collies, etc.), the edge of the liver may not even extend to the 13th rib. In older dogs, the liver may be more ventrally and caudally located than in younger ones. Regardless of its position, the caudal ventral border of the liver should come to a relatively sharp point. The caudal margin of the caudate lobe of the liver may be identified cranial to the right kidney in obese dogs. It can be recognized because of its triangular shape and position adjacent to the cranial pole of the right kidney. The appearance of the liver in cats is similar to that in dogs; however, in obese cats a large amount of fat may accumulate in the area of the falciform ligament (ventral and caudal to the liver) and may markedly displace the liver dorsally (Fig. 3–7). This radiographic appearance tends to falsely suggest that the liver is abnormally small. On the ventrodorsal view, the liver is frequently hard to delineate because many structures are superimposed over it. It is bordered cranially by the diaphragm. The caudal border is located at the level of the cranial wall of the nondistended stomach. The liver should extend to both lateral body walls, but in

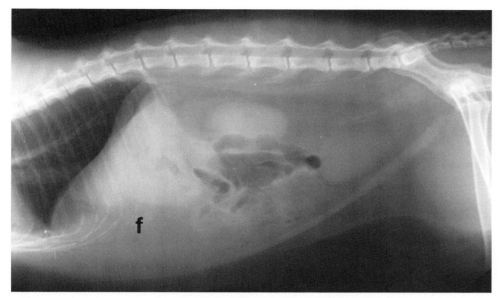

Figure 3–7. A 4-year-old female domestic short-haired cat with a 2-day history of vomiting. The lateral view revealed marked accumulation of fat in the region of the falciform ligament (*black f*), which separated the normal liver from the ventral body wall. The cat responded to symptomatic therapy. **Diagnosis:** Obesity.

obese animals there may be fat between the body wall and the liver. The gallbladder, while located slightly to the right of the midline and in the cranial ventral area of the liver, is not routinely seen on survey abdominal radiographs because there are rarely significant amounts of fat between it and the surrounding hepatic lobes. In the cat, the ventral margin of the gallbladder may be seen on the lateral radiograph as an oval structure extending ventrally beyond the ventral liver margin.

The liver is not always accessible to ultrasound scanning because a portion of it may be obscured by the overlying stomach. In dogs with deep thoracic conformation, the liver may be cranial to the last rib and relatively inaccessible to scanning. Scanning through the intercostal spaces may be prevented by the overlying lung. The entire liver should be examined systematically starting on one side and sweeping across to the other. This may require using an approach in which you start beneath the costal arch on one side and progress across the abdomen to the other side. The liver can be recognized during an ultrasound examination because of its position anterior to the stomach and posterior to the diaphragm. When the liver architecture is abnormal, identification of the bright echogenic line of the diaphragm is a reliable indicator of the liver's position. The liver is less echogenic (blacker) than the spleen and more echogenic (whiter) than the kidney. The architecture of the liver is composed of a uniform texture, which is interrupted by short, highly echogenic, paired parallel lines surrounding an anechoic lumen representing the portal veins and anechoic linear structures representing the hepatic veins (Fig. 3–8). The resulting pattern is heteroechoic with the uniformly echogenic hepatic cells interrupted by the portal and hepatic vein echoes. The hepatic and portal veins should be approximately the same size. The intrahepatic biliary ducts, extrahepatic bile ducts, and hepatic arteries are not evident on an ultrasound examination because they are too small. The gallbladder varies considerably in size; however, its ovoid shape is easily recognized and distinguished from the hepatic vein and caudal vena cava.[6–9] Usually, the gallbladder wall is poorly visualized or not identified. When visible, the gallbladder wall is normally 2 to 3 mm thick. Wall thickness and visibility varies with transducer frequency and placement. High frequency transducers directed perpendicular to the gallbladder wall are recommended when gallbladder wall measurements are desired. Measurement of the wall closest to the transducer is recommended.[9] A small amount of sediment may be identified in a normal fasting

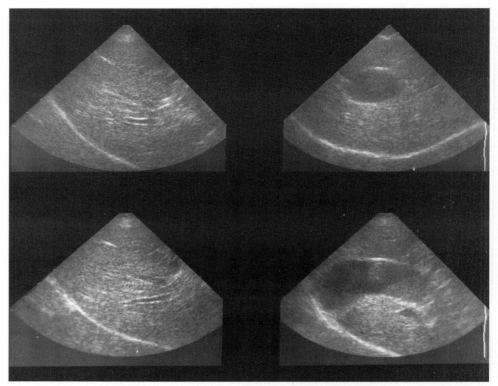

Figure 3–8. Longitudinal sonograms of the liver of a 4-year-old castrated male basset hound with a history of abdominal pain of 2 days' duration. The liver is normal. The gallbladder is slightly distended most likely because the animal has not eaten recently. The diaphragm can be seen as a hyperechoic curved line. The walls of the portal veins are hyperechoic. **Diagnosis:** Normal liver.

animal. A double gallbladder has been reported as an incidental finding in cats. This produces a bilobed appearance to the gallbladder. The gallbladder may be bilobed, attached at the neck, or arise from separate cystic ducts.[10]

In obese animals, the falciform fat may interfere with attempts to obtain a good image of the liver, and unless the sonographer is careful may even be confused with the liver. The echogenicity of the falciform fat in comparison to the liver can vary from being hyperechoic, to hypoechoic, or isoechoic. The architecture of the falciform fat is usually more uniform than that of the liver. It also contains more numerous hyperechoic linear streaks, which are closer together than the hyperechoic walls of portal veins. Liver lobes are more moveable during respiration while the falciform fat is more stationary. A hyperechoic line may be visible at the interface between the liver and falciform fat. Identifying the architecture of the liver adjacent to the diaphragm and scanning caudally toward the falciform fat is usually helpful in recognizing the difference in architecture between the falciform fat and the liver even when the liver is small.

Slice thickness artifacts are frequently encountered when examining the liver. The right kidney, gallbladder, and fat in the porta hepatis can create the illusion of hepatic masses.[11] Careful examination by moving the transducer in all directions will facilitate recognition of these artifacts.

Stomach

The stomach can be divided into four parts. The cardia is the point where the esophagus joins the stomach, the fundus is the portion of the stomach to the left and dorsal to the cardia, the major portion of the stomach is the body, and the pylorus (which includes the pyloric antrum and pyloric canal) is that portion of the stomach to the right of the midline and extending cranially to the pyloric sphincter. In the dog, the cranial wall of the stomach is in contact with the liver, except for a portion of the cardia which touches the left diaphragmatic crus. The position of the caudal wall depends on the amount of material or gas contained within the stomach; normally this should not extend caudal to L4. The angle the stomach assumes reflects the liver size. On the lateral view, a line drawn between the cardia and pylorus should be parallel to or more upright (vertical) than the 12th intercostal space. The appearance of the stomach depends on the type and volume of gastric content. If the stomach contains both fluid and air, as is usually the case, a right lateral recumbent radiograph will have the fluid in the pyloric portion of the stomach and the air in the fundus. The pylorus will appear radiographically as a round tissue density in the midventral portion of the abdomen just caudal to the liver and the cardia. The fundus will be seen as an air-containing structure dorsal to the pylorus and caudal to the liver. In a left lateral recumbent radiograph, the pylorus will contain air and the cardiac and fundic portions of the stomach will contain fluid.[1] The pylorus is usually located cranial to the level of the fundus. On the ventrodorsal view, the stomach extends from nearly the left lateral body wall across the midline to the area of the right lateral body wall. In the ventrodorsal view, the body of the stomach will contain gas and the cardia and pylorus will contain fluid. In the dorsoventral view, the fluid will be in the body and the cardia and pylorus will contain air. The pylorus is usually located cranial to the level of the cardia. The appearance of the stomach in the cat is very similar to that of the dog. The main difference is that on the ventrodorsal view the cat's pylorus is approximately on the midline. It is very difficult to evaluate gastric wall thickness on survey radiographs, because the apparent thickness depends on the degree of gastric distension as well as the amount and type of gastric contents. If the gastric wall appears thickened on survey radiographs, air or contrast should be administered in order to confirm this abnormality. Rugal fold thickness varies with the degree of gastric distension. Normal gastric fold thickness is reported to range from 1 to 8 mm in dogs ranging in weight from 2 to 50 kg.[12] Alteration in the shape of the stomach with or without gastric wall thickening is a more significant abnormal finding than alteration in stomach size.

The ultrasound appearance of the stomach varies with the content and degree of distension. Peristalsis can be observed. The stomach may be scanned in both longitudinal and transverse planes extending from the cardia on the left to the pylorus on the right. The stomach wall thickness varies from 3 to 5 mm with larger breeds having a thicker wall. Five layers may be identified starting with a hyperechoic serosa, a hypoechoic muscularis, a hyperechoic submucosa, a hypoechoic mucosa, and the hyperechoic lumen or mucosal surface (Figs. 3–9 and 3–10). The luminal gas produces reverberation artifacts, which are useful in identifying the stomach. The rugal folds may be identified if the stomach is relatively empty but they disappear when the stomach is distended. Fluid and gas may be seen swirling around within the stomach as a result of normal peristalsis. Water may be administered by stomach tube in order to improve examination of the gastric wall.[8,13]

Pancreas

The pancreas is immediately caudal to the stomach and medial to the duodenum. The pancreas has two portions: (1) the left lobe (limb), which is immediately caudal to the stomach and extends from the gastroduodenal junction to the cardia; and (2) the right lobe, which is immediately medial to the descending duodenum and extends caudally from the gastroduodenal junction. In normal animals, the pancreas usually cannot be identified radiographically because of its small dimensions and the large number of superimposed structures of similar density. In a very fat cat, a triangular soft tissue density may be observed on the ventrodorsal view just caudal to the stomach and medial to the spleen. This may represent the tip of the left limb of the pancreas.

Identifying the pancreas during an ultrasound examination is a challenge even for the expert ultrasonographer. This organ can be identified in a cooperative small

Figure 3–9. Longitudinal sonograms of the stomach of a 10-year-old spayed female Yorkshire terrier with a history of mammary tumors. The abdominal ultrasound was performed to investigate the possibility of abdominal metastasis. The dog was clinically normal. The stomach is normal. The gastric wall is well defined and uniform in thickness. Gas can be identified within the stomach. The five layers of the gastric wall can be identified with the hypoechoic mucosa and muscularis and the hyperechoic serosa, submucosa, and mucosal or lumenal surface. **Diagnosis:** Normal stomach.

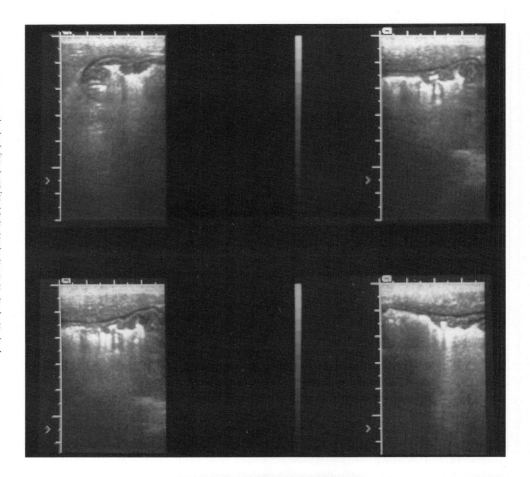

Figure 3–10. Longitudinal (A) and transverse (B,C,&D) sonograms of the stomach of a 12-year-old castrated male cat with a history of hematochezia and a palpable abdominal mass. The stomach is normal. The distinct layers of the stomach wall are not as defined as in the dog, however the wall is uniform in width. Gas is evident within the gastric lumen creating the reverberation artifact which is visible. **Diagnosis:** Normal stomach.

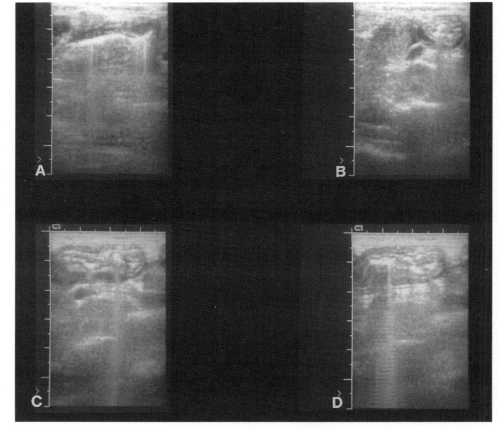

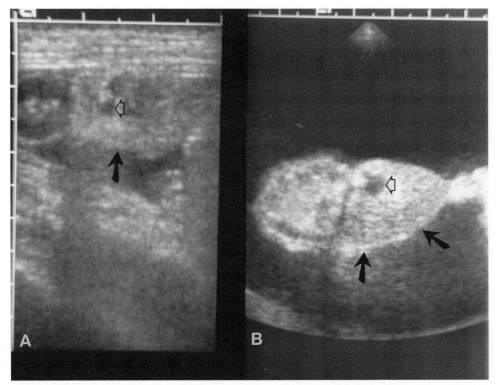

Figure 3–11. Transverse sonograms of a 5-year-old male miniature poodle (A) and an 11-year-old castrated male Doberman pinscher (B). The pancreas is visible as an echogenic, somewhat triangular shaped structure (*arrows*) adjacent to the duodenum. A small amount of peritoneal fluid is present in the poodle's abdomen while a large amount of peritoneal fluid is present in the abdomen of the Doberman. This has caused the difference in the echogenicity of the pancreas in these two dogs. An oval hypoechoic structure is evident in the pancreas adjacent to the duodenum (*small arrows*). This represents the pancreatoduodenal vein. **Diagnosis:** Normal pancreas.

patient when using a high frequency transducer or in animals with peritoneal fluid. Infusion of 60 ml of isotonic saline per kilogram body weight into the peritoneal cavity has been recommended in order to visualize the pancreas. No complications were encountered with this technique.[14] The pancreas is usually isoechoic when compared to the mesentery, similar in echogenicity to abdominal fat, and hyperechoic when compared to the liver (Figs. 3–11 and 3–12).[8,14,15] It is most often identified adjacent to the duodenum and pylorus. An oval hypoechoic structure, which represents the pancreatoduodenal vein, may be identified within the pancreas adjacent to the duodenum. In normal animals, identification of the pancreas is best accomplished in the transverse plane so that its position relative to the duodenum and stomach can be documented. The right kidney, which is located dorsal to the pancreas, can also be used as a landmark.[14]

Spleen

Usually, the spleen is clearly visible as a homogeneous tissue density. Its normal size varies. On the lateral view, the canine spleen usually is seen as a triangular density just caudal and slightly ventral to the stomach or liver. This is a cross-sectional view of the body of the spleen. If the spleen is adjacent to and touches the liver, the lack of contrasting density between them will make exact identification difficult. If the spleen is positioned along the length of the left body wall, the cross section may not be apparent in the lateral radiograph. In some cases, the head of the spleen, which appears as a triangular density just caudal to the stomach, may be seen in the dorsal part of the abdomen superimposed on or dorsal to the shadow of the right kidney. On the ventrodorsal view, the spleen usually is seen as a triangular tissue density on the left side just caudal and slightly lateral to the stomach and cranial and slightly

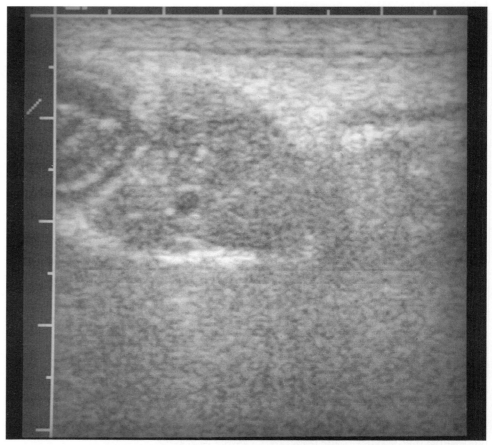

Figure 3–12. Transverse sonogram of the duodenum and pancreas of a 12-year-old spayed female dog with a history of icterus, hepatomegaly, and splenomegaly. The pancreas is normal. The oval hypoechoic area is the pancreatoduodenal vein. The pancreas is triangular in shape and similar in echo intensity to the surrounding normal fat. **Diagnosis:** Normal pancreas, lymphosarcoma.

lateral to the left kidney. If the spleen is positioned so that it crosses the midline, it will be difficult to visualize its full length. If it is positioned along the left body wall, the entire length of the spleen may be visible. The variable locations of the spleen are caused by its relatively lax attachment to the stomach by the gastrosplenic ligament (Fig. 3–13). The spleen of the cat differs from that of the dog in that it is usually smaller and somewhat less variable in both size and position. The body of the spleen may not be identified on the lateral view, and its head may be seen as a small triangular tissue density just caudal and dorsal to the stomach. Frequently, the entire extent of the spleen may be seen on the ventrodorsal view.

The spleen is easily identified during an ultrasound examination. It is located on the left side, caudal or lateral to the stomach. It is moveable and often extends into the caudal abdomen and across the midline to the right side. It may be adjacent to the liver, lateral to the stomach, may extend into the caudal abdomen along the left lateral abdominal wall, or may cross the midline caudal to the stomach or cranial to the urinary bladder. The size of the spleen varies; when it is small it may be difficult to find. This is especially true in cats. The spleen is hyperechoic when compared to the liver and renal cortex. It has a uniform homogeneous architecture. The splenic capsule may be evident as a bright marginal line, although this varies depending on the angle with which the ultrasound beam strikes the spleen (Fig. 3–14).[7,16] In an animal with peritoneal fluid, the capsule is much more apparent. The splenic veins can be identified as anechoic structures that enter the spleen along its medial border. These can be followed as they branch within the splenic parenchyma. In normal

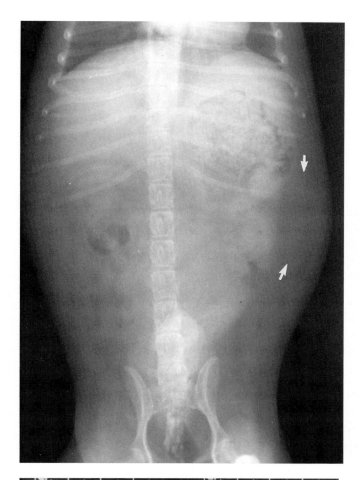

Figure 3–13. A 3-year-old male West Highland white terrier with a 1-day history of anorexia. The ventrodorsal view revealed that the spleen lay along the left lateral body wall (*white arrows*). This is one of the many positions that the spleen may normally assume. **Diagnosis:** Normal abdomen.

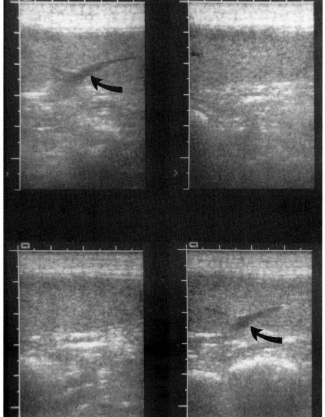

Figure 3–14. Transverse sonograms of the spleen of a 5-year-old female mixed breed dog who presented for abdominal sonographic evaluation because of the presence of a mast cell tumor on the right stifle. The spleen is normal. The splenic veins can be identified extending to the margin of the spleen (*arrows*). **Diagnosis:** Normal spleen.

dogs, a hyperechoic area may be identified at the splenic margin adjacent to the splenic veins. This is the result of mesenteric fat within splenic capsular invaginations. Splenic arteries are rarely seen although they may be detected by Doppler ultrasound. The shape of the spleen will vary depending on the orientation of the spleen to the ultrasound beam. It is usually seen as a thin, flat triangle; however, if the beam is oriented along the long axis of the spleen it can appear as a wider structure. The spleen should be examined in both longitudinal and transverse planes. The spleen is useful as an acoustic window for evaluating the left kidney. Imaging the kidney through the spleen provides a comparison for echogenicity of both structures.

Kidneys

The appearance and location of the kidneys in dogs are affected by the animal's age, posture, and general body condition. The kidneys are usually apparent, but the intestines may be superimposed over them and may obscure some or all of their perimeter. The right kidney is identified less frequently than the left because it is less moveable and is in contact with the liver. The kidneys become more movable and, as the dog ages, will become more ventrally and caudally located. When positioned in lateral recumbency, the dependent kidney moves cranially and the nondependent kidney droops becoming more visible and more bean-shaped. The extent of this movement or drooping is variable.[9,17] The kidneys also move a distance of approximately 1 vertebral body with respiration. The right kidney extends from T12 to L1, while the left lies in the area from L1 to L3. On the lateral view, the right kidney is dorsal and cranial to the left kidney and may be superimposed over the gastric and/or splenic shadows. Frequently, the cranial pole of the right kidney is not seen because it is nestled within the renal fossa of the caudate process of the caudate lobe of the liver. At this site, there is little or no fat to provide contrast between the two organs. On the ventrodorsal view, the right 13th rib superimposes on the pelvis of the right kidney. As on the lateral view, it is often difficult to see the cranial pole of the right kidney on the ventrodorsal view. The left kidney is seen lateral to the spine at the level of L3 just medial and caudal to the spleen. The normal length of the canine kidney is approximately 2.5 to 3.5 times the length of L2.[18] Although the normal width (from the medial to lateral borders) and depth (from the dorsal to ventral borders) of the kidney are less commonly quantified, these parameters should be evaluated subjectively. The left kidney, which is somewhat movable within the retroperitoneal space, may orient itself on the ventrodorsal projection at such an angle that its apparent length is shorter than its actual length. In the average dog (12–20 kg), the kidney measures 6 to 9 cm long, 4 to 5 cm wide, and 3 to 5 cm thick.

In the cat, both kidneys are located at the level from L1 to L4, with the right kidney usually slightly cranial to the left. On the lateral view of the cat, the kidney shadows may be superimposed on each other in the dorsal midabdomen or the right kidney may be slightly cranial and dorsal to the left kidney. The area of overlap of renal shadows may be interpreted incorrectly as a small kidney. On the ventrodorsal view of the cat, it is usually easier to see the entire perimeter of the kidneys. The right kidney in the cat is located lateral to the spine and completely caudal to the right 13th rib. The left kidney is usually parallel to the right or just slightly caudal to it. The normal length of the kidney in the cat is approximately 2.0 to 3.0 times the length of L2.[18] In the cat, the average kidney measures 3.8 to 4.4 cm long, 2.7 to 3.1 cm wide, and 2.0 to 3.5 cm thick.

If the kidneys are palpable, they can be identified easily during an ultrasound examination. If they are small or contained within the margins of the rib cage, locating them may be more difficult. The size of the kidney may be measured accurately provided the transducer is positioned carefully to produce a symmetrical image of the kidney. Renal volume can be computed, however this parameter is not particularly useful.[19–21] The normal renal pelvis and proximal ureter as well as the renal vein can be identified when high frequency transducers are used. The ureter can rarely be traced beyond the renal pelvis. Interlobar, arcuate, and interlobular arteries are usually not visible although they can be examined using color flow or Doppler ultrasound.

The appearance of the kidneys is influenced by the animal's size as well as by the transducer and machine used. Anatomic detail identified when examining small co-operative dogs using high frequency transducers may not be detected in examinations of large, deep-chested obese dogs. The kidneys are usually examined in three planes: longitudinal (along a frontal plane), transverse, (at right angles to a mid-sagittal plane), and sagittal. These planes are referenced to the kidney and not to the patient. The orientation of the kidney to the transducer markedly alters its appearance, and artifacts can be created when oblique planes are used. The renal cortex, renal medulla, and renal pelvis can be identified consistently. The renal cortex is brighter than the medulla with an echo intensity slightly less than that of the liver and markedly less than the echo intensity of the spleen. The renal medulla has a few internal echoes but appears more homogenous and hypoechoic relative to the cortex. It is common for individuals performing ultrasound examinations for the first time to misinterpret the echo intensity of the renal medulla as hydronephrosis. The renal pelvic recesses (diverticulae) appear as bright, evenly spaced, round or linear echoes. This appearance is most likely the result of the presence of renal pelvic fat and the interlobar arteries. The renal pelvis or ureter may be seen. Fat within the renal hilus produces a hyperechoic region (Fig. 3–15).[22–24]

The renal cortex of the cat is markedly hyperechoic when compared to the

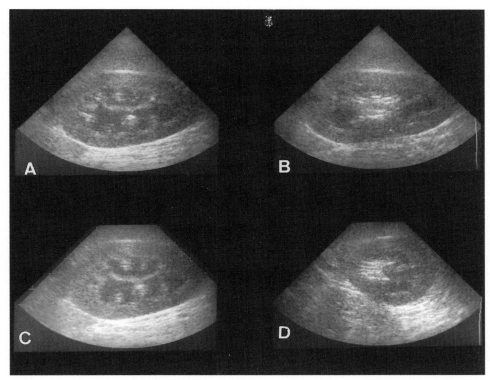

Figure 3–15. Longitudinal (A,B,&C) and transverse (D) sonograms of the left kidney of a 3-year-old male mixed breed dog. The dog was clinically normal. The kidney is normal. The cortex is hypoechoic relative to the adjacent spleen which provides an acoustic window for examination of the kidney. The renal pelvic recesses contain fat and appear as hyperechoic regions in the center of the kidney. The renal medulla is hypoechoic relative to the renal cortex. In the transverse sonogram (D) the renal hilus is hyperechoic because of the fat which is present. The renal pyramid can be seen as a "V"-shaped hypoechoic structure extending into the hyperechoic hilar fat. Retroperitoneal fat provides a bright line which outlines the kidney. **Diagnosis:** Normal kidney.

medulla, because of the presence of fat within the cortex. Cortical echogenicity is more variable in cats than in dogs. A linear hyperechoic zone observed within the medulla of the cat's kidney has been associated with the presence of microscopic deposits of mineral within the tubules in a zone between the corticomedullary junction and the renal crest (Fig. 3–16). The length of the kidney in cats ranges from 3.0 to 4.3 cm.[25–27]

During the ultrasound examination, the transducer is moved cranially and caudally along the kidney in order to obtain a series of transverse scans, or medially and laterally (or dorsally and ventrally) to obtain a series of longitudinal scans. The spleen may be positioned between the left kidney and the body wall providing an acoustic window for examination of the kidney. The right kidney may be examined through the liver, however the ribs may cast acoustic shadows that obscure portions of the right kidney.

Ureters

The ureters in both the dog and cat extend caudally from the kidneys to the bladder, traversing the retroperitoneal space slightly ventral to the lumbar muscles and slightly lateral to the vertebral column. Normally, because of their small size the ureters are not visible; however, it is helpful to know their course through the abdomen in order to detect conditions such as ureteral calculi. The abdominal portion of the ureter is retroperitoneal in location and lies adjacent to the psoas muscle. Within the pelvic cavity it enters the genital fold in the male and the broad ligament in the female. The ureters tunnel through the bladder wall and empty into the bladder at the ureteral orifice onto converging ridges (urethral columns). These columns continue as ridges (plica urethra) and meet to form the urethral crest, which projects into the urethra. In the male, this terminates at the colliculus seminalis.

The proximal ureter may be identified during an ultrasound examination providing the patient is cooperative and a high frequency transducer is used. The proximal ureter forms a "Y" extending along both sides of the renal crest. With good resolution, peristalsis may be evident in the proximal ureter just beyond the renal pelvis, however the normal ureter cannot be traced beyond the pelvis. Mild to moderate renal pelvic dilation occurs secondary to intravenous fluid administration, and this dilation can be observed during the ultrasound examination in normal dogs.[28] The ureter must be distinguished from the renal artery and vein. This can be done

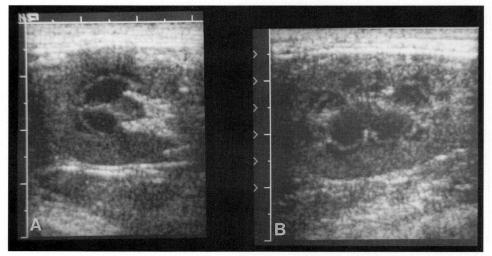

Figure 3–16. Transverse (A) and longitudinal (B) sonograms of the left kidney of a 5-year-old castrated male cat with a history of vomiting and icterus of 1-week duration. There is a thin hyperechoic line visible within the renal medulla. This is a normal finding in some cats. It is due to accumulation of mineral within the renal medulla. **Diagnosis:** Normal kidney.

using Doppler to determine which is the artery and vein. In addition, the renal vessels branch and enter the kidney away from the renal crest (more dorsal and ventral than the ureter in the transverse view), while the ureter branches directly on the renal crest.

Ovaries

In the female, the ovaries are immediately caudal to the kidneys. They are not identifiable radiographically.

The ovaries are difficult but not impossible to identify during an ultrasound examination. They can be found adjacent to the caudal pole or just caudal to the kidneys. The ovaries are hypoechoic and partially obscured by surrounding fat. Their round shape and position just caudal to the kidneys make their identification possible (Figs. 3–17 and 3–18). Small anechoic cysts and developing follicles have been identified. A lateral scanning plane, rather than a ventral approach, may facilitate localization and examination of the canine ovaries.[29]

Adrenal Glands

Usually, the adrenal glands are not identified radiographically. In older cats, the adrenal glands may become mineralized and therefore evident on the abdominal radiograph. This is apparently an aging change and is not associated with clinical signs.

Identification of the normal adrenals using ultrasound requires a high resolution transducer and a cooperative patient. The left adrenal can be identified in most dogs, while finding the right adrenal is more difficult. The left adrenal lies adjacent to the aorta just cranial to the left kidney. The adrenal may be found by imaging the left kidney in a longitudinal plane and then moving or rolling the transducer toward the midline until the aorta is identified. The adrenal gland will be located adjacent

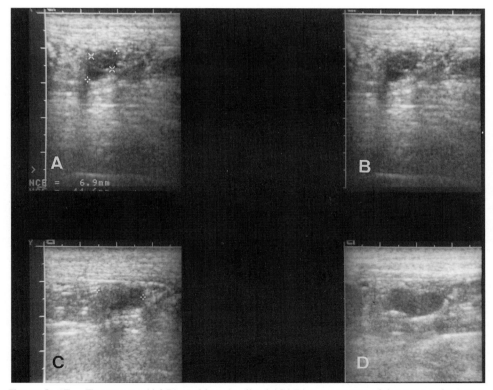

Figure 3–17. Transverse (A&B) and longitudinal (C&D) sonograms of the ovary of a 4-year-old female mixed breed dog with a history of lethargy, weight loss, delayed puberty, and delayed estrus. The left ovary is visible as a hypoechoic somewhat oval shaped structure. The architecture and size are normal. **Diagnosis:** Normal ovary.

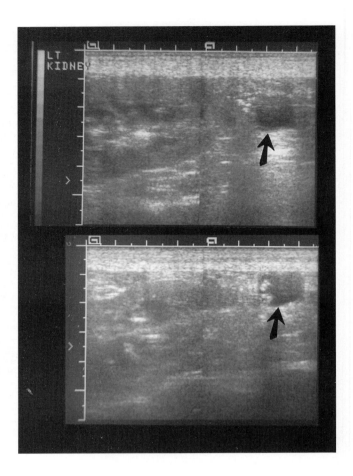

Figure 3–18. Longitudinal sonograms of the left and right kidney and ovary of a 9-year-old female mixed breed dog with a history of chronic pericardial effusion. The ovaries can be identified as oval hypoechoic structures (*arrows*) caudal to the kidneys. The ovaries appear slightly enlarged but their architecture is normal. **Diagnosis:** Normal ovaries.

to the left lateral aspect of the aorta just cranial to the origin of the left phrenicoabdominal artery. An alternate method of finding the left adrenal consists of imaging the aorta transversely and tracing it caudally to the origin of the phrenicoabdominal artery just cranial to the left kidney. The adrenal may be oriented slightly obliquely to the aorta; therefore, the transducer must be manipulated until the complete adrenal gland is identified in a longitudinal plane. The adrenal is frequently masked by overlying intestines, and gentle pressure using the transducer may be required to displace these intestinal loops away from the adrenal gland.[30] The right adrenal may be imaged by identifying the caudal vena cava in a longitudinal plane and moving the transducer toward the right kidney at the level of the cranial pole. The vena cava may be imaged in the transverse plane and followed cranially and caudally at the level of the kidney until a cross section of the adrenal is found. Placing the transducer on the right dorsolateral abdomen in a longitudinal orientation and identifying the vena cava and the aorta helps to locate the right adrenal, which will be in the plane of the caudal vena cava. The adrenals are extremely variable in size and shape (round, oblong, oval, or triangular). In some dogs, the adrenal gland appears bipartite or peanut-shaped with an echo intensity similar to renal medulla. In some patients, a distinction can be made between the hypoechoic cortex and hyperechoic medulla (Fig. 3–19). The cranial and caudal poles are often asymmetrical. The length of the adrenal glands may vary from 15 to 30 mm, the width varies from 4 to 20 mm, and the thickness varies from 3.5 to 11 mm.[31] Introduction of normal saline into the peritoneal cavity was not helpful in improving visualization of the adrenal glands.[14]

Small Intestine

The small intestines are visible on radiographs because of the contrast provided by fat within the mesentery and omentum and the luminal content. The degree to

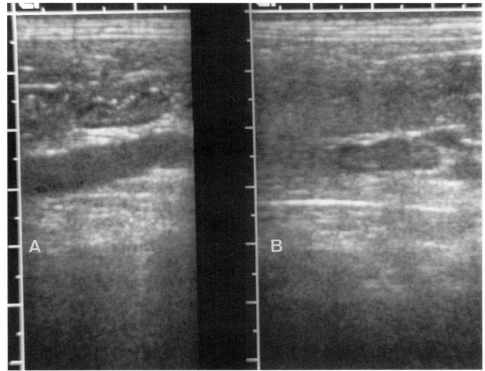

Figure 3–19. Longitudinal sonograms of the left (A) and right (B) adrenal glands of an 11-year-old male poodle who presented with a history of chronic urinary tract infections. Both adrenal glands are normal in size and shape (*arrows*). The aorta is visible deep to the left adrenal gland. The hypoechoic adrenal cortex and hyperechoic medulla are visible bilaterally but more clearly identified in the left adrenal gland. **Diagnosis:** Normal adrenal glands.

which their serosal surface can be identified depends upon the amount of fat present within the peritoneal cavity. The intestines should contain either fluid or air. Non-digestible material, such as bone, may also be present within the small intestines. The small intestines are curvilinear when seen longitudinally and round when seen in cross section. With the exception of the descending duodenum, the locations of the various parts of the small intestine are quite variable in both the dog and cat. On the lateral view, the duodenum leaves the pylorus in a cranial direction and immediately curls tightly in a right dorsal direction to become directed caudally at a level just dorsal to the midabdomen. The duodenum then follows a relatively straight course from its turn to the level of L4 or L5. At this position it turns to the left and becomes the transverse duodenum, which is difficult to identify radiographically. This extends for a short distance across the midline where it turns again to head cranially as the ascending duodenum. On the ventrodorsal view, the origin of the duodenum may be seen extending cranially for a very short distance before it curves tightly right and assumes a caudal direction. The descending duodenum may take a slightly diagonal orientation with the cranial extent lying along the right lateral abdominal wall and the caudal extent being slightly to the right of the midline. The position of the descending duodenum in the cat is similar to that of the dog except that it originates just to the right of the midline on the ventrodorsal view. Specific identification of the position of the transverse and ascending duodenum as well as specific portions of the jejunum and ileum is very difficult because of the movable nature of these structures. They are distributed around the root of the mesentery, which extends caudoventrally from the level of L2 following the course of the cranial mesenteric artery. Most of the mesenteric lymph nodes are found in this area but normally are not apparent radiographically. The small intestine normally contains gas or fluid unless bone or other material has been eaten. Most of the gas present comes from ingestion. The diameter of the normal small intestine varies, but generally it should be no wider than the width (or height) of a lumbar vertebral body. Evaluation of small intestinal wall thickness cannot be made accurately without a contrast study, because the apparent thickness will depend on the degree of distension and the nature of the intestinal contents.

With ultrasound, the descending duodenum can be traced from the pylorus, has a relatively consistent position along the right lateral abdominal wall, and has a thicker mucosa than other portions of the intestinal tract. The ileum can sometimes be traced to the ileocecocolic junction; however, the specific portions of the small intestines cannot always be distinguished with ultrasound. The lumen of the small intestines always contains some gas bubbles and therefore can be recognized as a hyperechoic linear or curved structure. The wall of the small intestine can be identified and, although the layers of the wall are the same as the stomach, in most cases all five layers cannot be distinguished. Usually the hyperechoic lumen and the hyperechoic serosa can be identified, with the mucosa, submucosa, and muscularis appearing as a single hypoechoic structure. The intestines should be scanned in both longitudinal and transverse planes. The wall thickness (normally 2–4 mm), luminal content, and bowel shape should be examined (Fig. 3–20).[8,13] Although the intestines should be examined in a systematic fashion, a single intestinal loop usually can be followed for only a short distance because of interference from other gas-filled loops. Peristalsis should be observed within the small intestines.

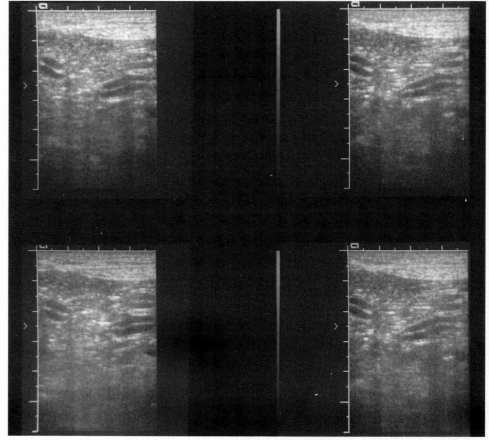

Figure 3–20. Sonograms of the abdomen of a 2-year-old spayed female Welsh corgi with a history of polyuria, polydipsia, and vomiting for 1 month. There are several loops of small intestine visible in both longitudinal and transverse sections. These intestines are normal. The lumen is visible as a centrally located hyperechoic line. The wall is hypoechoic with a hyperechoic serosal surface. Wall thickness is 2 to 3 mm. **Diagnosis:** Normal small intestines.

Large Intestine

The large intestine (colon) begins with the cecum. Although its position is somewhat variable, the cecum is usually located in the midabdomen ventral to L3 or L4 and slightly to the right of the midline in the dog. The cecum frequently contains gas and may be apparent as a spiral or comma shaped structure on both the lateral and ventrodorsal views. The cecum of the cat is much smaller, not spiraled, and less frequently identified on survey radiographs. It is slightly more cranial in the abdomen with its usual location ventral to L2 or L3. In both the dog and cat, the ileocolic lymph nodes are located at the ileocecocolic junction but are not visible radiographically. Cranial to this site, there is a short ascending colon that extends cranially from the cecum and a transverse colon that crosses the midline from the right to the left and connects the ascending colon to the descending colon, which extends caudally to the rectum. The transverse colon in both animals is located immediately caudal to the stomach and, when seen on the lateral view in an end-on projection, may appear as a round tissue density if it is filled with fluid, a round radiolucency if it is filled with gas, or a granular mixture of fluid and gas if it contains fecal material. On the ventrodorsal radiograph, the descending colon is usually on the left of the midline extending caudally along the lateral abdominal wall. On the lateral radiograph, the colon is usually located in the middle third of the abdomen. The position of the colon varies depending on its content. It may be on the right side in some normal animals and may take an irregular course through the abdomen when distended with air or filled with fecal material. In some normal dogs the colon appears tortuous, particularly at the region of the junction between the transverse and descending colons. The distal colon may be deviated to the right or the left by a distended urinary bladder. The normal colon diameter is usually no more than 2 to 3 times that of the small bowel. The colon may be completely empty or filled with fluid and therefore appear as a tissue-dense tube, completely gas-filled and appear as a radiolucent tube, completely distended with fecal material and appear as a tube ranging in density from tissue to bone, or a combination of the above. Because of this high degree of variability, it is difficult to recognize colonic lesions without the aid of special procedures.

The colon can be identified during an ultrasound examination, however most of its structure is obscured by the highly echogenic nature of its content.[8,13] Gas and fecal material are so highly echogenic that the details of the colon wall are obliterated. The size and position of the colon and the absence of peristalsis enable the ultrasonographer to recognize it and distinguish it from small intestines. When the colon is empty, the mucosal folds may be visible resulting in a wrinkled appearance of the wall of the colon. Although the normal colon wall is approximately 2 to 3 mm in width, it will appear thinner when the colon is distended. In the transverse plane, the colon usually appears as a semicircle because the gas within the lumen shadows the far wall. In the longitudinal plane, the colon appears as an echogenic line. If the colon is fluid-filled, the far wall will be evident and the tubular nature of the bowel can be recognized. The three portions of the colon can be recognized because of their position within the abdomen.

Urinary Bladder

The urinary bladder, a teardrop-shaped tissue-dense organ, is normally seen immediately cranial to the pelvic brim (or prostate in the male) and varies in size depending on the amount of urine it contains. The cranial border of the normal urinary bladder rarely extends cranial to the umbilicus. The degree of urinary bladder distension usually reflects the fact that the animal has not had the opportunity to urinate, and it is hazardous to evaluate bladder function based solely on bladder size. When the bladder size is correlated with the patient's history (i.e., a markedly distended bladder in an animal that has just urinated would suggest bladder atony or urinary obstruction), some functional information can be gleaned from the radiograph.

The urinary bladder is ovoid with a cranial blunt vertex, a rounded middle portion (or body), and a neck that leads to the urethra. In the female dog and in both male and female cats, the bladder normally has a long gradually tapering neck. In the male dog, the bladder neck is shorter, tapers more abruptly, and is closer to the pelvic brim. All of the bladder is covered by peritoneum except the bladder neck, which is retroperitoneal. This is important when evaluating patients for bladder trauma, because rupture of the bladder caudal to the neck will result in retroperitoneal fluid, while rupture of other portions of the bladder will produce peritoneal fluid. The bladder should be uniformly tissue-dense; however, air bubbles may be observed in the bladder of a normal dog or cat that has been catheterized or less often in one that has had a cystocentesis.

Ultrasound is ideally suited for examination of the urinary bladder.[32] Even a small bladder not detected by abdominal palpation or radiographs can be identified using ultrasound. The anechoic urine contrasts well with the echogenic bladder wall (Fig. 3–21). Compression of the abdominal wall by transducer pressure frequently distorts the bladder's shape. Ultrasound artifacts, such as slice thickness and reverberation, can create the appearance of cellular material within the bladder. The bladder wall can be measured. The thickness of the bladder wall varies with bladder distension. A focal thickening of the bladder wall has been described at the trigone area where the ureter enters the bladder. (Fig. 3–22).[33] When the specific gravity of the urine in the bladder is different from the specific gravity of the urine in the ureter, swirling may be observed secondary to propulsion of urine from the ureter into the bladder (Figs. 3–21 and 3–23). This may be observed more readily using color-flow Doppler; however, if the urine contains highly cellular or crystalline material these jets may be observed during routine ultrasound examinations.

Ultrasound can be used for guidance when performing a cystocentesis. The needle tip can be observed as it penetrates the bladder (Fig. 3–24).

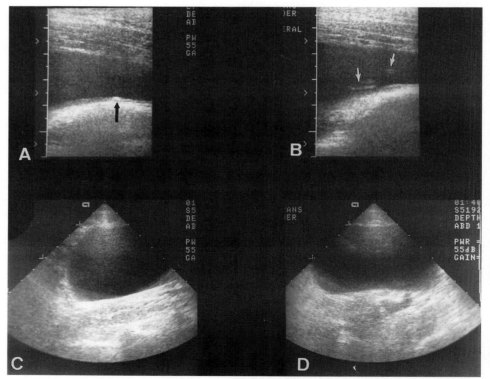

Figure 3–21. Longitudinal (A,B,&C) and transverse (D) songrams of the bladder of a 1-year-old castrated male boxer with a history of weight loss and diarrhea of 3 months' duration. The bladder is normal. The bladder wall is poorly seen because of the degree of bladder distension. The ureteral orifice is evident (A) (*arrow*). The echoes within the bladder lumen (B) (*arrows*) represent turbulence of the urine associated with a ureteral jet. Other echoes within the bladder are artifacts due to electronic noise and reverberation. **Diagnosis:** Normal bladder.

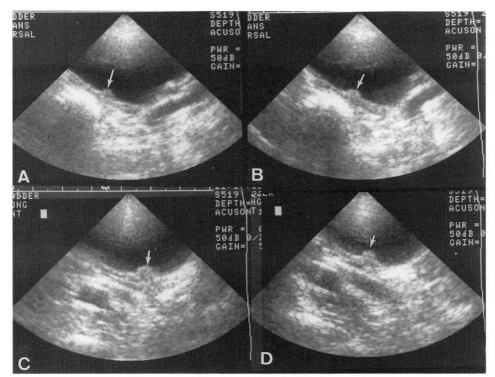

Figure 3–22. Transverse (A&B) and longitudinal (C&D) sonograms of the urinary bladder of a 13-year-old male Doberman pinscher who presented for reevaluation of bladder polyps, which had been removed surgically 3 years previously. There is a smooth convex bulge on the mucosal surface of the urinary bladder (*arrows*). This is in the region of the bladder trigone and represents the normal ureteral papillae. This could be mistaken for a bladder wall mass. **Diagnosis:** Normal bladder.

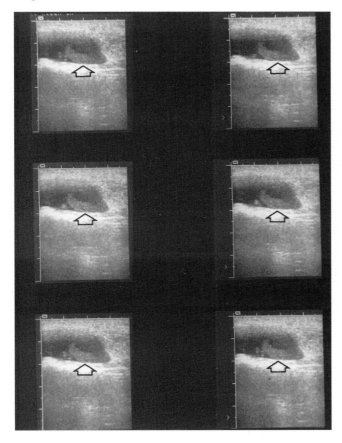

Figure 3–23. Transverse sonograms of the urinary bladder of a 6-year-old spayed female mixed breed dog with a history of chronic urinary tract infection. An echogenic swirl of urine has created the turbulence visible in the dorsal left side of the urinary bladder (*arrows*). This is the result of urine being propelled into the bladder lumen from the ureteral papillae. This occurs when the specific gravity of the urine within the bladder is different from that which is in the ureter. This is a normal phenomenon and has been termed a ureteral jet. **Diagnosis:** Ureteral jet.

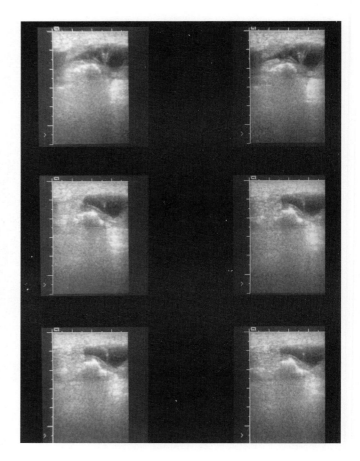

Figure 3–24. Transverse sonograms of the urinary bladder of a 12-year-old male cocker spaniel with a history of chronic diarrhea and hypoalbuminemia of 2 months' duration. A cystocentesis was performed using ultrasound guidance. In the initial images the needle is visible penetrating the bladder wall and pushing a "V"-shaped fold of bladder mucosa into the bladder lumen. As the puncture progresses the mucosa is penetrated and in the last image the tip of the needle becomes visible in the center of the bladder. This indenting of the bladder mucosa is often responsible for a failure to obtain urine during a cystocentesis. Ultrasound guidance is extremely valuable when the bladder is small or cannot be palpated. **Diagnosis:** Ultrasound guided cystocentesis.

Uterus

The body of the uterus is located between the urinary bladder and the colon. It is not seen routinely in the normal nongravid female. In fat patients, the uterine body may be seen as a tubular soft tissue structure located between the colon and the bladder or superimposed upon the urinary bladder.[34]

Hysterography has been used for evaluation of uterine abnormalities. Catheterization of the cervical canal is followed by slow injection of iodinated contrast. Intrauterine pressure is monitored during the contrast injection, and the injection is terminated when the pressure reaches 100 mm Hg. This technique has been used on a limited basis mostly because of the difficulty in catheterization.[35,36] Ultrasound is much more useful than hysterography for evaluation of uterine abnormalities.

The uterine body may be identified during an ultrasound examination. It can be identified either dorsal or dorsolateral to the urinary bladder (Fig. 3–25). It is usually easier to detect it when examining the bladder in a transverse plane. It appears as a round heteroechoic structure with a very small hyperechoic lumen. It may also be examined in a longitudinal axis, however orienting the transducer to the uterine body is more difficult. The uterus must be distinguished from adjacent loops of intestine and this is difficult anterior to the urinary bladder.

Prostate

In male dogs, the prostate is immediately caudal to the urinary bladder and completely surrounds the urethra. Normally, the prostate does not extend cranial to the pelvic brim. In chondrodystrophic breeds, it is common to see some of the prostate's perimeter cranial to the brim of the pelvis. When the bladder is distended it may pull the prostate cranially. Criteria for normal prostatic size have been published but are not used routinely because of the somewhat cumbersome methodology.[37] It is usu-

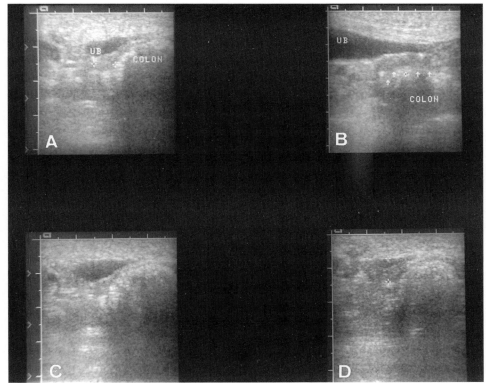

Figure 3–25. Transverse (A,C,&D) and longitudinal (B) sonograms of the caudal abdomen of a 6-year-old female dachshund with a history of vomiting, anorexia, pancytopenia, and splenomegaly. The uterus is visible as a hyperechoic oval or tubular structure dorsal to the urinary bladder and to the right (A,C,&D: +) or dorsal (B: *small white arrows*) to the colon. This represents a normal uterus. **Diagnosis:** Normal uterus.

ally adequate to determine if there is prostatic enlargement based on a subjective evaluation of the prostate's size relative to that of the dog's abdomen. In a medium size dog (15–25 kg), the prostate is approximately 1.5 to 3.0 cm in diameter. In the male cat, the prostate is a very small accessory sex organ located just caudal to the urinary bladder. It covers the urethra on only three sides and is not normally seen.

The prostate can be examined and measured ultrasonographically.[38,39] Usually, it is easiest to identify the prostate by locating the urinary bladder in a transverse plane and then moving the transducer caudally following the bladder until the bladder narrows at the neck and then disappears. The prostate can then be identified as a uniformly heteroechoic (similar in echo intensity to the spleen), round or bilobed structure surrounding the bladder neck or urethra. The median raphe may not be obvious, and the gland may appear more round than bilobed. A wall or capsule surrounding the prostate is usually not evident. The urethra may be seen as an anechoic round or linear structure, but this is uncommon. Small anechoic areas within the prostate probably represent small intraprostatic cysts. These are more common in older intact dogs, and whether they are normal or abnormal is debatable. It is difficult to see the prostate if it is intrapelvic.[38,39] Rectal palpation may be used to displace the prostate out of the pelvic canal making it more accessible to ultrasound examination. Tilting the patient head-down may move the prostate out of the pelvic canal. As the bladder distends, the prostate will be pulled anteriorly out of the pelvic canal and this may permit prostatic evaluation. In large dogs, an intrapelvic prostate may be examined by placing the transducer within the rectum. Ultrasound evaluation of prostatic size is subjective.

Testicles

The testicles are not usually evaluated radiographically, however they should be evaluated using ultrasound. The normal testicle is uniformly heteroechoic and is hyperechoic when compared to most abdominal structures. The mediastinum testes produces a central hyperintense line with some slight shadowing. The tail of the epididymis is anechoic or hypoechoic (Fig. 3–26).[40]

Abdominal Vasculature

Within the abdomen certain vascular structures may be seen in some normal animals. In animals with large amounts of fat, the aorta and in some cases the caudal vena cava may be seen on the lateral view. They can be recognized because of their linear shape and position. The aorta is slightly ventral to the spine and branches at the level of L5 (the deep circumflex iliac arteries) and at the level of L6–L7 (the external iliac arteries). The caudal vena cava runs obliquely from the caudal dorsal abdomen in a cranioventral direction toward the liver.

Vascular anatomy can be examined using ultrasound. The caudal vena cava and the aorta and their branches, the hepatic veins, and the portal vein can be detected and examined. In most vessels, flow can be observed when high resolution transducers are used. Flow can be quantitated using Doppler ultrasound. The aorta and caudal vena cava can be examined in both longitudinal and transverse planes. The aorta is dorsal and slightly to the left of the caudal venal cava. The aortic pulsations can be observed. The wall of the aorta is slightly thicker than that of the caudal vena cava, but in smaller dogs the wall usually is not identified.[41] Aortic pulsations may not be readily apparent and may be transmitted to the caudal vena cava making discrimination between these vessels difficult. Compression of the vessels using the ul-

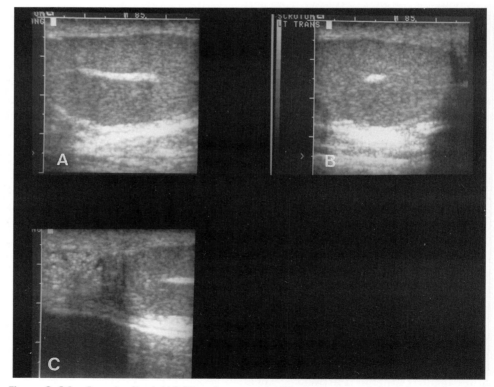

Figure 3–26. Longitudinal (A&C) and transverse (B) sonograms of the left testicle of a 6-year-old male bullmastiff with a history of abnormal ejaculate and low sperm counts. The testicle is normal. The hyperechoic centrally located structure is the mediastinum testes. The architecture of the testicle is uniform. The epididymis is evident in the longitudinal section (C). **Diagnosis:** Normal testicle.

trasound transducer helps discriminate between the aorta and the vena cava because the cava is more easily compressed.[41] The celiac and cranial mesenteric arteries can be detected if the stomach and intestines are relatively empty. They can be followed a short distance from their origin before being obscured by intestines. The phrenicoabdominal artery can be identified just cranial to the left kidney and is used as a landmark to locate the left adrenal gland. The renal arteries may be seen at their origin, however they are rarely seen in the renal hilus. Renal arteries can be detected using Doppler even though they cannot be identified specifically. The terminal branches of the aorta can be seen most readily when the aorta is followed in the transverse plane. The splitting of the aorta into several round vessels can be identified. These branches are more difficult to follow in the longitudinal plane. It is difficult to follow the vessels beyond the inguinal ring. The caudal vena cava is wider than the aorta and lacks the pulsations observed in the aorta. The wall of the vena cava can be identified in some larger dogs. The renal and splenic veins can be identified in association with these organs but cannot be traced to the caudal vena cava. The vena cava may be followed in the transverse or longitudinal planes to the liver where the hepatic veins can be observed to join the vena cava. The portal vein can be traced from the confluence of the mesenteric veins to the liver where it branches. The presence of hyperechoic walls helps to identify the portal vein. The portal vein, hepatic vein, and extrahepatic bile ducts come together at the porta hepatis. It is sometimes difficult to recognize the difference between these structures. The echogenicity of the walls of the portal vein is helpful in recognizing the portal branches. Doppler is sometimes necessary to distinguish between these three structures. Portal blood flow can be measured using pulsed Doppler. An overestimation of portal flow usually results. A scanning plane through the right 11th or 12th intercostal space is recommended.[42] Doppler can be used to examine intra-abdominal arteries and veins. The examination is technically difficult in an awake unsedated animal. The value of this technique is unproven in veterinary medicine.

GASTROINTESTINAL SYSTEM

SPECIAL PROCEDURES: GENERAL CONSIDERATIONS

The abdominal organs are affected by many lesions which exert their pathologic effect at a physiologic or anatomic level not discernible by survey radiography. These lesions may be identified by one or more special (contrast) procedures. Many different special procedures may be performed to evaluate the abdominal organs. Recommended methods for these procedures vary; however, the principles of interpretation are the same regardless of technique. The described methods of performing the procedures are those preferred by the authors.

PERITONEAL CAVITY

Positive-Contrast Peritonography and Pneumoperitoneum

Radiographic definition of peritoneal structures or the diaphragm may be improved by the use of either a positive-contrast peritoneogram or pneumoperitoneum.[43] These procedures were used infrequently before ultrasound became available and are even less commonly used now. The pneumoperitoneum is performed by placing a needle or catheter through the abdominal wall and inflating the peritoneal cavity with gas. Carbon dioxide (CO_2) or nitrous oxide (N_2O) are preferred because they are more soluble and more quickly absorbed; room air is safe and may be used. The amount of gas needed varies, but the abdomen should be tympanitic after inflation. The radiographic position used varies with the structure of interest. Positioning should cause the air to surround the organ of interest based on the fact that air will rise to the highest point within the abdomen. For example, if the right lateral liver lobe is of interest, the preferred positioning would be either a lateral with the left side down so that the air would rise to the right side or a ventrodorsal view performed using a horizontally directed x-ray beam and having the animal held in an erect standing position (i.e., with the forelimbs elevated). If a diaphragmatic hernia is suspected, a minimal amount of gas should be used because of the risk of pneumothorax. Positive contrast peritonography is most useful when peritoneal fluid is present. The contrast will mix with the fluid and outline the soft tissue-dense abdominal viscera. Positive contrast peritonography can also be used for evaluation of the integrity of the diaphragm; however, these procedures are used infrequently because ultrasound is a much easier technique.

Selective Abdominal Compression

Both normal and abnormal structures within the abdomen can be obscured by overlying intestines. Selective abdominal compression is a technique that utilizes a wooden spoon or paddle to isolate these structures by displacing the intestines away from the area of interest.[2,3] With the animal in lateral or dorsal recumbency, the structure of interest is palpated and isolated from the intestines. A radiolucent wooden spoon or paddle is placed over the structure to hold it in place and prevent the intestines from moving back into the area. The individual who is performing the examination can then remove his/her hand and the radiographic exposure can be made. The portion of the abdomen that is of interest will be compressed or thinner than normal; therefore, the radiographic technique must be reduced to compensate for the reduced thickness. As in any technique that requires someone to be in the x-ray room at the time of the x-ray exposure, protective devices such as lead gloves and aprons must be worn. In addition, the x-ray beam must be collimated to the area of interest rather than exposing the whole abdominal area. This technique can be used very effectively to displace the intestines away from the kidney when a renal or ureteral calculus is suspected, to isolate the uterine horns or body, or to isolate an intestinal mass which can be palpated but cannot be identified because of overlying gas or ingesta-filled bowel.

PORTAL BLOOD FLOW

Operative Mesenteric Portography, Splenoportography, and Cranial Mesenteric Arteriography

Several special procedures are available to evaluate portal blood flow to the liver. These include the operative mesenteric portogram, the splenoportogram, or the venous washout phase of the cranial mesenteric arteriogram.[44–46] The splenoportogram is performed by introducing a needle or catheter into the body of the spleen, preferably near the origin of the splenic veins. At this time, a manometer may be attached to the system to determine splenic pulp pressure (a reflection of the pressure in the portal system). After this, water-soluble iodinated contrast media (at a dose of 1–2 cc/kg) is injected as rapidly as possible, and a radiograph is taken as the last part of the injection is completed. Placement of the needle within the spleen and stability of the needle during the contrast injection to ensure that the contrast is injected into the spleen and not into the peritoneal cavity are the major difficulties in this procedure. Another method of demonstrating these structures is the operative mesenteric portogram. In this procedure, a laparotomy is performed and a mesenteric vein is cannulated with an 18-gauge intravenous catheter. Iodinated water-soluble contrast media is injected at a dose of 1 cc/kg body weight, and radiographs are taken as the last part of the injection is delivered. This technique requires intraoperative radiographs or multiple closures and reopenings of the abdominal incision. The third method uses the venous phase of an injection of contrast into the cranial mesenteric artery.[46] Because fluoroscopy is required and the detail of the venous phase is sometimes poor, this method is performed infrequently. Of the three techniques, operative mesenteric portography currently is the technique used most frequently. Transcolonic portography using a radio-isotope has become popular as a screening procedure for the detection of portosystemic shunts. This technique requires the use of a scintillation (gamma) camera and usually is only available at referral centers.

GALLBLADDER

Cholecystography

Cholecystography is occasionally performed to visualize the gallbladder.[47–49] This may be done for a questionable location of the gallbladder (e.g., suspected diaphragmatic hernia) or if obstruction to bile flow is suspected. The use of this procedure in biliary obstruction is quite limited, because the liver handles the contrast media in the same manner that it handles bilirubin. Therefore, in icteric animals it is quite unlikely to opacify the gallbladder in an adequate manner, because the liver will regurgitate both bile and contrast media and prevent accumulation of the contrast within the gallbladder. Both oral and intravenous contrast agents have been used in dogs and cats. Oral cholecystography has been performed in dogs using calcium ipodate at a dose of 150 mg/kg body weight. In cats, oral cholecystography has been performed using iobenzamic acid at a dose of 50 mg/kg and iodopate at a dose of 150 mg/kg. Radiographs are obtained 12 to 14 hours following contrast administration. Intravenous cholecystography has been performed in dogs using iodipamide at a dose of 0.5 mg/kg and in cats at a dose of 1 ml/kg. Although the contrast may be seen in the gallbladder as early as 15 minutes post injection, radiographs are usually obtained 60 minutes post intravenous injection.

Percutaneous cholecystography has been performed safely in dogs.[50] A needle is placed into the liver under fluoroscopic guidance and radiopaque water soluble contrast is injected as the needle is withdrawn. The gallbladder is identified by flow of contrast into the lumen. The gallbladder is monitored as it is filled with contrast material, and filling is continued until the contrast flows into the common bile duct and reaches the duodenum. Aspiration of the contrast and bile is performed before the needle is removed from the gallbladder. Twenty to 30 ml of contrast is usually required for average size dogs (11–25 kg). A similar technique can be used for cholangiography, in which the contrast is identified within an intrahepatic bile duct or hepatic vein as the needle is withdrawn using fluoroscopy. These techniques are of limited value and are available only at centers that have fluoroscopic equipment.

Although the gallbladder and bile ducts can be evaluated using ultrasound, limited functional information can be obtained. Sincalide, a synthetic cholecystokinin, has been used to induce gallbladder emptying in order to obtain some functional information and distinguish between obstructive and nonobstructive biliary disease. The drug is injected intravenously at a dose of 0.04 µg/kg, and the response of the gallbladder is monitored using ultrasound. Normal dogs and dogs with nonobstructive biliary disease reduce the volume of the gallbladder by 40% within 1 hour, while obstructed dogs reduced their gallbladder volume less than 20%. Side effects to the injection were not reported.[51]

GASTROINTESTINAL SYSTEM

Gastrointestinal Series

Non-contrast radiographs should always precede a GI contrast study. This approach may save you the effort, the patient the discomfort, and the owner the expense of a contrast study. Even if non-contrast radiographs were obtained several hours or a day before, they should be repeated. The most commonly performed special study of the GI tract is the GI (barium) series. This is indicated when the animal has exhibited clinical signs of GI disease that have failed to respond to symptomatic treatment or has other findings (e.g., history of ingestion of foreign matter, suspicious palpation of the abdomen, etc.) which suggest that anatomic evaluation of the GI tract may be helpful in elucidating the problem. The presence of diarrhea with no other GI sign is rarely an indication to perform a GI series. The most common mistakes made when performing a GI contrast study are improper patient preparation, administering too little contrast, and obtaining too few radiographs after contrast administration. The patient's GI tract should be empty before contrast administration, because food and fecal material can mimic or obscure lesions. This is achieved by withholding all food for at least 12 hours and using laxatives and/or enemas. If necessary, dogs may be sedated with an intravenous dose of 0.1 to 3.0 mg of acetylpromazine unless contraindicated by other factors (e.g., a history of seizures).[8,52] Cats may be sedated by the intravenous injection of 10 mg of ketamine or by intramuscular injection of ketamine (12 mg/lb); acepromazine/ketamine (0.1 mg/lb, 6 mg/lb); or ketamine/valium (6 mg/lb, 0.2 mg/lb).[53,54] A 25% to 40% weight/volume suspension of barium (we do not recommend the use of iodine-containing water-soluble contrast media for this purpose) is administered by orogastric or nasogastric intubation at a dose of 5 to 8 ml/lb. Although others have recommended smaller dosages, it is our experience that the most common problem with this study is the use of an inadequate dose, which fails to distend the GI tract completely. Commercially premixed products are preferred to barium powder that requires mixing with water, because the suspending agents in commercially prepared products seem to produce superior mucosal detail, more uniform passage, and a more stable suspension. Both ionic and non-ionic water-soluble iodine-containing contrast media are used by some veterinarians because they will pass more rapidly through the GI tract.[8,55] The presumed advantage of more rapid transit by the water-soluble iodine-containing contrast media is far outweighed by the disadvantage of the very poor contrast and detail these products provide.[8,56,57] These agents do not coat the mucosa very well, and the ionic agents may also irritate the gastric mucosa and cause vomiting. Furthermore, as the contrast media passes through the intestine, the hyperosmolar ionic agents draw body fluids into the intestine. This results in a decreasing density throughout the study and systemic dehydration, which may be dangerous in an already dehydrated patient. The use of water-soluble agents is recommended when bowel rupture is suspected because of the potential for granulomatous peritonitis caused by free barium in the abdominal cavity. While this is a valid consideration, the possibility of misdiagnosis (because of poor contrast density) in cases of minimal leakage from small defects in the bowel, coupled with the opportunity to flush any leaked barium from the abdomen at laparotomy, leads us to recommend the use of barium for almost all studies.

Instillation by stomach tube requires certainty that the tube is positioned in the stomach. Careful palpation of the esophagus after placing the stomach tube is required. Even in cats, the orogastric tube can be palpated to distinguish it from the trachea if care is exercised. Use of a stomach tube is superior to oral instillation, because it is common for animals to expectorate a portion of the barium as well as to inhale some of the barium as they struggle. They also tend to swallow large amounts of air at the same time. Gastric intubation ensures that the stomach will receive a proper dose of barium so that it is adequately distended.

It has been reported that the normal time for barium to reach the colon after instillation is 180±90 minutes in the dog and 30 to 60 minutes in the cat.[52,54,58–60] In dogs, radiographs should be taken immediately after the barium has been administered and at intervals of 15 minutes, 30 minutes, 1 hour, 2 hours, 3 hours, and periodically thereafter until the barium reaches the colon. In the cat, barium passes through the normal GI tract more rapidly and therefore radiographs should be taken at 0 minutes, 10 minutes, 20 minutes, 30 minutes, 1 hour, and hourly thereafter until the barium reaches the colon and the stomach is empty. Four views (ventrodorsal, dorsoventral, and left and right recumbent laterals) should be taken immediately after contrast administration because different portions of the stomach are profiled in each view. At least a ventrodorsal and lateral view should be taken at each time thereafter. If this is impossible, the ventrodorsal view is preferred because it minimizes superimposition of structures and allows for evaluation of the majority of the stomach. In the normal animal, gastric contractions will be apparent and will alter the gastric shape over time. An open pylorus is rarely seen radiographically because, compared to gastric mixing, pyloric opening is relatively infrequent and of short duration. The length of time required for complete gastric emptying varies; however, a marked delay in beginning the passage of significant amounts of contrast agent from the stomach implies a pyloric outflow obstruction. Gastric emptying may be prolonged in nervous patients. These animals will usually resume normal peristalsis if left in a quiet environment for a few minutes. There is a great deal of variation in gastric emptying times among normal dogs so most figures given are useful only as crude estimates. Although each individual dog is consistent there is considerable variation from dog to dog.

Mixing food with barium to evaluate gastric emptying serves no useful purpose. In most cases, the liquid barium will separate from the food and transit the intestines while the food remains in the stomach until it becomes liquefied. Although gastric emptying time following administration of barium food mixture is fairly consistent for an individual dog, a large variation is observed among dogs. Variation in total gastric emptying time from 5 to 14 hours has been reported.[59,61]

In the normal intestinal tract, the contrast passes through in a relatively organized fashion. The loops are smooth-walled and uniformly distended with a few constrictions representing normal peristalsis. A fimbriated or brush border may be present. A normal pattern of symmetrical oval contractions, termed a "string of beads," has been described in the duodenum of the normal cat. Irregularities in the duodenum of the dog consisting of one or more crater like lesions result from the presence of gut-associated lymphoid tissue (GALT, Peyers patches).[8,54]

Often lesions of the stomach will be seen clearly on the ventrodorsal or dorsoventral view and not on the lateral view. The paramount principle in evaluating a GI series is the repeatability of a lesion at least on multiple radiographs if not multiple positions. Thus, a study that has a limited number of radiographs may be nondiagnostic. If a structure appears abnormal on one film but does not remain constant in appearance on at least the same view throughout the series, it should be regarded as spurious and the study should be considered normal. The GI series is a poor evaluator of physiologic function and is a more accurate evaluator of gross anatomic change. The large intestine should not be evaluated with the GI series. This is because of the lack of colon distension. To evaluate the colon radiographically a pneumocolon, barium enema, or double contrast enema should be performed.

Double Contrast Gastrogram

In most instances the stomach can be evaluated adequately by the GI series; however, the double contrast gastrogram is recommended for those conditions requiring evaluation of relatively minor anatomic changes.[8,62–64] Because of the use of glucagon, this procedure may be contraindicated in animals with diabetes mellitus. Fluoroscopy is recommended but not required to perform this procedure. The patient should be anesthetized or heavily tranquilized. Immediately prior to the procedure, glucagon is injected intravenously (0.1 mg for small dogs to 0.35 mg for large dogs) after which a 100% weight/volume barium suspension is administered via a stomach tube at a dose of 1.5 to 3.0 ml/kg. Following this, the stomach is distended with air until it is tympanitic (approximately 20 ml/kg) upon percussion. Immediately after the contrast agents have been administered, a minimum of four views (ventrodorsal, dorsoventral, left lateral, and right lateral) are taken and additional oblique views may be needed to ensure that every gastric surface is fully evaluated.

Pneumocolon

The easiest radiographic special procedure for the evaluation of the colon is the pneumocolon.[8,65] Preparation of the abdomen is not as important as it is for the GI series. The procedure is performed by inserting a catheter or syringe tip through the rectal sphincter and injecting 1 to 3 ml of air per kilogram of body weight. Lateral and ventrodorsal views are then exposed. Based on the appearance of the radiographs, more air may be added as needed. The technique is useful for evaluating the colon and rectum for intraluminal, intramural, and extraluminal lesions. It can be used to demonstrate the cranial extent of a mass or stricture that narrows the lumen of the colon too much for passage of an endoscope. It is also useful for identifying the location of the colon and distinguishing it from distended small intestines.

Barium Enema/Double Contrast Enema

Evaluation of the colon may also be accomplished by the barium or double contrast enema. Preparation of the colon using multiple enemas or laxatives is essential because the colon must be emptied prior to the study. Fecal material within the lumen of the colon may mimic or obscure a lesion. This contrast technique is rarely used because evaluation of the colon using a rigid or flexible colonoscope or proctoscope is relatively easy. Colonoscopy has the advantage of directly visualizing lesions, determining their extent, and potentially obtaining a biopsy or cytological specimen. If the lesion is not accessible with the equipment available and a pneumocolon will not provide sufficient information, a contrast enema is indicated. The patient must be anesthetized. A 15% to 20% weight/volume barium suspension is instilled at a dose of 22.2 ml/kg via a cuffed enema tube.[8,66] Lateral and ventrodorsal views should be taken. The barium is then drained from the colon, which is then insufflated with an equal volume of air to create a double contrast enema. Lateral and ventrodorsal radiographs are taken.

ABNORMAL FINDINGS

GENERAL ABDOMEN

Body Wall

Radiographic changes in the size or shape of the body wall are limited to either increases or decreases in thickness or disruption of continuity. Increases in body wall thickness may be focal or diffuse. In focal thickening, the diagnosis may be suggested by the density. If the thickened portion is fat-dense, a lipoma is the probable diagnosis. If the thickened portion is tissue-dense, a tumor, abscess, or granuloma may be present. Occasionally, mammary or other abdominal wall tumors will contain calcified densities. This may occur in association with mixed mammary tumors or soft tissue osteosarcomas. The mammary glands may appear as focal areas of soft tissue density peripheral to the body wall (Fig. 3–27). When body wall thickening is present, the regional lymph nodes that drain the area should be evaluated for enlargement, which would suggest tumor metastasis. Diffuse thickening of the body wall suggests the possibility of infection, edema, or hemorrhage. If enlarged, the inguinal lymph nodes may be observed as an oval soft tissue density ventral to the caudal abdominal wall. Either traumatic or developmental defects in the body wall, through which abdominal contents herniate, may not be readily seen, but the displaced abdominal viscera will usually be apparent (Fig. 3–28). Decreased density within the abdominal wall may occur in association with a hernia when intestines are present within the hernia or when subcutaneous emphysema is present. The intestines can be recognized by their curvilinear shapes, while the subcutaneous emphysema tends to be more linearly or irregularly shaped.

The abdominal wall can be evaluated using ultrasound, although it is rarely necessary. When a hernia is present, the defect in the abdominal wall can be identified by tracing the normal structures that surround the defect. This makes recognition of the defect easier. Mineral structures, gas, and intestines can be identified within a hernia. Ultrasound is much better at detecting the presence of the urinary blad-

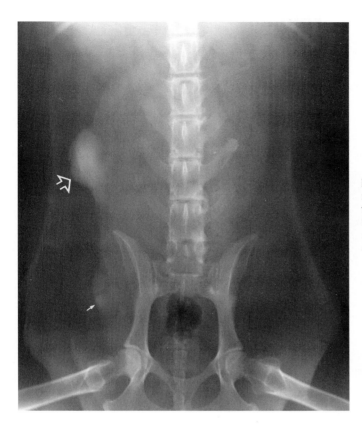

Figure 3–27. A 12-year-old female golden retriever with masses on the ventral body wall. The ventrodorsal view revealed a highlighted tissue density mass (due to the fact that the mass was surrounded by air) on the right of the midline (*open white arrow*). A normal nipple is also apparent (*small white arrow*). **Diagnosis:** Ventral hernia.

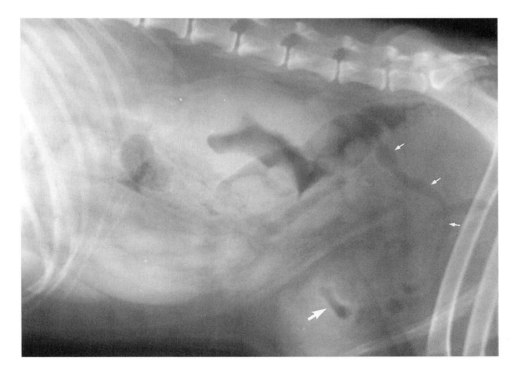

Figure 3–28. A 14-year-old neutered male mixed breed dog with gagging for 2 days. There are multiple gas-filled bowel loops (*large white arrow*) ventral to and crossing (*small white arrows*) the normal line of the ventral body wall. **Diagnosis:** Ventral hernia.

der within a hernia than is radiography. Ultrasound is very useful for detecting foreign bodies within the soft tissues. Objects such as wood, glass, or plastic, which may be tissue-dense and therefore not detected radiographically, can be readily identified as hyperechoic structures that shadow. Enlarged inguinal lymph nodes are usually round or oval and hypoechoic.

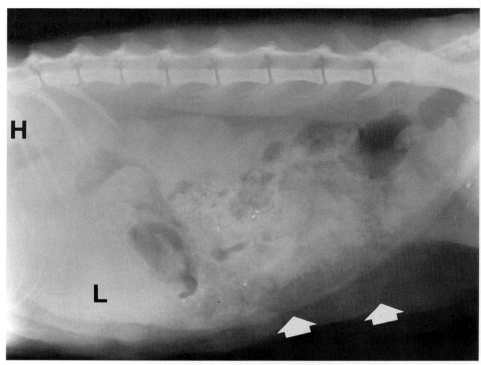

Figure 3–29. A 7-year-old male Siamese cat with anorexia and vomiting for 4 days and pain upon abdominal palpation. There is a mottling of tissue density in the normally homogenous density of the abdominal fat. This is readily apparent in the fat pads ventral to the abdominal wall (*white arrows*). Also noted is hepatomegaly (*black* L) and hydrothorax (*black* H). Differential diagnoses include steatitis or neoplasia with abdominal carcinomatosis and thoracic metastases. **Diagnosis:** Steatitis (the cat had been on an all tuna diet).

Peritoneal Cavity

The ability to identify viscera within the peritoneal cavity radiographically results from the presence of abdominal fat. Loss of detail in the peritoneal cavity may be focal or diffuse and may be associated with cachexia, youth, carcinomatosis, steatitis, peritonitis, or hydroperitoneum (Fig. 3–29). A small amount of peritoneal fluid is normally present in puppies and kittens. Hydroperitoneum may be caused by feline infectious peritonitis, right-sided heart failure, bacterial infection, urine as a result of rupture of the urinary tract, hypoproteinemia, portal hypertension, or hemorrhage. Hydroperitoneum may be present in any degree, ranging from minimal with just slight blurring of the edges of the abdominal viscera to marked causing a homogeneous tissue density throughout.

Occasionally, free air may be seen within the abdomen. The most common cause is previous surgery. In experimental dogs, the duration of pneumoperitoneum ranged from 7 to 34 days depending mostly on the volume of air administered.[67] Air may be present in readily visible amounts for up to 10 days, and in minimal amounts for up to 30 days after surgery in normal animals. Penetrating wounds of the abdominal wall and rupture of a hollow viscus (stomach or intestine) may result in free peritoneal air. Spontaneous pneumoperitoneum (i.e., not associated with surgery or ruptured viscus) is rare. It has been reported subsequent to gastric volvulus with or without splenic necrosis.[68] With severe intestinal distension secondary to ileus, air may diffuse into the peritoneal cavity across the thin intestinal wall. The presence of pneumoperitoneum is recognized by identifying air density dissecting between normal structures and often outlining the individual liver lobes, the abdominal side of the diaphragm, or the nondependent kidney. Increased definition of the serosal surfaces of the intestines may be evident. Air bubbles and linear or triangular air patterns may be seen. These are most readily recognized in areas of the abdomen that do not normally contain small intestines such as around the liver, lateral to the

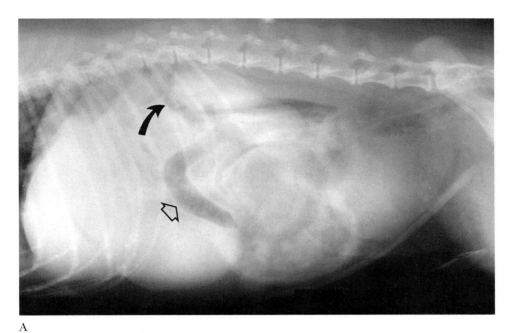

A

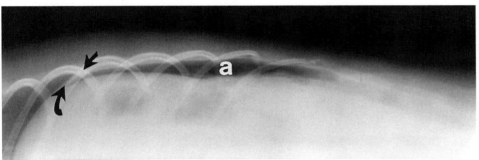

B

Figure 3–30. A 7-year-old male West Highland white terrier with vomiting and anorexia for 3 days. (A) The lateral view revealed a moderate loss of normal abdominal detail consistent with a hydroperitoneum. There is a mildly dilated loop of small intestine (*open black arrow*). Close scrutiny revealed the suggestion of air density in the region of the kidneys (*solid black arrow*). (B) The left lateral decubitus revealed the presence of free abdominal air (*white a*), which outlines the tissue dense diaphragm (*between black arrows*) against the air density of the lung. Differential diagnoses include rupture of an intestinal structure, infection of the abdominal cavity with a gas-forming organism, or iatrogenic pneumoperitoneum (secondary to surgery). **Diagnosis:** Pneumoperitoneum and peritonitis secondary to a ruptured small intestinal leiomyosarcoma.

spleen, and dorsal to the colon. If the diagnosis is questionable, a left lateral decubitus view (a radiograph taken with horizontal x-ray beam with the patient in left lateral recumbency) should be taken to show the air between the liver and right lateral body wall (Fig. 3–30). A right lateral decubitus view may also be used, however gas within the stomach may be mistaken for free peritoneal air.

Occasionally, one or more small, round structures with calcified rims ("egg shell" calcification) will be seen. These structures, if not associated with any abdominal organ, are probably mesenteric cysts (cholesterol cysts) which are free in the peritoneum and are of no pathologic significance (Fig. 3–31). Occasionally, blood vessel walls may be calcified. These appear as pairs of thin linear calcific densities following the paths of the major arteries. These findings may be the result of advanced renal failure, hyperadrenocorticism, hyperparathyroidism, or atherosclerosis (Fig. 3–32).

Unless present in massive amounts, fluid within the peritoneal cavity facilitates the ultrasound examination (Fig. 3–33). If marked distension of the abdomen has

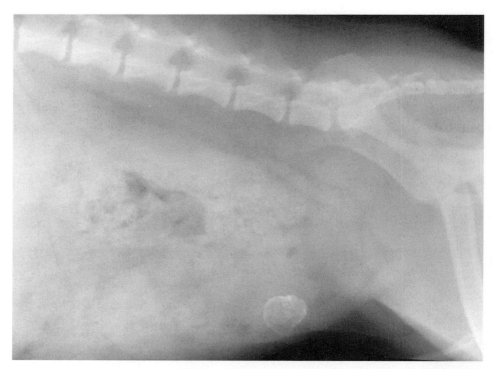

Figure 3–31. A 5-year-old male Lhasa apso with vomiting for 3 days. There is a structure with calcified borders ("egg shell" calcification) in the caudal ventral abdomen. Differential diagnoses include mesenteric cyst, cystic calculus, or intestinal foreign body. On the ventrodorsal view the structure was not located within the bladder or small intestine. **Diagnosis:** Mesenteric cyst (the dog's vomiting resolved with symptomatic treatment).

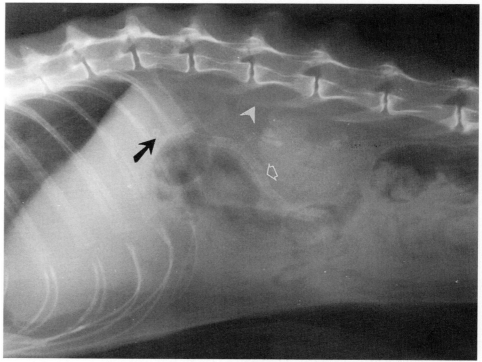

Figure 3–32. A 13-year-old castrated Persian cat with chronic renal disease. There are fine linear calcifications outlining portions of the celiac (*black arrow*), cranial mesenteric (*open white arrow*), and renal arteries (*solid white arrowhead*). Differential diagnoses include calcification due to chronic renal failure, hyperadrenocorticism, or atherosclerosis. **Diagnosis:** Arterial wall calcification due to chronic renal failure.

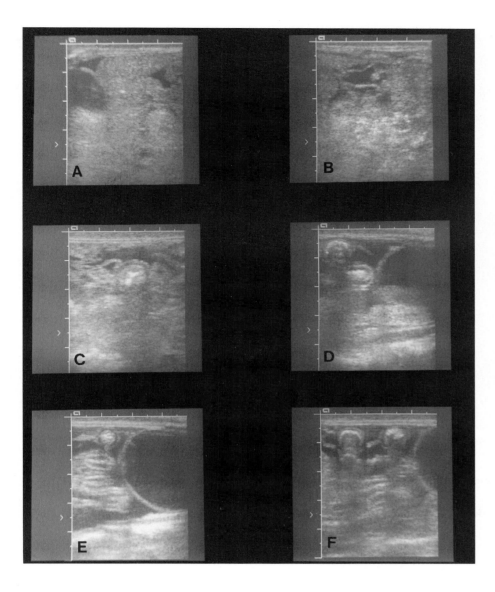

Figure 3–33. Sonograms of the abdomen of a 14-year-old castrated male cat with a history of abdominal distension and a palpable abdominal mass. There is anechoic free peritoneal fluid throughout the abdomen. This can be seen outlining the spleen and gall bladder (A), the folds of the mesentery and omentum (B), several intestinal loops (C,D,E,&F) and the urinary bladder wall (D,E,&F). **Diagnosis:** Ascites, lymphosarcoma.

occurred, removal of the fluid is recommended because the patient will be more comfortable and will breathe less rapidly and the abdominal wall will be more compressible allowing the placement of the transducer closer to the structure of interest. In an experimental study in dogs, ultrasound was more sensitive than radiography in detecting abdominal fluid. As little as 2 ml of fluid per pound of body weight could be detected using ultrasound, while at least 4 ml of fluid per pound of body weight were required before the fluid could be detected radiographically.[69] The nature of the abdominal fluid cannot be determined using ultrasound; however, if the fluid contains a large number of cells these can be recognized and fibrin strands can also be identified. In most instances, the ultrasound examination provides guidance for abdominocentesis. Peritoneal masses or granulomas can be detected using ultrasound. These may be observed as heteroechoic structures on the parietal peritoneum attached to the body wall or may be seen on the serosal surface of abdominal viscera. Abdominal abscesses may produce an irregularly defined hypoechoic mass with little or no through-transmission. A definitive diagnosis based solely on the ultrasound examination is rarely possible.[70]

Ultrasound examination of calcified abdominal masses is often unrewarding. The mineral produces shadowing, which obscures the internal structure of the mass (Fig. 3–34).

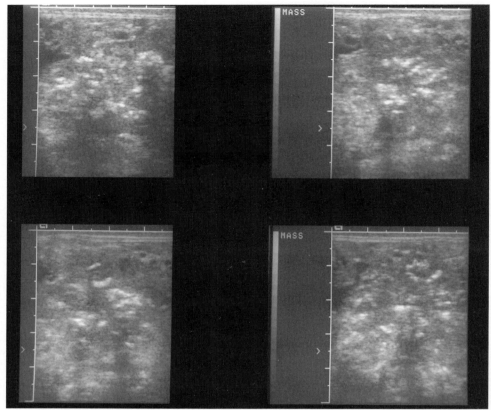

Figure 3–34. Longitudinal sonograms of the midabdomen of a 14-year-old castrated male cat with a history of anorexia and weight loss of 4 months' duration. The cat was FeLV +. There is a heteroechoic mass identified in the midabdomen. This mass contains many hyperechoic foci of varying size. The mass was not associated with the GI tract. This is indicative of a mesenteric mass with mineral foci within the mass. **Diagnosis:** Lymphosarcoma.

Air within the peritoneal cavity may be detected during the ultrasound examination. It is hyperechoic and creates a reverberation (comet tail) artifact (Fig. 3–35). Important features that identify the presence of free air are its location away from the intestines and its movement with changes in the animal's position.

LIVER

Radiographic Abnormalities

DENSITY CHANGES

Radiographic lesions of the liver are frequently nonspecific, but they will support diagnoses indicated by other data. Density changes in the liver are uncommon; however, calcifications and air accumulations have been described. The liver may be partly or almost completely calcified in end stage liver disease, abscess, tumor, hematoma, or cyst (Figs. 3–36 and 3–37). While the most common pattern of calcification is punctuate or stippled, the calcification may also appear as larger aggregations or an egg shell pattern. Choleliths (gallstones) are usually composed of bile pigments and may not be radiographically apparent; however, those that are partially or completely calcified may be seen on non-contrast radiographs (Fig. 3–38). In one study of dogs with clinical signs of cholelithiasis, 48% had radiopaque stones that could be identified on noncontrast radiographs.[71] Usually, choleliths are not clinically significant because they rarely obstruct the flow of bile. Gas densities may

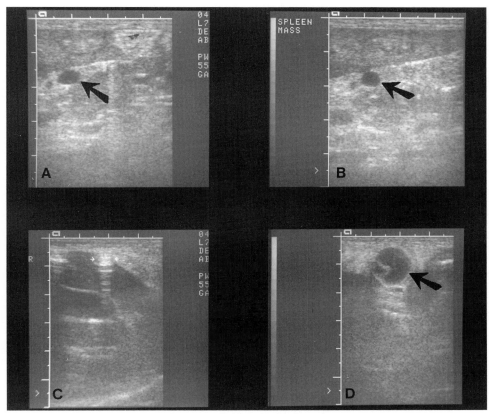

Figure 3–35. Transverse sonograms of the spleen (A&B), cranial abdomen (C), and caudal abdomen (D) of an 11-year-old Tibetan terrier with a history of chronic vomiting and melena. There are oval shaped hypoechoic masses visible medial to the spleen and in the caudal abdomen (*arrows*). These represent enlarged abdominal lymph nodes. There is a focal area of increased echo intensity in the cranial abdomen adjacent to the body wall (C). There is a reverberation artifact associated with this lesion (*white arrows*). This is indicative of free intraperitoneal air. **Diagnosis:** Lymphosarcoma, intraperitoneal air secondary to bowel perforation.

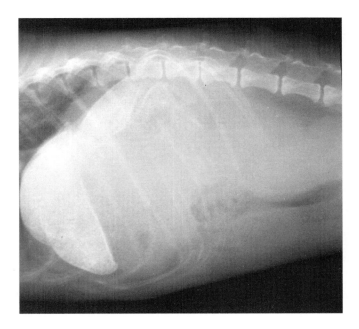

Figure 3–36. A 3-year-old female poodle with vomiting, anorexia, and icterus. There is a homogeneously stippled pattern of calcification involving all the liver lobes. There is poor abdominal detail and minimal soft tissue over the vertebrae consistent with cachexia. **Diagnosis:** Hepatic calcification.

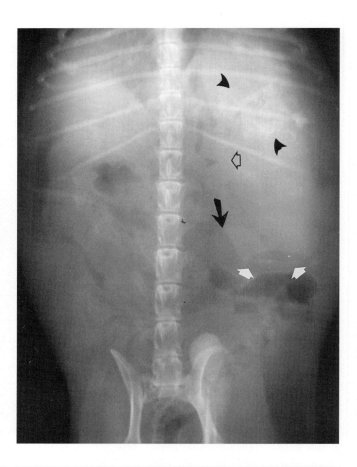

Figure 3–37. An 8-year-old male mixed breed dog with a 4-day history of anorexia and vomiting. There is enlargement of the left lateral liver lobe which extends caudally to the level of L4 (*white arrowheads*). The mass has displaced the left kidney caudally (*black arrow*) and the cardia and fundus of the stomach medially (*open black arrow*). There are multiple areas of calcification within the cranial portion of the liver mass (*black arrowheads*). Differential diagnoses include primary liver tumor with calcification, metastatic tumor with calcification, or extraskeletal osteosarcoma arising within the liver. **Diagnosis:** Extraskeletal osteosarcoma of the left lateral liver lobe.

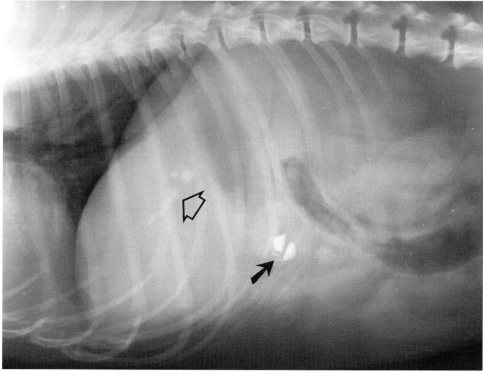

Figure 3–38. A 10-year-old neutered female mixed breed dog with hematuria for 1 week. While there are no radiographic findings pertinent to the urinary tract there are multiple calcific densities in the gallbladder (*open black arrow*). There are a few mineral-dense structures in the pylorus of the stomach. These are ingested small bone chips (*solid black arrow*). **Diagnosis:** Gallstones (the hematuria resolved after treatment with antibiotics).

be seen within the liver parenchyma and within and around the gallbladder and bile ducts (Figs. 3–39 and 3–40). This may be the result of infection of the liver or gallbladder by anaerobic gas forming organisms or, in diabetic patients, because of infection of these structures by organisms capable of fermenting glucose and producing CO_2 as a by-product.[72] The linear shape of the air densities when they are within the bile ducts or gallbladder wall or the oval shape of the air density when it is within the gallbladder permit recognition of this condition. When the gas is within an abscess or necrotic tumor, the air will be more irregularly shaped. Identification of the

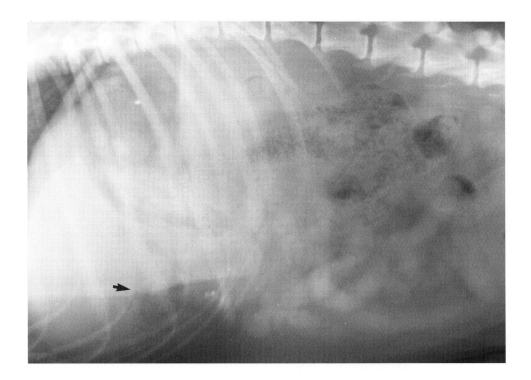

Figure 3–39. A 9-year-old male standard poodle with vomiting and pyrexia. There is an area of irregular gas density seen within the cranial ventral portion of the liver (*black arrow*). Differential diagnoses include abscess either with a glucose fermenting organism in diabetes mellitus or a *Clostridium sp.* **Diagnosis:** *Clostridium sp.* abscess.

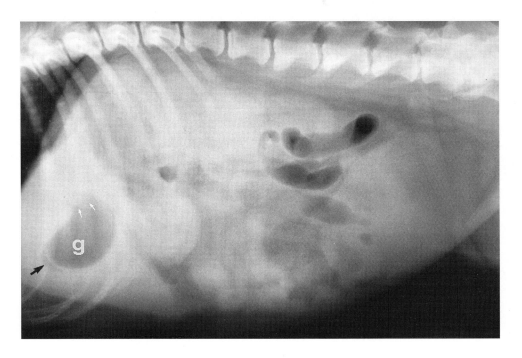

Figure 3–40. A 4-year-old male English bulldog with anorexia and vomiting for 3 days. The lateral radiograph revealed gas in the gallbladder (*white g*) and in the immediately adjacent space (*black arrow*). Close scrutiny revealed a round tissue-dense structure in the neck of the gallbladder (*white arrows*) which proved to be a stone. **Diagnosis:** Cholelith with emphysematous cholecystitis and pericholecystitis due to infection with *Clostridium sp.*

gas on two views is essential to confirm its position within the liver. Confusion with gas within the stomach is possible; however, the air contained within the liver will be fixed in position when the animal is moved while the gas within the stomach will change its position.

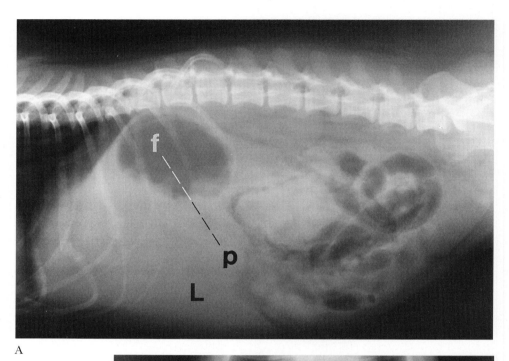

A

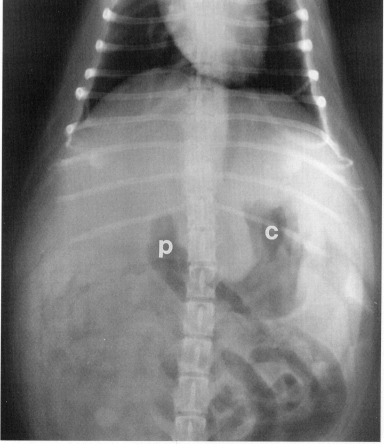

B

Figure 3–41. A 6-year-old female poodle with chronic polyuria and polydipsia. (A) On the lateral view there is extension of the caudal ventral border of the liver well beyond the chondral arch (*black L*) and increased angulation (i.e., an angle greater than that of the intercostal spaces) of the stomach from the fundus (*white f*) to the pylorus (*black p*). (B) On the ventrodorsal view, the pylorus (*white c*) of the stomach is displaced medially. **Diagnosis:** Generalized hepatomegaly (in this case secondary to diabetes mellitus).

SIZE CHANGES

The most common radiographic change in the liver is an increase in size. Because the normal appearance varies greatly depending on the animal's breed and body condition, recognition of pathology can be difficult. The length of the liver, as measured from the most cranial point on the diaphragm to the caudal-most point on the ventral liver, has been correlated with liver volume in normal dogs.[73] Whether this measurement is useful or practical in patients has not been established. There are several radiographic changes that indicate hepatomegaly. The greater the number of changes that can be identified the more reliable the diagnosis of hepatomegaly becomes. On the lateral view, the radiographic signs of diffuse hepatomegaly include increased angulation of the gastric shadow (increased caudal displacement of the pylorus relative to the cardia and fundus), extension of the ventral hepatic border beyond the 13th rib and chondral cartilages, and rounding of the hepatic borders (Fig. 3–41). On the ventrodorsal view, there may be displacement of the pylorus toward the midline by the right liver lobes, displacement of the cardia toward the midline by the left hepatic lobes, and caudal displacement of the stomach, small intestines, and right kidney. Although hepatic enlargement will displace the spleen caudally, the spleen is normally quite moveable; therefore, the position of the spleen is a poor indicator of the presence of hepatomegaly. Generalized hepatomegaly is a nonspecific finding for which the differential diagnoses include hepatitis; fatty infiltration (either primary or secondary to diseases such as diabetes mellitus); hyperadrenocorticism (due to hepatic accumulation of glycogen); passive congestion; hypertrophic nodular cirrhosis; primary neoplasia (such as lymphosarcoma, mast cell tumor, hepatocellular carcinoma, carcinoid, or bile duct carcinoma); and metastatic neoplasia.

Enlargement of specific hepatic lobes may be more difficult to identify than generalized hepatomegaly. In some instances, a pneumoperitoneum may be useful in reaching a definitive diagnosis by clearly outlining the size and shape of a liver lobe. Enlargement (or masses) of the left lateral lobe may cause displacement of the cardia of the stomach to the right on the ventrodorsal view and dorsally on the lateral view (Fig. 3–42). The small intestine and spleen may be displaced caudally on both views. Enlargement of the right lateral lobe may cause the duodenum to be displaced medially on the ventrodorsal view and dorsally on the lateral view (Fig. 3–43). Enlargement of the caudate lobe may produce a tissue-dense mass in the dorsal, cranial portion of the abdomen. If the caudate process of this lobe is affected, the right kidney may be displaced caudally from its normal position (the 13th rib crossing the right kidney at the level of renal pelvis) (Fig. 3–44). Pneumoperitonography may be particularly helpful in outlining the borders of the caudate lobe. Differential considerations in all of these instances should include primary neoplasia (hepatocellular carcinoma, carcinoid, or bile duct carcinoma); metastatic neoplasia; torsion; incarceration; or benign lesions (hepatic cyst, abscess, or unusually large area of nodular hyperplasia).

Occasionally, a liver may appear smaller than normal. Because many animals have livers that appear small without clinical signs or biochemical abnormalities, it is difficult to define the exact measurements that should be considered pathological. The liver often appears smaller in deep-chested dogs (Afghan hounds, Irish setters, etc.) than in dogs with shorter, squarer thoracic conformation. The position of the stomach close to the diaphragm is usually a sign of a small liver. In the lateral radiograph, the stomach may be angled in a caudodorsal to cranioventral direction. In those cases where the liver is quite small, the differential diagnoses should include hypotrophic cirrhosis or fibrosis (Fig. 3–45). These may be found in association with portosystemic shunts as well as toxic, metabolic, inflammatory, or idiopathic causes.

SHAPE CHANGES

Abnormalities in liver shape are a significant sign of liver disease and may occur in the absence of hepatomegaly. Only some of the conditions that produce hepatomegaly will alter the contour of the liver. Irregular, lumpy liver margins may be

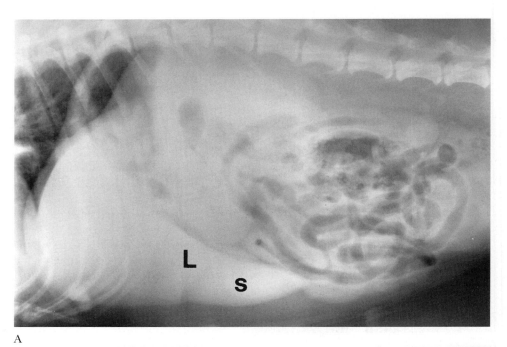

A

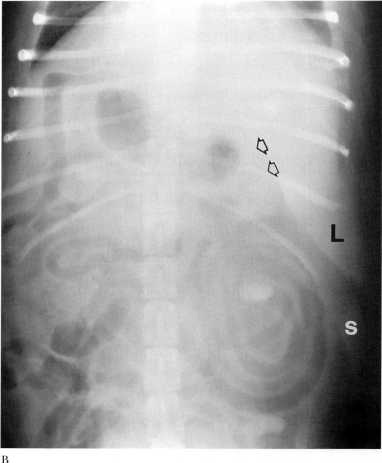

B

Figure 3–42. A 9-year-old female, mixed breed dog with a 3-week history of anorexia. (A) There is extension of the liver caudal to the chondral arch (*black L*). The spleen (*black s*), seen adjacent to the liver, obscures the liver's caudal border. (B) The left lateral lobe of the liver (*black L*) extends caudal to its normal position and has displaced the spleen (*white s*) caudally and the fundus of the stomach medially (*open black arrows*). Differential diagnoses included primary or metastatic liver tumor, nodular hyperplasia, or granuloma. **Diagnosis:** Left lateral liver lobe hepatoma.

caused by neoplasia, abscess, cyst, cirrhosis, or nodular hyperplasia (Fig. 3–46). Smooth rounding of the liver edges is a nonspecific finding suggesting hepatic swelling. The radiograph tends to underestimate alterations in liver shape; therefore, if the liver appears irregular on a radiograph the degree of change that is present will be marked.

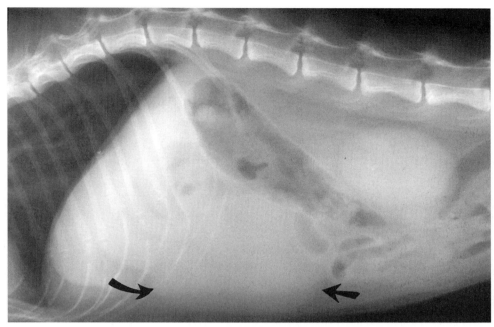

A

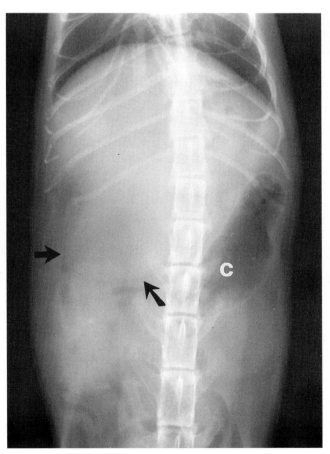

B

Figure 3–43. A 3-year-old female domestic short-haired cat with no clinical problems brought to the clinic for an ovario-hysterectomy. Physical examination revealed a palpable mass in the cranial abdomen. (A) There is a smooth bordered tissue density mass extending from the liver caudally beyond the chrondral arch (*black arrows*). (B) The ascending and transverse colon (*white c*) are displaced to the left and caudally by the right-sided abdominal mass (*black arrows*). Differential diagnoses include hepatic neoplasia (primary or metastatic), granuloma, or hepatic cyst. **Diagnosis:** Hepatic cyst arising from the right lateral liver lobe.

POSITION CHANGES

The position of the liver is maintained by the tight coronary, triangular, and falciform ligaments between the liver and the diaphragm. Liver lobes may be displaced

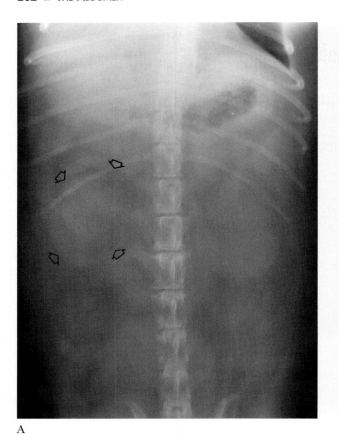

A

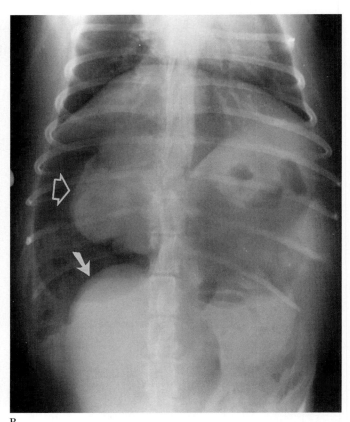

B

Figure 3–44. A 9-year-old female Cairn terrier with a 4-week history of vomiting and partial anorexia. (A) on the ventrodorsal view the right kidney (*open black arrows*) is displaced caudally from its normal position where the 13th rib would bisect it at the renal pelvis. This is suggestive of an enlargement of the caudate process of the caudate liver lobe. (B) On the dorsoventral pneumoperitoneum (this position was used to float the gas into the area of interest), the caudate process of the caudate lobe of the liver (*open white arrow*) shows marked rounding and irregularity. The right kidney (*solid white arrow*) is also seen. Differential diagnoses include hepatic neoplasia (primary or metastatic) or granuloma. **Diagnosis:** Caudate liver lobe hepatoma.

by diaphragmatic hernia or less commonly by torsion.[74] A hernia itself may cause no dysfunction; however, scarring of the diaphragmatic defect may put pressure on hepatic vessels and cause clinical signs some time after the original injury. Another possible result of trauma to the liver is fracture of one or more liver lobes. This is not readily detectable radiographically; however, there usually will be hemorrhage, which causes a loss of detail in the hepatic area. Pleural fluid, pleural or pulmonary masses, or tension pneumothorax may put pressure on the diaphragm and move the liver caudally. This can be recognized easily and should not be mistaken for hepatomegaly.

Ultrasound Abnormalities

SIZE CHANGES

It is difficult to measure the size of the liver objectively, because only a small portion of the liver can be seen during an ultrasound examination, and hepatomegaly is a function of liver volume rather than liver area.[75] A scheme has been proposed that utilizes a single linear measurement from the tip of the ventral liver lobe to the diaphragm. In normal dogs, this measurement correlated with liver mass.[76] Whether this technique will be useful in abnormal dogs is not established. A graph of normal measurements correlated with body weight has been published.[77] A subjective impression may be gained, and this often forms the basis for the impression that the liver is enlarged. If the liver occupies the entire cranial abdomen and can easily be

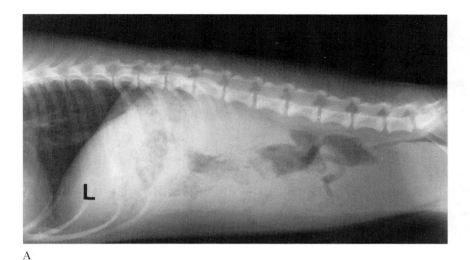

A

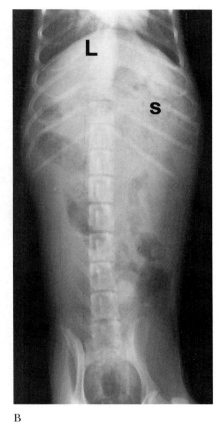

Figure 3–45. A 1-year-old male bichon frise with dementia after eating. (A) The liver (*black L*) is very small and the angle of the stomach is directed cranially. There is poor detail due to a lack of abdominal fat. (B) The liver (*black L*) is small and the stomach (*black s*) is displaced cranially. **Diagnosis:** Small liver due to portosystemic shunt.

B

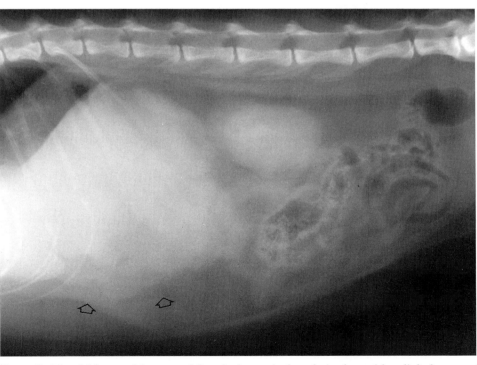

Figure 3–46. A 10-year-old neutered female domestic short-haired cat with a slight lump and mass on the left elbow. Physical examination revealed a palpably irregular cranial abdominal mass. The lateral radiograph revealed moderate hepatomegaly and clearly irregular ventral borders of the liver (*open black arrows*). Laparotomy revealed multiple hepatic masses. **Diagnosis:** Hepatic cystadenoma.

identified caudal to the last rib on both the left and right sides, there will be little argument that the liver is enlarged. In some patients, the liver is more easily identified on the left side than on the right. This does not necessarily indicate that the liver is enlarged. Focal enlargement of the liver may cause displacement of other organs, however this is also difficult to recognize during an ultrasound examination. As is the case for evaluation of the liver size radiographically, rounding of the liver margin detected during an ultrasound examination may be used as an indicator of hepatomegaly. Recognizing a small liver presents a similar problem. In some dogs, the liver will be contained within the rib cage, and because of gas within the stomach and overlap from the caudal lung lobes it will be almost totally inaccessible to ultrasound examination. This does not indicate that the liver is small. Radiography is preferred to ultrasound for determining liver size.

SHAPE CHANGES

Alterations in contour of the liver can be recognized using ultrasound. These changes can be observed if the margins of the liver are carefully examined. Oblique or off-axis views may be helpful in evaluating the contour of the liver. Minor irregularities can be detected and any irregularity should be considered abnormal. Rounded liver margins may be observed when the liver is enlarged. Although a common cause of these irregularities is tumor, this can also occur with cirrhosis and nodular regeneration.

CHANGES IN ECHO INTENSITY AND PATTERN

The echo intensity and pattern of the liver parenchyma are the most important features of the liver. The liver is usually hypoechoic when compared to the spleen and slightly hyperechoic when compared to the kidney. This relative echogenicity can be used provided the spleen and kidney are normal. With experience, a subjective impression of the "brightness" of the liver may be gained, however this subjective impression is not totally reliable. The alteration in echogenicity of the liver may be diffuse or focal. Focal changes are easier to detect because the surrounding hepatic parenchyma will be normal. Diffuse changes are not easily detected and may be artifactual.[78] A diffuse increase in echogenicity of the liver is nonspecific and may occur as a result of lymphosarcoma, fatty infiltration, fibrosis (cirrhosis), or steroid hepatopathy (Figs. 3–47 and 3–48).[79] A diffuse decrease in echogenicity may be associated with diffuse neoplasia (i.e., lymphoma) and hepatic congestion. Hepatitis may be hyperechoic, hypoechoic, or heteroechoic depending on the stage or severity of

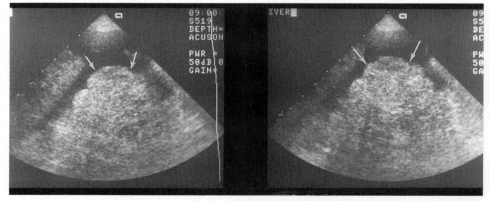

Figure 3–47. Longitudinal sonograms of the cranial abdomen of an 8-year-old Labrador retriever who presented with a history of ascites and lethargy of 10 days' duration. There is anechoic peritoneal fluid. The liver is small, hyperechoic, and irregular in contour (*arrows*). The architecture of the liver is abnormal appearing uniformly granular. This is indicative of chronic liver disease with cirrhosis or fibrosis and ascites. **Diagnosis:** Cirrhosis of the liver. A cause was not determined.

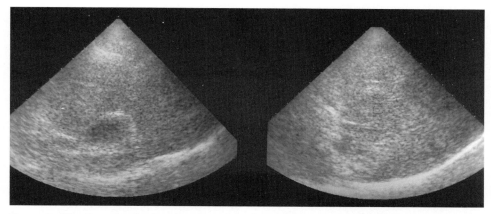

Figure 3–48. Longitudinal sonograms of the liver of a 3-year-old spayed female Great Dane with a history of lethargy, anorexia, icterus, vomiting, and melena. The architecture of the liver is coarse with loss of the normal portal vein echoes. This is indicative of diffuse liver disease which may be due to chronic fibrosis or cirrhosis. **Diagnosis:** Cirrhosis of the liver secondary to toxin.

the disease. Focal changes in hepatic echo intensity may result in lesions that are hyper- or hypoechoic, or a combination of the two.[78,80]

If it is mild, a fatty infiltration of the liver may not produce radiographic changes. In some patients, diffusely increased echogenicity with liver enlargement may be recognized. An increased attenuation of the sound beam may be associated with fatty infiltration of the liver and may create a false impression that the liver is hypoechoic in its deeper portion. In cats, the ultrasound finding of a liver that was hyperechoic when compared with the echo intensity of the falciform fat was the best criterion for diagnosis of severe hepatic lipidosis. Blurring of vascular margins and increased attenuation of the ultrasound beam were also observed; however, in this study of 10 cats with clinical signs of hepatobiliary disease, these changes were also observed in one cat with cholangiohepatitis and one cat with hepatic fibrosis.[81] Hepatic lipidosis may produce a focal rather than a diffuse hyperechoic lesion (Fig. 3–49). This is rare.

Focal changes in echogenicity may be poorly defined or well defined. Both solid and cystic lesions may be identified. These focal changes are also somewhat nonspecific and may occur in association with lymphoma, primary or metastatic neoplasia, abscesses, or nodular hyperplasia (Figs. 3–50, 3–51, and 3–52).[78–80,82,83] Focal anechoic lesions with well-defined walls and distal enhancement are most likely hepatic cysts. Although some tumors, abscesses, and hematomas may appear anechoic these lesions more often have internal echoes, a less distinct or irregular wall, and do not show posterior enhancement. Hypoechoic lesions may be nodular hyperplasia, tumors, abscesses, or hematomas. Hyperechoic lesions may be due to nodular hyperplasia, tumor, abscess, hematoma, foreign body, gas, or mineral. The presence of shadowing or reverberation artifact is helpful in recognizing the foreign body, gas, or mineral that produces these artifacts and distinguishes them from nodular hyperplasia, tumors, abscess, or hematoma, which do not produce such artifacts. Examination of abdominal radiographs is extremely helpful in determining if gas or mineral densities are present. Mineral densities that are not associated with the gallbladder or bile ducts can be associated with granuloma, abscess, hematoma, or neoplasia. Air may be observed within a hepatic abscess or neoplasia. Mixed hyperechoic and hypoechoic lesions are also non-specific and may result from any of the conditions discussed so far. Multifocal hyperechoic or hypoechoic lesions may be due to tumor or infection (Figs. 3–53, 3–54, 3–55, and 3–56). A specific pattern labeled a "target" or "bulls eye" lesion has been associated with metastatic tumors. These lesions have a bright center (resulting from tumor necrosis) and a hypoechoic rim (resulting from the tumor itself). Biopsy or fine needle aspirates are usually required to determine the nature of most focal hepatic lesions.

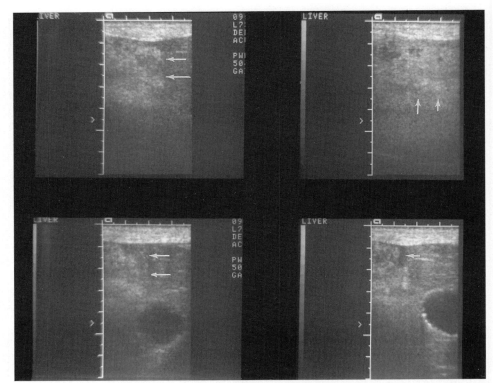

Figure 3–49. Transverse sonograms of the liver of a 10-year-old female mixed breed dog with a history of elevated liver enzymes and a mass arising from the lateral thoracic wall. A poorly defined hyperechoic lesion is noted in the ventral portion of the liver (*arrows*). This could represent a tumor or infection. A biopsy of the liver was performed and a histologic diagnosis of lipidosis was made. **Diagnosis:** Focal hepatic lipidosis.

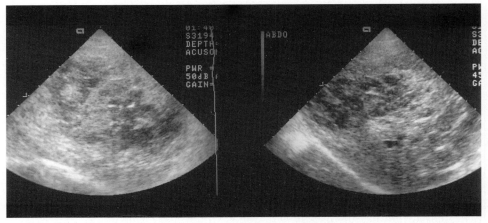

Figure 3–50. Longitudinal sonograms of the liver of an 11-year-old spayed female golden retriever with a history of anemia and lethargy. The dog had a splenectomy previously for a splenic hemangiosarcoma. There is a poorly marginated heteroechoic mass within the liver. This is most likely neoplastic. **Diagnosis:** Hemangiosarcoma.

Ultrasound is superior to radiography for evaluation of the gallbladder and bile ducts. The size of the gallbladder is extremely variable in normal animals, and almost any animal that has not been fed for a while or is anorectic will have a large gallbladder. Differentiation between intrahepatic and extrahepatic biliary obstruction may be possible. Dilated anechoic tubular structures radiating outward from the porta hepatitis combined with a small gallbladder is indicative of intrahepatic biliary obstruction. The bile ducts appear similar to hepatic veins (their walls are anechoic);

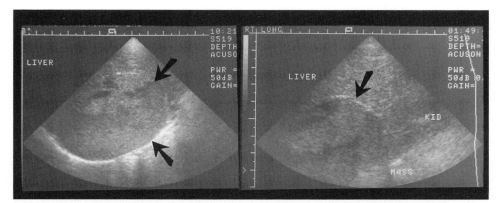

Figure 3–51. Longitudinal sonograms of the liver of a 10-year-old spayed female mixed breed dog with a history of polyuria, polydipsia and hepatomegaly of 3 months' duration. There is a heteroechoic well defined mass (*arrows*) within the caudate lobe of the liver. This is indicative of a liver tumor. **Diagnosis:** Hepatoma.

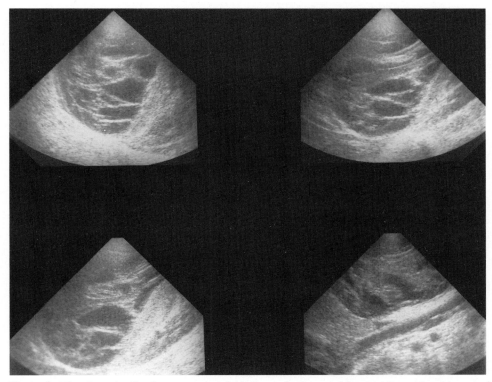

Figure 3–52. Longitudinal sonograms of the liver of a 4-year-old rottweiler with a history of a chronic intermittent left axillary abscess which occurred after a dog fight. There is a septated heteroechoic mass noted in the region of the right caudate liver lobe. This mass could be a hematoma, abscess or tumor. **Diagnosis:** Hematoma.

however, when obstructed they are more numerous, more curved, and have a more irregular branching pattern than the hepatic veins (Fig. 3–57). Extrahepatic biliary obstruction would result in an enlarged gallbladder with dilation of both intrahepatic and extrahepatic bile ducts. Experimentally, the common bile duct becomes enlarged within 24 hours following duct ligation, and the peripheral intrahepatic ducts may be identified by 5 to 7 days following obstruction.[84] The degree of intrahepatic duct dilation in experimental dogs varied, and therefore the size of the dilated ducts allows only a rough estimate of the duration of the biliary obstruction. The extrahepatic ducts appear as dilated tortuous tubular structures around the porta hepatis.

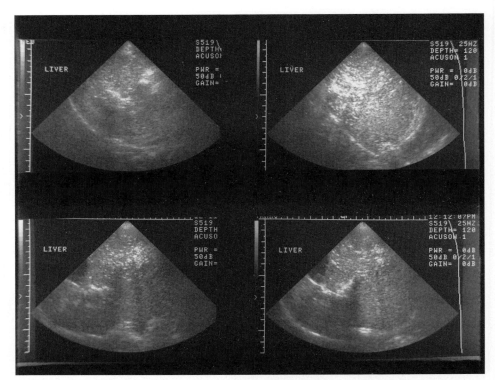

Figure 3–53. Longitudinal sonograms of the liver of a 6-year-old male Bedlington terrier who presented with a history of polyuria, polydipsia, elevated liver enzymes, and leucocytosis. There are multiple hyperechoic foci scattered diffusely throughout the liver. This could be the result of mineralization, however shadowing is not evident. It most likely represents diffuse neoplasia. **Diagnosis:** Bile duct carcinoma.

Figure 3–54. Transverse (A&B) and longitudinal (C&D) sonograms of the liver of a 6-year-old castrated male Himalayan cat with a history of pyrexia, vomiting, and hepatomegaly of 2 months' duration. The liver contains multiple poorly defined hypoechoic lesions. These could represent tumors or abscesses. **Diagnosis:** Suppurative hepatitis.

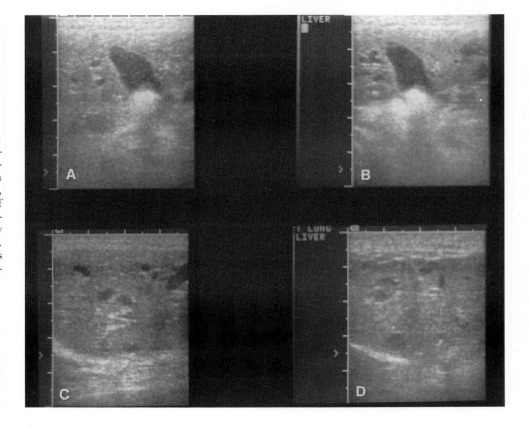

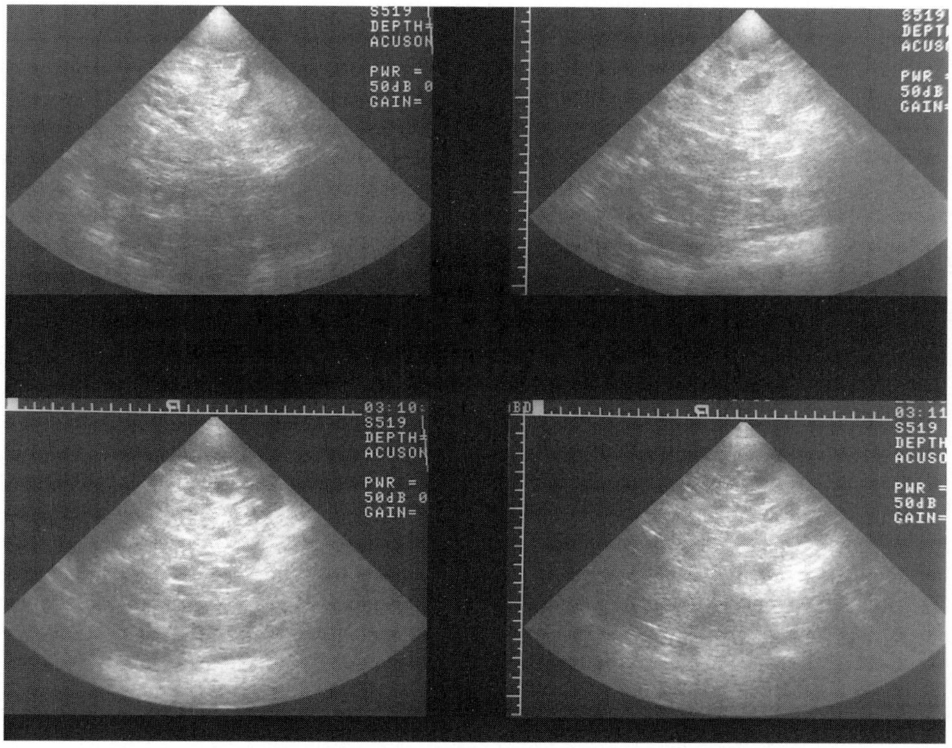

Figure 3–55. Transverse sonograms of the liver of a 8-year-old male rottweiler with a history of vomiting and diarrhea of 2 weeks' duration. There are multiple hypoechoic lesions of various sizes scattered diffusely throughout the liver. These may represent metastatic neoplasia or multiple abscesses. **Diagnosis:** Metastatic carcinoma.

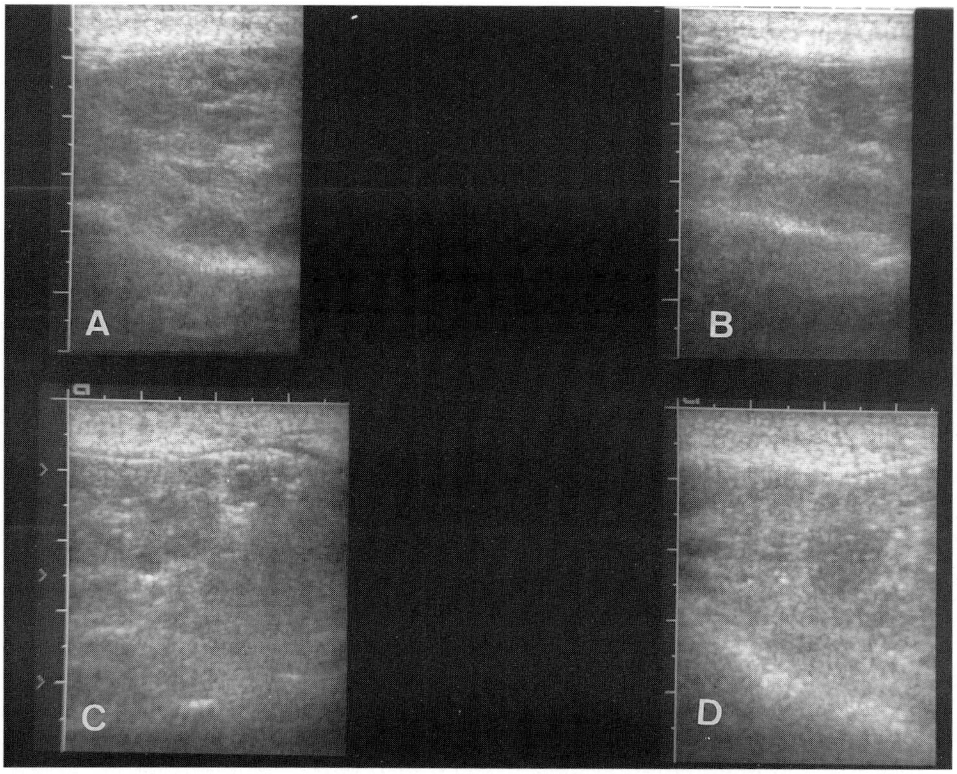

Figure 3–56. Transverse (A&B) and longitudinal (C&D) sonograms of the liver of a 15-year-old male Jack Russell terrier with a history of vomiting, azotemia, and hepatomegaly of 3 weeks' duration. There are multiple hypoechoic lesions scattered diffusely throughout the hepatic parenchyma. These most likely represent diffuse neoplasia. Infection could also produce similar lesions. **Diagnosis:** Metastatic adrenal carcinoma.

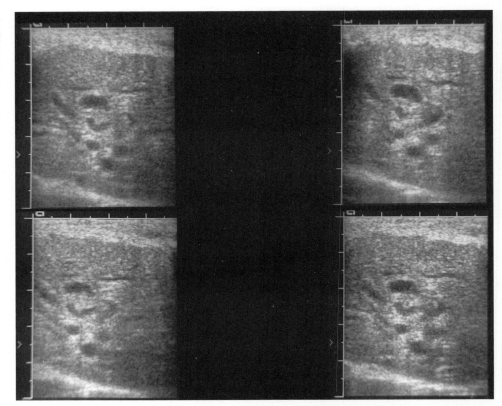

Figure 3–57. Longitudinal sonograms of the liver of a 13-year-old spayed female cat with a history of chronic pancreatitis. There are multiple tortuous hypoechoic linear structures throughout the liver. These represent dilated bile ducts most likely secondary to biliary obstruction. **Diagnosis:** Biliary obstruction secondary to chronic pancreatitis.

If the gallbladder cannot be identified during an ultrasound examination, it may be obscured by gas within the stomach or small intestines. In humans, a gallbladder that has a lumen completely filled with gallstones may be difficult to identify. The shadows produced by the stones will obscure the gallbladder, however the presence of the shadow indicates the position of the gallbladder.

Biliary pseudocyst (biloma) may occur as a complication of liver biopsy or following abdominal trauma. An anechoic cystic structure separate and distinct from the gallbladder may be seen during the ultrasound examination.[85]

The thickness of the gallbladder wall can be evaluated during an ultrasound examination, but the value of that information is questionable. The gallbladder wall will become thicker when the gallbladder is empty, however the exact measurement has not been established. Thickening of the gallbladder wall may occur secondary to cholecystitis or edema (Fig. 3–58). Gallbladder edema may occur secondary to right heart failure or hypoproteinemia.[9] Patients with liver flukes or cholangiohepatitis may have thickened irregular gallbladder walls. Gallbladder neoplasia is uncommon; however, sessile or polypoid masses may occur within the gallbladder secondary to cystic hypertrophy of mucus-producing glands within the gallbladder wall (Fig. 3–59).

The gallbladder wall may become hyperechoic secondary to mineralization or gas accumulation. Radiographs are useful in discriminating between these conditions. Gallbladder wall mineralization may produce shadowing, while reverberation artifacts (comet tails) may be observed when air is present. Calcification may occur within the gallbladder wall as a result of chronic inflammation or tumor. Air may be present within the gallbladder or bile ducts secondary to emphysematous cholecystitis. This will produce a hyperechoic gallbladder wall which causes shadows. Reverberation artifacts may be present, and these will be a clue to the fact that the echoes

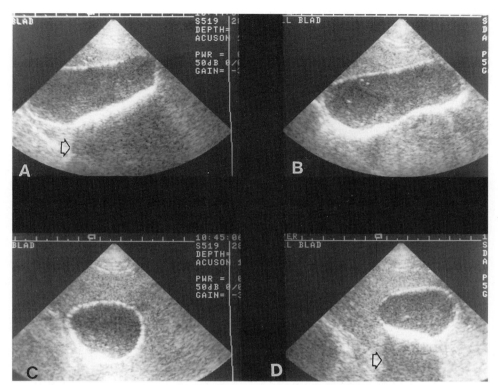

Figure 3–58. Longitudinal (A&B) and transverse (C&D) sonograms of the liver a 12-year-old spayed female German shepherd dog who presented for evaluation of chronic epistaxis. The gallbladder is slightly distended, the gallbladder wall is slightly thickened and hyperechoic, and there is echogenic material in the dependent portion of the gallbladder. There is shadowing evident deep to this echogenic material (*arrows*). This represents small gall stones. **Diagnosis:** Cholecystitis with mineralized material (gall stones) within the gallbladder.

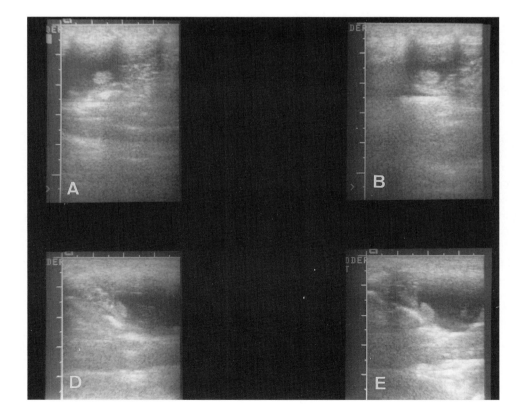

Figure 3–59. Transverse (A&B) and longitudinal (C&D) sonograms of the gallbladder of a 3-year-old male miniature poodle with a history of elevated liver enzymes and chronic dermatitis of 6 months' duration. There is a hyperechoic mass within the gallbladder. This mass is fixed in position. **Diagnosis:** Polyp within the gall bladder.

are associated with air. As with calcified densities, an abdominal radiograph will confirm the diagnosis. If the air or mineral is in the gallbladder wall rather than free within the lumen of the gallbladder, it will remain fixed in position despite changes in the patient's position. Rotating the patient while observing the movement of the hyperechoic structures will help discriminate between air or mineral in the gallbladder wall or within the lumen.

Cholelithiasis may be seen as an incidental finding in many animals.[86] These stones may be large and well-defined or may consist of a sand- or sludge-like material (Figs. 3–58, 3–60, and 3–61). They may form a hyperechoic layer within the de-

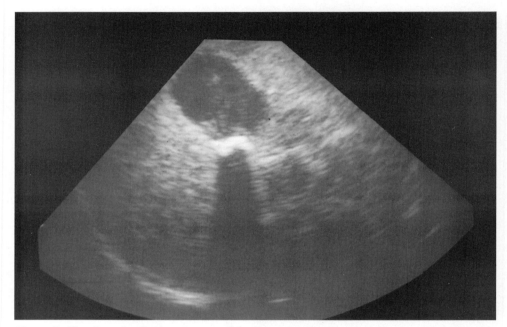

Figure 3–60. Longitudinal sonogram of the liver of a 13-year-old male schnauzer with a history of depression, anorexia, and bloating. A hyperechoic structure is evident in the dependent portion of the gallbladder. There is shadowing deep to this structure. This represents a mineralized gallstone. **Diagnosis:** Cholelithiasis.

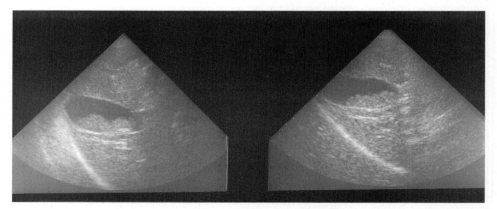

Figure 3–61. Longitudinal sonograms of the gallbladder of a 13-year-old spayed female pit bull with a history of hematuria which was secondary to a transitional cell carcinoma of the bladder. The dog was undergoing chemotherapy. There is echogenic material within the dependent portion of the gallbladder. This changes appearance with repositioning of the dog. This is helpful in confirming that the material is within the gallbladder and is not a slice thickness artifact. Transverse sonograms (not illustrated) are also important to document that the material is within the gallbladder. This represents inspissated bile or sludge within the gallbladder. This is a common incidental finding. **Diagnosis:** Inspissated material within the gall bladder.

pendent portion of the gallbladder or may be wedged within the gallbladder and remain fixed in position. Gallstones are usually hyperechoic and may or may not cause shadows. They will change their position within the gallbladder with changes in patient position. Sludge or inspissated bile is commonly seen in asymptomatic patients. Reverberation or slice thickness artifacts may project echoes into the gallbladder. These can be recognized if the ultrasonographer is aware of their occurrence and uses caution in examining the gallbladder in both longitudinal and transverse planes.

PORTOSYSTEMIC SHUNTS

Several contrast procedures may be useful when portosystemic shunts are suspected. Regardless of the method used, the portal vein should be seen branching into several hepatic radicals (Fig. 3–62). After passing through the liver, the contrast medium should enter the hepatic vein and then pass into the caudal vena cava. Shunts may go from the portal vein to the azygous vein, perirenal veins, perineal venous structures, or caudal vena cava (whether from posthepatic portal caval shunts or a persistent patent ductus venosus) (Figs. 3–63 and 3–64). Identification of the presence of portal radicals is important as a prognosticator for successful surgical intervention in animals with shunts. The presence of portal radicals suggests that partial or complete ligation of the shunt(s) will probably be helpful.

Portosystemic shunts can be detected using ultrasound if the patient is cooperative and the stomach is not too distended.[87,88] The portal vein and caudal vena cava must be identified and traced cranially or caudally. The shunt vessel may be observed connecting the portal vein and the vena cava. The portal vein and caudal vena cava

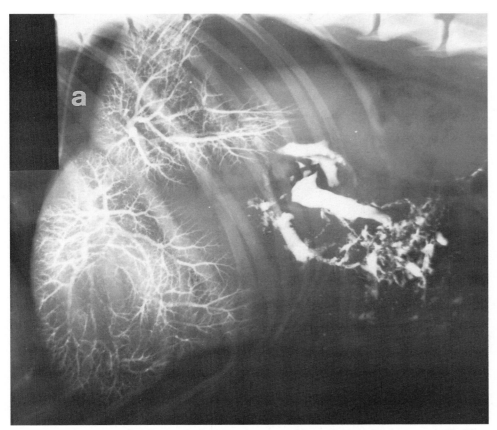

Figure 3–62. A lateral radiograph showing the normal hepatic portal veins as opacified by a portogram. There is a marked pneumoperitoneum (i.e., free abdominal air between the liver and diaphragm identified by *white a*) due to the surgical procedure required to gain access to the portal vein. **Diagnosis:** Normal portogram.

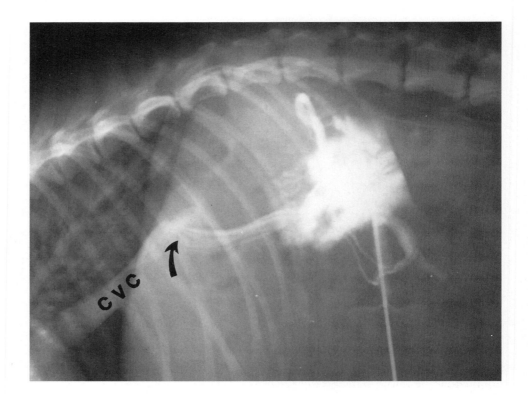

Figure 3–63. A 2-year-old female bichon frise with occasional seizures and periods of stupor after eating. The spleno-portogram revealed direct flow of portal blood to the liver and the presence of a short straight shunt (*black arrow*) directly to the caudal vena cava (*black cvc*). Differential diagnoses include extrahepatic portocaval shunt or persistent patent ductus venosus. **Diagnosis:** Persistent patent ductus venosus.

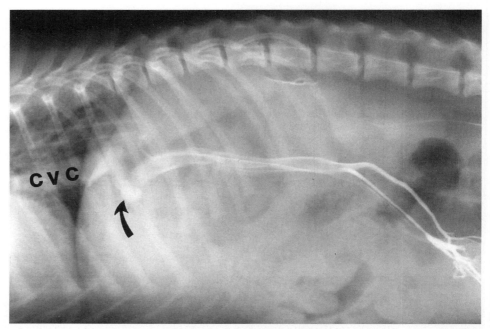

Figure 3–64. A 2-year-old male Yorkshire terrier with postprandial depression and occasional seizures. Survey radiographs had revealed a small liver. The operative mesenteric portogram revealed a solitary shunt going from the portal vein directly to the caudal vena cava. The shunt vessel (*black arrow*) is clearly caudal to the caudal border of the liver and goes directly to the caudal vena cava (*black cvc*). An esophageal stethoscope is seen in the caudal esophagus. The renal pelves and ureters are seen due to contrast excretion from prior injections of contrast media during this study. **Diagnosis:** Solitary extrahepatic portocaudal vena caval shunt. No hepatic vessels were seen. This suggested a poorer than normal prognosis for shunt ligation; however, partial ligation of the shunt resulted radiographically in increased hepatic blood flow and a resolution of clinical signs.

are close together in the porta hepatis, and caution must be used when examining this area to ensure that a shunt is not diagnosed incorrectly. Failure to identify the shunt does not exclude the diagnosis. Alteration in the course of the portal vein or tortuosity of the portal vein are suggestive of the presence of a shunt even though the communication is not obvious (Figs. 3–65 and 3–66). The diagnosis should be confirmed by other studies, such as portovenography or technetium transcolonic portography. Other shunts, such as portal azygous or portal renal, may be detected. At times, abnormally large or tortuous veins indicating the presence of a portosystemic shunt may be identified, although establishing their exact course may be difficult.

HEPATIC VENOUS CONGESTION

Enlargement of the hepatic veins can be identified during an ultrasound examination. In most cases, this is the result of hepatic venous congestion secondary to cardiac disease (right heart failure, pericardial disease, intracardiac mass). The veins will be large and many smaller branches will be visible extending to the margin of the liver. The evaluation is subjective; however, in most cases an experienced ultrasonographer has little difficulty recognizing the abnormality (Fig. 3–67).

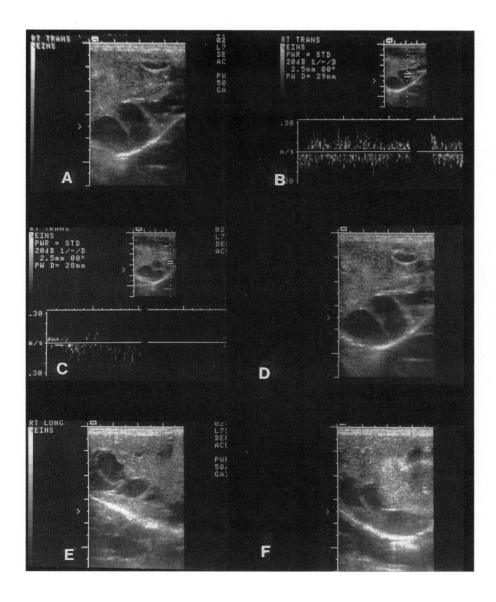

Figure 3–65. Transverse (A,B,&C) and longitudinal (D,E,&F) sonograms of the liver of a 3-month-old female mixed breed dog with a history of chronic diarrhea and hypoalbuminemia. There is an enlarged tortuous vein which extended from the portal vein to the caudal vena cava. This is indicative of a portosystemic shunt. **Diagnosis:** Extrahepatic portosystemic shunt.

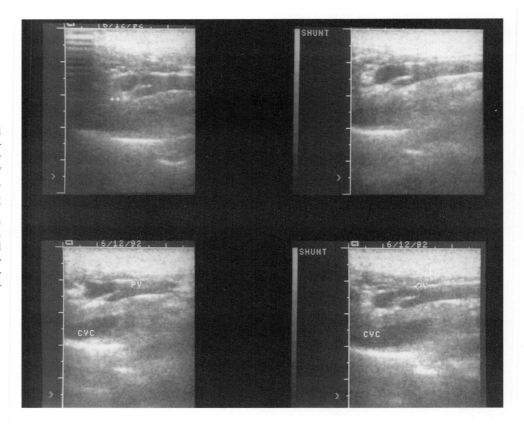

Figure 3–66. Longitudinal sonograms of the cranial abdomen of a 10-month-old male Yorkshire terrier with a history of stunted growth, dementia, and elevated liver enzymes. There is a large vessel (*small white arrows*) originating from the portal vein (PV) which communicated with the caudal vena cava (CVC). This is indicative of an extrahepatic portocaval shunt. **Diagnosis:** Extrahepatic portocaval shunt.

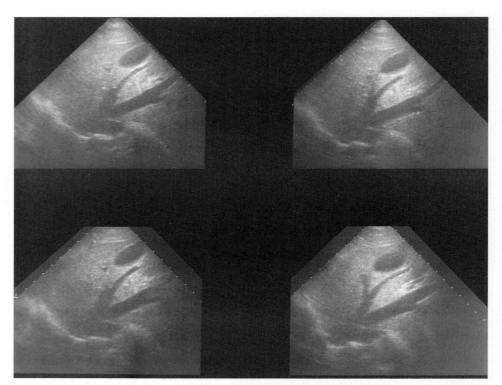

Figure 3–67. Longitudinal sonograms of the liver of a 5-year-old male mixed breed dog with a history of respiratory distress of 3 weeks' duration. There is marked hepatic venous distension. This is indicative of venous obstruction, which may be associated with an intrathoracic (cardiac or caudal mediastinal) mass, pericardial disease, or with right heart failure. **Diagnosis:** Right heart failure secondary to heartworms.

ARTERIOVENOUS FISTULA

Ultrasound has been used to document arteriovenous fistula in dogs. Anechoic, irregular, tortuous tubular structures were identified adjacent to or within the liver. Doppler examination demonstrated unidirectional flow within these structures.[89]

CIRRHOSIS

Doppler ultrasound has been used in the evaluation of experimentally induced cirrhosis.[90] Extensive extrahepatic portosystemic shunts were identified. Portal blood flow velocity was markedly reduced from a normal level of 18.1 mm/sec to 9.2 mm/sec. Mean portal blood flow was also reduced from 31 cc/min/kg to 17.2 cc/min/kg. Large incident angles can introduce significant velocity errors, and in some dogs it is impossible to attain a proper incident angle (60°–72°). In these dogs, accurate measurement of portal blood flow cannot be obtained. Qualitative as well as quantitative information may be obtained from portal Doppler ultrasound. This includes determination of patency of the portal vein and direction of flow, evaluation of portosystemic shunts, recognition of arteriovenous malformations, and discriminating between dilated bile ducts and hepatic vessels.

STOMACH

Density Changes

Gastric lesions may be recognizable on survey radiographs providing the stomach is filled with air and does not contain a large amount of food. Foreign bodies and masses may protrude into the lumen and may be apparent. Because of this air:mass interface, these tissue-dense lesions will have very discrete borders (Fig. 3–68). If a

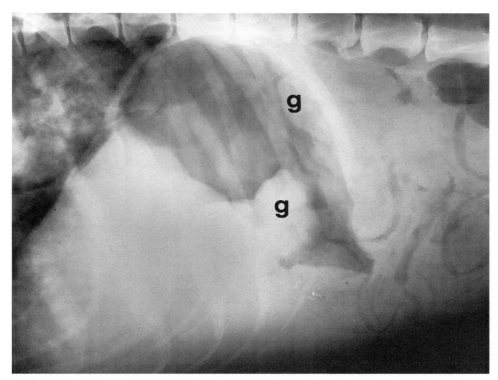

Figure 3–68. A 6-year-old male Great Dane with weight loss for 3 months and vomiting and diarrhea for 3 days. There are large, irregular tissue-dense masses outlines by air in the stomach (*black g*). The caudal lung lobes revealed a nodular interstitial pattern infiltrate. Differential diagnoses include neoplasia or granuloma. **Diagnosis:** Tuberculosis with gastric, hepatic, and pulmonary involvement.

foreign body is metal-dense, the possibility of lead or zinc should be considered. This is particularly important in the stomach because gastric acid may solubilize lead and zinc and cause metal intoxication. Zinc toxicity has been associated with ingestion of nuts, bolts, zinc containing ointments, and pennies minted after 1982.[91] Food in the stomach may disguise the presence of foreign matter. If food or granular material is present in the stomach of an animal that has a history of total anorexia or vomiting multiple times, this density most likely represents a foreign body. Food in the stomach, particularly if surrounded by air, may mimic the appearance of foreign bodies. Some foreign bodies may appear radiolucent if they are of a fat-dense material (e.g., some rubber balls) or have air-filled centers (e.g., seeds, nuts, or pits) and are surrounded by gastric or intestinal fluid (Fig. 3–69). Calcification of the submucosa, appearing as a fine linear calcification parallel to the mucosal border, may be seen with chronic renal failure (Fig. 3–70).

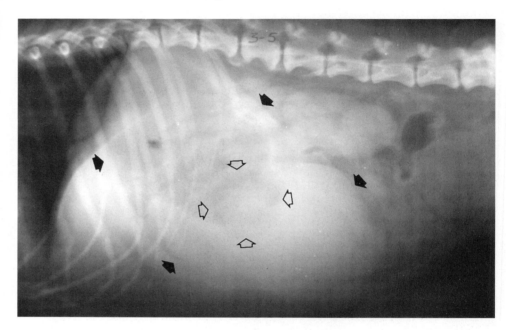

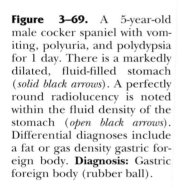

Figure 3–69. A 5-year-old male cocker spaniel with vomiting, polyuria, and polydypsia for 1 day. There is a markedly dilated, fluid-filled stomach (*solid black arrows*). A perfectly round radiolucency is noted within the fluid density of the stomach (*open black arrows*). Differential diagnoses include a fat or gas density gastric foreign body. **Diagnosis:** Gastric foreign body (rubber ball).

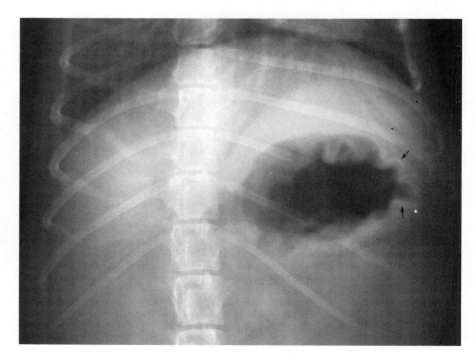

Figure 3–70. A 13-year-old male miniature poodle with chronic polyuria and polydipsia and vomiting for 4 days. There is a fine line of calcification (*black arrows*) seen within the stomach wall which parallels the rugal folds. This is consistent with calcification of the gastric submucosa secondary to the vasculitis and gastritis induced by renal failure. **Diagnosis:** Renal gastritis.

Size, Shape, or Position Changes

Changes in the size of the stomach may also be an important sign of dysfunction. Although it is normally a distensible organ, the caudal border of the stomach should not extend beyond the level of L4. Severe distension of the stomach may be due to excess gas, food, or fluid within the stomach. Occasionally, a dog will simply overeat (particularly young dogs) and the resultant gastric dilation will cause clinical signs (Fig. 3–71). Gastric dilation in an anorectic or vomiting dog may indicate some form of pyloric outflow obstruction or gastric dilation/volvulus. Gastric volvulus is rotation of the stomach around its long axis. The degree of rotation may vary from as little as 90° to 360°, or more. The most common is a 180° rotation. The degree of gastric dilation will vary (Figs. 3–72 and 3–73). The classic appearance on a survey radiograph is a segmented or compartmentalized ("double bubble") stomach on the lateral view. The rugal folds of the cardia and fundus will be seen ventral and caudal to the pylorus. If identifiable, the duodenum will be seen residing in a dorsoventral orientation cranial to the body of the stomach. The rugal folds may be seen to the right and caudal to the smooth-walled pylorus. Right and left lateral recumbent radiographs are helpful in diagnosing this condition because, in contrast to the normal dog, fluid will be evident in the pylorus when the dog is in left lateral recumbency and gas will be in the pylorus when the dog is in right lateral recumbency. The spleen may be enlarged and displaced from its normal position. Failure to identify the normal stomach in a dog with a dilated, fluid-dense esophagus may indicate gastroesophageal intussusception.

Only a few diseases that affect the stomach are not recognizable on survey radiographs, especially if the stomach contains air or air is administered to the patient by stomach tube. Most radiographic changes seen with these diseases affect either the mucosa or wall of the stomach and these structures can be delineated by air. If a portion of the stomach is difficult to evaluate due to the presence of normal gastric fluid, positional maneuvers, which take advantage of the gravitational effect on

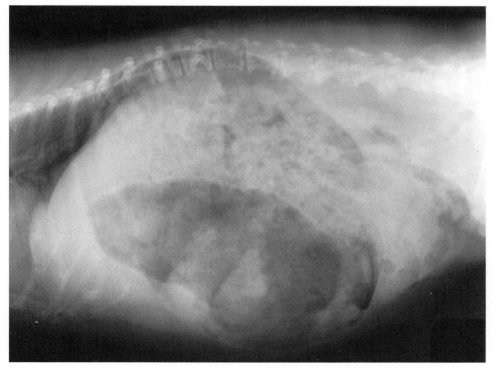

Figure 3–71. A 12-year-old neutered female dachshund with acute abdominal distension. The lateral view revealed that the stomach is severely distended with food and gas. Differential diagnoses include gastric distension from overeating, gastric outflow obstruction, or gastric distension with volvulus. There is no segmentation of the stomach or displacement of the pylorus from its normal position. **Diagnosis:** Acute gastric distension.

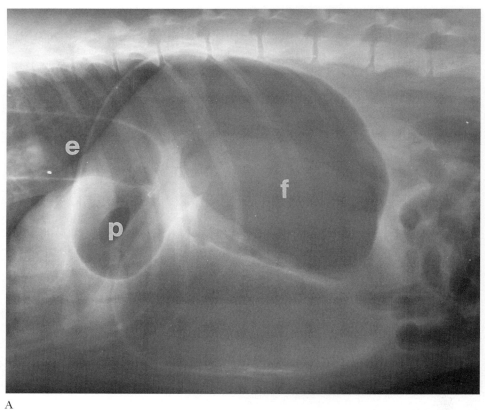

A

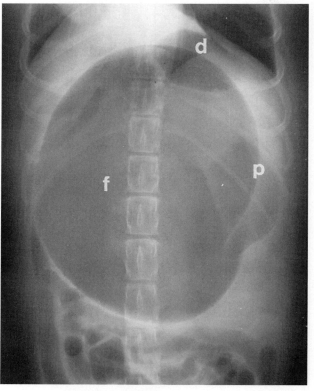

B

Figure 3–72. A 5-year-old spayed Siberian husky with acute abdominal distension. (A) On the lateral view there is marked gaseous distension of the stomach and esophagus (*white e*). There is a segmented appearance to the stomach caused by its twisting. The pylorus (*white p*) is seen cranial to the fundus (*white f*). (B) On the ventrodorsal view the pylorus (*white p*) and duodenum (*white d*) are seen left of the midline and appear cranial to the fundus (*white f*) which is seen right of the midline. **Diagnosis:** Gastric dilation/volvulus.

air and fluid, can be used to define that portion of the stomach. Gastric masses, such as tumor, granuloma, or gastrogastric intussusception, may be identified on non-contrast radiographs when air is present within the stomach.[92] Using both right and left lateral, sternal, and dorsal recumbent radiographs, air within the stomach can

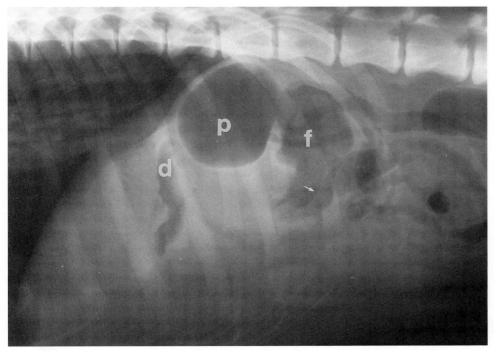

A

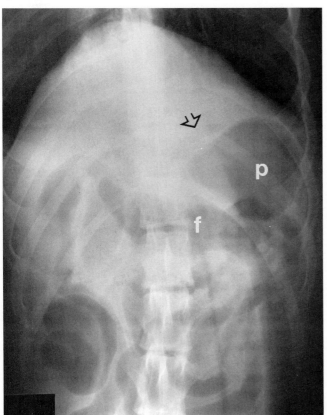

B

Figure 3–73. A 1-year-old male Great Dane with retching for 2 days. (A) On the lateral view a tubular gas density (duodenum–*white d*) is oriented dorsoventrally just caudal to the liver. Immediately dorsal and caudal to this is a smooth bordered, gas-filled structure (the pylorus of the stomach–*white p*). Just caudal to this is a gas-filled structure (fundus of the stomach–*white f*) that has tissue-dense pillars (rugae–*white arrow*). (B) On the ventrodorsal view the gastric fundus (*white f*) and pylorus (a smooth walled, gas-filled structure–*white p*) is seen in the left cranial portion of the abdomen. Immediately cranial and extending to the right of this is the duodenum (a tubular gas-filled structure–*open black arrow*). Immediately caudal to the fundus and extending to the right is the gastric cardia. **Diagnosis:** Gastric volvulus.

be manipulated to define all areas of the stomach. This will often allow for a diagnosis to be made and saves the cost of a GI series. As with a contrast study, it is important to identify the lesion on multiple radiographs in order to be confident that the abnormality observed is not merely an artifact. Infiltrative lesions of the gastric wall, such as tumors or granulomas, may interfere with normal gastric distention and may alter the shape of the stomach. Although shape alteration is usually the result of gastric wall lesions, incarceration of the stomach by the omentum can also alter the stomach's shape because it will interfere with gastric distention. Some of these diseases may only be identified using either the GI series or double contrast gastrogram. Some gastric diseases, such as nonulcerative gastritis, rarely have recognizable changes even on contrast gastrography, and confirmation of the diagnosis requires endoscopy or biopsy.

The GI Series

For complete evaluation of the stomach during the GI series, ventrodorsal, dorsoventral, and right and left lateral radiographs should be taken initially, and at least a ventrodorsal and a lateral view should be taken thereafter as the study progresses (Fig. 3–74). The choice of which views to take (right vs left lateral, dorsoven-

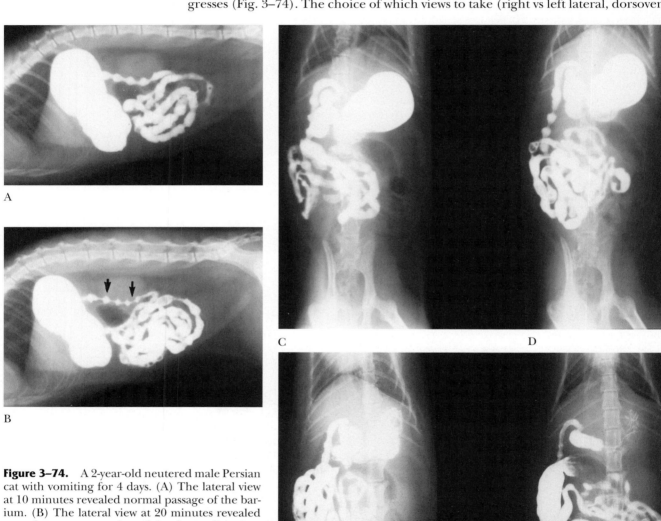

Figure 3–74. A 2-year-old neutered male Persian cat with vomiting for 4 days. (A) The lateral view at 10 minutes revealed normal passage of the barium. (B) The lateral view at 20 minutes revealed some hypersegmentation of the descending duodenum ("string of pearls"–*black arrows*). (C) The ventrodorsal view at 10 minutes revealed a normal study. (D) The ventrodorsal view at 20 minutes was normal. (E) The ventrodorsal view at 30 minutes revealed opacification of most of the small intestine. (F) The ventrodorsal view at 1 hour revealed that the barium had reached the colon. The amount of barium that remained within the stomach was within normal limits. **Diagnosis:** Normal GI series.

tral vs ventrodorsal) may be determined by which position the animal is most comfortable in or by which view shows a suspicious abnormality. It is very important that multiple views are taken during the study, because the most important diagnostic criterion is the repeatability of a lesion.

During the normal GI series the stomach should be larger at the cardia and should taper through the fundic area to the pylorus. The rugal folds, more prominent in the cardia and fundus, are directed mainly in a cranio-lateral to caudo-medial orientation. At the pylorus they become smaller and are directed toward the right side. There may be a slight irregularity to the otherwise smooth gastric wall at the gastroesophageal junction, which is located slightly to the left of the midline on the cranial surface. This is sometimes quite prominent in normal cats.

Because the normal stomach makes frequent mixing or propulsive motions, the stomach should have different shapes on the multiple views taken during the GI series. If the shape of the stomach fails to change, it either indicates gastric atony, which will be associated with gastric dilation, or infiltration of the gastric wall, which will usually not have marked gastric distension (Fig. 3–75). This radiographic appearance has been referred to as a "leather bottle" stomach because the shape of the stomach may be reminiscent of a leather wineskin. While all infiltrative lesions must be considered, the most likely diagnosis is lymphosarcoma. Other differential diagnoses would include eosinophilic gastritis, gastric adenocarcinoma, gastric fibrosis, mycotic lesions, or various less frequently seen neoplasms.

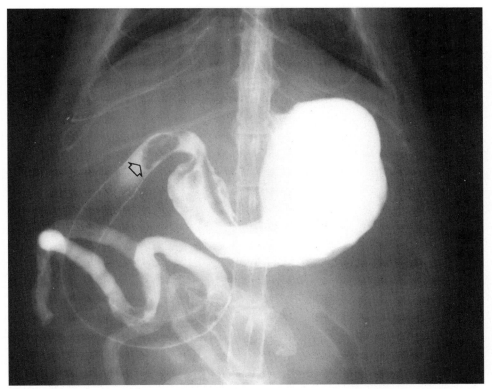

Figure 3–75. A 7-year-old female Siamese cat with vomiting for 2 weeks. Survey radiographs revealed no abnormalities. The ventrodorsal view of the GI series revealed a slightly narrowed distal body and pylorus of the stomach. There are no indications of any gastric constriction due to peristaltic or mixing motions, nor were any indications seen on other views. There is an intraluminal mass in the proximal duodenum (*open black arrow*) which partially obstructs the lumen. The gastric findings are indicative of an infiltrative process. The duodenal mass could be either a foreign body or neoplasm. Differential diagnoses of the stomach lesion include lymphosarcoma, adenocarcinoma, diffuse granuloma, or chronic inflammatory disease. **Diagnosis:** Diffuse lymphosarcoma of the stomach and focal lymphosarcoma of the duodenum.

GASTRIC WALL THICKENING

The normal gastric wall is smooth and uniform and is a few millimeters thick when the stomach is fully distended. It may be much thicker if the stomach is not distended. The gastric wall thickness may be somewhat difficult to perceive in animals that do not have adequate body fat to allow identification of the serosal surface of the stomach. In these instances, thickening may be suggested if there is an unusual decrease in the size of the stomach lumen or if the stomach does not distend uniformly when filled with air. While gastric wall thickening is frequently due to gastric neoplasia, granulomatous diseases or other infiltrative disease should also be considered in the diagnosis. The types of gastric neoplasia include adenocarcinoma, lymphosarcoma, and leiomyosarcoma. While these lesions may resemble each other, the diagnosis frequently can be suggested based on the pattern of change and clinical information. Adenocarcinoma of the stomach usually presents as a diffuse thickening of the gastric wall. Adenocarcinomas rarely have masses that protrude or extrude from the gastric wall. There is a tendency to develop ulcers within the thickened gastric wall (Fig. 3–76). An important factor to note when evaluating the lesion for possible treatment by gastrectomy is that the tumor usually extends in the subserosa well beyond the area that is recognizable radiographically. Lymphosarcoma usually presents as a more focal mass than adenocarcinoma, or as a very diffuse lesion with only minimal to moderate wall thickening but with a lack of motility (Fig. 3–77). Leiomyosarcoma tends to present as a mass that extends out from the gastric wall and does not affect the lumen. Leiomyosarcoma may also appear as a distinct mass within the stomach lumen. An infection that should be considered in cases with gastric wall thickening is phycomycosis (zygomycosis).[93] The lesion is most often found within the pyloric portion of the stomach. Zygomycosis occurs most often in the southern and southwestern United States. In boxers, thickening of the gastric rugae has been associated with eosinophilic gastritis.[94] The condition is not limited to this breed. Thickening of the rugal folds with normal gastric

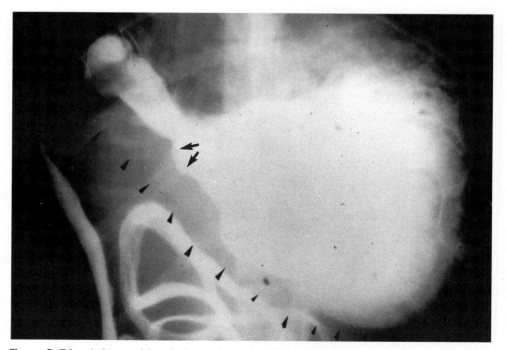

Figure 3–76. A 6-year-old male basset hound with vomiting for 4 weeks and hematemesis and melena for 3 days. The ventrodorsal view revealed a thickened gastric wall (*black arrowheads*) with a deep ulcer (*black arrows*). Differential diagnoses include neoplasia (adenocarcinoma, lymphosarcoma, other neoplasms) or granuloma. **Diagnosis:** Gastric adenocarcinoma with an ulcer.

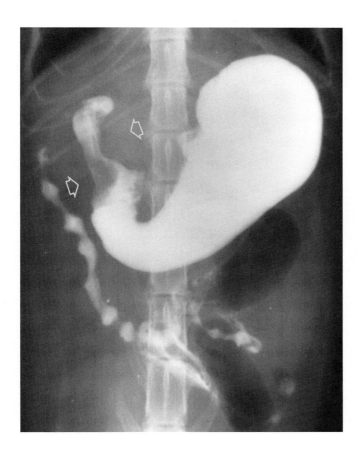

Figure 3–77. A 10-year-old neutered male Persian cat with chronic vomiting. There is marked thickening of the gastric wall (*open white arrows*) with restriction of the lumen in the pylorus. This is seen on multiple views. Circumferential mural lesions such as this have differential diagnoses of lymphosarcoma, adenocarcinoma, granulomas. **Diagnosis:** Lymphosarcoma.

wall thickness has been reported with chronic hypertrophic gastritis.[95,96] Rugal fold thickening may also be observed in uremic gastritis and in chronic gastritis of any etiology. The size of the gastric rugal folds varies with gastric distension, and a marked increase in gastric rugal fold size is required in order to be confident that the rugal folds are abnormal. Determination of rugal fold thickness is subjective, and although the ratio of normal rugal fold height to interrugal fold distance is reportedly 2:1 this measurement is rarely used. The best method of confirming a diagnosis of gastritis is by endoscopy.

ULCERS

On occasion, gastric ulcers may be visible on the non-contrast radiographs, but in most cases a GI series or preferably a double contrast gastrogram are needed. Gastric ulcers will appear as protrusions of the barium either into or through the gastric wall. The ulcers may be secondary to neoplasia, the result of excess gastric acid secretion caused by gastrinoma (Zollinger-Ellison syndrome), or secondary to administration of aspirin or other non-steroidal anti-inflammatory drugs (Fig. 3–78). Benign ulcers usually will have much less associated gastric wall thickening than will malignant ulcers, but differentiation between the two types is very difficult. Ulcers are diagnosed more easily by gastroscopy.

GASTRIC OUTFLOW OBSTRUCTIONS

A single radiograph represents a short interval in the process of normal gastric peristalsis. For that reason, fluoroscopy is important when evaluating pyloric outflow problems. The pylorus remains open briefly, and only a small portion of each bolus passes through the pylorus with the greatest fraction remaining in the stomach. Pyloric stenosis, pyloric spasm, intramural gastric neoplasm and granulomas, mucosal hypertrophy, and extraluminal masses may interfere with gastric emptying. Pyloric

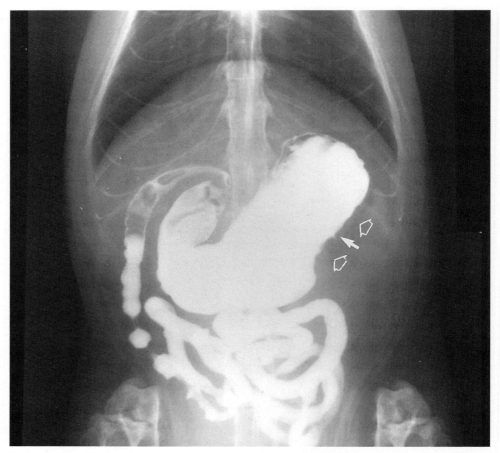

Figure 3–78. A 12-year-old castrated Siamese cat with vomiting for 2 months. There is thickening of the gastric wall in the area of the greater curvature (*open white arrows*). Within this area there is a small ulcerated area in which the barium extends into the mass (*small white arrow*). Differential diagnoses include ulcerated neoplasia or granuloma. **Diagnosis:** Small ulcer in area of inflammation. Examination of the pancreas at autopsy revealed an islet cell tumor. The presumptive final diagnosis was gastrinoma with gastric ulceration.

stenosis and mucosal hypertrophy produce smooth, usually circumferential, narrowing of the pylorus. Tumors and granulomas usually have irregular mucosal surfaces and/or are asymmetric with a smooth mucosal surface. Retention of significant volumes of barium within the stomach from several minutes (more than 30) to hours after administration is suggestive of gastric outflow obstruction. The morphologic reasons for this may not be clearly delineated by the GI study but may include polyps, gastric mucosa hypertrophy, which can act as a valve, or hypertrophy and/or spasticity of the pyloric sphincter. Gastric polyps in the pyloric region will appear as small filling defects protruding into the lumen near the pyloric sphincter (Fig. 3–79). These may function as a ball valve causing the outflow obstruction. Hypertrophy of the muscular layer of the pylorus and proximal duodenum may not be apparent radiographically; however, concentric rings of hypertrophy, which appear as circular, smooth, ridge-like filling defects encircling the pyloric outflow region with the lumen coming to a sharp point (parrot's beak sign), may be identified (Fig. 3–80). Hypertrophy of the gastric mucosa may not be identifiable radiographically but can cause outflow obstruction.[97] Mucosal hypertrophy may be symmetrical or asymmetrical and may be evident only when a wave of peristalsis pushes the contrast material into the pylorus. When this occurs, the normal pylorus should be convex on both the cranial and caudal aspect. Mucosal hypertrophy may produce a concavity or flattening on one side. This should be evident in more than one radiograph during the GI series.

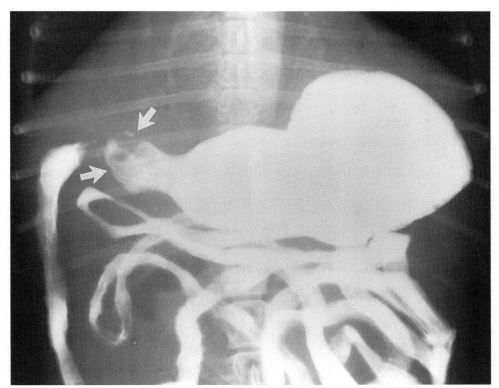

Figure 3–79. A 10-year-old female miniature schnauzer with a 1-week history of vomiting. There is an irregularly-shaped tissue-dense mass in the pylorus on all ventrodorsal views of this series (*white arrows*). Differential diagnoses include polyps, leiomyosarcoma, or granulomas. **Diagnosis:** Pyloric polyps.

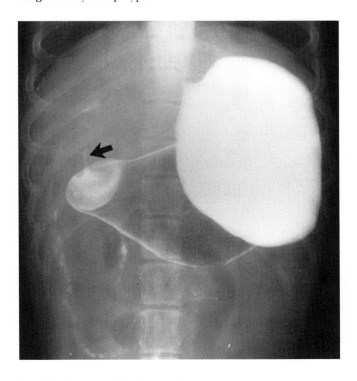

Figure 3–80. A 4-year-old female poodle with projectile vomiting for 3 weeks. The ventrodorsal view shows a round "donut-shaped" ring of muscular hypertrophy at the pylorus which is covered with a minimal amount of barium. The narrowed pyloric outflow tract is also visible as a faint, narrow stream of barium extending rostrally (*black arrow*). These findings were present on all ventrodorsal views. Differential diagnoses include pyloric muscular hypertrophy, neoplasia, or granuloma. **Diagnosis:** Pyloric muscular hypertrophy.

Double Contrast Gastrography

ULCERS

The double contrast gastrogram is most helpful in evaluating the stomach for benign ulcers, but it is also useful in evaluating some mass lesions.[64,74] Benign gastric ulcers, which may be difficult to detect on a standard GI series, may become more readily apparent in the double contrast study. When evaluating this study, the effects of gravity on the contrast media and the normal gastric anatomy must be considered (Fig. 3–81). If located on a non-dependent surface, the ulcer(s) will be seen as lines running in directions other than the normal gastric rugal folds; on dependent projections, the barium will puddle in the ulcer crater (Fig. 3–82).

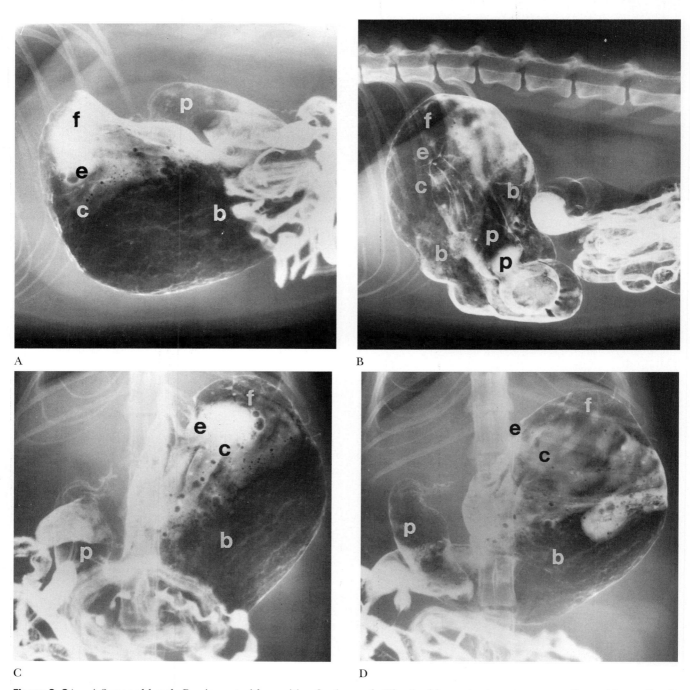

A

B

C

D

Figure 3–81. A 2-year-old male Persian cat with vomiting for 1 month. The double contrast gastrogram performed immediately after a standard GI series was normal on all views: (A) left lateral, (B) right lateral, (C) ventrodorsal, and (D) dorsoventral. The various regions of the stomach that are visible on each view are labeled (c) cardia, (e) esophagogastric junction, (b) body, (f) fundus, and (p) pylorus. **Diagnosis:** Normal stomach on both double contrast gastrogram and endoscopic examination.

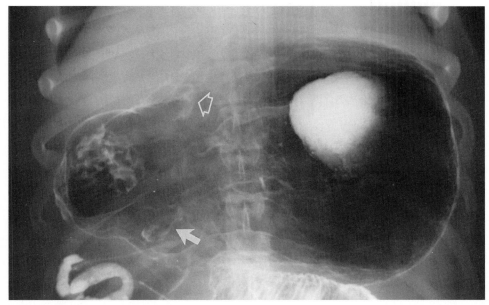

Figure 3–82. A 9-year-old male giant schnauzer with vomiting for 1 week and melena and hematemesis for 2 days. The ventrodorsal double contrast gastrogram (performed immediately after a GI series which was normal) revealed an irregularly oval-shaped structure outlined by a thin line of barium just to the right of the midline and on the caudal wall of the stomach (*solid white arrow*). A similar lesion is poorly outlined on the cranial body wall of the stomach (*open white arrow*). The pylorus is tightly closed in this view and the normal mucosal folds are coated with barium. **Diagnosis:** Benign gastric ulcers.

INTRAMURAL AND INTRALUMINAL LESIONS

The double contrast gastrogram may be helpful in evaluating some cases of gastric carcinoma or other gastric wall masses, particularly if the masses are small or not located on one of the surfaces that is seen clearly on the regular GI series (Fig. 3–83). The contrast or air can be used to highlight the lesion by positioning the patient so that the lesion is dependent (surrounded by barium) or up (surrounded by air). The position of a filling defect during a double contrast gastrogram is helpful in distinguishing between intramural and intraluminal objects. Intraluminal objects will move freely within the gastric lumen and will therefore move with the barium during the double contrast examination. Intramural objects will remain fixed in location and will therefore be outlined with air on one view and with barium on the (180°) opposite view.

Abnormal Gastric Ultrasound

The stomach can be evaluated from left to right in a systematic fashion in both the longitudinal and transverse planes. Gastric wall symmetry can be observed and wall thickness can be measured, wall layers can be identified, extent of a wall lesion can be determined, and peristaltic activity observed.[13,98] The lumen of the stomach also can be evaluated provided the stomach contains fluid without a large amount of air or ingesta. In some animals, it may be necessary to fill the stomach with fluid to facilitate the ultrasound examination. This is rarely necessary but can be accomplished easily without sedation of the patient.

Thickening of the gastric wall is the most common sonographic abnormality seen.[98] It must be interpreted cautiously because false-positive examinations have occurred.[99] Gastric wall thickening may be local or diffuse and symmetrical or asymmetrical. Both tumors and granulomas produce local asymmetrical thickening with

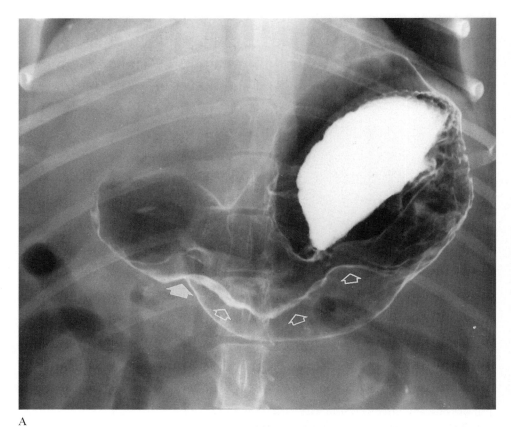

A

Figure 3–83. (A) An 11-year-old female mixed breed dog with chronic vomiting for 2 months. The ventrodorsal double contrast gastrogram revealed an irregular ridge of tissue in the body of the stomach, the whole surface of which was outlined by barium (*open white arrows*). This ridge of tissue extended to blend in with the normal serosal border (*solid white arrow*). This indicated a thickening of the gastric wall. Differential diagnoses include gastric neoplasia (particularly adenocarcinoma) or granuloma. **Diagnosis:** Gastric adenocarcinoma. (B) A 13-year-old female Dandie Dinmont terrier with previous laminectomy for disc extrusion (the reason the large gauge wire is superimposed over the spine), multiple partial gastrectomies for gastric mass resections (fine metal staples in gastric wall extending cranial and caudal from the *black arrow*), and a splenectomy performed along with the first gastrectomy due to the extension of the mass into the gastrosplenic ligament. The ventrodorsal double contrast gastrogram revealed an area of marked narrowing of the gastric body (due to the previous surgeries—*solid black arrow*). A small mural mass is seen on the caudal wall of the body of the stomach; it protrudes into the lumen of the stomach (*white arrows*). This mass has been followed for 2 years by sequential radiographs which show no change in its size. Histology of the previously resected masses revealed granulomatous reaction. **Diagnosis:** Recurrent gastric granuloma with no increase in size for 2 years.

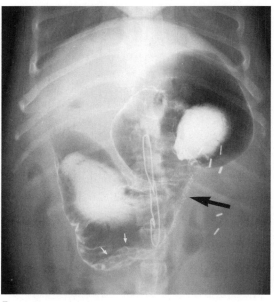

B

disruption of the layers of the gastric wall (Fig. 3–84). Generalized thickening may occur with either inflammatory disease or infiltrative neoplasia (Fig. 3–85). Infiltrative neoplasia may disrupt the gastric wall and interfere with identification of the wall layers to a greater extent than inflammatory disease.[98] Gastric lymphoma has various manifestations; however, in cats a transmural circumferential lesion with disruption of the normal gastric wall architecture, decreased echogenicity, and local interference with peristalsis was the most common form observed.[100,101] Lymph node involvement was commonly identified.

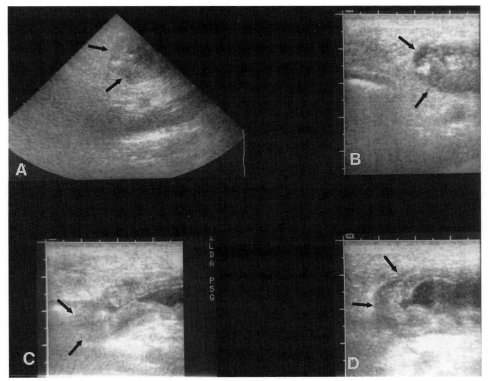

Figure 3–84. Transverse (A) and longitudinal (B,C,&D) sonograms of the pylorus of a 6-year-old miniature poodle with a history of chronic gastric distension, anemia, and hypoproteinemia. The pylorus is markedly thickened and irregular (*arrows*). This is indicative of a focal inflammatory or infiltrative lesion. **Diagnosis:** Gastric carcinoma.

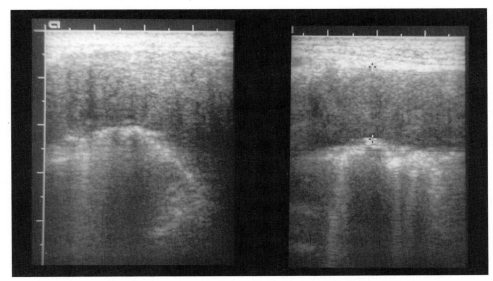

Figure 3–85. Transverse sonograms of the stomach of a 3-year-old male mixed breed dog with a history of vomiting of 3 months' duration. The gastric wall is markedly thickened. The architecture is abnormal and the individual layers cannot be identified. The hyperechoic region with the comet tail artifacts identifies the gastric lumen and the hyperechoic fat adjacent to the body wall identifies the outer margin of the stomach wall. The calipers (+) were used to measure the gastric wall thickness, which was 1.4 cm. This represents a neoplastic or infectious lesion. **Diagnosis:** zygomycosis.

Intramural masses may be detected and may produce discrete rounded or lobulated lesions, which may be outlined by fluid within the gastric lumen. Localizing the mass to a distinct layer of the stomach is difficult. Most gastric masses are heteroechoic and characterizing the mass as neoplastic or inflammatory is not possible. Observing the motion of the mass with change in position of the patient or gastric peristalsis is useful in determining whether the mass is intramural or intraluminal. Intramural lesions will be fixed in position despite peristalsis or changes in patient position. Intramural masses may also interfere with normal wall movement during peristalsis.

It is more difficult to recognize diffuse gastric wall thickening. If the gastric wall diameter exceeds the normal range of 3 to 5 mm, the wall layers should be examined to see if they are asymmetrically widened or disrupted, and the gastric wall should be observed carefully during peristalsis to determine if there is a segmental loss of motility. Thickening of the gastric wall may be localized to a specific layer and this may be helpful in determining what disease is present.[98] Localized thickening of the gastric wall with a focal loss of peristalsis may be observed in association with pancreatitis. Recognition of the lesion within the pancreas will help to determine that the gastric wall thickening is secondary. Craters or defects may be identified within the thickened stomach wall when gastric ulcers are present.

Pyloric outflow obstruction may be recognized during the ultrasound examination. Symmetrical or asymmetrical thickening of the pylorus or a mass may be observed. Hypertrophic pyloric gastropathy produces a uniform thickening of the hypoechoic muscular layer of the pylorus. The extent of pyloric wall thickening varies from 9 to 19 mm with the thickness of the muscularis ranging from 3.0 to 5.4 mm. Gastric distension and vigorous peristalsis were also observed.[102]

A thickened gastric wall, thickened rugal folds, and loss or decreased definition of the normal gastric wall layers were identified ultrasonographically in dogs with uremic gastritis. A hyperechoic line identified at the mucosal-luminal junction was associated with gastric mineralization.[103]

Foreign bodies may be identified using ultrasound. Most foreign bodies will be hyperechoic, will have sharply defined margins, and will shadow.[98,104] Foreign bodies will readily move within the stomach with changes in the patient's position. Chunks of dry dog food may have a similar appearance, however their large number and uniform size will make them easily recognizable.

Gastrogastric intussusception was identified during an ultrasound examination. A spiraled, tapered echogenic mass was seen in the gastric fundus. The pyloric antrum and the body of the stomach could not be identified.[92]

PANCREAS

Density Changes

Pancreatic lesions are frequently difficult to define radiographically. Although several radiographic findings have been described in association with pancreatitis, it is our experience that none of the radiographic findings are reliably present and the absence of these findings in any specific case should not preclude the diagnosis of pancreatitis.[105,106] The most commonly seen radiographic change is an apparent haziness and loss of detail in the cranial right- and/or midabdomen. This change must be interpreted cautiously, because most animals have poor detail in this area due to the large number of contiguous and adjacent fluid-dense structures. The proximal duodenum may be dilated and fixed in diameter in response to the local inflammation. A similar rigidity may be observed in the gastric wall adjacent to the left limb of the pancreas. In the ventrodorsal radiograph, the proximal duodenum may be displaced toward the right lateral abdominal wall and the pylorus may be displaced toward the midline. This widens the angle or curve between the pylorus and proximal duodenum. The transverse colon may be displaced caudally away from the

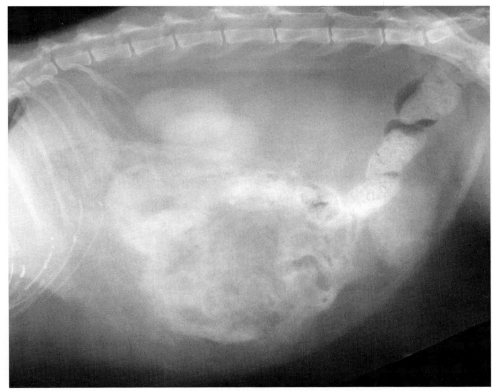

Figure 3–86. A 6-year-old female domestic short-haired cat that had chronic periodic anorexia and vomiting. The lateral radiograph revealed a loss of detail throughout the entire abdomen and is mostly apparent in the cranial areas. Differential diagnoses include carcinomatosis, pancreatitis, or steatitis. **Diagnosis:** Chronic relapsing pancreatitis with saponification of mesenteric fat.

stomach and may be either distended and fixed in diameter or completely empty. In severe pancreatitis, there may also be a haziness throughout the entire abdomen (Fig. 3–86).

Pancreatic Masses

Both pancreatic neoplasia and pancreatic abscess produce identical radiographic changes. Pancreatic pseudocyst has been reported in the dog and cat. It will produce a mass in the region of the pancreas. Pancreatic masses such as carcinoma, cyst, abscess, or "bladder" formation may involve the duodenum or stomach wall (Fig. 3–87).[106,107] These lesions produce radiographic changes similar to pancreatitis; occasionally, however, the outline of the mass may be observed. The mass may interfere with normal gastric or duodenal peristalsis producing a fixed or rigid wall. The lesions may distort the shape of the stomach or intestine and may be difficult to distinguish from intramural lesions. The transverse colon may be displaced caudally, and the descending duodenum may be displaced laterally due to a mass effect from the inflammation, build-up of scar tissue in the pancreatic area, or from the pancreatic mass itself.[108]

In chronic pancreatitis, punctate calcifications may occur in the pancreatic area due to saponification of mesenteric fat by pancreatic enzymes.[109] Either pancreatic tumors or abscesses may have areas of calcification.

Ultrasound of Pancreatic Abnormalities

The descending duodenum and right kidney are used as landmarks to locate the right limb of the pancreas, and the stomach is used as a landmark to locate the left limb.[15] When the pancreas is easily recognized as a hyperechoic structure adjacent

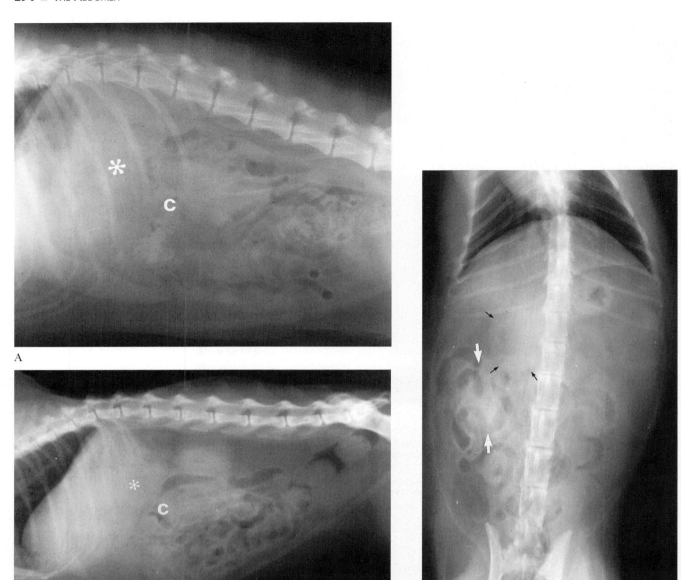

Figure 3–87. (A) A 7-year-old male miniature schnauzer that vomited five times the previous day. The dog has experienced multiple similar bouts. Palpation revealed abdominal tenderness. The lateral radiograph revealed an ill-defined tissue density (*white **) caudal to the stomach which displaces the transverse colon (*white c*) caudally. Differential diagnoses include pancreatic mass, splenic mass, or mass arising from the caudal gastric wall. **Diagnosis:** Pyogranuloma of the pancreas due to chronic relapsing pancreatitis. (B) A 5-year-old male domestic short-haired cat with vomiting for 1 week and a palpable cranial abdominal mass. The lateral radiograph revealed a tissue-dense mass (*white **) between the stomach and the transverse colon (*white c*). (C) The ventrodorsal view of the cat revealed a mass (*black arrows*) just to the right of the midline and cranial to the right kidney (*white arrows*). Differential diagnoses include chronic pancreatitis, pancreatic neoplasia, or pancreatic bladder. **Diagnosis:** Pancreatic bladder.

to the stomach and duodenum, it is probably enlarged.[8] Pancreatitis, pancreatic abscess, and pancreatic adenocarcinoma produce similar ultrasound abnormalities.[108] In experimental dogs, free peritoneal fluid in the pancreatic region, dilation and thickening of the wall of the duodenum, and an inhomogeneous mass were identified 24 to 48 hours after induction of acute pancreatitis.[110,111] In dogs with acute pancreatitis, the pancreatic duct may enlarge and be as big as the pancreatoduodenal vein. Ultrasound is an extremely valuable diagnostic tool for identifying pancreatitis in dogs and cats. Pancreatitis can result in decreased echogenicity of the pancreas relative to the normal surrounding mesenteric fat. This results from hemorrhage, edema, or necrosis. Fat saponification associated with chronic pancreatitis may produce an increase in echogenicity within the mesentery. The pancreas may be either hyperechoic, hypoechoic, or both. A mass may be observed adjacent to the duodenum or greater curvature of the stomach. This mass can usually be distinguished from the normal mesentery and omentum because it is more well-defined and usually has areas of hyperechoic, hypoechoic, or anechoic tissue within it (Figs. 3–88 and 3–89). Duodenal or gastric wall thickening with limited peristalsis may be observed. Extrahepatic biliary obstruction may occur as a result of inflammatory obstruction of the common bile duct.[112] Differentiating between pancreatic abscess and pancreatic neoplasia is difficult. Chronic pancreatitis may rarely produce focal areas of mineralization, and these areas may be detected as hyperechoic foci which shadow. Biliary distention may occur secondary to pancreatic lesions, but its presence is not useful in discriminating between tumor and abscess.

Pancreatic pseudocysts can be recognized as well-defined anechoic lesions with distant enhancement and a few internal echoes.[113] Aspiration of the pseudocyst using ultrasound guidance can be performed. Dilation of the pancreatic duct may be mistaken for a pseudocyst.

Insulinomas may be detected using ultrasound. They appear as hypoechoic well-defined nodules that may be identified within the hyperechoic mesenteric fat in the pancreatic region. The pancreas itself may not be identified. Lymph node metastasis may be indistinguishable from an insulinoma.

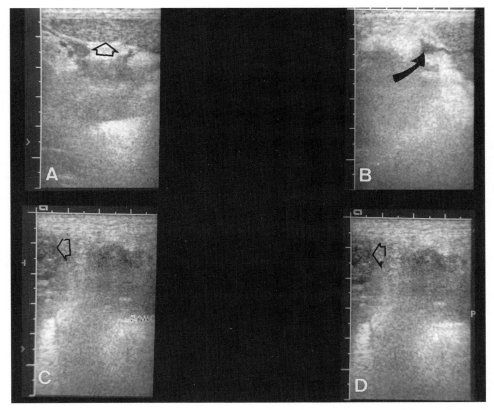

Figure 3–88. Transverse sonograms of the cranial abdomen of a 4-year-old spayed female schnauzer with a history of acute abdominal discomfort and abdominal pain. There is a heteroechoic mass surrounded by hyperechoic fat which extends from the spleen (A: *open arrow*) to the duodenum (C&D: *open arrows*). There is a small amount of free peritoneal fluid (B: *closed arrow*). This is indicative of pancreatitis or a pancreatic mass. **Diagnosis:** Pancreatitis.

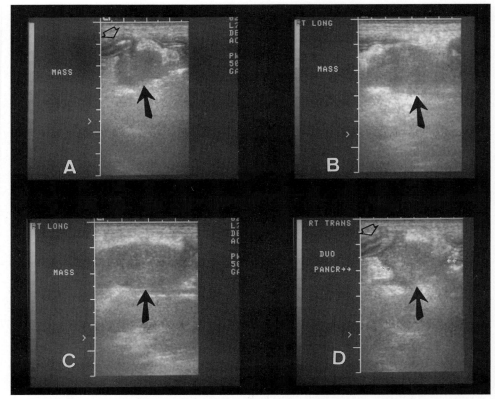

Figure 3–89. Transverse (A&D) and longitudinal (B&C) sonograms of the cranial abdomen of a 2-year-old spayed female cocker spaniel who presented with a history of lethargy and cranial abdominal pain. There is a heteroechoic mass in the cranial abdomen (*arrows*) medial to the duodenum (*small arrows*). The tissue around this mass appears hyperechoic. This is indicative of a pancreatic tumor or abscess. **Diagnosis:** Pancreatic abscess.

SMALL INTESTINES

Density Changes

Small intestinal lesions may be detected on survey radiography by an abnormal density within the intestinal lumen. The bowel will normally contain fluid (tissue density), food (which may contain tissue and bone density), or air. Air contained within the GI tract is usually the result of aerophagia.[54] Occasionally, a segment of small bowel may contain material that has the density and pattern of feces (a mixture of tissue and bone density). This is usually indicative of small bowel obstruction with desiccation of material trapped proximal to the obstruction (Fig. 3–90). The bowel may contain metal or mineral-dense material, which may indicate ingestion of toxic materials (e.g., lead, zinc); excretion of contrast agents (due to bile and small intestinal excretion of intravenous contrast media in a patient with severe renal failure); medications (e.g., kaopectate, pepto bismol, zinc oxide); or foreign bodies (e.g., metal oxide coated recording tapes, coins, needles, staples) (Figs. 3–91 and 3–92).

On rare occasions, gas may accumulate within the bowel wall. This produces a double line that outlines the intestine. The double line will be present on both sides of the lumen. The outer serosal surface is usually smooth while the inner mucosal surface is more undulant. This has been associated with necrosis of the wall caused by a loss of the normal blood supply.[8] Mesenteric thrombosis, severe bowel wall trauma, and infiltrating neoplasms may cause this radiographic change. Infection with a gas producing organism may produce emphysema of the bowel wall. This occurs most often in the colon and has been observed in the stomach. It has not been reported in the small intestines.

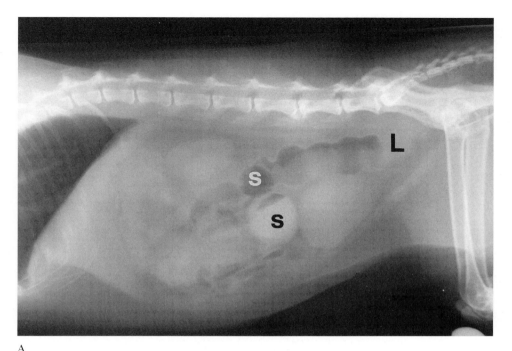

A

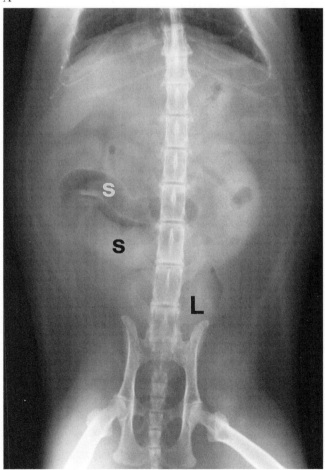

B

Figure 3–90. A 16-year-old neutered male Siamese cat with vomiting for 6 weeks. (A) The lateral view revealed feces in the descending large intestine (*black L*), which extends cranially. Superimposed on the colon is a dilated, gas-filled loop of small intestine (*white s*), which goes on to become a loop that contains material of the same density as feces (*black s*). (B) On the ventrodorsal view the feces-filled large intestine (*black L*) is seen to the left of the spine. The gas-filled small bowel loop (*white s*) is seen going from just to the left of L4 to near the right lateral body wall where it curls ventrally and now contains material with density the same as feces (*black s*). Differential diagnoses include a small intestinal obstruction (because adenocarcinoma is a frequent cause for small bowel obstruction in older Siamese cats this would be the most likely cause) or a very redundant and tortuous colon being mistaken for small bowel. **Diagnosis:** Adenocarcinoma of the jejunum.

Position Changes

The location of the small intestine is constantly changing due to intestinal peristalsis. This is one of the reasons that detection of focal abnormalities of the small in-

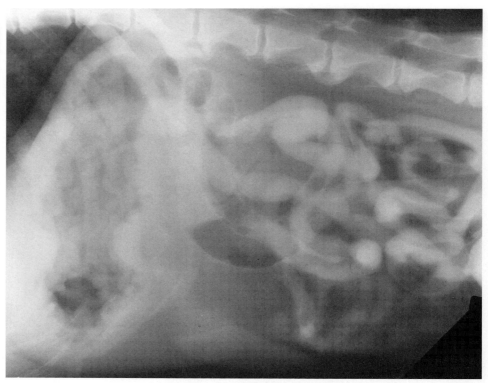

Figure 3–91. An 11-year-old male Saint Bernard that had been given an excretory urogram the day before this radiograph. That examination revealed poor excretion of the contrast media. This lateral abdominal radiograph revealed a nearly homogeneous metallic density throughout the small intestine with occasional gas bubbles. Secondary to the kidney, the routes of excretion of contrast media are through the bile and directly by the small intestinal lining cells. **Diagnosis:** Excretion of contrast media via secondary routes into the intestine.

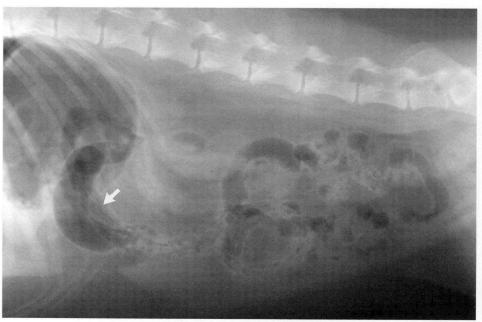

Figure 3–92. A 5-year-old spayed Siberian husky with vomiting for 1 day. There is plication (bunching upon itself) of the small intestine and eccentrically positioned, vaguely triangular gas bubbles in the intestinal lumen. Close examination revealed fine, linear mineral-dense structures (*white arrow*) in the intestinal lumen. **Diagnosis:** Linear foreign body due to ingestion of recording tape.

testine is difficult. Small bowel displacement is usually a function of passive movement in response to changes in size and shape of other abdominal organs. This displacement is an important radiographic change used to determine which abdominal organ is abnormal. Displacement of the intestines into the pleural cavity indicates a diaphragmatic hernia, while identification of the intestines in the pericardial sac indicates a peritoneopericardial diaphragmatic hernia. Displacement of the small bowel into various other hernia sacs (e.g., femoral, ventral, paracostal, or perineal) may also be noted (Fig. 3–93). The small intestine may twist around the root of the mesentery. This will cause the small bowel to be both dilated and in an abnormal location.[114] With linear foreign bodies, the small intestine is characteristically gathered upon itself and often collecting on the right side of the abdomen. The intestines may have an abnormally large diameter and a pattern of frequent serosal undulations or plications. Frequently, there are small, teardrop-shaped gas bubbles due to the shape the bowel assumes as it attempts to pass the foreign body (Fig. 3–94).[115] The extent to which these findings will be present depends on the diameter and length of the linear foreign body. Some yarns or ropes that have large diameters may not plicate the intestines. Small intestinal adhesions secondary to peritonitis may also result in a gathering of the small intestines into a localized area.

Size and Shape Changes

The size and shape of the small bowel is variable depending on content and motility. The most significant size change is dilation. The small bowel diameter normally should be less than the width of a lumbar vertebral body (as viewed on the ventrodorsal projection) or should not exceed the diameter of the large intestine. Distention of the small intestine with air, fluid, or food is termed *ileus*. Two types of dilation (ileus) are seen: dynamic and adynamic. In dynamic ileus some peristalsis is present and both normal size and dilated small bowel loops will be present (Fig. 3–95). This usually is the result of partial or incomplete intestinal obstruction. With complete obstruction all of the bowel proximal to the obstruction will dilate eventually; the distal bowel will be empty or normal in size. Because 6 to 8 hours are

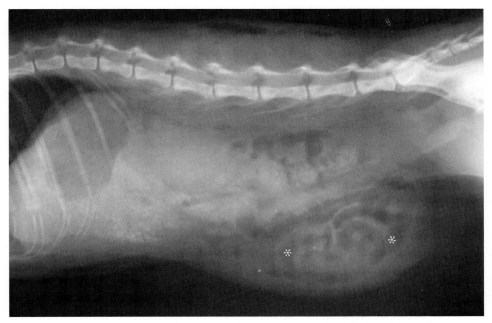

Figure 3–93. A 5-year-old female domestic short-haired cat that was in a fight with a German shepherd dog. There is a ventral tissue mass that contains multiple gas-filled loops of small intestine (*white **). Also present is an extensional fracture/luxation involving L3 and L4 and subcutaneous emphysema in the dorsal soft tissues. **Diagnosis:** Ventral hernia, fracture/luxation of L3–L4, and subcutaneous emphysema.

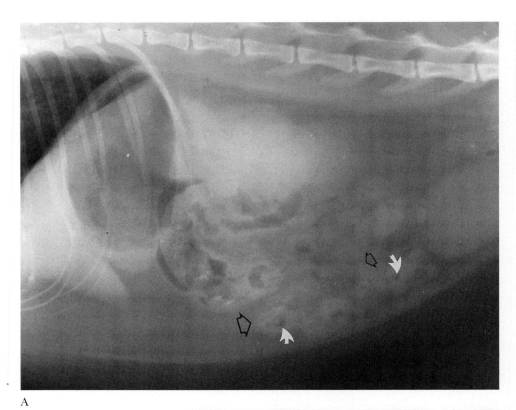

A

Figure 3–94. A 6-year-old neutered female short-haired cat with vomiting (6 to 8 times per day) and complete anorexia for 2 days. (A) There is marked plication (bunching upon itself) of the small intestine which is seen most easily in the ventral areas (*open black arrows*) and multiple, small, eccentrically-positioned, vaguely triangular-shaped gas bubbles (*white arrows*). (B) The plication of the small intestine (*open black arrows*) and characteristic gas pattern is seen. The majority of the small bowel is present on the right side of the abdomen. **Diagnosis:** Small intestinal linear foreign body (sewing thread).

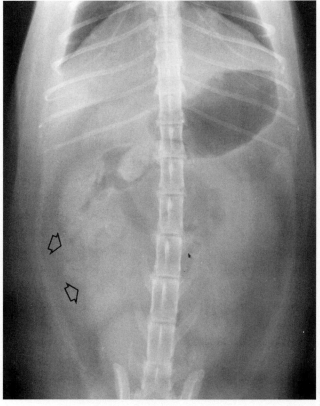

B

required to empty the bowel distal to the obstruction, some gas or feces may be present in these loops for a time after the obstruction is complete. The intestines proximal to a complete obstruction often distend with air and fluid while the intestines proximal to an incomplete (partial) obstruction often distend with undi-

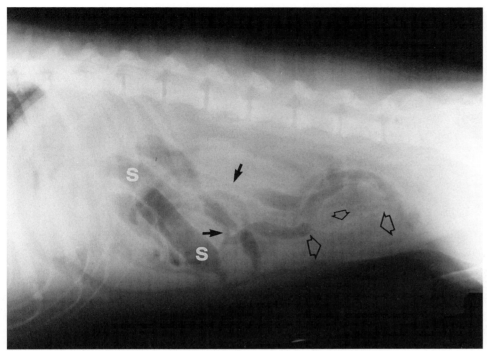

Figure 3–95. A 4-year-old male Labrador retriever with vomiting (4 to 5 times per day) for 2 days. The lateral radiograph revealed marked dilation of some of the gas-filled loops (*white s*) and of some of the normal-sized loops (*solid black arrows*) of the small intestine. This is indicative of a dynamic ileus. Differential diagnoses include foreign body, neoplasia, or inflammation. Careful examination revealed an area with density slightly greater than that of the rest of the small intestine and a characteristic pattern of very small gas lucencies which are aligned in rows (*open black arrows*). **Diagnosis:** Dynamic ileus secondary to a corncob foreign body.

gestible material, such as bone and hair, and appear to be filled with food or fecal-dense material. The intestine proximal to the obstruction may be dilated to many times its normal diameter (Fig. 3–96). In partial small bowel obstruction, the degree of small bowel dilation is often less than that associated with complete obstruction.

In adynamic ileus there will be no evidence of peristaltic contractions. Adynamic ileus is typified by the uniform dilation of all of the affected small bowel and is most commonly the result of the administration of parasympatholytic drugs, vascular compromise (infarction), peritonitis, pancreatitis, severe enteritis (e.g., parvo virus), and prolonged small bowel obstruction.

In situations where the complete bowel obstruction is in the proximal descending duodenum, the dilation of the small bowel may not be apparent because of the short length of involved intestine. The stomach will become markedly distended with fluid and gas due to reverse peristalsis, which moves the fluid and gas from the duodenum back into the stomach. These cases may be more apparent if both right and left lateral recumbent views are taken (Fig. 3–97).

Obstructions may be caused by foreign bodies, torsion, volvulus, strangulation (such as from displacement through a rent in the mesentery), intussusception, adhesions, granulomas, or neoplasms. Although some foreign bodies are opaque and readily evident on the radiographs, many are tissue-dense and not identified because they are surrounded by fluid within the intestines. Nuts or seeds may contain air within their centers or may have mineral density in their shells and may therefore be evident on the radiograph. Although a "coiled spring" appearance has been described in association with intussusception, this change is rarely evident. In most cases, the cause of the intestinal obstruction will not be evident on the non-contrast radiograph. If there are non-contrast radiographic findings indicative of intestinal obstruction, a GI series is not indicated. In these patients, the lack of peristalsis that

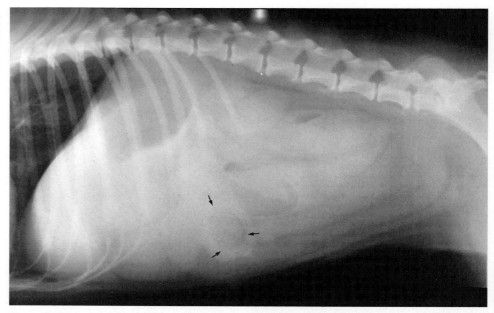

Figure 3–96. A 3-year-old female miniature poodle with a 5-day history of vomiting. The lateral radiograph revealed that virtually all identifiable loops of the small intestine are uniformly dilated (adynamic ileus). Close scrutiny revealed a relative radiolucency with the shape of a fruit pit (*black arrows*). **Diagnosis:** Intestinal foreign body (apricot pit) with adynamic ileus.

produced the ileus will prevent the contrast from reaching the point of obstruction. This is more often the case in complete rather than in incomplete obstruction.

GI Series

The GI series may be helpful in defining and delineating lesions of the small intestine. Although some radiographic changes may be more often associated with tumor or infection, all may be observed in either condition. A GI series rarely results in a specific diagnosis and most often confirms the presence of a lesion within the intestines, which must be biopsied in order to establish a specific diagnosis.[116] The GI series can be normal despite the presence of disease. As with the stomach, the paramount criterion of a positive finding is its repeatability. The small intestine should normally appear as a smooth tube on the GI series. The contrast should pass through the intestines in a column with some areas of constriction associated with peristalsis. A brush border is normal.

MUCOSAL PATTERNS

There are a large number of normal mucosal patterns ranging from a thin streak of barium ("string sign") to a roughly cobbled pattern.[117] The only clearly abnormal mucosal pattern on the GI series is flocculation of the barium. This is a granular appearance of the contrast medium (Fig. 3–98). It may be caused by poorly mixed barium suspensions, prolonged passage times, instillation of the barium into large volumes of gastric fluid, by disease causing the presence of excess mucus or hemorrhage in the intestines, or, perhaps, by a change in the intestinal pH.[8] When flocculation is present, infiltrative bowel diseases or malabsorption syndromes should be considered: lymphangiectasia, chronic enteritis, plasmacytic/lymphocytic enteritis, eosinophilic enteritis, or lymphosarcoma.

MAJOR CLASSIFICATIONS OF CHANGE

Lesions that radiographically affect the small intestine may be considered to be diffuse or focal and either intraluminal, mural, or extramural.

Diffuse intestinal diseases include inflammation, diffuse neoplasms, immune disease, lymphangiectasia, or hemorrhagic gastroenteritis. Focal intestinal diseases include fungal granuloma and neoplasia.

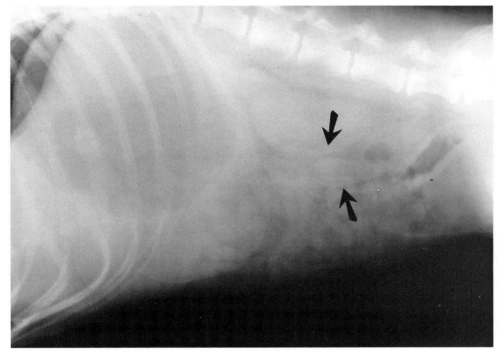

A

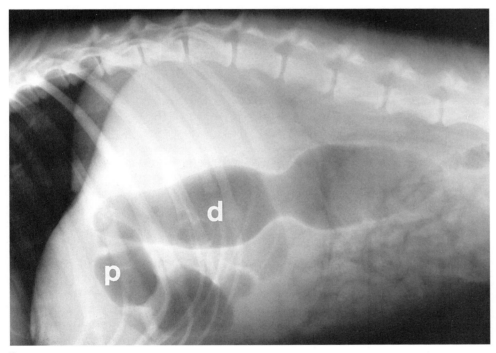

B

Figure 3–97. A 4-year-old female miniature poodle with a 2-day history of vomiting. (A) On the right recumbent lateral view there is moderate fluid distension of the stomach. Close scrutiny revealed a fluid dilated loop of small intestine (*black arrows*). (B) The left recumbent lateral view causes the air in the stomach to go to the pylorus (*white p*) and duodenum (*white d*), which revealed marked dilation of the descending duodenum. The severity of dilation indicates complete blockage of the duodenum. Differential diagnoses include foreign body or neoplasia. **Diagnosis:** Duodenal foreign body (ball).

Intraluminal. If intraluminal lesions are relatively small in diameter and short in length, there may be little change in size or shape of the small intestine. On the GI series, the only findings may be narrow linear filling defects within the lumen. These

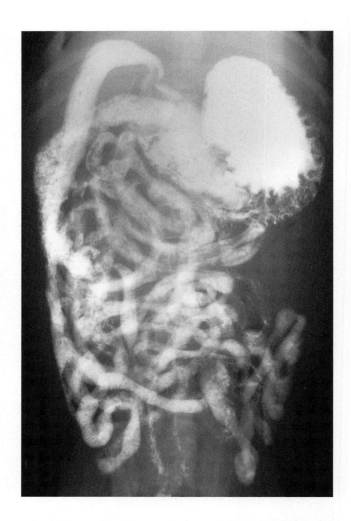

Figure 3–98. A 1-year-old male German shepherd dog with chronic diarrhea. The ventrodorsal view revealed a granular, nonhomogeneous appearance to the barium (flocculation) within the small intestine. This is most consistent with a malabsorption syndrome. Differential diagnoses include lymphangiectasia, eosinophilic gastroenteritis, lymphosarcoma of the small intestine, and chronic enteritis. **Diagnosis:** Lymphangiectasia.

may be due to ascarids, tape worms, or linear foreign bodies of short length. In cases of relatively narrow diameter, long, linear foreign bodies, the GI series may reveal a small intraluminal filling defect with plication or displacement of the small bowel (Fig. 3–99A). In cases where the linear foreign body is relatively wide, the intraluminal filling defect will be seen but plication will not be significant (Fig. 3–99B). Most commonly, intraluminal lesions may be identified because the intestine is dilated at a focal site in both the ventrodorsal and lateral views with a smooth and somewhat gradual zone of transition between the normal diameter and the distension (Fig. 3–100). These lesions usually result in some degree of intestinal obstruction. These range from partial (those seen with baby bottle nipples that allow fluid and air to pass) to complete obstructions (seen with very large foreign bodies). While foreign bodies are the most common intraluminal lesions, other considerations must include neoplasms that extend into the lumen. Most intraluminal objects will allow the passage of contrast on all sides, while tumors that protrude into the intestinal lumen will have at least one point of attachment to the wall. Careful evaluation of the contrast column in all views may be required in order to discriminate between luminal objects and those that arise from the intestinal wall. In many cases, laparotomy will be required to determine the exact nature of the lesion.

Mural. Mural lesions can be categorized as those with thickening, those that have ulcerations of the intestinal walls, or those with both. The normal bowel wall thickness varies depending on whether it is at rest or actively involved in a peristaltic movement. With full luminal distension and at rest, the bowel wall is normally a few millimeters thick. The presence of thickened walls suggests infiltrative disease. The most common cause is adenocarcinoma. Adenocarcinoma usually causes a concen-

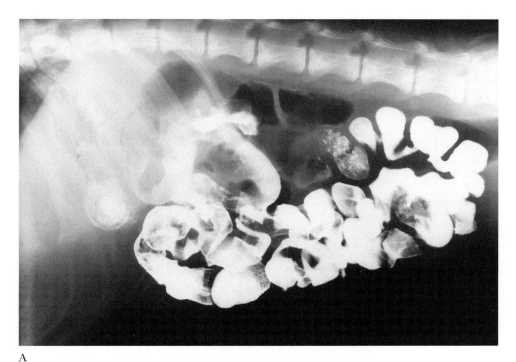

A

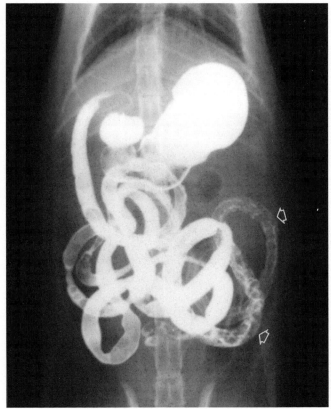

B

Figure 3–99. (A) A 1-year-old male coonhound with anorexia, depression, vomiting, and diarrhea for 2 weeks. The 30-minute lateral view revealed marked plication of the majority of the small intestine. This appearance is most consistent with a linear foreign body of small to intermediate diameter. **Diagnosis:** Small intestinal linear foreign body (sewing thread). (B) A 3-year-old neutered male domestic short-haired cat with vomiting and anorexia for 2 days. The survey radiographs revealed no abnormalities. The ventrodorsal view taken at 30 minutes into the GI series revealed mild dilation of the small intestine and an irregular lucent filling defect which extends over a significant length of small intestine and is best seen in the loops in the left portion of the abdomen (*open white arrows*). No plication is seen. Linear foreign bodies that have a wide diameter do not cause the bowel to plicate but rather act as any other foreign body that causes a partial small intestinal obstruction. **Diagnosis:** Small intestinal linear foreign body (athletic shoelaces).

tric narrowing of the intestinal lumen and thickening of the wall over a length of a few centimeters, which leads to an area of nearly compete intestinal obstruction (Fig. 3–101). The normal bowel proximal to the lesion may be dilated. The diameter of the bowel distal to the lesion is usually normal. Lymphosarcoma may occasionally present with concentrically thickened intestinal walls, but more commonly it extends

Figure 3–100. A 3-year-old male cocker spaniel with vomiting for 2 days. Survey radiographs revealed a distended stomach and normal intestinal shadows. The GI series revealed a large intraluminal mass (filling defect in the barium column) in the proximal duodenum partially obstructing the intestine. This is seen on both (A) the lateral and (B) ventrodorsal views. Due to the location of this obstruction in the proximal duodenum there is no dilation of the majority of the small bowel. **Diagnosis:** Duodenal foreign body (sponge rubber ball).

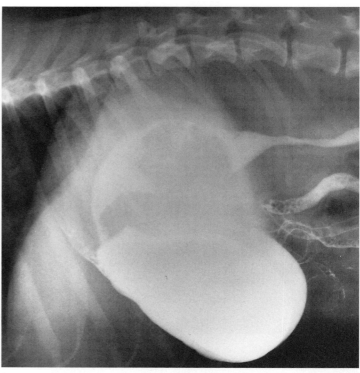

A

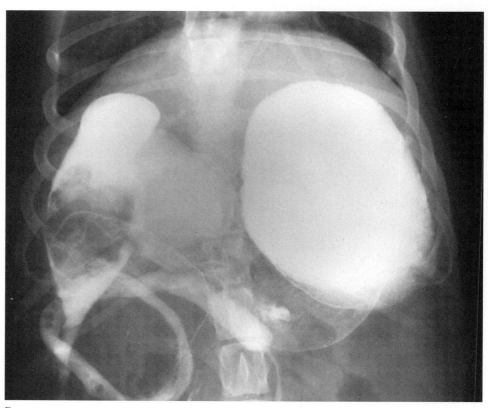

B

over several centimeters and is not completely circumferential. In dogs, lymphosarcoma may appear as irregular, small, focal asymmetric thickened areas of the small intestinal wall that have neither a concentric pattern nor result in obstruction (Fig. 3–102). This may be difficult to differentiate from some normal variations but the

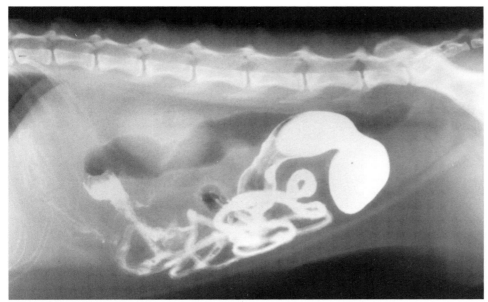

A

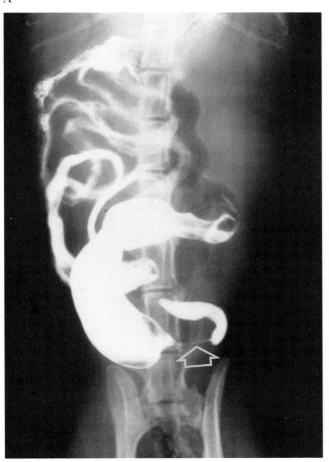

B

Figure 3–101. An 8-year-old. castrated Siamese cat with vomiting for 2 months. (A) The lateral view shows dilation of the small intestine but the cause of this is not readily apparent. (B) On the ventrodorsal view, at 4 hours (delayed passage time), there is dilation of the ileum, which ends abruptly due to a concentric restriction of the lumen. A thin stream of barium is seen extending for approximately 2 cm to a normal-sized portion of ileum (*open white arrow*). Differential diagnoses for a focal concentric lesion include adenocarcinoma, lymphosarcoma, or granuloma. **Diagnosis:** Adenocarcinoma of the ileum.

repeatability of the lesion is a strong clue. In cats, the more common presentation of lymphosarcoma is thickening of the intestinal walls with luminal dilation. Involvement of the lymph nodes at the ileocolic junction with minimal radiographic changes is also frequently seen. There may be an obstruction proximal to the lesion with dilation of the small bowel.

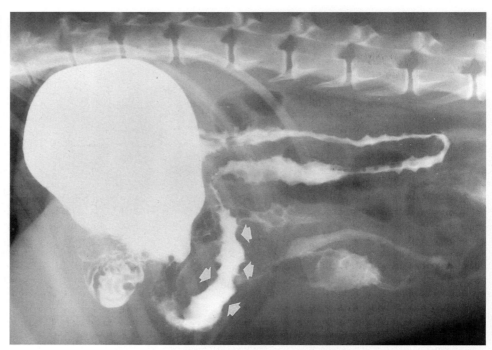

Figure 3–102. A 9-year-old spayed mixed breed dog with anorexia for 5 days and melena for 2 days. There are areas of marked irregularity to the mucosal border in the small bowel (*white arrows*) suggesting the presence of submucosal accumulation of abnormal cells. This appearance was consistent on all views. Differential diagnoses include any infiltrative small bowel disease such as lymphosarcoma, eosinophilic enteritis, plasmacytic/lymphocytic infiltrative disease, fungal enteritis, etc. **Diagnosis:** Lymphosarcoma of the small intestine.

The other form of mural disease is ulceration. An ulcer may be seen during a contrast study as a "crater-like" or linear outpouching of the contrast column. The intestinal wall may be thickened. A ring-shaped radiolucent defect with a central contrast containing portion may also be observed when the ulcer is chronic. This diagnosis is particularly difficult to establish in the dog's duodenum due to the normal presence of pseudoulcers (Fig. 3–103). Representing areas between accumulations of gut-associated lymphoid tissues (Peyer's patches) in the descending and transverse duodenum, pseudoulcers are seen radiographically as outpouchings of the barium from the normal duodenal lumen.[118] They are typically on the antimesenteric surface. This may be of little help radiographically, because the bowel may rotate on its normal axis and make identification of the mesenteric attachment difficult. Pathologic ulcers may occur with or without concurrent mural thickening. One of the more common causes of small intestinal ulceration is mast cell tumor. This is frequently associated with intestinal wall thickening and is most commonly seen in the duodenum. Non-steroidal anti-inflammatory drugs may also cause intestinal ulceration. Another cause of intestinal ulceration that is rarely seen is the Zollinger-Ellison syndrome. This syndrome (hypergastrinemia secondary to a pancreatic tumor producing gastrin) results in increased production and subsequent dumping of gastric acid into the duodenum. The radiographic changes show multiple ulcerations and ileus of the affected segment (Fig. 3–104). A third possible cause of ulceration is trauma from ingestion of foreign material.

Ulcers may also be identified in conjunction with diffuse or focal mural diseases. The presence or absence of ulceration is not helpful in distinguishing between inflammatory and neoplastic diseases.

Extramural. Extraluminal masses may result in a "thumb print" sign on the small bowel. This appears as a narrowing of the intestinal lumen on one view and a widening of it on the other view, much as would appear if one were to press a thumb onto

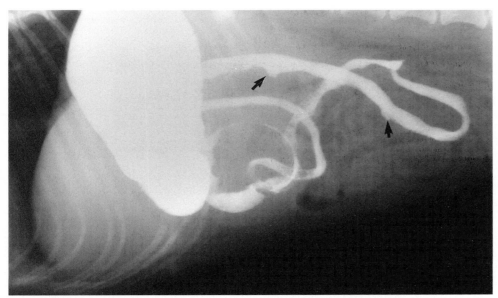

Figure 3–103. A 1-year-old female miniature schnauzer with occasional vomiting. The 15-minute lateral view of the GI series revealed two areas in the descending duodenum of out-pouching of the barium from the apparently normal lumen border (*black arrows*). Differential diagnoses include pseudoulcers (normally present small depressions in the mucosa of the duodenum of the dog) or true ulcerative disease. **Diagnosis:** Pseudoulcers.

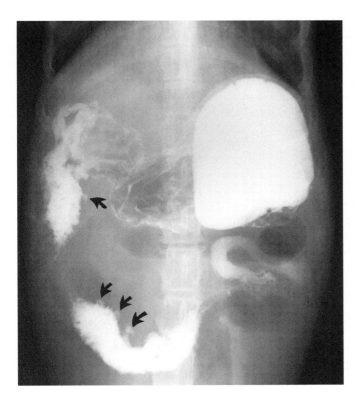

Figure 3–104. A 6-year-old spayed German shepherd dog with vomiting for 6 days. There is marked dilation and irregularity of the descending and transverse duodenum as well as multiple ulcers extending well beyond the normal intestinal serosal border (*black arrows*). Differential diagnoses include ulcers due to mast cell tumor, gastrinoma (Zollinger-Ellison syndrome), or idiopathic causes. **Diagnosis:** Duodenal ulcers (secondary to gastrinoma causing hypersecretion of gastric acid).

a distensible tube. Often the mucosal surface over these lesions is smooth. Ulceration or irregularity of the mucosal surface indicates that the lesion is intramural. Extramural lesions are usually not due to disease of small bowel origin but indicate impingement by other structures. One example of this type of lesion is the presence of adhesions from previous abdominal surgery (Fig. 3–105). Enlarged ileocolic lymph

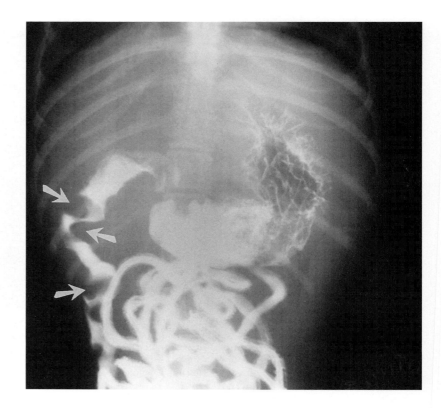

Figure 3–105. A 6-year-old male basenji with vomiting (2 to 3 times per day) for 3 days. The dog had undergone a laparotomy for an jejunal foreign body 5 weeks prior. Survey radiographs revealed no abnormalities. The ventrodorsal view of the GI series revealed 3 areas (*white arrows*) where the bowel is displaced and narrowed. On the lateral view these areas appeared slightly widened. This is most consistent with an extramural process affecting the small intestine. Differential diagnoses include adhesions obstructing the intestine or masses adjacent to the intestine causing partial obstruction. **Diagnosis:** Multiple adhesions compressing the duodenum.

nodes may produce an extramural compression of the ileum or cecum. An extraluminal mass may arise from the intestinal wall and extend outward to spare the intestinal lumen from compression. This type of finding is typical of intestinal leiomyosarcoma. These masses may contain gas densities if their centers become necrotic and develop a communication with the intestinal lumen (Fig. 3–106). Extraluminal masses may occasionally cause intestinal obstruction, but rarely is the obstruction complete and in most cases the contrast readily passes around the mass.

Ultrasound of Small Intestinal Abnormalities

Ultrasound can be used to evaluate the size, shape, and wall thickness of the small intestine.[13,98] Usually, only three layers of the wall can be seen. Thickening of the small intestine can be detected most easily when the thickening is asymmetric. The normal intestinal wall width ranges from 2 to 3 mm.[13] The wall of the duodenum is normally slightly thicker than the rest of the small intestine and may be up to 4.5 mm thick. Variation in bowel wall thickness and diameter occurs in association with normal peristalsis. Because peristalsis can be observed during the ultrasound examination, the change in bowel diameter can be observed directly and dilation of the intestines can be documented. A lack of peristalsis associated with intestinal dilation would be indicative of ileus. This can be recognized during the ultrasound examination.[98] The major problem in detecting small intestinal distention is distinguishing between the small intestine and the colon. The presence of active peristalsis indicates that the bowel is small rather than indicating the large intestine. The position of the colon is usually fixed, and the course that the colon follows is usually straighter than the small intestine. These are helpful although they are not completely reliable features. Intraluminal, intramural, and extramural lesions can be detected using ultrasound. Intraluminal objects can be observed surrounded by mucus or normal intestinal content. Most foreign objects are hyperechoic and shadow (Fig. 3–107).[98,104] They may be masked by the presence of air within the intestinal lumen, but in most cases manipulation of the bowel using the transducer or changing the patient's position will improve visualization of the intraluminal object. Ultrasound is superior to

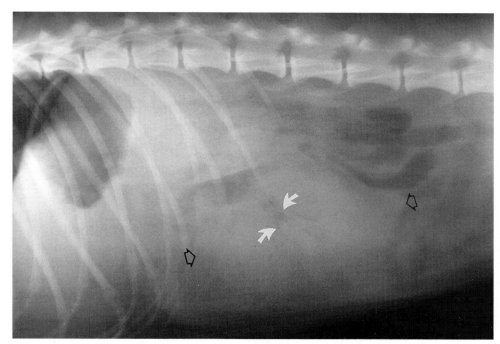

Figure 3–106. A 13-year-old female poodle with anorexia for 1 week and a palpable abdominal mass. There is a large ventral midabdominal mass (*open black arrows*) with fine linear gas densities (*white arrows*) extending into it. There is no intestinal dilation. Differential diagnoses include nonluminal intestinal mass, splenic mass, or mesenteric lymph node enlargement. **Diagnosis:** Small intestinal leiomyosarcoma.

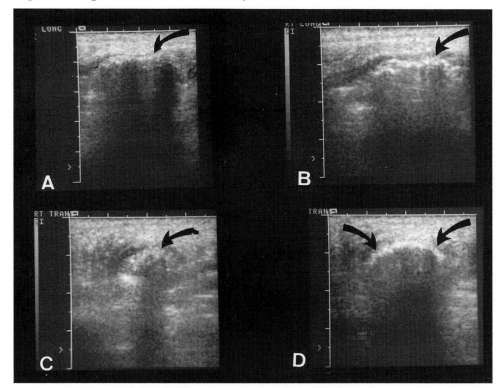

Figure 3–107. Longitudinal (A&B) and transverse (C&D) sonograms of the midabdomen of an 8-year-old spayed female silky terrier with a history of chronic vomiting and a palpable midabdominal mass. There is a hyperechoic curvilinear structure in the abdomen (*arrows*). This structure shadows and appeared to be associated with the GI tract. This most likely represents a foreign body but could also represent mineralization of the bowel wall. **Diagnosis:** GI foreign body.

non-contrast radiography for detecting GI tumors. Intramural lesions can be detected as the bowel is examined in both longitudinal and transverse planes, and the lesion can be localized to a specific layer of the intestine. Intestinal neoplasms are most often heteroechoic but contain hyperechoic or anechoic regions and may protrude into the lumen or from the serosa. If they are intraluminal, they may be outlined by fluid or ingesta within the intestine. If they protrude from the serosal surface, they may distort the shape of the intestines producing angular gas shadows rather than the normal oval or smooth linear shadows seen normally. Some masses may become quite large, and it may be difficult to determine that they are associated with the bowel. Many masses are eccentric to the bowel lumen and careful thorough examination may be required to confirm or identify the intestinal loops passing through or adjacent to the mass. The presence of gas within an abdominal mass should be seen as an indication that the mass is bowel associated (Fig. 3–108).[119] In cats, intestinal lymphosarcoma produces a transmural hypoechoic lesion that interferes with normal peristalsis.[100] Lymph node enlargement is frequently seen in association with the intestinal lesion.[101] Most extramural lesions displace the intestines; therefore, there will be no alteration in intestinal shape nor will there be gas within the mass.

Intussusception can be identified using ultrasound (Fig. 3–109).[98,120] In addition to the dilation of the intestines and lack of peristalsis, the intussusception itself can be identified as a multilayered lesion, which appears as linear streaks of hyperechoic and hypoechoic tissue in long section and as a series of concentric rings when viewed in cross section.

Enteric duplication cysts have been detected using ultrasound.[121] A "cyst-like" mass

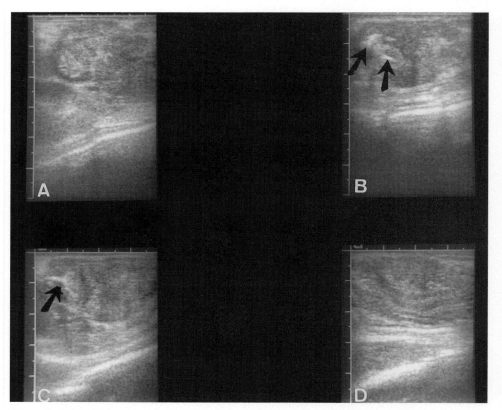

Figure 3–108. Transverse (A,B,&C) and longitudinal (D) sonograms of the abdomen of a 14-month-old castrated male Siamese cat with a history of anorexia and lethargy of 2 months' duration. A mass was palpable in the midabdomen. There is a heteroechoic abdominal mass with an eccentrically located hyperechoic region (*arrows*), which represents the intestinal lumen. This is indicative of a bowel associated mass. **Diagnosis:** Feline infectious peritonitis.

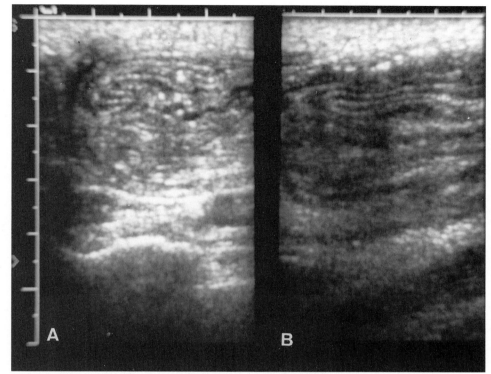

Figure 3–109. Transverse (A) and longitudinal (B) sonograms of the midabdomen of a 1-year-old male mixed breed dog who presented with a history of vomiting and anorexia of 1 week's duration. There is a multilayered series of alternating hyperechoic and hypoechoic bands visible. This is indicative of an intussusception. **Diagnosis:** Intussusception.

partially encircling and sharing a wall with a segment of small intestines was described. The wall of the mass had three layers, with a hyperechoic inner and outer layer surrounding a hypoechoic central layer. The hypoechoic central layer was continuous with the hypoechoic muscular layer of the adjacent normal intestine. Diffuse mobile echoes were identified within the lumen of the cyst. The cysts did not communicate with the intestines and peristalsis was not observed within the cysts.

LARGE INTESTINE

Size Changes

The normal colon may be empty or may contain air, fluid, or fecal material. It varies in size and position depending on the amount and type of material present. Normally, the colon is no more than three times larger than the small bowel. When the colon is severely distended, differential diagnoses should include colonic obstruction, megacolon, or obstipation (Fig. 3–110).

The colon can become distended if the animal is well trained and not allowed to go outside to defecate. Therefore, the size of the colon must always be evaluated relative to the patient's history or physical examination. If a colonic obstruction is present, the colon will become markedly distended; however, the small intestines will usually remain normal.

Congenital short colon has been reported in the dog and cat. In these patients, the cecum was located on the left and there was no demarcation of the ascending, transverse, and descending colon.[122] The colonic mucosa was smooth, suggesting that the condition was congenital rather than secondary to chronic colitis. Chronic colitis can also produce a short colon, however mucosal irregularities should also be present.

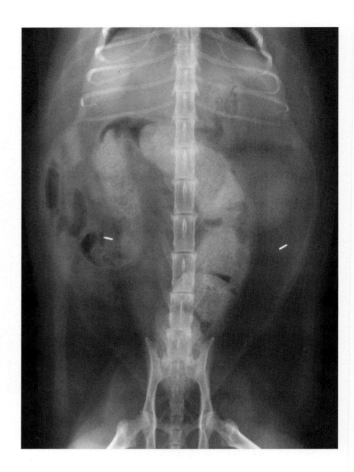

Figure 3–110. A 7-year-old neutered female domestic short-haired cat with straining to defecate for 2 weeks. There is a large amount of stool in the large intestine which distends it. The stool is nearly bone density, which indicates that it is dehydrated. Differential diagnoses include obstipation of idiopathic causes or secondary to such things as old pelvic fractures, damage to the cauda equina, or colon obstruction. **Diagnosis:** Idiopathic obstipation.

Density Changes

Density changes are almost exclusively limited to the presence of foreign matter (e.g., stones or metallic material) or obstipation with the presence of fecal material, which may become nearly bone-dense. In cases of exocrine pancreatic insufficiency, the colon may be filled with fluid-dense stool that is mixed with many gas bubbles. Rarely, gas may accumulate within the colon wall secondary to chronic colitis because of gas producing bacteria, such as *Clostridia*, and will be visible radiographically as linear lucent streaks.[123,124] Calcification of the colon or rectal wall may be seen in association with some neoplasms. Metallic foreign bodies may be present in the lumen or may rarely become embedded in the wall of the colon.

Position Changes

The cecum and ascending colon have a relatively constant position within the abdomen. In a small percentage of dogs (and occasionally in cats), the colon will be reversed from its normal position without generalized situs inversus being present. In both species, the transverse colon is usually found immediately caudal to the stomach on the ventrodorsal view. If the transverse colon is displaced caudally, a pancreatic or splenic mass may be present. Colonic displacement to the left can occur secondary to pancreatic or right renal masses or with intussusception of the distal small intestine and/or cecum into the ascending and transverse colon. Torsion may cause gross alteration in the normal location of the colon with marked distention of the colon with gas. Fortunately, this is uncommon. As the colon passes through the pelvic canal, displacement from the midline on the ventrodorsal view may indicate a pelvic canal mass (perineal hernia or pararectal tumor). On the lateral view the colon may be ventrally displaced as it passes through the cranial portion of the pelvic canal. This usually indicates enlargement of the sublumbar (external iliac, internal iliac, and coccygeal) lymph nodes or other caudal retroperitoneal mass (extension of a pelvic canal neoplasm). Dorsal colonic displacement in this area indicates a ventral mass that is usually due to prostatic enlargement or urethral tumor. Both dorsal and ventral narrowing may occur in cases of prostatic carcinoma with metastasis to the sublumbar lymph nodes or may be due to a tumor or stricture within the wall of the colon. Because the position of the colon varies normally depending on its content, displacement of the colon from its normal position indicates that the area from which the colon is displaced should be examined carefully. If a mass is not seen displacing the colon, then the displacement is a normal variation.

The dog's cecum often contains gas. It is not always identifiable, however, in a dog with a history of chronic tenesmus. Failure to identify the cecum may indicate cecal inversion.

Special Procedure Findings

Many colonic diseases are apparent only by direct examination (by endoscopy) or by use of contrast radiography (pneumocolon or barium enema). The fiberoptic endoscope is usually more accurate than most radiographic special procedures for evaluation of the colon. The major exception occurs when luminal narrowing or stricture does not permit passage of an endoscope.

Either pneumocolon or barium enema may be used to evaluate the colon. The most difficult problem is being certain that normal colonic content is not mistaken for an intraluminal or intramural mass. In most inflammatory colonic diseases, there is no radiographically apparent change. Lymphocytic plasmacytic colitis may produce diffuse thickening of the colon wall. In severe cases of ulcerative colitis, the colon wall will appear thickened and extensions of the barium column into the thickened wall may be observed.[125] Inflammation may predispose to intussusception. The most common site for intussusception in the dog is the ileocolic junction. In some cases, both the terminal ileum and cecum may be involved. In most cases, there will be dynamic ileus of the small bowel. Radiographically, there may be an apparent tissue-dense mass within a gas-filled loop of colon on survey films. The folded edematous intestinal mucosa produces a pattern that has been described as a "coiled spring" when outlined by the gas-filled colon. More frequently, the diagnosis requires a contrast study of the colon. The contrast must be administered retrograde, because the ileus will prevent contrast that is administered orally from reaching the site of the obstruction. The classic appearance is of a tube within a tube (intussusceptum into intussuscipiens) (Fig. 3–111). A variant of the intussusception is an inversion of the cecum. When this happens, the cecum inverts into the colon and

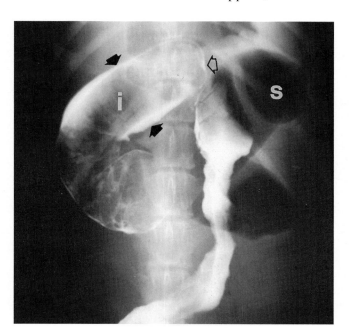

Figure 3–111. A 1-year-old male coonhound with vomiting and anorexia for 3 days and a palpable midabdominal mass. Survey radiographs revealed poor abdominal detail due to cachexia and a dynamic ileus. The barium enema revealed dilated, gas-filled small intestinal loops (*white s*). There is a tissue-dense mass within the ascending and transverse large intestine (*white i*), which is outlined by a thin line of barium (*black arrows*) surrounding it. Close scrutiny revealed a slight depression in the border of the mass at its tip in the transverse colon (*open black arrow*). Differential diagnoses include intussusception, intracolonic neoplasm, or foreign material. **Diagnosis:** Ileocolic intussusception.

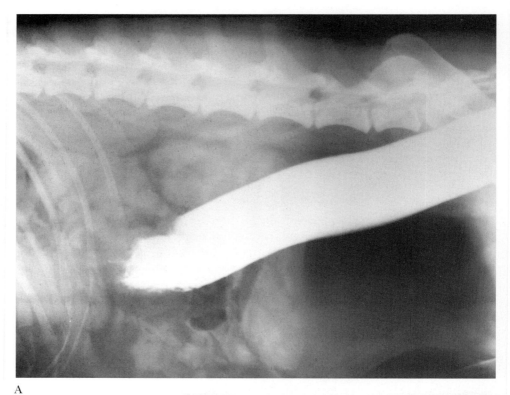

A

Figure 3–112. A 9-year-old male golden retriever with diarrhea for 6 weeks. Survey radiographs revealed no abnormalities. (A) The lateral view of the barium enema revealed constriction of lumen at the junction of the transverse and descending large intestine. This "napkin ring" of tissue or "apple core" appearance of the barium is indicative of a mural lesion. (B) The ventrodorsal view shows the patent but severely restricted intestinal lumen through this area (*open black arrow*). Differential diagnoses include carcinoma or granuloma. **Diagnosis:** Adenocarcinoma of the large intestine.

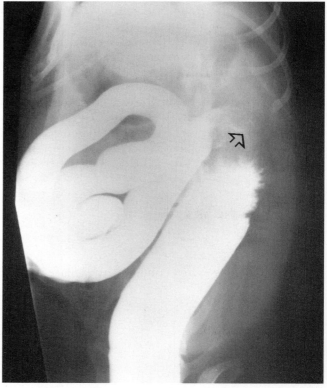

B

causes some degree of blockage at the ileocolic junction.[126] The shape of the cecum, which is seen as a tissue-dense mass surrounded by air or barium within the lumen of the colon, permits recognition of this lesion. The inverted cecum may not completely interfere with passage of contrast into the colon from the small intestines, therefore the cecal inversion may be diagnosed during an upper GI series.

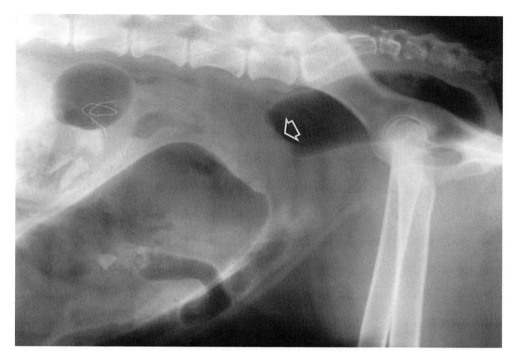

Figure 3–113. A 10-year-old female standard poodle with dyschezia for 4 months and hematochezia for 1 week. On the survey radiographs there was a suspicious tissue density in the distal descending large intestine and marked distension proximal to this. The lateral view of the pneumocolon revealed that the rectum is normal. There is a tissue-dense mass involving the descending large intestine with a small defect in its middle suggestive of a residual lumen (*open white arrow*). Proximal to the mass, the large intestine is severely dilated. Differential diagnoses include neoplasia (adenocarcinoma) or granuloma. **Diagnosis:** Adenocarcinoma of the distal large intestine.

Tumors and granulomas may produce intramural colonic lesions that may be evident as thickening of the colonic wall or as tissue-dense masses protruding into the lumen. These can often be recognized without the administration of contrast, thus relying on the normal contrast afforded by the gas within the lumen of the colon. Adenocarcinoma may produce a circumferential intramural lesion (Figs. 3–112 and 3–113). The colon may be dilated with air, fluid, or feces cranial to the lesion. Rectal administration of air or barium will outline the extent of the lesion when an endoscope cannot be passed through the area of narrowing. The mucosa is often irregular and/or ulcerated. Strictures may also produce circumferential narrowing, however they usually have a smooth mucosal surface. In most cases, biopsy is required to make a specific diagnosis.

Extramural masses may compress or displace the colon but usually do not distort the mucosal margin. Prostatic enlargement may compress the colon, and stump pyometra may produce a smooth indentation of the colon. Enlarged ileocolic lymph nodes can produce a mass adjacent to the colon or cecum. Some degree of small intestinal obstruction may also occur. The mass will not alter the smooth mucosal surface of the cecum or colon. Perirectal tumors (perianal masses or metastases) may affect the colon but usually are apparent without contrast studies.

Ultrasound of Colonic and Cecal Abnormalities

The colon does not lend itself to ultrasound examination very well because it usually contains air. The colon wall can be evaluated by ultrasound, and although layers cannot be detected the thickness of the wall can be determined. Diffuse thickening of the colon wall may be observed in inflammatory and infiltrative disease such as infectious or lymphocytic plasmacytic colitis (Figs. 3–114 and 3–115). The ultrasound findings are non-specific. Focal areas of thickening and heteroechoic masses

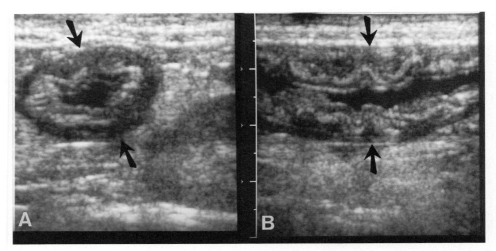

Figure 3–114.   Transverse (A) and longitudinal (B) sonograms of the colon of a 2-year-old spayed female domestic short hair cat who presented with a history of 1 month of depression, anorexia, vomiting, and dyschezia with large amounts of mucus in the feces. The wall of the colon is markedly thickened (*arrows*). This is indicative of an inflammatory or infiltrative lesion. The entire descending colon was involved. **Diagnosis:** Lymphocytic plasmacytic colitis.

Figure 3–115.   Transverse (A&B) and longitudinal (C&D) sonograms of the colon of a 2-year-old male boxer with a history of bloody diarrhea of 4 months' duration. The colon wall is markedly thickened. The thickening appears to be mainly within the mucosa. The mucosal surface is irregular. The lesion involved the entire colon from the rectum to the cecum. This may be associated with inflammatory or infiltrative disease. **Diagnosis:** Ulcerative colitis.

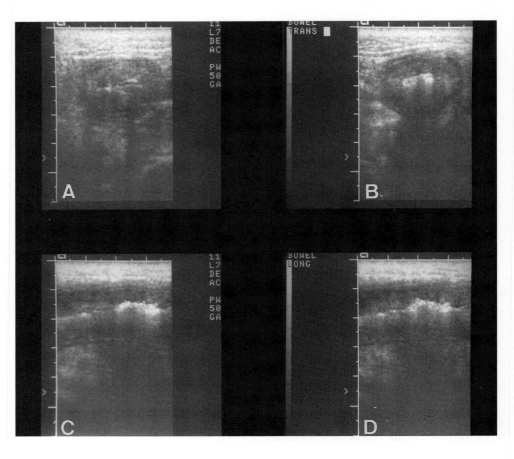

may also be detected. These may be neoplasms or granulomas. The terminal colon and rectum are hidden from ultrasound examination by the pelvic canal. Transrectal ultrasound may be used to evaluate the rectum, however the information that can be gained about the colon wall is minimal.

In rare cases, the cecum can be identified separately from the colon. Cecal inversion may produce a structure within the colon that is similar to an intussusception.

In long axis views, linear streaks of hyperechoic and hypoechoic tissue will be seen, and in transverse views a series of concentric rings may be observed. The length of the cecal inversion will be shorter than most intussusceptions.

URINARY SYSTEM

Diseases of the urinary tract can be categorized into those affecting the upper urinary tract (kidneys and ureters) and those affecting the lower urinary tract (bladder and urethra). These structures can be evaluated radiographically and the findings may be specific in some diseases.

SPECIAL PROCEDURES: TECHNIQUES

EXCRETORY UROGRAPHY

Several safe, rapid, and simple special procedures can be used to evaluate the urinary tract. The excretory urogram (EU), also referred to as an intravenous pyelogram (IVP), is used to evaluate the size, shape, position, and density of the kidneys.[127–132] The quality of the study is affected by two major factors: (1) glomerular filtration—because the contrast medium is passively filtered by the glomerulus, a decrease in filtration will decrease the amount of radiopaque material excreted and therefore decrease the density of the study; and (2) urine specific gravity—because reabsorption of water within the tubules increases the concentration and therefore increases the density of the contrast within the kidney and ureter.[127,133,134] The renal tubules cannot reabsorb the contrast medium; therefore, the greater the ability of the renal tubules to resorb water, the greater the contrast medium concentration and resultant visualization of the collecting system. While there are no absolute contraindications to this study, there are several precautions to consider including dehydration, diabetes, known allergy to iodine, Bence-Jones proteinuria, and combined renal and hepatic failure.[135,136] Anaphylactic shock is extremely unlikely in animals (in humans this occurs in approximately 1 of every 10,000 examinations), however a cutaneous reaction (hives) occurs on occasion. If this reaction has occurred in the past, the study should be avoided. Dehydration has been associated with adverse reactions and acute renal failure. In animals with multiple myeloma, the EU should be performed cautiously because Bence Jones proteins may precipitate in the renal tubules as a reaction to the contrast media.[128,137] If the study is needed, it can be performed despite the presence of Bence Jones protein or high levels of any urinary protein, provided that the patient is well hydrated and a fluid diuresis continues after the contrast is injected. In humans, diabetics are considered to be at increased risk for contrast reaction. This may also be the result of, or exacerbated by, dehydration. Contrast induced acute renal failure has been documented in the dog and cat.[137,138] In any contrast reaction, the patient should be fluid diuresed and observed. The degree of renal dysfunction is not a factor in predicting undesirable reactions, because the contrast media may be excreted by alternate routes if the animal has minimal or no renal function. The most common reaction is retching and/or vomiting, which usually occurs during or immediately following the contrast injection, is transient, and results in no long-term problem.

As is the case for all abdominal special procedures, the abdomen should be prepared by withholding food for at least 12 hours prior to the study and by administering laxatives and enemas to remove fecal material from the colon.[128,139] Abdominal radiographs should be obtained before contrast injection to ensure that the GI tract is empty and to serve as a pre-contrast baseline radiograph. The study is performed by injecting an intravenous bolus of iodinated water-soluble contrast media with an iodine content equivalent to 660 mg iodine per kg body weight (300 mg/lb body weight).[128,134] Ionic contrast agents have been used safely in animals for many years. In a high risk patient such as a diabetic dog or a dog with multiple myeloma, a non-ionic contrast agent may be used. These agents have a reduced toxicity, however they are more expensive than the ionic agents and are not totally without risk of contrast induced renal failure.

Anesthesia or sedation may be used to help in positioning the patient for radiography. This is not necessary for a cooperative patient, but it reduces the radiation exposure to the individuals positioning the patient and does not increase the risk of the study. Animals that are tranquilized or anesthetized may still retch or vomit following contrast administration. Although not proven, there appears to be a reduced incidence of post contrast administration vomiting if tranquilizers are used.

Immediately after contrast injection, ventrodorsal and lateral radiographs should be taken. Lateral and ventrodorsal radiographs should be taken 5, 10, 20, and 30 minutes after injection. The sequence and timing of the radiographs is determined by the information that is provided by the urogram. If the position of the kidneys is the only information desired, a single radiograph taken immediately following contrast administration may be sufficient. If the position of the ureters relative to the urinary bladder is of interest, then several radiographs may be required. Some authors recommend the routine use of abdominal compression to block the ureters, interfere with ureteral peristalsis, and distend the renal collecting system.[139] We do not routinely perform compression, but we recommend it when adequate visualization of the collecting system is not present on the 10-minute films. With isosthenuria or hyposthenuria even abdominal compression may not result in adequate anatomic detail. If the urine concentration of contrast being excreted is reduced as a result of reduced urine specific gravity, a second or third intravenous injection of contrast material can be administered.[128] A contrast dose that exceeds 1980 mg iodine per kg body weight (900 mg/lb) does not seem to offer any additional benefit because the contrast agent itself produces an osmotic diuresis. There is no correlation between serum urea nitrogen level and the quality of the excretory urogram.[140]

Excretion of the contrast material will affect the urinalysis resulting in an increase in urine specific gravity, false-positive urine protein determinations, alteration in cellular morphology, and the presence of unusual appearing crystals.[141,142] Growth of some bacterial species is inhibited by the presence of contrast within the urine.[143] Because of these factors, and because a higher contrast dose may be required if the urine specific gravity is low, a urinalysis and urine culture should be obtained before administration of the contrast material.

The contrast study is complete when the questions raised by the history, physical examination, or initial radiographs are answered. This may require a single radiograph or multiple radiographs obtained over a long period of time. Combining the excretory urogram with a pneumocystogram may be necessary, especially when ectopic ureters are suspected.

Although not documented in animals, the presence of contrast material may increase the echo intensity of the kidneys, and the diuresis that results from contrast administration may cause ureteral dilation, which could be mistaken for mild hydronephrosis during an ultrasound examination. For that reason, the ultrasound examination usually precedes the contrast study.

CYSTOGRAPHY

Examination of the bladder may be accomplished by several special procedures (e.g., the positive-contrast cystogram, pneumocystogram, or double contrast cystogram).[144-146] For these procedures, it is important to ensure that the colon and small bowel are not filled with fecal material. Food deprivation and the administration of laxatives at least 12 hours prior to the study are advised. It is usually necessary to perform one or more enemas immediately prior to the study to evacuate the distal colon; however, allow sufficient time for the colon to empty because a fluid-filled colon may distort the shape of the bladder.

Complications resulting from cystography are rare. Trauma to the bladder or urethra may result from catheterization—infection may be introduced into the bladder if the catheterization is not performed carefully. Rupture of the urinary bladder should not occur if the bladder is inflated slowly and inflation is stopped when the distended bladder can be palpated or if the animal shows evidence of pain or discomfort during bladder inflation.

If ultrasound examination of the bladder is expected, this should precede cystography. Air within the bladder will interfere with ultrasound examination, and bubbles within the contrast may also degrade the ultrasound image.

DOUBLE CONTRAST CYSTOGRAPHY

In most clinical situations, the double contrast cystogram is the preferred technique to study the urinary bladder, because it provides the best evaluation of the mucosal surface.[147] In performing this procedure, the bladder is catheterized, all urine is removed, and the bladder is distended with a gas such as CO_2, N_2O, or air. Although the bladder should be fully distended to evaluate the bladder wall properly, a determination that the bladder is normal can be made without complete distention and distention can mask signs of mild to moderate cystitis.[147,148] The volume of gas needed to maximally distend the bladder varies with the individual and the disease. Bladder palpation is required to judge when adequate distension has been achieved. After insufflation with gas, a small amount of radiopaque contrast media (0.5 cc for a cat to 3.0 cc for a large dog) is instilled through the urinary catheter. After instillation of both contrast agents, three exposures are recommended: either a right or left lateral and two obliques. If it is practical to take only two views, the lateral and ventrodorsal views should be performed. Superimposition of the vertebral column over the urinary bladder reduces the value of the ventrodorsal view.

POSITIVE-CONTRAST CYSTOGRAPHY

When frank hematuria is present or bladder rupture is suspected, the pneumocystogram and double contrast cystogram are contraindicated. This is due to the possibility of a fatal air embolism, as has been reported following pneumocystograms in patients with hematuria.[149,150] A positive-contrast cystogram (PCC) or EU is recommended. Other considerations when choosing a special procedure for evaluating suspected bladder rupture include the difficulty in observing free peritoneal air with hydroperitoneum and the superiority of the PCC in delineating the point of bladder rupture. To perform a PCC, all urine should be removed from the bladder and it should be maximally distended with dilute contrast media—50 ml of water-soluble iodinated contrast diluted with 250 ml of saline. As with the double contrast cystography the lateral and oblique views are recommended, but the lateral and ventrodorsal are adequate if the oblique views are not practical.

Normal Cystogram

The normal bladder is ovoid with a tapering neck, which is longer in the female dog and in the cat than in the male dog. The bladder wall is uniform in diameter. A contrast puddle should be evident in the center of the dependent portion of the bladder when a double contrast cystogram has been performed. Air or contrast may reflux into the ureters or renal pelvis following bladder distention.[151–153] This is a normal finding. However, in the presence of cystitis, vesicoureteral reflux may predispose the animal to pyelonephritis.

RETROGRADE URETHROGRAPHY

Retrograde urethrography may infrequently reveal prostatic pathology, but the study has little value as a routine procedure for the evaluation of prostatic disease.[154]

We do not routinely recommend this procedure for evaluation of the prostate. Ultrasonography provides an easier and more thorough examination of the prostate.

The retrograde urethrogram will evaluate the entire urethra. Water-soluble radiopaque contrast medium is used at a dose of 0.5 cc/kg (0.25 cc per pound) with a maximum volume per injection of 20 cc for the largest male dogs. The study should be performed carefully to avoid air bubbles in the contrast media, as these may be mistaken for radiolucent calculi. A catheter with a balloon near the tip (e.g., Foley) is recommended. The tip of the catheter should be positioned just beyond the urethral papilla in the female and just caudal to the os penis in the male. The injection should be made manually with as much force as is easily obtained, and the radiograph should be exposed as the last portion of contrast is injected. Both lateral and ventrodorsal views should be taken—the ventrodorsal in the male should be slightly obliqued to prevent superimposition of the distal and proximal urethra. Distension of the urinary bladder prior to retrograde urethrography is not recommended.[139,144,155–165]

Sedation or anesthesia are not required but are recommended to reduce the chance that the patient will move during the contrast injection. In addition, sedation or anesthesia helps reduce the possibility of infection by facilitating urethral catheterization.

Trauma to the urethra and post catheterization infection are the only complications resulting from contrast urethrography.[163,166,167] Contrast material may gain access to the systemic circulation if rupture or ulceration of the urethral mucosa is present. This is not a problem if positive contrast material is used; however, when air has been used deaths from air embolism have occurred.[149,150]

Vaginourethrography

In female dogs and cats, especially when ectopic ureters are suspected or the animal is too small for urethral catheterization, vaginourethrography may be performed. This study is performed by placing a Foley or other balloon-tippped catheter into the vagina distal to the urethral papillae and injecting contrast into the vagina. The urethra will usually fill with contrast as well. A nontraumatic forceps usually is required to close the vagina, keep the catheter in place, and prevent contrast leaking to the outside. This technique can also be used for the evaluation of urethral rectal fistulas or rectovaginal fistulas. Anesthesia may be required to keep the patient from struggling during catheter and forceps placement or contrast injection.

Normal Retrograde Urethrogram

In the male canine, the urethra is uniform in width except for a slight narrowing at the pelvic brim, bladder neck, and at the ischial arch. The prostatic urethra is often wider than the rest of the urethra and an indentation of the urethra may be present dorsally because of the colliculus seminalis.[168] Reflux of a small amount of contrast into the prostate is normal.[154,162] The urethra of the male cat is narrowest in the penile portion. The urethra of the female dog and female cat is short and wide and tapers to the external sphincter.[145,146]

ABNORMAL FINDINGS

KIDNEYS

Renal abnormalities may involve changes in size, shape, position, and/or density. The criteria for normal kidney length (2 to 3 times the length of L2 in the cat and 2.5 to 3.5 times the length of L2 in the dog) have been defined.[18] Subjectively, the width should be in proportion to the length. Because the left kidney in the dog is fairly mobile, it may not be positioned at right angles to the x-ray beam. This may result in a foreshortened image. The kidneys are normally "kidney-bean shaped" with regular (smooth) borders.

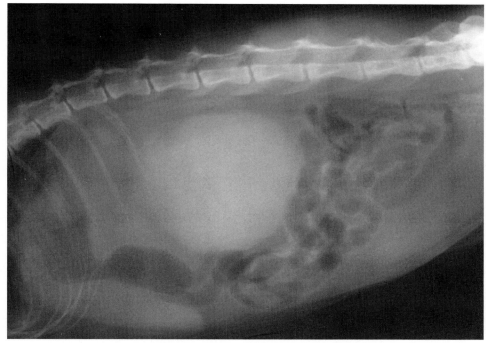

A

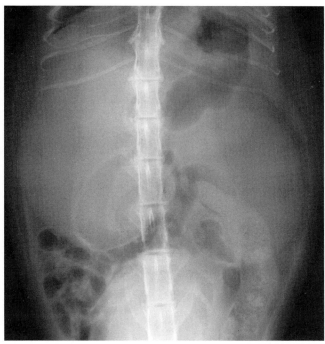

B

Figure 3–116. A 5-year-old female Siamese cat with anorexia and vomiting for 4 days. (A&B) The kidneys are bilaterally enlarged and regularly shaped. Differential diagnoses include lymphosarcoma, FIP, bilateral obstructive nephropathy, perirenal cysts, bilateral renal tumors, acute pyelonephritis, or polycystic renal disease. **Diagnosis:** Perirenal cysts.

When the kidney is evaluated radiographically, changes in the size, shape, symmetry, and the number of kidneys involved may be correlated to develop a table of differential diagnoses. Because many diseases have multiple manifestations, they appear on several lists.

Size and Shape Changes
BILATERAL, LARGE, REGULAR (FIG. 3–116)

Feline. Lymphosarcoma, feline infectious peritonitis (FIP), perirenal cysts, bilateral ureteral obstruction (hydronephrosis), bilateral tumors (primary or metastatic), bilateral acute pyelonephritis, polycystic, amyloidosis.

Canine.   Bilateral ureteral obstruction (hydronephrosis), bilateral acute pyelonephritis, bilateral tumors (primary or metastatic), lymphosarcoma, amyloidosis, polycystic, lipidosis secondary to diabetes mellitus, ethylene glycol toxicity, myeloma.

BILATERAL, LARGE, IRREGULAR (FIG. 3–117)

Feline.   FIP, lymphosarcoma, bilateral tumors (primary or metastatic), acute pyelonephritis, polycystic.

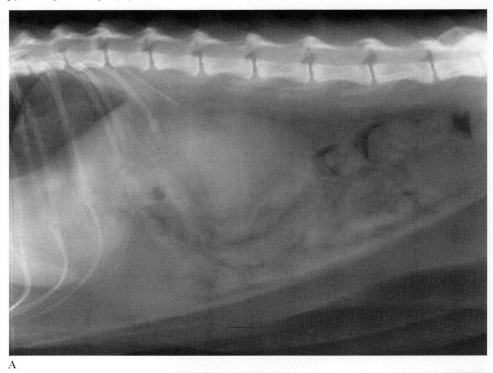

A

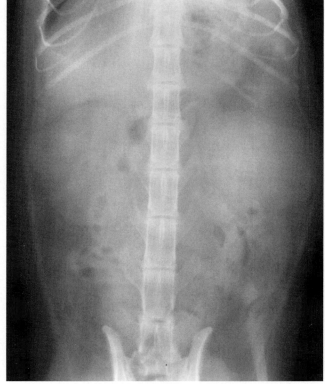

B

Figure 3–117.   A 7-year-old male domestic short-haired cat with chronic vomiting. (A&B) The kidneys are bilaterally enlarged and irregularly shaped. Differential diagnoses include lymphosarcoma, bilateral renal tumors, polycystic disease, or acute pyelonephritis. **Diagnosis:** Lymphosarcoma.

Canine. Lymphosarcoma, acute pyelonephritis, bilateral tumors (primary or metastatic), polycystic.

BILATERAL, SMALL, REGULAR (FIG. 3–118)

Feline. Chronic interstitial nephritis (CIN), hypoplasia (congenital).
Canine. CIN, dysplasia, hypoplasia.

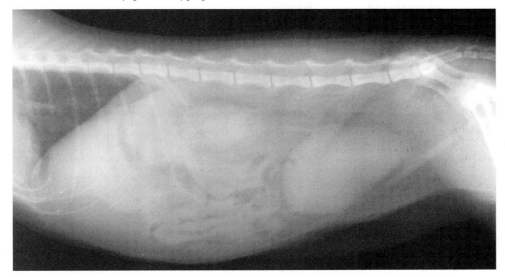

A

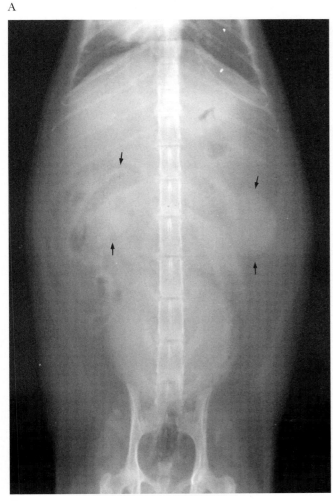

B

Figure 3–118. An 11-year-old neutered male domestic short-haired cat with gradual weight loss, polyuria, and polydipsia for 2 months and vomiting for 2 days. (A&B) The kidneys are bilaterally small and regularly shaped (*black arrows*). Differential diagnoses include CIN, chronic pyelonephritis, or renal hypoplasia. **Diagnosis:** Chronic interstitial nephritis.

BILATERAL, SMALL, IRREGULAR (FIG. 3–119)

Feline. CIN, infarcts, chronic pyelonephritis.
Canine. CIN, infarcts, chronic pyelonephritis, dysplasia.

UNILATERAL, LARGE, REGULAR (FIG. 3–120)

Feline. Compensatory hyperplasia, ureteral obstruction, acute pyelonephritis, FIP, lymphosarcoma, tumor (primary or metastatic), pyonephrosis, perirenal cyst, renal vein thrombosis.
Canine. Ureteral obstruction, tumor (primary or metastatic), acute pyelonephritis, compensatory hyperplasia, renal vein thrombosis, lymphosarcoma, pyonephrosis, myeloma, amyloidosis.

UNILATERAL, LARGE, IRREGULAR (FIG. 3–121)

Feline. FIP, tumor (primary or metastatic), lymphosarcoma, cyst, abscess.
Canine. Adenocarcinoma, lymphosarcoma, metastatic neoplasia, cyst, abscess.

UNILATERAL, SMALL, REGULAR (FIG. 3–122)

Feline. Congenital hypoplasia, CIN.
Canine. CIN, congenital hypoplasia.

UNILATERAL, SMALL, IRREGULAR (FIG. 3–123)

Feline. CIN, chronic pyelonephritis, multiple infarcts.
Canine. CIN, chronic pyelonephritis, multiple infarcts.

UNILATERAL, SMALL, CONTRALATERAL LARGE (FIG. 3–124)

Feline and Canine. Unilateral chronic pyelonephritis or congenital hypoplasia and contralateral compensatory hyperplasia.

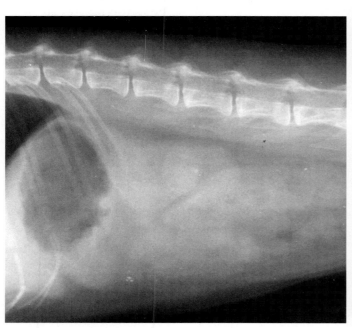

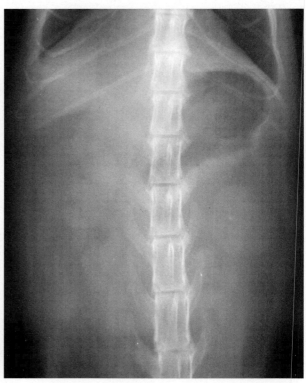

A   B

Figure 3–119. A 6-year-old neutered female domestic short-haired cat with lethargy and anorexia for 1 month. (A&B) The kidneys are bilaterally small (the left kidney is even smaller than the right kidney) and markedly irregular in shape. Differential diagnoses include CIN, chronic pyelonephritis, or renal infarcts. **Diagnosis:** Chronic pyelonephritis.

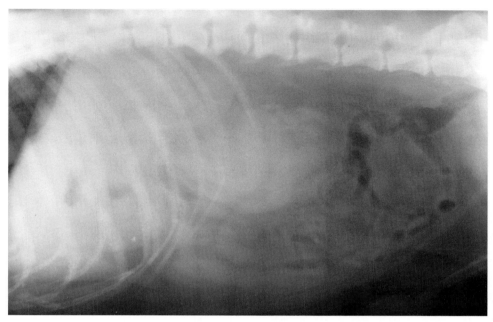

A

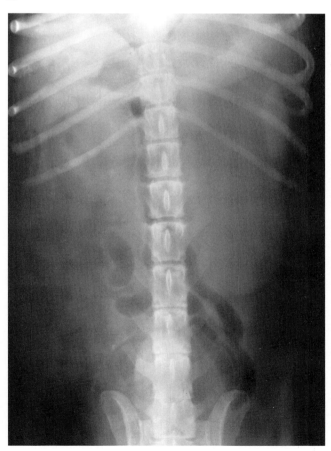

B

Figure 3–120. A 12-year-old male cocker spaniel with vomiting for 3 weeks. (A&B) The left kidney is large with regular and smooth margins. Differential diagnoses include obstructive nephropathy, neoplasia, acute pyelonephritis, pyonephrosis, compensatory hyperplasia, or renal vein thrombosis. **Diagnosis:** Left renal hydronephrosis of unknown etiology.

NORMAL SIZE AND SHAPE

Feline and Canine. Acute tubular nephrosis, calculi, kidney rupture, acute pyelonephritis, neoplasia, amyloidosis. The fact that the kidneys are normal in size can never be used as evidence that renal disease is not present.

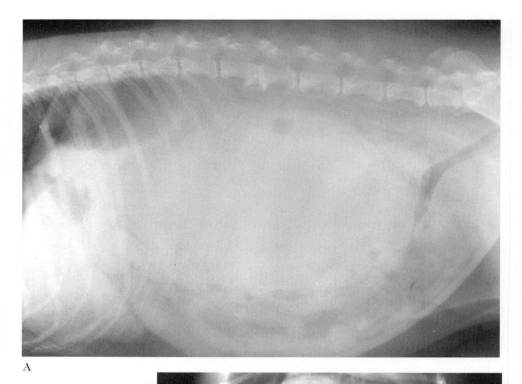

A

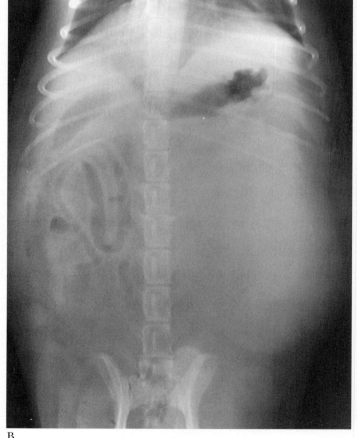

B

Figure 3–121. A 7-year-old male mixed breed dog with hematuria for 1 month. (A&B) The left kidney is very large and irregularly shaped. The right kidney, while difficult to visualize, is normal in size and shape. Differential diagnoses include neoplasia, renal cyst, or renal abscess. **Diagnosis:** Nephroblastoma (see Fig. 3–95).

Density Changes

Changes in renal density may also be seen. Renal parenchymal calcification may occur as a result of primary nephrocalcinosis, osseous metaplasia or dystrophic calcification of a neoplasm, infarct, or abscess.[74,169] Primary nephrocalcinosis may be as-

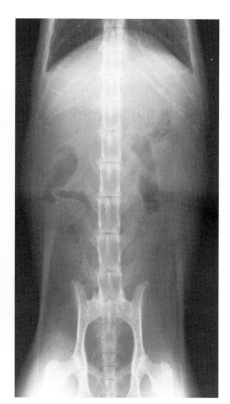

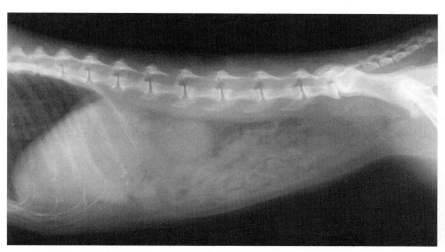

A

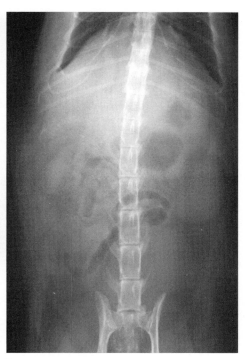

Figure 3–122. A 14-year-old neutered female domestic short-haired cat with vomiting. (A&B) The left kidney is small and regular-shaped. The right kidney is normal. Differential diagnoses include hypoplasia, CIN, or chronic pyelonephritis. The cat responded to symptomatic therapy. **Diagnosis:** Hypoplasia of the left kidney.

B

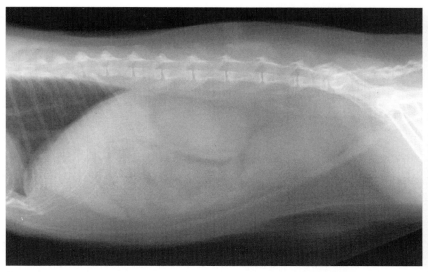

A

Figure 3–123. A 12-year-old neutered female domestic short-haired cat with anorexia for 3 days. (A&B) The right kidney is small and irregularly shaped. The left kidney is within normal limits for size and shape. Differential diagnoses include chronic pyelonephritis, CIN, or multiple renal infarcts. **Diagnosis:** Chronic pyelonephritis.

B

sociated with disorders of calcium and phosphorus metabolism such as hypervitaminosis D, primary or secondary hyperparathyroidism, excess or unbalance of calcium and phosphorus in the diet, and Cushing's disease. Osseous metaplasia has been described in association with hydronephrosis. Nephrocalcinosis may also result

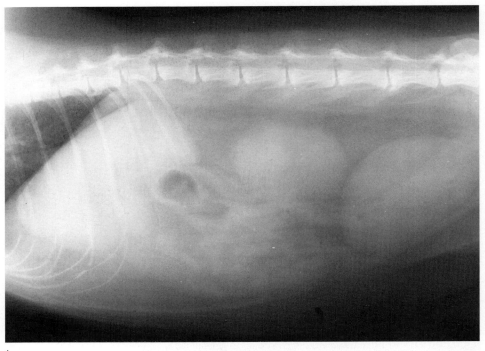

A

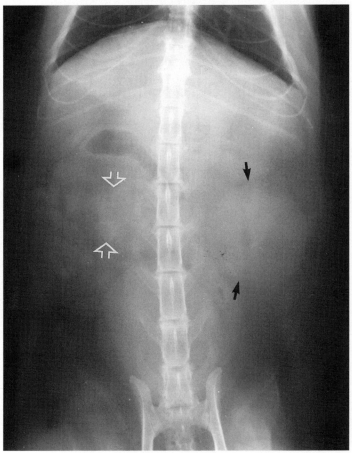

Figure 3–124. A 10-year-old male domestic short-haired cat with tenesmus and vomiting. (A&B) The right kidney is small and irregularly shaped (*open white arrows*). The left kidney is large and regularly shaped (*black arrows*). Differential diagnoses include unilateral chronic pyelonephritis or congenital hypoplasia and contralateral compensatory hypertrophy. **Diagnosis:** Chronic pyelonephritis of the right kidney and hypertrophy of the left.

B

from chronic renal failure as well as being a cause of chronic renal failure. These conditions usually cause the deposition of calcium salts on the pseudopapillae. These present as pyramidal (inverted "V") or linear densities. Mineralization of the renal parenchyma at the cortical medullary junction may also occur and will pro-

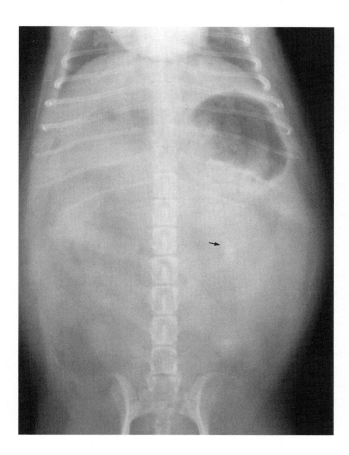

Figure 3–125. A 4-year-old female Maltese with occasional seizures. The ventrodorsal radiograph revealed a calcific density shaped like a renal pelvis within the left renal pelvis (*black arrow*). This location was confirmed on the lateral view. **Diagnosis:** Left renal calculus.

duce a pattern of fine parallel lines at the cortical medullary junction. Vascular mineralization may also be seen. The vessels can be recognized because of their linear shape and location. Usually, parallel lines representing the vessel walls are seen. Dystrophic mineralization of the renal parenchyma secondary to neoplasia, infarct, abscess, or hemorrhage usually results in a poorly defined area of mineralization within the renal parenchyma away from the renal pelvis. The pattern of mineralization usually is less structured than that seen in renal parenchymal mineralization and does not conform to renal anatomy. Another cause of increased density is renal calculi. These may be large or small and will be recognized as oval or irregularly shaped densities in the renal pelvis. They may become large and conform to the shape of the renal pelvis (staghorn calculi) and may even replace most of the renal parenchyma (Fig. 3–125). It is sometimes difficult to discriminate between renal calculi and parenchymal mineralization. An excretory urogram or an ultrasound examination may be helpful in distinguishing between these two conditions. Calculi will produce filling defects during the excretory urogram and may cause hydronephrosis with a dilated renal pelvis and urine evident surrounding the stone. This can also be seen during the ultrasound examination.

Mineralized material within the GI tract may be mistaken for renal mineralization. Mineralization must be identified on both lateral and ventrodorsal radiographs to be certain that it is associated with the kidneys. If there is a suspicious density, additional radiographs to include oblique views and abdominal compression may be used. Repeating the radiographs after a few hours often allows the densities to change position if they are associated with the GI tract.

Position Changes

An uncommon finding on survey radiographs is the presence of a kidney in an inappropriate position. Both kidneys in the cat and the left kidney in the dog are fairly mobile. As a dog ages, and especially in obese dogs, both kidneys become more moveable and are often found caudal and ventral to their usual position. In the dog, caudal displacement of the right kidney is associated with enlargement of the caudate liver lobe. Adrenal masses may displace the kidney caudally and laterally while ovarian masses may displace the kidney cranially. Retroperitoneal masses can also displace the kidney from its normal position. Displacement of one or both kidneys in either the dog or cat may be the result of a congenital anomaly or traumatic avulsion from the normal location. Congenital ectopia may be seen with the kidney most often located in the caudal abdomen just cranial to the bladder.

Excretory Urography

The EU (IVP) is the radiographic method for evaluating abnormalities of the kidneys and ureters that are not apparent on the survey radiographs.[127,129,130,170–176] The study may be divided into two distinct phases. The first phase is the nephrogram stage—usually seen on the radiographs exposed within the first few minutes after contrast injection (Figs. 3–126A and 3–127A). During this phase, contrast is distributed evenly throughout the renal intravascular compartment and to some extent within the renal tubules.[177] Homogenous opacification ("blush") of the kidneys occurs due to the relatively large fraction of total blood volume that goes to the kidney. This is the ideal phase for evaluation of the renal size and shape. In some studies, a difference in density between renal cortex and medulla will be seen and a cortical medullary ratio may be determined. The second phase of the study is the pyelogram (Figs. 3–126B and 3–127B). During this phase, the collecting structures and renal pelvis should be seen. This is usually visualized on the radiographs taken 5 and 10 minutes after contrast injection.

Although not usually considered a phase of the excretory urogram, the vascular anatomy can sometimes be identified during an excretory urogram if the patient is

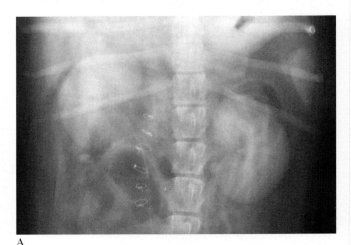

A

B

Figure 3–126. An 11-year-old female Jack Russell terrier with polycythemia. (A) On the radiograph made immediately after injection of the contrast media there is homogeneous opacification of the renal parenchyma. The other abdominal organs are also highlighted due to the contrast media in the vascular compartment. This is the nephrogram phase of the EU in which the contrast media is mainly in the vascular compartments and renal tubules. (B) The radiograph taken 30 minutes after injection revealed clearly defined diverticulae of the collecting system, which contain contrast media (*black arrow*) and pseudopapillae (tissue spaces between the diverticulae) (*white arrow*) as well as pelvic sinuses (*small black arrowhead*) and proximal ureters (*small white arrowhead*). This is the late pyelogram phase of the EU. **Diagnosis:** Normal EU.

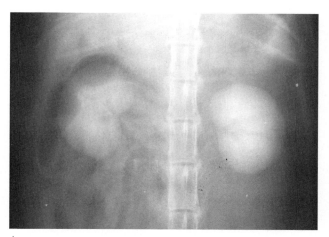

A

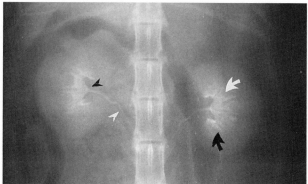

B

Figure 3–127. A 10-year-old neutered female domestic short-haired cat with hematuria and cystic calculi. (A) On the radiograph made immediately after contrast media injection there is homogeneous opacification of the kidneys. This is the nephrogram. (B) The radiograph taken 15 minutes after contrast injection revealed clearly defined diverticulae (*black arrow*), pseudopapillae (*white arrow*), pelvic sinus (*small black arrowhead*), and proximal ureters (*small white arrowhead*). This is the pyelogram phase. **Diagnosis:** Normal EU.

positioned for radiography before the contrast is injected, the contrast is injected rapidly, and the radiographic exposure is made approximately 10 seconds after the contrast injection is completed. Often the renal artery and vein can be identified in this radiograph. The nephrogram phase will follow this vascular phase very quickly.

In the dog, the normal kidney has a small, triangular-shaped pelvic sinus and evenly spaced, regular pelvic recesses (diverticulae). The lobar renal arteries (the first branches from the renal arteries) may be seen as linear radiolucencies lying within the diverticulae. In many normal dogs, the diverticulae may not be readily apparent. In instances where it is necessary to visualize the diverticulae, or where opacification of the kidney is poor, it may be useful to apply a tight, constricting bandage circumferentially around the caudal abdomen to occlude the ureters by compression. This will induce a mild iatrogenic hydroureter and hydronephrosis, which may make the renal outline and collecting structures much more apparent (Fig. 3–128). Although glucagon has been used to achieve renal pelvic and ureteral dilation, we do not recommend its use. The pseudopapillae (renal structures between the diverticulae) should come to relatively sharp points. Occasionally, the kidney is projected at an angle such that the two sets of diverticulae are seen separately (Fig. 3–129). In the cat, some irregularity in nephrographic density may occur due to the cortical impressions of the subcapsular veins.

Evaluation of the excretory urography is simplified if the criteria for categorizing survey images are used.

BILATERAL, LARGE, REGULAR

Feline and Canine

LYMPHOSARCOMA. The EU may reveal generalized renal enlargement with normal collecting systems and only a slight decrease in opacification. Focal radiolucent areas within the parenchyma (focal filling defects) are a less frequent manifestation

Figure 3–128. A 5-year-old neutered male cocker spaniel with swollen joints, cystic calculi, and enlarged lymph nodes. (A) The EU revealed a suggestion of normal collecting structures but visualization was incomplete. (B) An abdominal compression ("belly band") study more clearly revealed that the collecting structures were normal. **Diagnosis:** Normal EU (the dog had multicentric lymphoma which did not involve the kidneys).

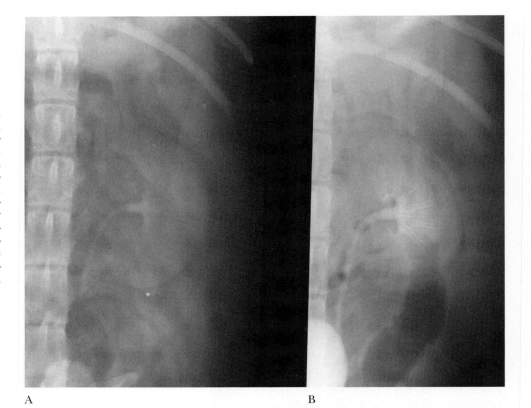

A   B

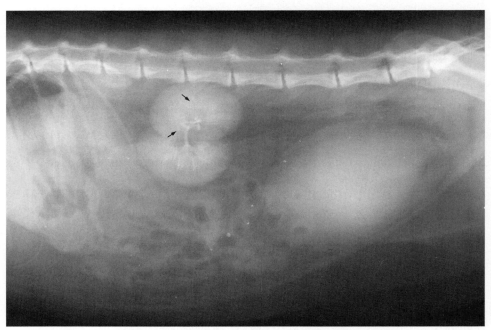

Figure 3–129. A 7-year-old male domestic short-haired cat with polyuria and polydipsia. The lateral view of the left kidney during the EU revealed an oblique view of the kidney such that both sets of diverticulae (*black arrows*) were distinctly visible. **Diagnosis:** Normal EU.

of renal lymphoma (Fig. 3–130). Changes in the collecting system are rare, however the focal form of the disease may compress a part of the collecting system.

FIP.   The appearance is very similar to that seen with lymphosarcoma except that the focal form is more common. The focal areas of radiolucency will usually be smaller in size than those seen with lymphosarcoma. The collecting system is rarely affected.

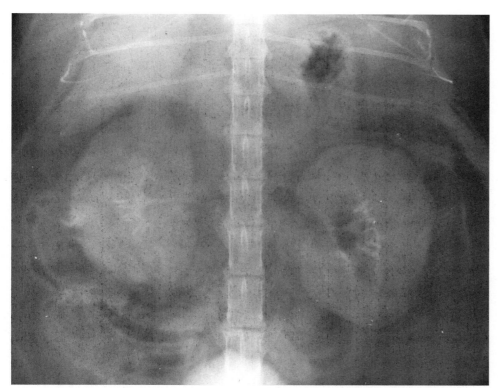

Figure 3–130. A 9-year-old neutered male domestic short-haired cat with polyuria and poly-dipsia for 2 months and palpably enlarged kidneys. The kidneys are enlarged and irregular. The collecting structures are within normal limits. Differential diagnoses include lymphosarcoma, FIP, polycystic kidney disease, or bilateral renal tumors. **Diagnosis:** Lymphosarcoma.

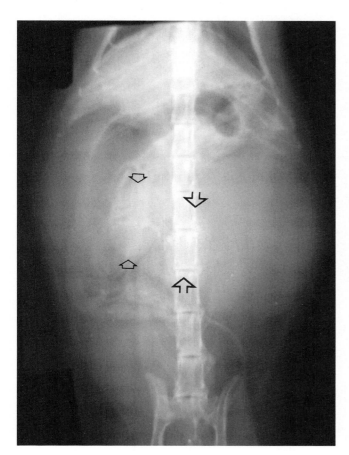

Figure 3–131. A 9-year-old neutered male domestic short-haired cat with palpably enlarged kidneys but no clinical signs. Survey radiographs revealed bilaterally enlarged, regularly-shaped kidneys. The EU revealed bilaterally small, regular kidneys (the left is superimposed over the spine–*open black arrows*) with large accumulations of fluid between the kidneys and the renal capsules. **Diagnosis:** Perirenal cysts.

PERIRENAL CYSTS.   Although the renal shadow is enlarged on the non-contrast radiograph, the kidneys themselves are usually small and slightly irregular in outline with normal opacification and normal or irregular collecting systems. There is usually some degree of contrast enhancement of the renal capsule, but the space between the kidney and the capsule may not be opacified (Fig. 3–131). In the later phases of the pyelogram, contrast may accumulate within the subcapsular cyst in a sufficient quantity to cause faint opacification.

HYDRONEPHROSIS.   The kidney usually is smoothly enlarged, the renal sinus is uniformly distended, and the diverticulae are smoothly and evenly expanded. In severe instances, the diverticulae may be enlarged so much that they are obliterated as separate structures and the entire renal pelvis becomes a smoothly marginated, dilated structure. In extreme cases, the renal parenchyma may be reduced to a shell surrounding the distended renal pelvis. On the immediate EU, linear opacifications may be seen radiating from the renal hilus to the periphery of the kidney. After opacification of the renal pelvis develops (which may take 24 hours or more), these

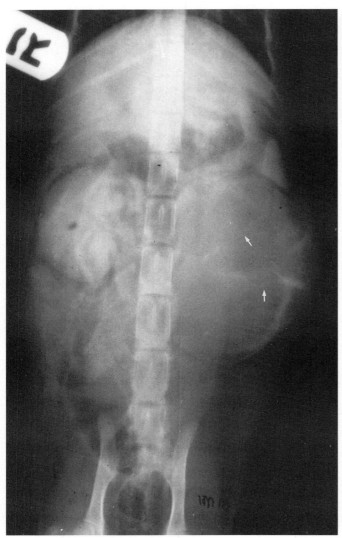

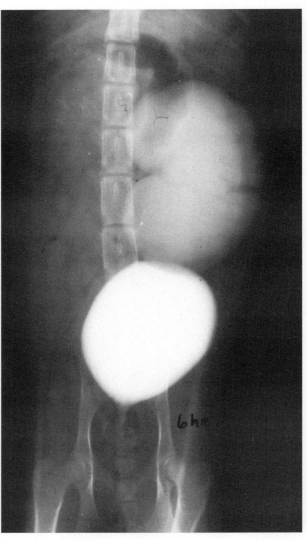

A

B

Figure 3–132.   A 1-year-old female domestic short-haired cat with a palpably enlarged left kidney detected on routine examination prior to ovariohysterectomy. (A) The 15-minute ventrodorsal view of the EU revealed minimal contrast enhancement to the structure except for a few linear radiodensities that radiated peripherally from the pelvis (*white arrows*). These represent renal blood vessels that were stretched. (B) The 6-hour ventrodorsal view revealed a markedly opacified kidney. This represented the delayed pyelogram of hydronephrosis. **Diagnosis:** Hydronephrosis of the left kidney.

may appear as linear lucencies radiating from the pelvis. These are the remaining intrarenal vascular structures (Fig. 3–132A). The pyelogram is markedly delayed due to the decreased rate of glomerular filtration (Fig. 3–132B).

BILATERAL RENAL TUMORS.   While renal tumors are usually unilateral lesions, they may be bilateral either due to metastasis from one kidney to the other, metastasis to both kidneys from a distant site, multicentric tumor, or systemic neoplasia (such as lymphoma). Irregular areas of increased density may be seen during the nephrogram phase due to variations in the vascularity of the neoplastic tissue and the presence of islands of functional renal tissue. The pyelogram may reveal distortion of the collecting system if the mass is focal. Complete obliteration or nonvisualization of the collecting structures may be seen if the lesion involves most of the renal parenchyma.

PYELONEPHRITIS.   Acute bilateral pyelonephritis presents as a normal to slightly diminished homogenous density during the nephrogram phase. Mild to moderate dilation of the diverticulae, renal sinus, and proximal ureters as well as blunting of the psuedopapillae may be seen in the pyelographic phase (Figs. 3–133 and 3–134).[171] The changes are usually irreversible and persist despite resolution of the infection.

ACUTE INTERSTITIAL AND GLOMERULAR NEPHRITIS.   The excretory urogram may be normal or may have slightly diminished homogenous density during the nephrogram phase. The pyelogram may be faint with a normal renal pelvis and normal pelvic recesses visible. Acute swelling of the kidney may cause compression of the renal pelvic recesses. This will persist despite properly applied abdominal compression.

POLYCYSTIC KIDNEYS.   The density during the nephrogram phase will generally be irregular due to obliteration of normal renal tissue by the cysts. Classically, there is

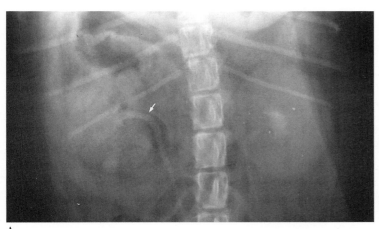

A

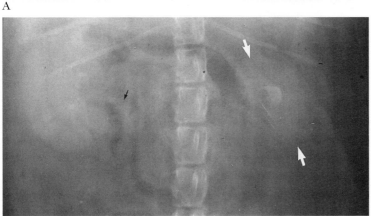

B

Figure 3–133. A 9-year-old female Shih Tzu with occasional vomiting, anorexia, and pyrexia. (A) There are bilaterally enlarged kidneys with shortened diverticulae, blunted pseudopapillae, dilated renal sinuses, and dilated proximal ureters (*white arrow*). **Diagnosis:** Acute pyelonephritis. (B) An EU performed 6 months later for a suspected recurrence of the original problem. There is marked decrease in size of the left kidney (*white arrows*) and dilation of the renal sinus. The right kidney is slightly enlarged with a poorly visualized but dilated renal sinus and proximal ureter (*black arrow*). The diverticulae are not seen. **Diagnosis:** Chronic pyelonephritis with scarring of the left kidney and acute pyelonephritis of the right kidney.

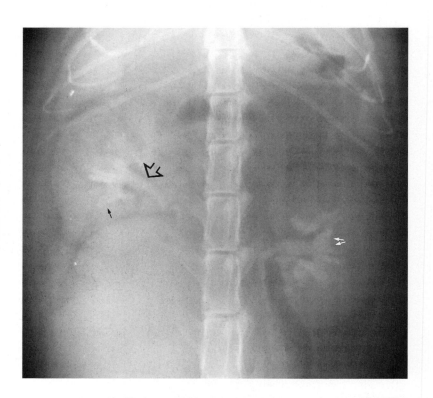

Figure 3–134. A 6-year-old neutered male domestic short-haired cat with anorexia, pyrexia, anemia, and pain upon palpation of the kidneys. Survey radiographs revealed slightly enlarged kidneys. The EU revealed mild renal enlargement, which is smooth and regular. The diverticulae are dilated (*small black arrow*), the pseudopapillae are blunted (*white arrows*), and the renal sinuses and proximal ureters are dilated (*open black arrow*). **Diagnosis:** Acute bilateral pyelonephritis.

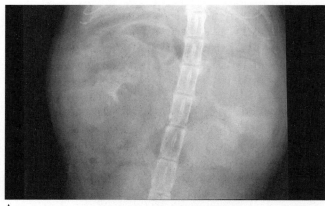

A

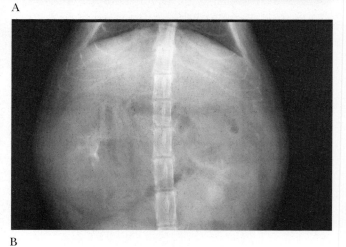

B

Figure 3–135. An 11-year-old neutered female domestic short-haired cat with polyuria and polydipsia for 6 weeks and palpably enlarged kidneys. Survey radiographs revealed that both kidneys were radiographically enlarged and had irregular borders. (A) The early stages of the EU reveal multiple foci of relative radiolucency separated by septae which are contrast enhanced. (B) The later stages show the multiple cysts more clearly and a distorted renal sinus. Differential diagnoses include polycystic kidney disease, bilateral multifocal renal tumors (metastatic or primary), lymphosarcoma, or FIP. **Diagnosis:** Polycystic kidney disease.

a fine rim of normally dense renal tissue surrounding the non-opacified cyst. The pyelogram may show distortion of the collecting structures if the cysts produce pressure upon them (Fig. 3–135).[178]

AMYLOIDOSIS.　The nephrogram is usually less opaque than normal. Frequently the pyelogram is difficult to see, but the collecting structures are usually normal in shape and size.[176]

ETHYLENE GLYCOL TOXICITY.　The nephrogram will reveal a smoothly marginated, mild to moderate enlargement of both kidneys. The nephrogram density may remain the same or increase in density throughout the study; the pyelogram either will not be present or will be poorly seen.[173]

LIPIDOSIS.　While there is no documentation in the veterinary literature that animals with diabetes mellitus are more likely to experience contrast media-induced renal failure, as is the case for humans, this possibility should be strongly considered in determining the need for the EU in suspected cases of renal lipidosis secondary to diabetes. If performed, the EU will appear normal except for the overall renal size.[172]

MULTIPLE MYELOMA.　Performing an EU in human multiple myeloma patients is not recommended because of the possibility of contrast media-induced renal failure. This reaction should be considered in animals as well. If an excretory urogram is performed, the nephrogram phase will show smoothly enlarged renal outlines with or without patchy areas of decreased density. The pyelogram phase will show normally shaped collecting structures that may have poor density.[130]

BILATERAL, LARGE, IRREGULAR

Feline and Canine.　The findings for diseases in this category (lymphosarcoma, FIP, bilateral renal tumors, acute bilateral pyelonephritis, amyloidosis, polycystic renal disease) are the same as described under *Bilateral, Large, Regular* except that the renal outlines are irregular.

BILATERAL, SMALL, REGULAR

Feline

CIN.　Renal opacification during the nephrogram phase usually is less than normal. The diverticulae may appear shortened or normal. The pelvic density is frequently less than normal.

HYPOPLASIA.　In this situation the EU will appear normal; however, all structures are proportionately smaller than normal.

Canine

CIN AND HYPOPLASIA.　The appearance of the EU is similar in both the dog and the cat.[179]

RENAL DYSPLASIA.　Renal opacification during the nephrogram phase is usually less than normal. The renal pelvis and pelvic recesses may not be visualized; however, when seen, they may be normal, small, or asymmetrically enlarged and distorted (Fig. 3–136).

BILATERAL, SMALL, IRREGULAR

Feline and Canine

CIN AND RENAL DYSPLASIA.　The appearance is similar to that discussed above, except the kidneys are irregular.

INFARCTS.　These usually show a normal urogram with one or more focal flattenings or indentations to the renal outline (Fig. 3–137). Renal pelvic structures will appear normal.

CHRONIC PYELONEPHRITIS.　The nephrogram phase may be normal or somewhat less dense than normal. Stretching and slight dilation of the renal sinus with loss or irregularity of the diverticulae may be seen (Fig. 3–138). Focal flattenings or indentations of the renal cortex peripheral to the areas of pelvic and pelvic recess irregularities may be present.

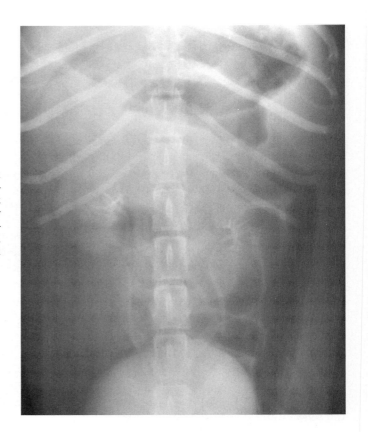

Figure 3–136. A 1-year-old female miniature schnauzer with vomiting, polydipsia, and polyuria. The kidneys were not identifiable on survey radiographs. The EU revealed that the left kidney was slightly smaller than normal and the right kidney was markedly smaller. The urinary collecting systems were normal. Differential diagnoses include congenital renal dysplasia, chronic pyelonephritis, or CIN. **Diagnosis:** Congenital renal dysplasia.

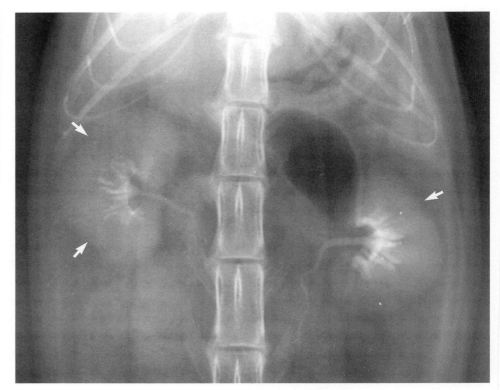

Figure 3–137. A 12-year-old male domestic short-haired cat with vomiting. The survey radiographs revealed slightly small, markedly irregular kidneys. The EU revealed slightly small renal outlines with focal flattening of the cortical borders (*white arrows*). The renal sinus and proximal ureter of the left kidney are slightly dilated. Differential diagnoses include multiple renal infarcts and/or chronic pyelonephritis. **Diagnosis:** Multiple renal infarcts with pyelonephritis of the left kidney.

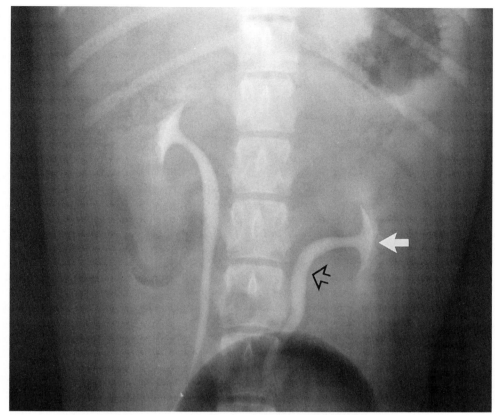

Figure 3–138. A 4-month-old female German shepherd dog with urinary incontinence since owned. Survey radiographs were normal. An EU performed after pneumocystography revealed normal size and shape of the kidneys. The renal sinuses were elongated and the diverticulae were not outlined which resulted in an appearance of the renal pelvis similar to a scimitar. The pseudopapillae are markedly blunted (*white arrow*). The proximal ureters are dilated (*open black arrow*). **Diagnosis:** Chronic pyelonephritis (the dog also had bilateral ectopic ureter).

UNILATERAL, LARGE, REGULAR

Feline and Canine. The urographic changes described in bilateral obstruction (hydronephrosis), hyperplasia, lymphosarcoma, FIP, and renal tumors (primary and metastatic) are the same in unilateral disease for the affected kidney.

PYONEPHROSIS. A rim of increased opacity with a relatively radiolucent center will be seen during the nephrogram. There will be no pyelogram (Fig. 3–139).

RENAL VEIN THROMBOSIS. Normal to reduced, but homogenous, opacification will be seen during the nephrogram. Usually, a pyelogram will not be seen.[74]

UNILATERAL, LARGE, IRREGULAR

Feline and Canine. The urographic changes described for bilateral cases of FIP and lymphosarcoma are the same in unilateral disease for the affected kidney.

PRIMARY AND METASTATIC NEOPLASIA. Irregular areas of increased density may be seen during the nephrogram phase. This is caused by variations in the vascularity of the neoplastic tissue and the presence of islands of functional renal tissue (Fig. 3–140). The pyelogram may reveal distortion of the collecting system if the mass is focal, or complete obliteration or nonvisualization of the collecting structures if the lesion involves most of the renal parenchyma (Fig. 3–141).

SIMPLE RENAL CYST. A smoothly marginated lucency with a well-defined circumferential rim of functional renal tissue will be seen during the nephrogram. Depending on the location of the cyst, the collecting system may be distorted (Fig. 3–142).

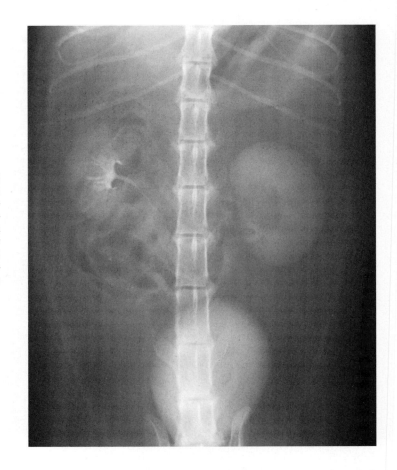

Figure 3–139. A 6-year-old male domestic short-haired cat with anorexia for 5 days, vomiting for 3 days, and pyrexia. Survey radiographs revealed a slight enlargement of the left kidney. The EU on the 15-minute ventrodorsal view revealed a normal right kidney. The left kidney shows a persistent nephrogram with a relatively radiolucent pelvis and faint traces of normal-sized diverticulae. Differential diagnoses include pyonephrosis or unilateral obstructive nephropathy. **Diagnosis:** Pyonephrosis.

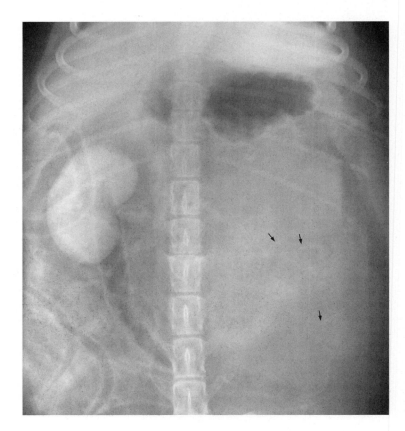

Figure 3–140. A 7-year-old male mixed breed dog with hematuria for 1 month. Survey radiographs revealed an enlarged, irregularly shaped left kidney (see Fig. 3–73). The nephrogram phase of the EU revealed wispy, irregular, opacified tubular structures (*black arrows*) within the left renal mass consistent with neovascularity associated with neoplasia. The right kidney had a flattened area in the cranial lateral margin suggesting a prior renal infarction. Differential diagnoses for the left renal mass included various forms of renal neoplasia. **Diagnosis:** Nephroblastoma.

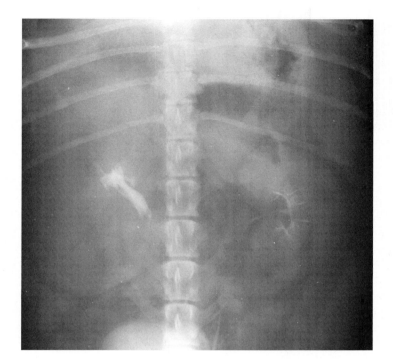

Figure 3–141. A 10-year-old male beagle with polydipsia and polyuria. There is a marked global, smooth enlargement of the right kidney with dilation of the renal pelvis, compression of the diverticulae (especially those draining the caudal pole), and obstruction of the ureter near the caudal pole. The left kidney and ureter are normal. Differential diagnoses include neoplasia (either primary or metastatic) with ureteral involvement or granulomatous disease. **Diagnosis:** Renal carcinoma with ureteral strangulation.

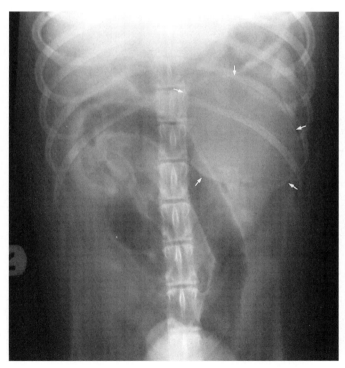

Figure 3–142. A 12-year-old male mixed breed dog with mild paraparesis. On physical examination an enlarged left kidney was palpated. Survey radiographs revealed that the cranial pole of the left kidney is enlarged. The EU revealed that the cranial pole of the left kidney is enlarged with a fine rim of contrast-enhanced renal tissue (*white arrows*) surrounding a relatively radiolucent mass. The cranial urinary collecting structures appear to be displaced caudally. Differential diagnoses include renal cyst, renal neoplasia, renal granuloma, or renal abscess. **Diagnosis:** Simple renal cyst.

UNILATERAL, SMALL, REGULAR

Feline and Canine. The urographic changes described in bilateral hypoplasia and CIN are the same in unilateral disease for the affected kidney.

UNILATERAL, SMALL, IRREGULAR

Feline and Canine. The urographic changes described in bilateral cases of CIN, chronic pyelonephritis, and renal infarcts are the same in unilateral disease for the affected kidney.

NORMAL SIZE AND SHAPE

Feline and Canine

ACUTE TUBULAR NEPHROSIS. Acute tubular nephrosis may be induced by excretory urography. The urographic findings are a nephrogram that persists or becomes progressively more dense with time. A pyelogram is not noted (Fig. 3–143). In such instances, treatment with intravenous fluids and diuretics should be instituted.

ACUTE PYELONEPHRITIS, INTERSTITIAL NEPHRITIS, AND GLOMERULAR NEPHRITIS. Depending upon the severity of the condition, the excretory urogram may be normal. If the condition is severe, a faint nephrogram and/or renal pelvic and ureteral dilation may be seen.

RENAL CALCULI. The nephrogram should appear normal and the pyelogram will reveal a radiolucent filling defect within the collecting system (see Fig. 3–164). If the calculus has caused obstruction, dilation of the renal sinus and possibly of the diverticulae may be seen. Because pyelonephritis is frequently seen in association with renal calculi, the changes associated with pyelonephritis may also be identified.

NEPHROCALCINOSIS. A normal to faint nephrogram may be present depending upon the extent of the renal parenchymal injury associated with the nephrocalcinosis. The pyelogram will be normal or slightly irregular, however filling defects will not be identified.

KIDNEY RUPTURE. The perirenal area will be hazy on survey radiographs. The EU will usually, but not necessarily, show extravasation of contrast media into the surrounding soft tissues.[172] The kidney may not excrete contrast. If the rupture is close to the renal pelvis, dilation of the pelvis and pelvic recesses may be present.

Functional Aspects of the Nephrogram

Evaluation of the nephrogram to perform a quantitative assessment of renal abnormalities has been suggested.[177] Renal perfusion abnormalities, glomerular dysfunction, intra- or extrarenal obstruction, renal tubular necrosis, and renal or systemic reactions to intravenous contrast administration may alter the nephrographic pattern of the excretory urogram. Standardization of the contrast dose and filming sequence is essential to be able to derive functional information from the contrast study. The time of maximum nephrographic density and the variations in density before and after maximum opacity are recommended to differentiate the disease processes. The evaluation has limited value. Several abnormal patterns have been

Figure 3–143. A 7-year-old female English pointer with polyuria and polydipsia for 2 weeks. (A) The immediate lateral view of the EU revealed a normal nephrogram. (B) The 20-minute view of the EU revealed that no collecting structures have become apparent nor that any contrast is seen in the bladder. The density of the kidney parenchyma is nearly the same as the immediate view. The nephrogram has remained persistent. **Diagnosis:** Acute renal failure.

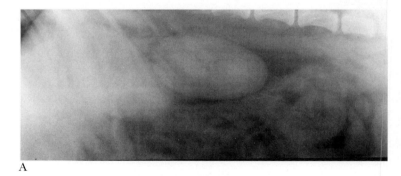

A

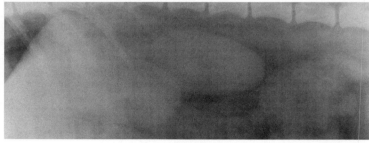

B

described. Although most of these patterns and their causes have been documented in humans, only a few have been recognized in dogs and cats.

A normal nephrographic density that is followed by a progressively increasing density or by a persistent density has been associated with contrast-induced systemic hypotension, acute renal obstruction, and contrast-induced renal failure. Poor nephrographic density followed by decreasing density has been associated with polyuric renal failure or an inadequate contrast dose. Poor initial density followed by increasing opacity has been associated with acute extrarenal obstruction, systemic hypotension, and renal ischemia. Poor initial density which does not decrease may occur with glomerular disease or severe interstitial or tubular disease.

Renal Ultrasound Abnormalities

SIZE

Calipers are part of most ultrasound machines and can be used to obtain direct and accurate measurements of the kidneys. All three renal dimensions can be measured and renal volume can be calculated.[19–21] Renal volumetric dimensions have not improved the accuracy of ultrasound in identifying renal abnormalities and, as a general rule, length, width, and height measurements are sufficient. The measurements will not be accurate unless the transducer is positioned perpendicular to the plane of the kidney. Measurements obtained using the ultrasound machine calipers are more accurate than radiographic measurements. Diuresis resulting from administration of contrast agents, diuretics, or intravenous fluid can cause minimal enlargement of the kidney, which can be detected and quantitated using the ultrasound calipers.[22,25,26,180] Whether detected by ultrasound or radiography, the differential diagnoses for renal enlargement is the same, however the ultrasound examination is capable of detecting smaller degrees of renal enlargement. Reduction in kidney size can also be detected using ultrasound. If the kidneys are extremely small, they may be hard to find. If the kidney is otherwise normal (there is no alteration in renal parenchymal echo intensity), a specific diagnosis cannot be made based solely on renal size alteration.

SHAPE

Distortion of the renal shape will be produced if the transducer is not oriented perpendicular to the kidney. This may be difficult to accomplish, especially when the kidney is positioned cranially under the rib cage. Ultrasound has been shown to be more sensitive than excretory urography and renal angiography for detecting slight alterations in renal contour caused by experimentally produced renal carcinoma.[181] Renal shape abnormalities are readily detected; however, depending on operator experience, both false-negative and false-positive results may be encountered. Contour irregularities are usually non-specific, but focal and global irregularities and unilateral or bilateral involvement can be detected and used to distinguish among renal diseases. The shape of the renal cortex and medulla can be evaluated and a determination can be made if the irregularity of the renal contour results from medullary or cortical disease.

POSITION

Renal masses and masses that displace the kidney can be identified using ultrasound.[182] The normal kidney can be readily identified and the characteristics of the mass that is displacing the kidney can be determined. The kidneys may be displaced from their normal position by the pressure that the operator exerts on the ultrasound transducer. This displacement should not be interpreted as a positional abnormality.

ECHO INTENSITY AND PATTERN

Echo intensity may be characterized as hyperechoic, hypoechoic, or anechoic. The echo intensity of the kidney is compared to adjacent structures, usually the liver and spleen. The kidney is normally hypoechoic relative to the spleen and liver, but comparison is only useful if the liver and spleen are normal.[182] The echo pattern may be uniform or heteroechoic. The renal medulla is hypoechoic relative to the renal cortex. At times the renal medulla appears almost anechoic. Ultrasound abnormalities may be described as hypo- or hyperechoic relative to normal renal cortex or medulla or relative to the opposite kidney. Ultrasound patterns and echo intensity are more specific for focal or multifocal renal abnormalities and less specific for diffuse renal disease.[182–185] Ultrasound has limited use in discriminating between benign lesions, such as abscesses or hematomas, and malignant lesions, such as adenocarcinoma.[183,184] The ultrasound findings may change with duration of disease. Renal tumors, hemorrhage, abscess, or infarct may produce hyperechoic, hypoechoic, or heteroechoic focal abnormalities depending on their duration (Figs. 3–144, 3–145, and 3–146).[182–184] Acute infarcts are hyperechoic and wedge shaped.[186] Similar lesions have been seen in experimental dogs with acute pyelonephritis.[187] Diagnosis may be difficult without biopsy or aspirate.

Intrarenal cysts or hydronephrosis produce anechoic lesions with well-defined near and far walls and through transmission.[182,184,185] Ultrasound can detect mild degrees of hydronephrosis with minimal renal pelvic or proximal ureteral dilation.[188]

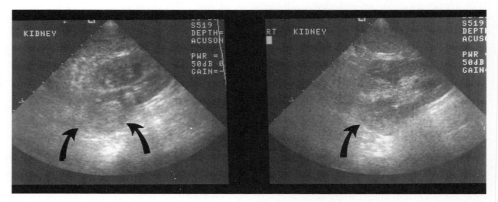

Figure 3–144. Longitudinal sonograms of the right kidney of a 16-year-old spayed female Doberman pinscher with a history of anorexia and vomiting for 2 weeks. The dog had a mass on the right rear foot. There is a heteroechoic mass associated with the renal cortex at the cranial aspect of the right kidney (*arrows*). This represents a renal tumor. **Diagnosis:** Metastatic melanoma.

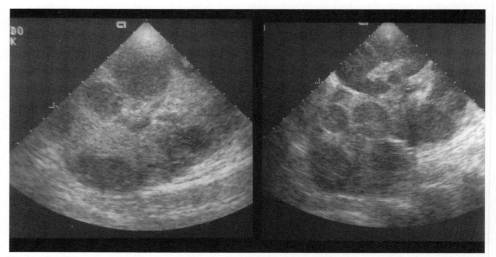

Figure 3–145. Longitudinal sonograms of the left kidney of a 10-year-old male rottweiler with a history of anorexia, vomiting and hematuria of 3 weeks' duration. The renal architecture is totally obliterated and replaced by multiple hypoechoic, somewhat oval-shaped lesions. This is indicative of renal neoplasia. **Diagnosis:** Metastatic carcinoma.

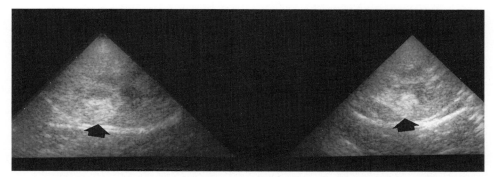

Figure 3–146. Longitudinal sonograms of the left kidney of a 3-year-old castrated male cat with a history of episodic hind limb paresis. There is a focal hyperechoic lesion at the corticomedullary junction in the cranial pole of the kidney (*arrows*). This most likely represents a renal infarct or focal area of infection. **Diagnosis:** Renal infarct secondary to hypertrophic cardiomyopathy.

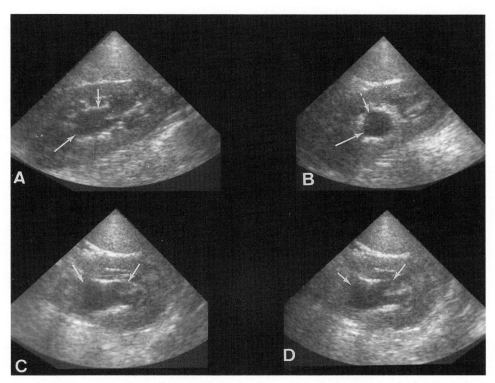

Figure 3–147. Longitudinal (A&B) and transverse (C&D) sonograms of the left kidney of a 5-year-old female rottweiler with a history of anorexia and pyrexia of 5 days' duration. There is moderate hydronephrosis with dilation of the renal pelvis (*arrows*). This may be secondary to infection or obstruction. **Diagnosis:** Hydronephrosis secondary to bladder wall thickening, lymphosarcoma.

The transverse view is more useful than the longitudinal view for this purpose. The ureter forms an anechoic "Y," which is centered on the renal crest and can be distinguished from the renal vein, which branches more toward the corticomedullary junction. As the ureter and renal pelvis dilate, they will appear progressively larger and will gradually replace the renal medulla and finally the entire renal cortex. The dilated renal pelvis will lose its "Y" shape and become wider, taking the shape of the renal pelvic recesses and eventually becoming a large oval (Figs. 3–147 and 3–148). With marked hydronephrosis, the renal vessels and associated fibrous tissue may appear as hyperechoic linear bands that stretch from the renal pelvis to the renal cortex (Fig. 3–149). Pyonephrosis may produce renal pelvic dilation, which appears similar to hydronephrosis. The fluid will usually be more echogenic, and the cellular

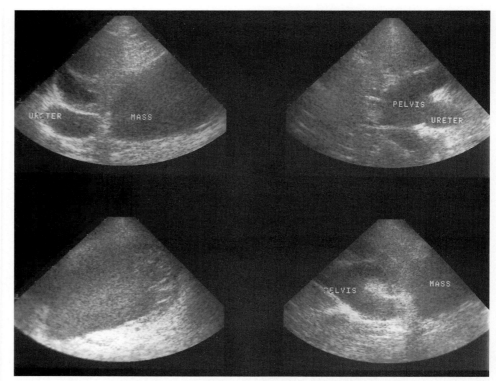

Figure 3–148. Longitudinal sonograms of the left kidney of a 13-year-old male coonhound with a history of vomiting and diarrhea of 4 weeks' duration. The ureter and renal pelvis are markedly distended. There is a heteroechoic mass which surrounds and obstructs the ureter. This is most likely neoplastic. **Diagnosis:** Retroperitoneal carcinoma with secondary hydronephrosis.

Figure 3–149. Longitudinal sonograms of the left kidney of a 12-year-old castrated male cocker spaniel with a history of vomiting and bloody diarrhea of 1 month's duration. There was a palpable abdominal mass. The left kidney has been replaced by an anechoic mass which contains hyperechoic linear septations. This is indicative of severe hydronephrosis. **Diagnosis:** Hydronephrosis.

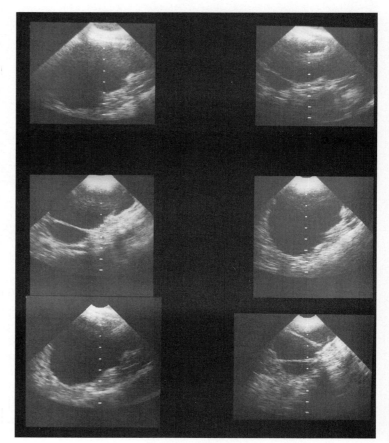

nature of the fluid can often be recognized by the motion of the cells within the purulent material contained in the renal pelvis. Aspiration of the renal pelvis using ultrasound guidance will provide a definitive diagnosis. Intrarenal cysts are anechoic, usually round, vary in size, may be septated, and are located within the renal parenchyma away from the renal pelvis. It is important to identify the cyst in both longitudinal and transverse planes in order to be certain it is in the kidney. The cysts may be single or multiple, large or small, and may protrude from the renal cortex or be located completely within the renal parenchyma (Fig. 3–150). Some tumors and abscesses appear cystic while some cysts contain echogenic material that may create the illusion that they are solid.[178,182,185] Aspiration or biopsy may be required for a definitive diagnosis.

Ultrasonography is more sensitive than excretory urography in detecting acute pyelonephritis. Renal pelvic and proximal ureteral dilation and a hyperechoic line along the renal crest have been described as the major findings. A uniformly echogenic renal cortex, focal hypoechoic or hyperechoic areas within the renal cortex, and hypoechoic focal lesions within the medulla have been observed (Figs. 3–151 and 3–152).[187]

Diffuse uniform hyperechoic patterns may occur in association with lymphosarcoma, feline infectious peritonitis, chronic interstitial nephritis, chronic pyelonephritis, chronic glomerulonephritis, renal dysplasia, renal mineralization, and with hemoglobin or hemosiderin deposits within the kidney (Figs. 3–150, 3–153, 3–154, and 3–155).

Diffuse uniform anechoic pattern will occur secondary to hydronephrosis. A diffuse heteroechoic pattern of hyperechoic and anechoic areas may be seen with polycystic kidney disease (Figs. 3–156 and 3–157).

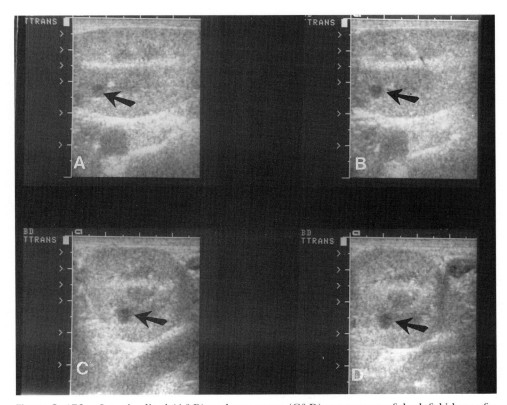

Figure 3–150. Longitudinal (A&B) and transverse (C&D) sonograms of the left kidney of a 9-year-old spayed female schnauzer with a history of chronic urinary tract infection and diabetes mellitus. There is a solitary anechoic lesion in the renal cortex (*arrows*) indicative of a renal cyst. The kidneys are diffusely hyperechoic with poor corticomedullary distinction. This is indicative of diffuse renal disease which may be secondary to chronic infection or infiltrative disease. **Diagnosis:** Solitary renal cyst, chronic pyelonephritis.

Figure 3–151. Transverse (A, B,&C) and longitudinal (D) sonograms of the left kidney of a 4-year-old male Great Dane with a history of hematuria of 4 months' duration. The renal architecture is markedly distorted with a large mass arising from the dorsal surface of the kidney (*arrows*). There is poor corticomedullary distinction within the more normal appearing portions of the kidney. This mass could represent a tumor or granuloma. A renal biopsy was performed, and *Escherichia coli* pyelonephritis with renal abscess was diagnosed. **Diagnosis:** Pyelonephritis with abscess.

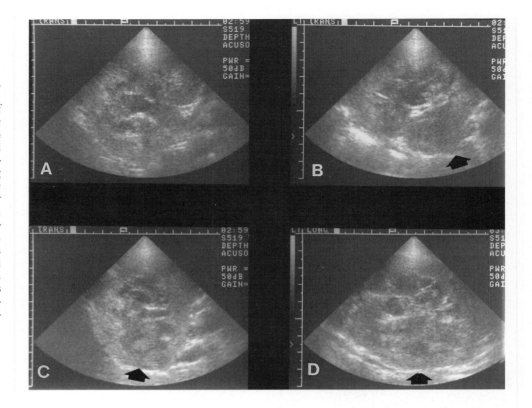

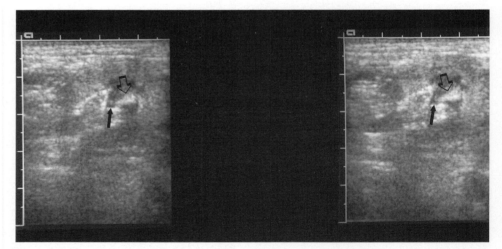

Figure 3–152. Transverse sonograms of the left kidney of a 9-year-old spayed female schnauzer with a history of urolithiasis of 3 months' duration. There is mild dilation of the renal pelvis (*solid arrows*). This may be secondary to obstruction or infection. There is a hyperechoic zone in the renal pelvis (*open arrows*). This is indicative of pyelonephritis. **Diagnosis:** Pyelonephritis.

Nephrocalcinosis may produce a diffusely hyperechoic kidney, but also can produce a hyperechoic band at the corticomedullary junction (Fig. 3–158).[189,190] This hyperechoic band has been referred to as the "medullary rim sign" and may also be seen with acute tubular necrosis, pyogranulomatous vasculitis, chronic interstitial nephritis, and hypercalcemia (Figs. 3–159 and 3–160).[190] Acoustic shadowing may or may not be present. Chronic renal failure may also produce a hyperechoic renal medulla. Ethylene glycol poisoning produces a similar hyperechoic medulla with a

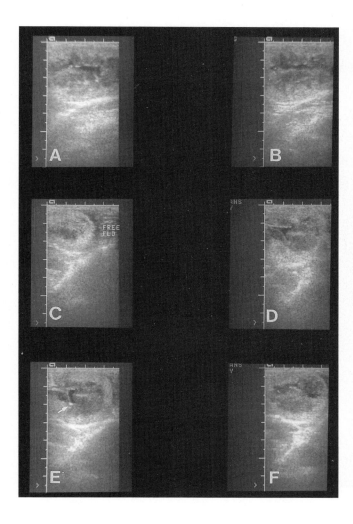

Figure 3–153. Longitudinal (A&B) and transverse (C,D,E,&F) sonograms of the left kidney of a 4-year-old castrated male Siamese cat with a history of polyuria, polydipsia, and palpably enlarged kidneys. The kidney is hyperechoic with poor corticomedullary distinction. The renal pelvis is dilated (*arrows*). There is peritoneal fluid (C). This findings are indicative of infiltrative or inflammatory renal disease. **Diagnosis:** Lymphosarcoma.

surrounding hypoechoic area. This has been termed the "halo sign" and is associated with a poor prognosis.[191]

Hyperechoic focal lesions within the renal pelvis may occur with renal calculi.[184] Renal calculi may or may not shadow, and it may be difficult to discriminate between renal calculi and renal pelvic mineralization. Identifying a dilated renal pelvis around the calculus may help in its recognition. The size of the renal calculus is important in determining whether or not it shadows; however, the amount and type of surrounding tissue will affect the stone's ability to produce a shadow. Thicker and less uniform surrounding tissue reduces the amount of shadowing. Chemical composition has little effect on the amount of shadowing.[192]

Small amounts of perirenal fluid (either retroperitoneal or subcapsular) may be detected using ultrasound. The exact location of the fluid may be difficult to define; however, if the fluid follows the contour of the kidney, it is probably subcapsular (Fig. 3–161). An anechoic zone will be observed around the kidney. The echo intensity of the kidney may be artifactually increased if a large amount of perirenal or peritoneal fluid is present.

URETERS

Normal ureters are not seen on radiographs because of their small diameter (1–2 mm). Few ureteral abnormalities are visible on survey radiographs, but radiodense calculi may be identified (Fig. 3–162). These vary in size and can be mistaken for

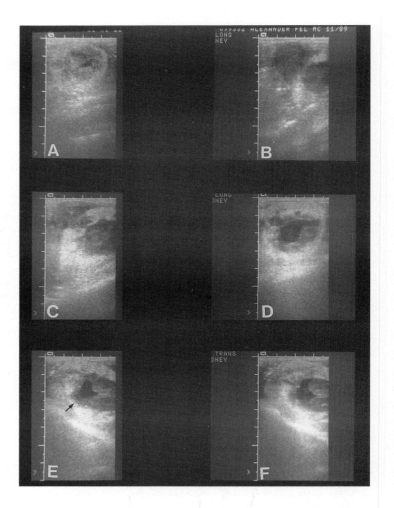

Figure 3–154. Transverse (A,E,&F) and longitudinal (B,C,&D) sonograms of the right kidney of a 4-year-old castrated male Siamese cat with a history of polyuria, polydipsia, and palpably enlarged kidneys. The renal pelvis is markedly dilated (*arrows*). The kidney is enlarged, irregularly shaped and contains both hyperechoic and hypoechoic regions. This is indicative of infiltrative renal disease. **Diagnosis:** Lymphosarcoma.

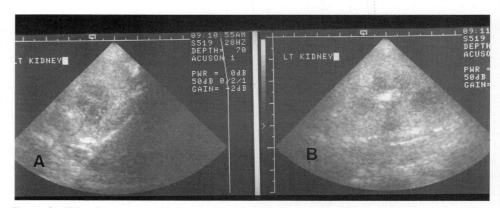

Figure 3–155. Transverse (A) and longitudinal (B) sonograms of the left kidney of a 9-year-old castrated male cat with a history of anorexia, weight loss, and icterus of 1 month's duration. The kidney is diffusely hyperechoic. This is indicative of inflammatory or infiltrative renal disease. **Diagnosis:** Lymphosarcoma.

mineral material within the GI tract; however, their position in the dorsal abdomen enables them to be identified as ureteral calculi. In most cases, renal calculi or cystic calculi will also be present, increasing the likelihood of ureteral calculi and making any mineralized density in the sublumbar or retroperitoneal area more suspicious. Ureteral calculi may be located anywhere from the renal pelvis to the trigone

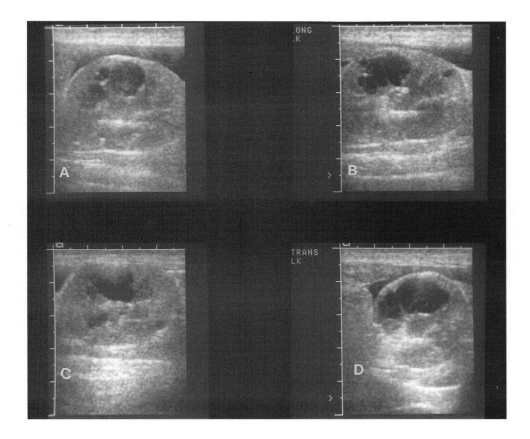

Figure 3–156. Longitudinal (A&B) and transverse (C&D) sonograms of the left kidney of a 5-year-old female Persian cat with a history of anorexia, diarrhea, hematuria, hypoglycemia, and hypoproteinemia of 6 months' duration. The size of the kidney is normal. There are several irregularly shaped hypoechoic and anechoic lesions visible within the renal parenchyma. There is poor corticomedullary differentiation. There is anechoic peritoneal fluid. These findings are indicative of polycystic renal disease with ascites. **Diagnosis:** Polycystic kidneys.

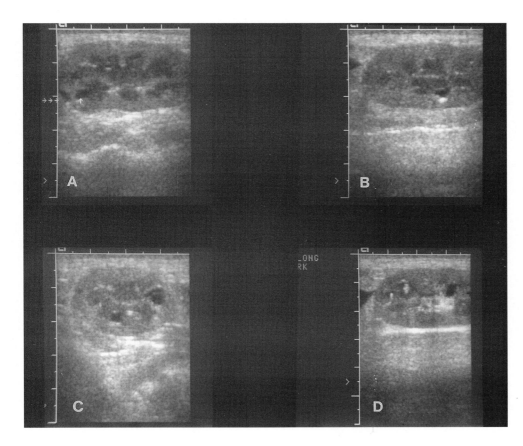

Figure 3–157. Longitudinal (A,B,&D) and transverse (C) sonograms of the right kidney of a 5-year-old female Persian cat with a history of anorexia, diarrhea, hematuria, hypoglycemia, and hypoproteinemia of 6 months' duration. The size of the kidney is normal, however the contour is slightly irregular. There are several irregularly shaped hypoechoic and anechoic lesions visible within the renal parenchyma. These findings are indicative of polycystic renal disease. There is a small amount of anechoic peritoneal fluid. **Diagnosis:** Polycystic kidneys.

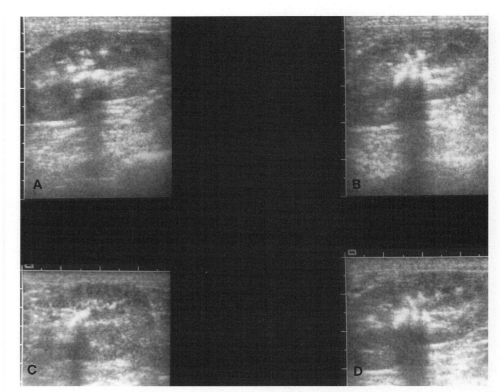

Figure 3–158. Longitudinal (A,B,&D) and transverse (C) sonograms of the left kidney of a 12-year-old bichon frise with a history of urinary tract infection of 3 months' duration. There are hyperechoic regions within the renal pelvis with shadowing. This is indicative of renal mineralization. **Diagnosis:** Renal mineralization.

Figure 3–159. Longitudinal (A&B) and transverse (C&D) sonograms of the left kidney of a 4-month-old female Great Dane with a history of fever, anorexia, depression, and reluctance to walk of 1 month's duration. The kidney is hyperechoic, and there is a hyperechoic band at the junction of the inner and outer renal medulla. This is indicative of renal tubular mineralization, acute tubular necrosis, pyogranulomatous vasculitis, chronic interstitial nephritis, and hypercalcemia. A somewhat similar pattern has been observed in ethylene glycol toxicity. **Diagnosis:** Acute tubular necrosis and renal mineralization associated with hypertrophic osteodystrophy.

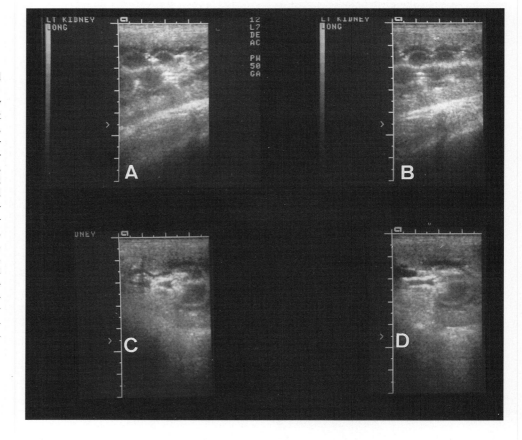

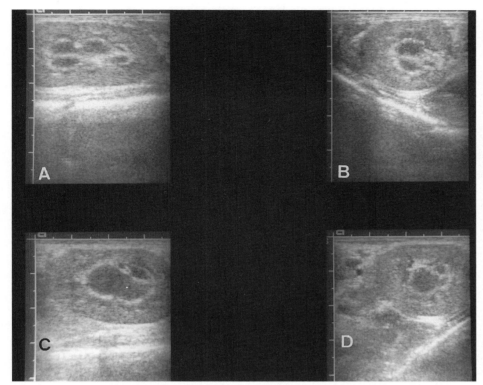

Figure 3–160. Longitudinal (A&C) and transverse (B&D) sonograms of the right kidney of a 14-month-old castrated male Siamese cat with a history of anorexia and lethargy of 2 months' duration. The renal cortex is hyperechoic, and there is a hyperechoic linear band at the corticomedullary junction. This can occur secondary to renal mineralization, acute tubular necrosis, ethylene glycol toxicity, chronic interstitial nephritis, and pyogranulomatous nephritis (FIP). **Diagnosis:** Pyogranulomatous nephritis (FIP).

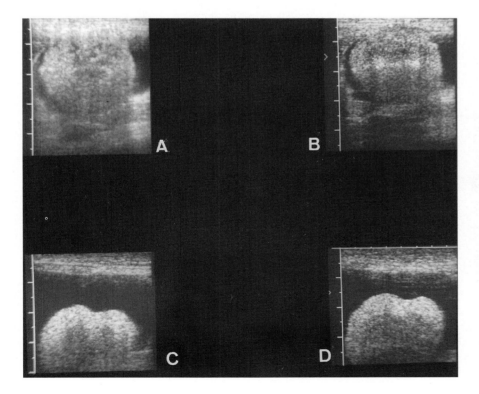

Figure 3–161. Transverse (A&B) and longitudinal (C&D) sonograms of the left kidney of an 8-year-old castrated male cat with a history of chronic abdominal distension. The kidney is small, hyperechoic, and surrounded by anechoic fluid. This fluid is limited to the area surrounding the kidney and is not present within the peritoneal cavity. These findings are indicative of chronic renal disease with perirenal fluid. **Diagnosis:** Chronic renal disease with subcapsular renal cyst.

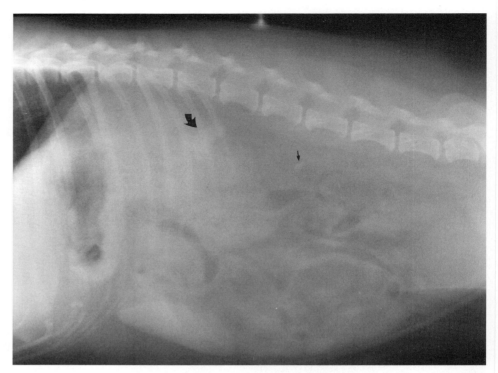

Figure 3–162. A 9-year-old female miniature pinscher with lethargy for 2 weeks and having an arched back, anorexia, and diarrhea for 2 days. The lateral radiograph revealed a calcific density, shaped like the renal pelvis, in the right renal pelvis (*large black arrow*). There is a calcified ureteral calculus seen ventral to L4 (*small black arrow*). Excretory urography revealed that the ureteral calculus was on the left side (see Fig. 3–98). **Diagnosis:** Left ureteral calculus and right renal calculus.

Figure 3–163. A 4-year-old female miniature poodle that was shot. The lateral radiograph revealed hydrothorax as well as the slug dorsal to T12. The colon and intestines are displaced ventrally by the retroperitoneal space, which is more tissue-dense than normal (it is usually fat density). Differential diagnoses include retroperitoneal hemorrhage or rupture of either a kidney or ureter with leakage of urine. **Diagnosis:** Ruptured right ureter (see Fig. 3–168).

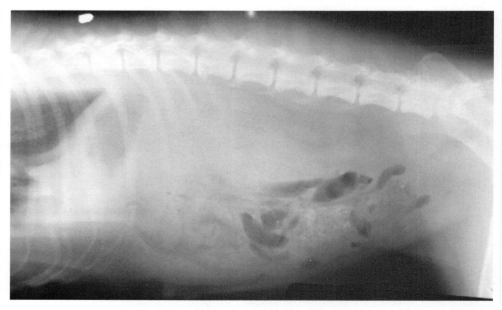

of the bladder. Retroperitoneal masses, which can be presumed to displace or encompass the ureters, may be seen. These produce a soft tissue swelling in the sublumbar or retroperitoneal space. The normal thin line of soft tissue density ventral to the vertebrae becomes thickened or irregular in contour. Retroperitoneal masses or swelling may also displace or obscure the kidneys. Ureteral rupture is not specifically identifiable on survey radiographs but may be suggested by the presence of haziness in the retroperitoneal space and loss of renal outline (Fig. 3–163). Retroperitoneal hemorrhage without ureteral damage is more common. This is seen in trauma cases associated with vertebral or pelvic fractures.

Excretory Urography

NORMAL FINDINGS

Excretory urography is helpful in defining ureteral lesions and is superior to ultrasound in this regard. In the normal EU, the ureters appear as narrow tubes extending from the renal pelvis to the trigone region of the bladder. The ureters exit the renal pelvis medially and curl caudally after a very short distance. It is unusual to see the entire length of the ureter on any one excretory urographic film. This is because ureteral peristalsis propels the urine to the bladder. The width of the ureter should vary due to ureteral peristalsis. As the ureters approach the bladder, they often extend slightly caudal to their bladder entrance site and curve back cranially just before entering the trigone.

ABNORMAL FINDINGS

The most common abnormality of the ureter(s) demonstrated by the EU is ureteral dilation. This is almost always due to ureteral obstruction. The site of the lesion is usually at the point where the ureteral size changes from dilated to normal. If only a portion of the ureter is dilated, ureteral calculi, periureteral masses, retroperitoneal fibrosis, ureteral tumor, or ureteral inflammation must be considered as differential diagnoses (Fig. 3–164). If the entire ureteral length is dilated, the lesion is probably located at the trigone of the bladder (Fig. 3–165). In some animals, most commonly in female dogs, the ureter(s) may be ectopic and may terminate in the

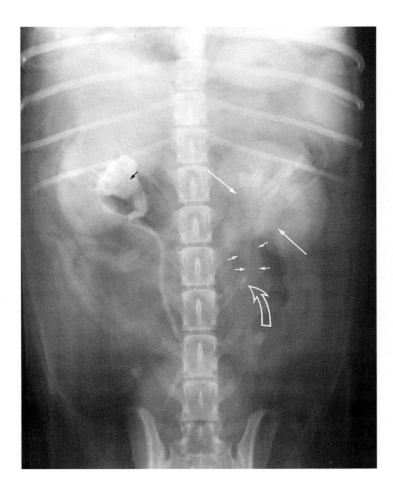

Figure 3–164. A 9-year-old female miniature pinscher with lethargy for 2 weeks, having an arched back, anorexia, and diarrhea for 2 days. Survey radiographs revealed a large calculus in the right renal pelvis and the suggestion of a calculus in the left ureter (see Fig. 3–96). The EU revealed a severely dilated right renal sinus with a central filling defect which is shaped similarly to the calculus (*black arrow*). The ureter distal to the pelvis is normal. The left kidney revealed a dilated renal pelvis and proximal ureter (*long white arrows*) as well as diverticulae. The ureteral dilation (*small white arrows*) ends at the level of the ureteral calculus (*open white arrow*). **Diagnosis:** Right renal calculus and left ureteral calculus with resultant proximal hydroureter and hydronephrosis.

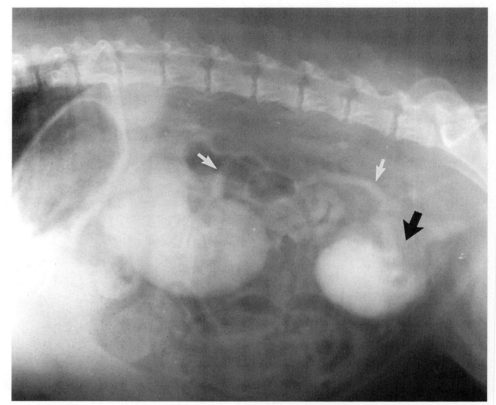

Figure 3–165. A 14-year-old female mixed breed dog with chronic hematuria. There is mild global enlargement of the left kidney and the collecting system of the kidney and the entire length of the ureter (*white arrows*). The right kidney is quite small with no discernible collecting structures. There is a large filling defect in the trigone region of the bladder (*black arrow*). Differential diagnoses for the right kidney include congenital hypoplasia or chronic atrophic pyelonephritis, those for the left kidney include obstructive uropathy or acute pyelonephritis and ureteritis, and those for the bladder include neoplasia or granuloma. **Diagnosis:** Transitional cell carcinoma of the bladder with obstruction of the left ureter and chronic atrophic pyelonephritis of the right kidney.

urethra or vagina (Figs. 3–166 and 3–167). Ectopic ureters are frequently dilated. If the position of the ureter relative to the urinary bladder cannot be determined, an excretory urogram combined with a double contrast cystogram is often helpful.[193–198]

An uncommon finding is the presence of a ureterocele.[130] This is a ureteral dilation that occurs between the serosa and mucosa of the bladder wall. It will appear as a small focal dilation of the ureter, and there may be apparent narrowing of the ureter as it empties into the bladder. The ureterocele will produce a round contrast-containing structure at the trigone and may produce a focal bladder wall mass or filling defect as the bladder fills with contrast. If ectopic ureter and/or ureterocele is considered likely (such as in a case of a young, incontinent female dog), it is helpful to distend the bladder with air and take multiple oblique views of the pelvic area in addition to the routine views. In some cases, the ureter will penetrate the bladder serosa, travel in the submucosa, and continue on to some distant site of termination without spilling urine into the bladder (Fig. 3–168). Ectopic ureter may be unilateral or bilateral. The presence of contrast within the urinary bladder does not rule out bilateral ectopic ureter, because the bladder may fill with contrast retrograde from the urethra. Repair of the ectopic ureter(s) usually requires surgical transplantation of the ureter(s) involved. Shortly after ureteral transplantation into the bladder there will be ureteral dilation. This is probably due to post surgical inflammation, which creates a temporary partial ureteral stenosis. This change usually will revert to normal condition over several months as the swelling subsides.

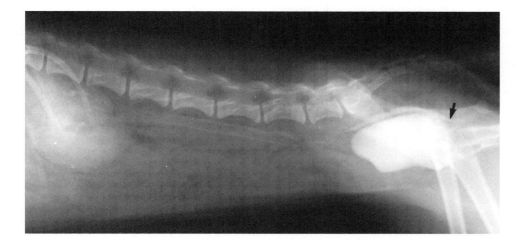

Figure 3–166. An 8-month-old female poodle with urinary incontinence since the owner adopted the dog (4 months). Survey radiographs were normal. The EU revealed the right ureter bypassed the normal site of entry into the bladder and extended on to enter into the vagina (*black arrow*). **Diagnosis:** Ectopic right ureter.

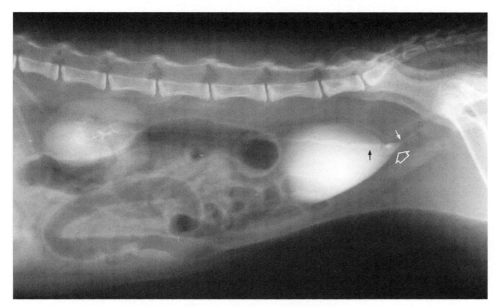

Figure 3–167. A 1-year-old neutered male domestic short-haired cat with incontinence since owned and cystitis for 3 months. Survey radiographs were normal. The EU revealed an ectopic right ureter (*black arrow*) which penetrated the serosa of the bladder in the trigone region and then dilated (ureterocele–*open white arrow*) and then entered directly into the urethra (*solid white arrow*) distal to the urinary sphincter. **Diagnosis:** Right ureteral ectopic with ureterocele.

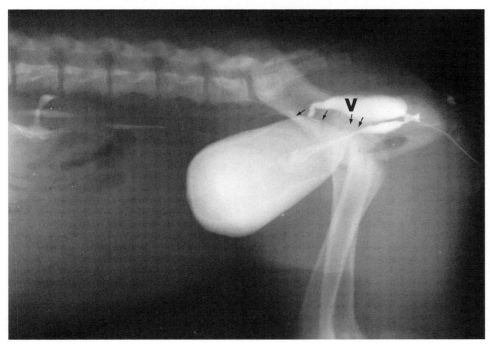

Figure 3–168. A 4-month-old female German shepherd dog with urinary incontinence. A positive-contrast cystogram and vaginogram (*black v*) have been performed. The EU revealed that the left ureter penetrates the serosa of the bladder, burrows through the submucosa, and then exits and extends on to enter into the urethra distal to the urinary sphincter (*black arrows*). **Diagnosis:** Ectopic left ureter.

The accumulation of contrast media in the retroperitoneal space identifies ureteral rupture. The greatest concentration of contrast media is noted at the level of rupture (Fig. 3–169). Ureteral dilation may accompany ureteral rupture. Contrast may also accumulate in the peritoneal cavity as a result of direct leakage or diffusion through the peritoneum.

Ultrasound of the Abnormal Ureter

The proximal ureter is the only portion of the ureter that can be identified unless the ureter is tremendously dilated. When the ureter is enlarged, it may be traced beyond the renal pelvis but it is often quickly obscured by the small intestines. The enlarged ureter may be identified adjacent to the urinary bladder. The ureter will appear as an anechoic linear, tubular, or "Y"-shaped structure. If the ureter is easily identified during an ultrasound examination, it is abnormal. Occasionally, a dilated ureter can be traced distally to the site of obstruction. In most cases, an excretory urogram will be required to determine the cause of the ureteral dilation. Dilation of the distal ureter may be identified as an anechoic or hypoechoic tubular structure extending laterally or dorsally from the bladder trigone. The opening into the bladder may be visible. Tracing the ureter proximally from the bladder is difficult.

Focal dilation of the ureter may occur secondary to trauma. This dilation may become large producing an anechoic "cyst-like" structure.[199] These structures are usually round or elliptical, show evidence of distant enhancement, have sharp margins, and may contain thin septa. Renal pelvic dilation is often seen in conjunction with these ureteral dilations. The lesion will fill with contrast if renal function and

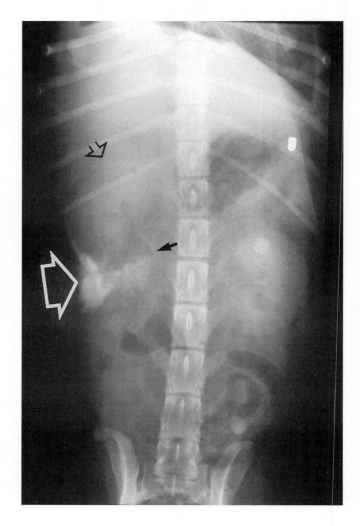

Figure 3–169. A 4-year-old female miniature poodle that was shot. Survey radiographs revealed an increased density in the retroperitoneal space, hydrothorax, and a slug lodged in the dorsal portion of the cranial left abdomen (see Fig. 3–162). The EU revealed a normal left kidney. The right kidney revealed a poor nephrogram (*open black arrow*). The proximal ureter (*solid black arrow*) is opacified and there is a large amount of contrast media free in the soft tissues immediately distal to it (*open white arrow*). Beyond this site the right ureter is not seen. **Diagnosis:** Ruptured right ureter caused by a gunshot wound.

ureteral flow is adequate, however this is not usually the case. Ultrasound guided drainage may be performed, and contrast can be injected into the dilation after urine drainage.

URINARY BLADDER

Normally, the bladder is a "teardrop-shaped" organ that is relatively firmly anchored by its ligaments and the urethra to the caudal abdominal and pelvic areas. The size of the bladder varies considerably because of its distensibility; however, normal bladders rarely extend cranial to the umbilicus. Although diseases with identifiable survey radiographic findings are uncommon (with the exception of cystic calculi), there are several changes in size, shape, density, or location that may be identified by contrast studies and correlated with sets of differential diagnoses.

Density Changes

Changes in density may affect the wall or contents of the bladder. Most cystic calculi are radiopaque, have irregular shapes, and are located in the "center" (most dependent portion) of the bladder (Figs. 3–170 and 3–171). The density of the calculi depends upon their size and their composition. While the structure of a stone is rarely diagnostic as to its composition, there are some strongly suggestive shapes. Calculi composed of silicates typically are shaped like the children's toy "jacks." If the calculus is very large and laminated, it is most likely composed of triple phosphates (struvite). However, struvite stones may form into a multitude of shapes. Oxalate calculi do not commonly assume any particular shape. Multiple small calculi (cystic sand) may be seen in cats and can be clinically significant (Fig. 3–172). A radiograph obtained using a horizontal x-ray beam with the patient standing may be useful in identifying small opaque calculi or sand, because this material will form layers in the urinary bladder thereby increasing their opacity. If not contaminated with calcium salts, two types of calculi, uric acid and cystine calculi, are usually radiolucent and not apparent on the survey film. Uric acid stones, if visible at all, will be

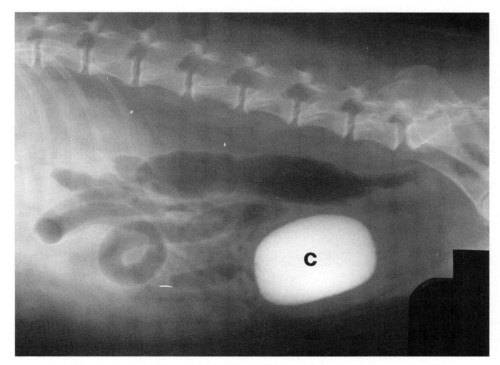

Figure 3–170. A 4-year-old female mixed breed dog with chronic hematuria and stranguria. Survey radiographs revealed a very large laminated calcium density in the bladder (*black c*). **Diagnosis:** Cystic calculus (triple phosphate).

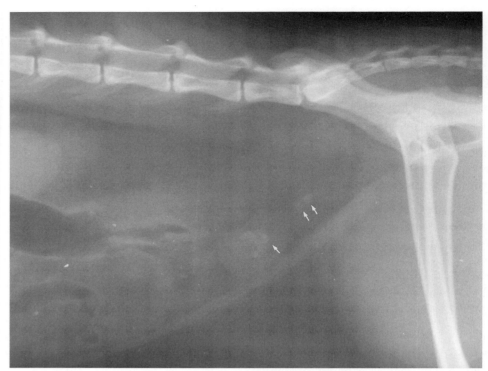

Figure 3–171. A 7-month-old female domestic short-haired cat with stranguria and pollaki-uria for 3 weeks. Survey radiographs reveal multiple poorly calcified calculi (*white arrows*) in the urinary bladder. **Diagnosis:** Multiple cystic calculi.

Figure 3–172. An 11-year-old male miniature schnauzer with chronic hematuria. There is a finely stippled calcific density in the entire bladder, which is most prominent in the center (most dependent portion–*black s*). There is also prostato-megaly. Differential diagnoses include cystic sand, calcifica-tion associated with neoplasia, or dystrophic calcification of bladder mucosa. **Diagnosis:** Multiple small cystic calculi (cystic sand).

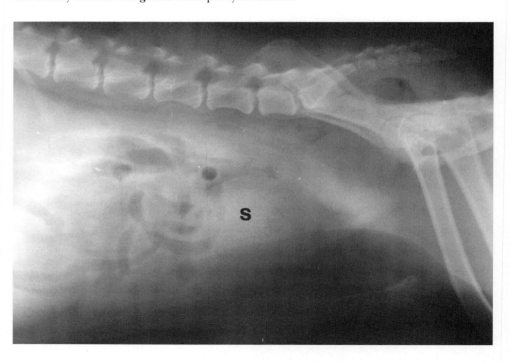

poorly calcified, relatively small, and frequently have an oblong appearance. Stru-vite calculi that are predominately composed of ammonium or magnesium phos-phate may also be nearly radiolucent. If radiolucent calculi are suspected, a double contrast cystogram or ultrasound examination is indicated.

Dystrophic calcification of the bladder mucosa may occur secondary to bladder inflammation or tumor. In chronic severe cystitis, such as that seen secondary to administration of cyclophosphamide, the bladder wall may appear as an "egg shell" type of calcification affecting only the mucosa (Fig. 3–173). In neoplasms, there may be focal areas of dystrophic calcification that usually appear as stippled or small foci of calcification in a limited portion of the bladder (Fig. 3–174). Focal areas of bladder mineralization may be differentiated from calculi because of their position. Calculi will tend to remain in the dependent portion of the urinary bladder and will move with changes in the patient's position. Calcification will be fixed in position and will be constant despite changes in the patient's position.[144] Differentiating small ureteral calculi, which are in the ureter at the trigone, from mineralization of the bladder wall can be difficult.

Gas densities may occasionally be seen in the bladder. The most common cause is the introduction of a small amount of air when the bladder is catheterized. This produces a small gas-dense bubble in the "center" (least dependent portion) of the bladder (Fig. 3–175). Emphysematous cystitis may occur: (1) in animals that have diabetes mellitus and a bladder infection caused by a glucose-fermenting organism such as *Escherichia coli*, or (2) in chronic cystitis where the mucosa become hypoxic and infection with a gas-forming organism such as *Clostridium sp.* occurs (Fig. 3–176).[144,200,201] The gas density will be seen in the submucosa and appears as linear streaking, air bubbles, or as a lucent halo outlining the bladder wall. There also may be accumulation of gas within the bladder; this will appear as a large radiolucent bubble in the "center" of the bladder or as multiple smaller bubbles. Air may dissect from the bladder mucosa into the retroperitoneal space or pelvic cavity.

Size Changes

Recognition of abnormal bladder size is difficult because of the high degree of normal variability. In some cases of chronic, partial, or nearly complete urinary obstruction, the bladder may be severely enlarged such that its cranial border extends

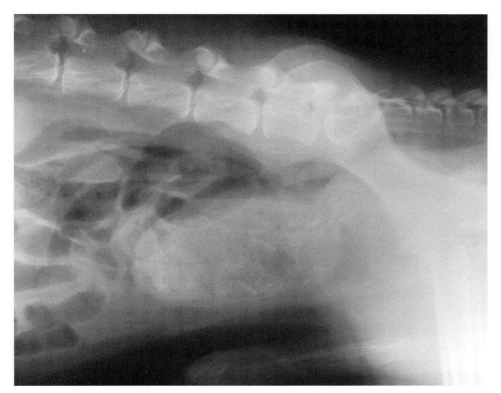

Figure 3–173. A 4-year-old male German shepherd dog with chronic cystitis and tetraparesis and urinary incontinence for 5 months. There is diffuse calcified plaque formation of the mucosa of the bladder and prostatic urethra. Differential diagnoses include dystrophic calcification of the mucosa or calcification associated with neoplasia. **Diagnosis:** Dystrophic calcification of urinary mucosa.

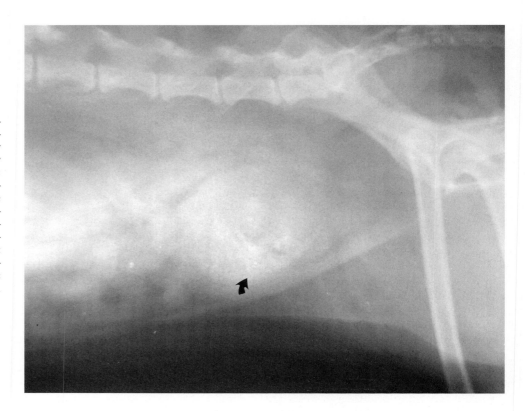

Figure 3–174. A 7-year-old female bichon frise with hematuria for 3 months. The survey radiograph revealed a finely stippled calcific density (*black arrow*) that is limited to the cranial and ventral portion of the bladder on the lateral recumbent view. Differential diagnoses include calcification associated with neoplasia, cystic sand, or dystrophic calcification of the mucosa. **Diagnosis:** Calcification associated with transitional cell carcinoma.

Figure 3–175. An 8-year-old male domestic short-haired cat with chronic cystitis. There are two round air densities in the center of the bladder (*black arrows*). These represent small air bubbles introduced by catheterization. Because the cat is in right lateral recumbency the air rose to highest level in the bladder; radiographically, this is in the center of the bladder. **Diagnosis:** Intravesicular air bubbles due to urinary catheterization.

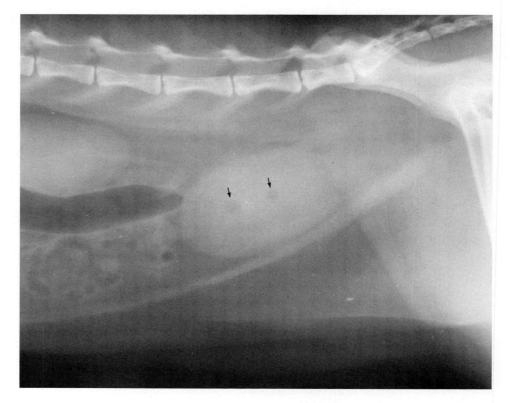

cranial to the umbilicus and the abdominal viscera are displaced cranially (Fig. 3–177). This may be extreme enough to suggest hydroperitoneum due to the homogenous tissue density in the majority of the abdomen; identification of displaced abdominal viscera precludes ascites as the diagnosis.

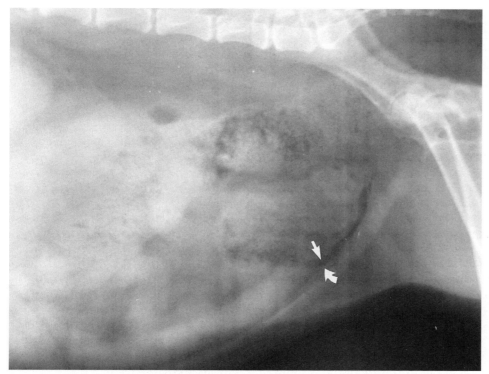

Figure 3–176. A 12-year-old female miniature poodle with chronic diabetes mellitus and pollakiuria for 2 weeks. The survey radiograph revealed a gas density dissecting between the serosa and mucosa (*white arrows*) of the bladder. Differential diagnoses include emphysematous cystitis due to glucose fermenting or anaerobic gas-producing bacteria. **Diagnosis:** *Eschericia coli* cystitis secondary to diabetes mellitus.

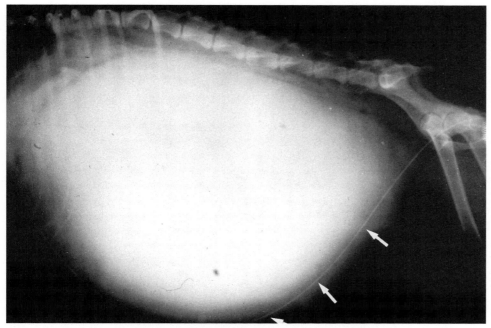

Figure 3–177. A 7-year-old female Norwegian elkhound with vaginal exudate. The lateral radiograph revealed a homogeneous tissue density throughout the majority of the abdomen. Scrutiny revealed that the intestines and other abdominal viscera have been displaced cranially. This indicated a large caudal abdominal mass. A urinary catheter (*white arrows*) was placed to define the bladder. Differential diagnoses include enlargement of the uterus, severe bladder distension, or mass arising from one of the caudal abdominal organs. **Diagnosis:** Severe bladder distention secondary to chronic granulomatous urethritis.

Shape Changes

Changes in bladder shape are rarely observed on survey films. Occasionally, the external surface may be distorted due to a congenital anomaly (urachal diverticulum), trauma (mucosal hernia), or bladder wall lesion (transitional cell carcinoma).

Location Changes

On survey radiographs the bladder may be seen in an abnormal location. The bladder may be displaced into the hernia sac in perineal, abdominal, or femoral hernias (Fig. 3–178). Positioning of the bladder within the pelvic canal ("pelvic bladder") has been associated with urinary incontinence; some animals with a pelvic bladder are continent. The significance of pelvic bladder and its relationship to incontinence is not clear.[202–204] Complete urethral transection distal to the urinary sphincter at the trigone of the bladder will result in the bladder retaining its normal size and shape but being cranially displaced within the abdomen (Fig. 3–179). Enlargement of the prostate can displace the bladder cranially.

Cystography

Evaluation of a cystogram should be performed by paying special attention to the location, shape, and integrity of the bladder; the thickness and regularity of the bladder wall; and the presence or absence of material within the contrast puddle on the double contrast cystogram.

Shape

Changes in the shape of the bladder may indicate the presence of a bladder diverticulum, persistent urachal remnant, or neoplasm. Diverticulae are protrusions of the lumen and cystic mucosa through a rent in the serosa. They will appear as either extensions of the gas or contrast media beyond the serosal border of the bladder but are contained within the bladder wall. These may be congenital or acquired as a result of trauma. The urachus normally involutes immediately after birth to become

Figure 3–178. (A) A 13-year-old female Siamese cat that was hit by a car. There is a loss of contiguity of the ventral abdominal stripe (rectus abdominis muscle) with a hazy density in the tissue swelling ventral to it (*white arrows*). The bladder is not identified in the abdomen. (B) The cystogram portion of the EU revealed that the bladder, along with some gas-containing loops of small intestine (*white arrow*), is incorporated into the hernia sac. **Diagnosis:** Urinary bladder and small intestine incorporated in traumatic inguinal hernia.

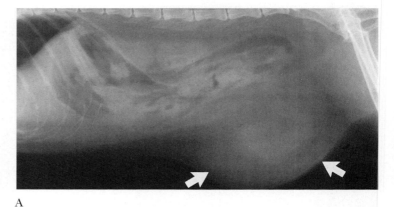

A

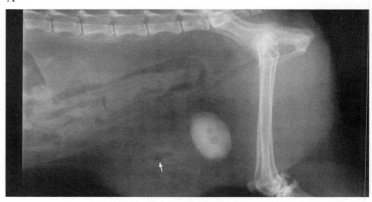

B

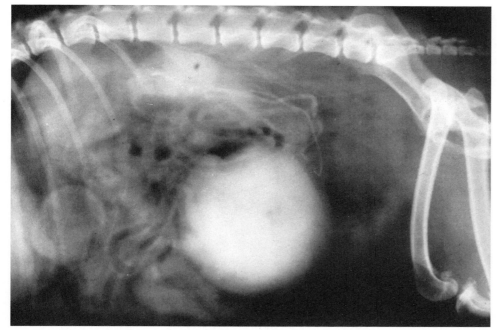

Figure 3–179. A 6-year-old female miniature poodle that was hit by a car. Survey radiographs revealed a right coxofemoral luxation and generalized loss of detail throughout the abdomen. Attempts to catheterize the bladder were unsuccessful. The EU revealed that the kidneys, ureters, and bladder were intact. However, the bladder, while normally distensible, is severely displaced cranially. **Diagnosis:** Avulsion of the urethra from the urinary bladder distal to the urinary bladder sphincter.

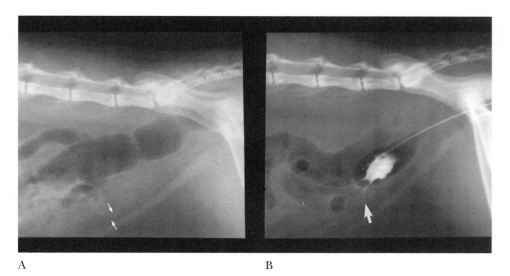

A   B

Figure 3–180. A 1-year-old neutered female domestic short-haired cat with urinary tract infections for the past 5 months. (A) There is a projection of a tubular-shaped, soft tissue density extending from the apex of the urinary bladder toward the umbilicus (*white arrows*). (B) The double contrast cystogram revealed contrast media within the tubular structure (*white arrow*). Differential diagnoses include persistent urachal remnant or cystic diverticulum due to other causes (trauma). **Diagnosis:** Persistent urachal remnant.

the middle ligament of the bladder. When this occurs, the cranial wall of the bladder remains regular and smooth. In some instances, involution is incomplete and the urachal remnant provides an outpouching of the bladder lumen on its cranioventral aspect (Fig. 3–180). Diverticulae and persistent urachal remnants provide an area for urine retention and stagnation. This situation predisposes to chronic cystitis.

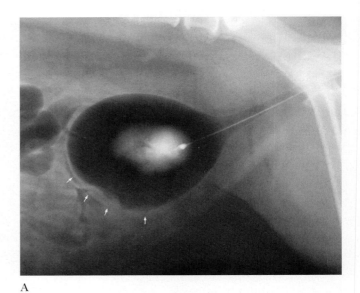

A

Figure 3–181. (A) A 10-year-old neutered female mixed breed dog with pollakiuria and hematuria for 2 months. Survey radiographs were normal. The double contrast cystogram revealed mild thickening of the cranial ventral portion of the bladder (*white arrows*). Differential diagnoses include cystitis, cystic neoplasia, or cystic granuloma. **Diagnosis:** Cystitis. (B) A 9-year-old male domestic short-haired cat with chronic hematuria. The lateral view of the positive-contrast cystogram revealed marked thickening of the cranial ventral part of the bladder. Contrast media has dissected partially through and under this mucosal thickening. **Diagnosis:** Cystitis with the dissection of contrast media into the submucosa. (C) A 5-year-old male Samoyed with chronic hematuria. The pneumocystogram revealed multiple, focal tissue densities projecting into the bladder lumen as well as marked thickening of the entire bladder wall. Differential diagnoses include polypoid cystitis or bladder neoplasia. **Diagnosis:** Polypoid cystitis.

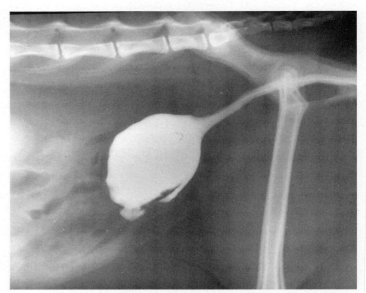

B

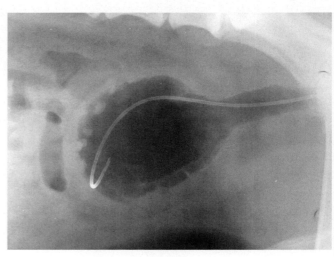

C

Infiltrative tumors may interfere with normal bladder distension and may alter the shape of the bladder. These also produce a mass within the bladder lumen that is much more easily detected on a cystogram than is the lack of bladder wall distensibility.

Bladder Wall Changes

Bladder wall changes are the most common cystographic abnormality. The normal bladder wall appears very smooth and consistent in thickness (approximately 1–2 mm). The appearance of even a few millimeters of increased thickness compared to the rest of the bladder wall is significant. Bladder wall thickening and irregularity, which is associated with the inflammation of cystitis, is usually seen in the cranial ventral aspect of the bladder (Fig. 3–181). This site is predisposed to change because it is normally the most dependent portion of the bladder; therefore, bacteria and other particulate matter tend to accumulate there. The entire bladder circumference may become thickened and irregular secondary to chronic inflammation. This is common in the sterile cystitis associated with cyclophosphamide therapy.[205–207] Bladder wall ulceration is most commonly associated with cystitis. The ulcers appear as small areas of contrast media adhering to the bladder wall (Fig. 3–182). The other major cause of bladder wall thickening is neoplasia. The most common tumor of the bladder is transitional cell carcinoma. This is usually focal in nature but may, on occasion, be generalized and diffuse. The mucosal surface may be smooth, but more commonly it is thrown up into folds with masses protruding into the lumen of the bladder. Occasionally, a focal tumor may cause bladder wall thickening on the cranial ventral aspect of the bladder making differentiation from cystitis difficult; however, tumor is more common at other sites, particularly the trigone (Fig. 3–183). Another tumor that may be identified radiographically is the botryoid rhabdomyosarcoma. This tumor is usually seen in young dogs (1–4 years of age) and is most commonly located on the dorsal surface of the trigone of the bladder. It consists typically of "cauliflower-shaped" fingers of tissue protruding into the bladder

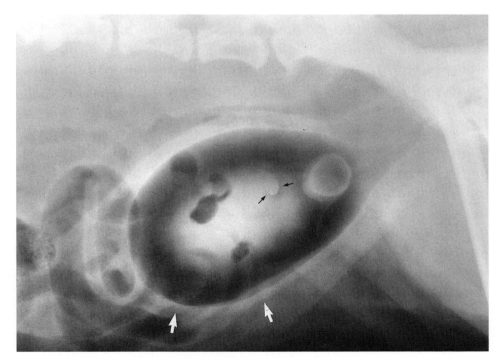

Figure 3–182. A 7-year-old female Yorkshire terrier with hematuria for 1 month. The survey radiographs were normal. A double contrast cystogram revealed an ulcer crater which retained contrast media when it was on the nondependent surface (*black arrows*). Differential diagnoses include cystitis or neoplasia with a mucosal ulcer. **Diagnosis:** Cystitis with a mucosal ulcer.

Figure 3–183. (A) A 14-year-old neutered female mixed breed dog with hematuria for 4 months. The EU revealed that there was a large sessile tissue density mass (*black arrows*) at the trigone of the bladder. Differential diagnoses include neoplasia (transitional cell carcinoma). (B) A 9-year-old neutered female Shetland sheepdog with hematuria for 4 weeks. A double contrast cystogram revealed multiple large, irregular masses within the bladder that have irregular surfaces and are associated with a thickened bladder wall. Differential diagnoses include bladder neoplasia, severe cystitis, or bladder granulomata. **Diagnosis:** Transitional cell carcinoma.

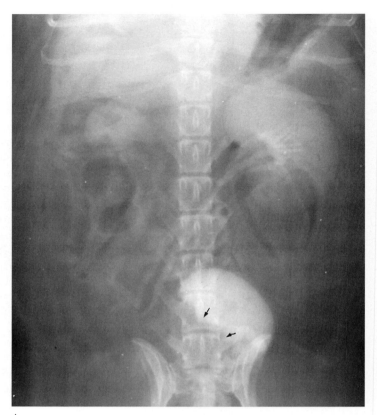

A

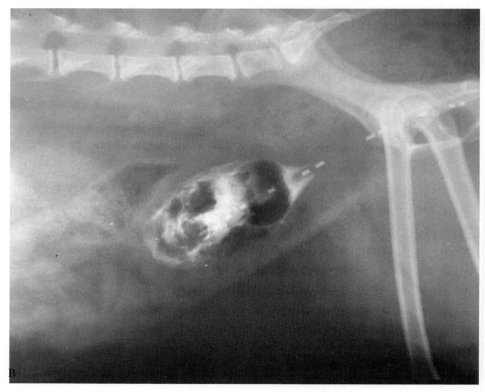

B

lumen (Fig. 3–184).[208] Other types of neoplasia (e.g., leiomyoma, leiomyosarcoma, polyp) may cause a smooth thickening of the wall, but there usually is some degree of mucosal irregularity and, more commonly, a mass protruding into the bladder lumen (Fig. 3–185).

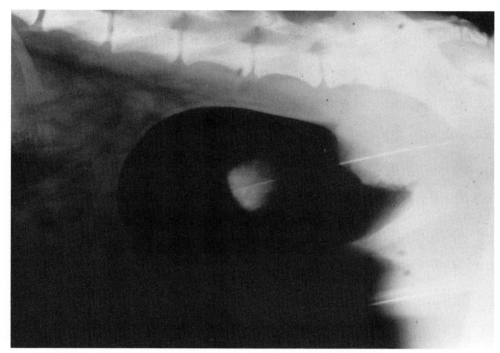

Figure 3–184. A 1-year-old male Irish setter with hematuria and stranguria for 5 months. Survey radiographs were normal. A double contrast cystogram revealed a cauliflower-like mass at the bladder trigone. Differential diagnoses include neoplasia or granuloma. **Diagnosis:** Embryonal rhabdomyosarcoma.

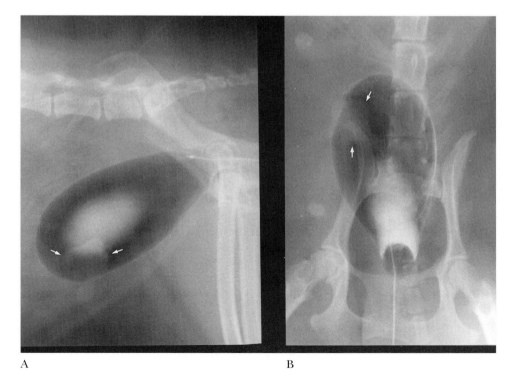

A   B

Figure 3–185. A 13-year-old female mixed breed dog with cystitis for 3 months. (A&B) There is a focal soft tissue mass present in the apex of the bladder (*white arrows*). There is minimal to no thickening of the bladder where it joins the borders of the mass. The surface of the mass is slightly irregular but not thrown into multiple folds. Differential diagnoses include neoplasia (benign-polyp or malignant-transitional cell carcinoma), adherent cystic blood clot, or granuloma. **Diagnosis:** Polyp in the urinary bladder.

Polypoid cystitis produces a generalized thickening of the bladder mucosa. Multiple smooth polypoid masses are evident throughout the entire bladder.[209] The fact that the entire bladder wall is usually involved helps to differentiate this condition from tumors.

Although it is usually easy to differentiate bladder tumor from chronic cystitis based on the location and appearance of the bladder wall irregularity, there are instances in which biopsy or urine cytology are needed for a definitive diagnosis. Lesions that are close to the area of the trigone should be evaluated by means of an excretory urogram in addition to the cystogram in order to determine the site of ureteral opening into the bladder. This is especially important if surgical removal of the bladder tumor is anticipated.

Another type of bladder wall change is a rupture or tear. This is usually due to trauma but occasionally is seen with other diseases. The tear will frequently develop a fibrin seal over the rent, which allows partial bladder filling. Eventually, bladder distension stretches the bladder wall and this exceeds the strength of the fibrin seal. A sequence of partial sealing and subsequent rupture develops; this releases urine into the abdominal cavity. To assess bladder rupture by cystography, one must produce adequate distension to test for a partial bladder seal. Positive-contrast cystography or excretory urography should be used instead of pneumocystography if rupture of the urinary bladder is suspected. Detection of air leakage in the presence of moderate or significant hydroperitoneum is difficult. The leak will be readily detected when a positive-contrast medium is used because there will clearly be positive-contrast distributed throughout the abdomen (Fig. 3–186). Bladder rupture may be retroperitoneal or into the pelvic cavity. In those cases, the positive contrast will be contained within the pelvic cavity or retroperitoneal space and may not diffuse into the peritoneal cavity.

Trauma to the bladder wall during cystography may result in injection of contrast material beneath the bladder mucosa. This produces a linear accumulation of contrast material which is fixed in position within the bladder despite changes in the patient's position.[167] It does not usually result in a serious injury to the bladder and the contrast is gradually absorbed.

Intraluminal Bladder Abnormalities

A double contrast cystogram (our generally recommended contrast procedure for evaluating the bladder) is the procedure of choice to determine the presence of material within the bladder. On the double contrast cystogram the contrast puddle should be evaluated carefully. Air bubbles, if present, will be radiolucent and usually are located at the periphery of the puddle (due to capillary action). If not on the periphery, the air bubbles usually are perfectly round (Fig. 3–187). Radiolucent calculi also produce filling defects. Usually, these are irregularly shaped, relatively small, and are found in the "center" of the contrast puddle (the most dependent portion of the bladder) (Fig. 3–188). Small radiolucent calculi may be overlooked in a pneumocystogram, but unless a large amount of positive contrast is used they are easily identified on a double contrast cystogram.[144] Blood clots may be seen in the center of the contrast puddle and may be round, wedge-shaped, or irregularly shaped filling defects with very smooth, distinct borders. They are usually larger (in some cases markedly larger) than most radiolucent calculi (Figs. 3–189 and 3–190). Blood clots will usually move with changes in the patient's position and this helps to distinguish them from tumors, which are fixed in location.[144] In cases where blood clots are noted with no other bladder abnormalities, the kidneys should be carefully examined because they are sometimes the source of the hemorrhage. Other material, such as strands of mucus or other cellular debris, may be noted. Mucus will usually produce thin linear filling defects. Cellular debris may produce small, amorphous filling defects (Fig. 3-191).

Several foreign bodies have been described within the urinary bladder. Some of these, such as air rifle pellets, are radiopaque and can be identified on the noncontrast radiograph. Others, such as fragments of urinary catheters or migrating plant

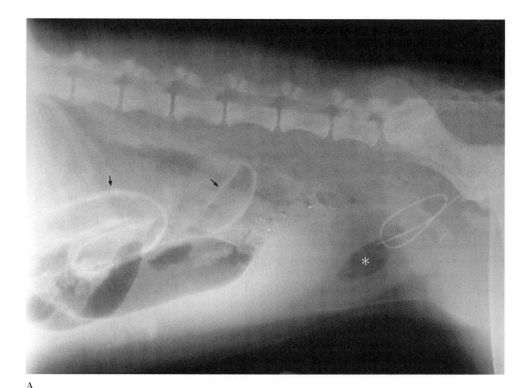

A

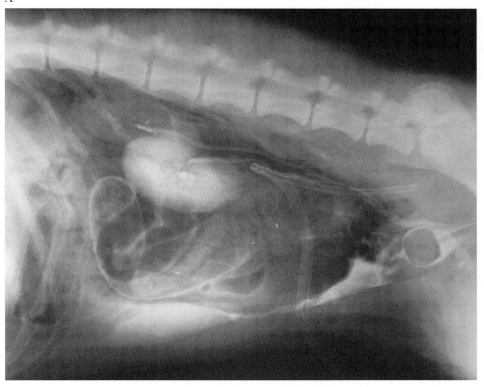

Figure 3–186. A 1-year-old female German shepherd dog that had been hit by a car. (A) There are fracture fragments from the pelvic floor cranial to the pubis. There is a generalized loss of contrast throughout the abdomen and there is a dynamic ileus. A catheter is in the urinary bladder and air has been instilled. A minimally distended, apparently intact bladder (*white **) is seen. Very careful examination revealed the serosal margins of some dilated small intestinal loops were apparent (*black arrows*)—this indicates leakage of air into the abdomen. (B) An EU, performed the next day after a Foley urinary catheter and an abdominal drain were placed, revealed obvious leakage of contrast media into the abdominal cavity from the urinary bladder. This demonstrated the superiority of positive-contrast techniques in assessing possible tears in the urinary tract. **Diagnosis:** Ruptured urinary bladder.

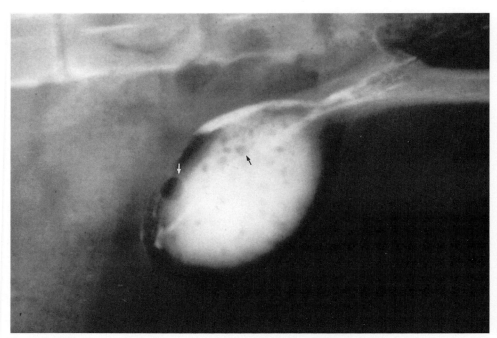

Figure 3–187. A 4-year-old female domestic short-haired cat with pollakiuria and hematuria for 2 weeks. The survey radiographs were normal. A double contrast cystogram was incorrectly performed by instilling contrast media followed by air. The study revealed multiple filling defects in the contrast media. Some are nearly perfectly round and on the periphery of the contrast, which suggests that they are air bubbles (*white arrow*). Others are somewhat irregular suggesting that they are radiolucent cystic calculi (*black arrow*). **Diagnosis:** Multiple radiolucent calculi.

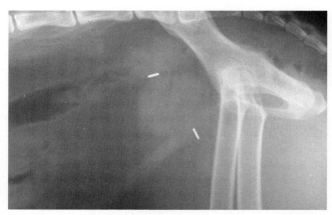

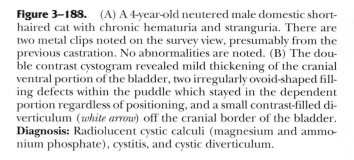

Figure 3–188. (A) A 4-year-old neutered male domestic short-haired cat with chronic hematuria and stranguria. There are two metal clips noted on the survey view, presumably from the previous castration. No abnormalities are noted. (B) The double contrast cystogram revealed mild thickening of the cranial ventral portion of the bladder, two irregularly ovoid-shaped filling defects within the puddle which stayed in the dependent portion regardless of positioning, and a small contrast-filled diverticulum (*white arrow*) off the cranial border of the bladder. **Diagnosis:** Radiolucent cystic calculi (magnesium and ammonium phosphate), cystitis, and cystic diverticulum.

A

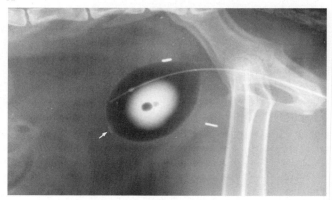

B

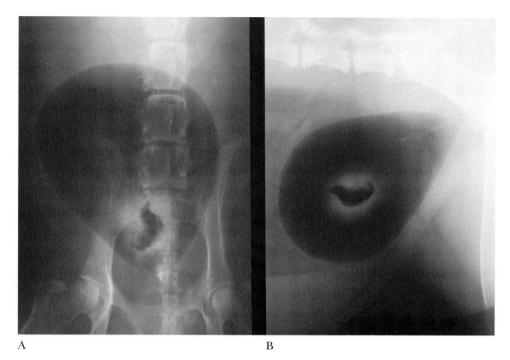

A   B

Figure 3–189. A 4-year-old female mixed breed dog with hematuria for 6 weeks. (A&B) The double contrast cystogram revealed a small filling defect within the contrast puddle on both views. This indicated that the mass is moveable within the bladder. The smooth borders and size suggest that a calculus is unlikely. Differential diagnoses include blood clot or calculus. **Diagnosis:** Intravesicular blood clot secondary to hematuria from a right renal adenocarcinoma.

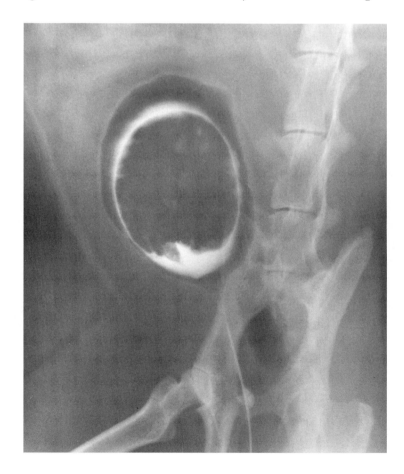

Figure 3–190. An 8-year-old neutered male Siamese cat with chronic hematuria. There is a very large filling defect within the center of the contrast puddle. The bladder wall shows moderate irregularity and thickening consistent with cystitis. Differential diagnoses include intravesicular blood clot, neoplasm, or radiolucent calculus. **Diagnosis:** Intravesicular blood clot secondary to hematuria due to cystitis.

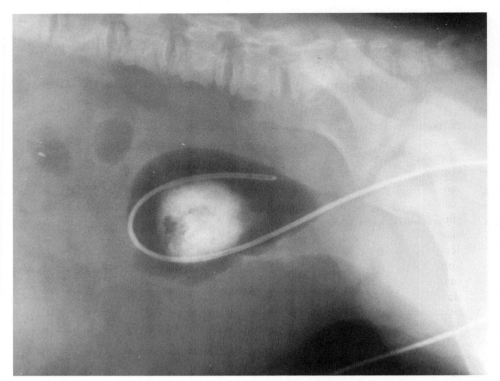

Figure 3–191. A 2-month-old male akita with hematuria and stranguria. There is mild thickening of the bladder with irregular mucosal thickening and small linear and round defects within the puddle of contrast media. Differential diagnoses include cystitis with intracystic debris or neoplasia. **Diagnosis:** Cystitis and intracystic debris (excess mucus and desquamated epithelium).

awns, can only be detected by cystography. Catheter fragments produce a filling defect within the contrast puddle during double contrast cystography. A pair of parallel radiolucent lines with contrast in the center (the catheter lumen) is typically seen with retained catheter fragments.[144] Although plant awns are uncommon, they will produce an irregularly shaped filling defect with distinct margins within the contrast puddle.

Position of the Urinary Bladder

Occasionally, the location of the bladder may not be apparent on the survey radiograph. This may be due to displacement of the bladder into a hernia, a very small bladder, or confusion of the bladder with other caudal abdominal masses. A cystogram may be helpful in these cases to clearly identify the location of the urinary bladder. A pneumocystogram is usually sufficient for this purpose. If the bladder is displaced into a hernia, the catheter should be passed carefully to avoid traumatizing the urethra. Retroflexion of the bladder can be recognized from the position of the urethra. The urethra will fold back upon itself and the vertex of the urinary bladder will be caudal to the bladder neck. Positioning of the bladder neck within the pelvic canal can be demonstrated during a contrast cystogram. If the bladder does not displace cranially as it is distended, the possibility of a pelvic bladder should be considered. The significance of this is controversial; however, in some female dogs it has been associated with incontinence.[202–204]

Ultrasound of the Abnormal Bladder

Ultrasound works best when the bladder is distended with urine, is within the abdominal rather than the pelvic cavity, and is not obscured by intestinal contents. It is ideally suited for evaluating the bladder wall and lumen.[32]

The bladder can be differentiated easily from other caudal abdominal masses such as the prostate, a retained testicle, lymph node, or uterus. On the other hand, it may be difficult to distinguish between the urinary bladder and a paraprostatic cyst. A careful ultrasound examination, however, usually identifies the cyst as a distinct structure separate from the urinary bladder. A uterus filled with fluid may also mimic a urinary bladder; however, identifying both uterine horns, multiple fluid-filled loops, or recognizing the tubular shape of the uterus will help discriminate between these structures.

The shape of the bladder is influenced by transducer pressure. Consequently, a careful examination of the bladder from all angles is important before a diagnosis of an abnormally shaped bladder is made. Bladder shape alteration is usually accompanied by bladder wall abnormalities, such as thickening or irregularity, so the diagnosis usually is not difficult.

Cystitis and tumors produce similar bladder wall abnormalities (Fig. 3–192). Cystitis may involve the entire bladder circumference and may produce a thickened bladder wall with a submucosal hypoechoic zone (Figs. 3–193, 3–194, and 3–195). More often, cystitis produces a focal bladder wall thickening at the cranioventral aspect of the bladder. A urachal diverticulum may be identified during the ultrasound examination as a focal defect in the bladder wall. The wall usually is thickened and irregular and the anechoic urine helps to define the defect. Most urachal diverticulae are small and detecting them using ultrasound and distinguishing them from cystitis is difficult. The fibrotic remnant of the closed urachus has been identified as a heteroechoic structure extending cranially from the bladder wall. This probably represented an abnormal urachus that was not patent at the time of the examination.

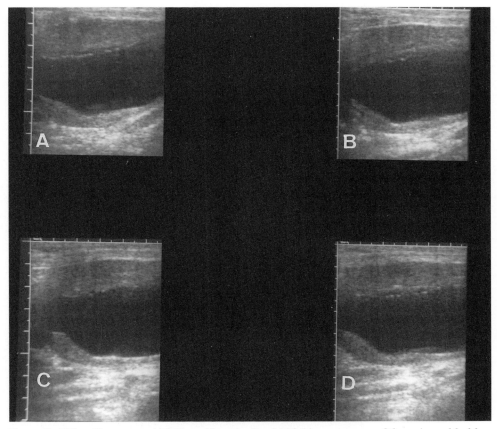

Figure 3–192. Transverse (A&B) and longitudinal (C&D) sonograms of the urinary bladder of a 5-year-old female rottweiler with a history of pyrexia and anorexia of 10 days' duration. There is marked thickening of the bladder wall. The entire bladder was involved. This is indicative of an inflammatory or infiltrative lesion of the bladder. **Diagnosis:** Lymphosarcoma.

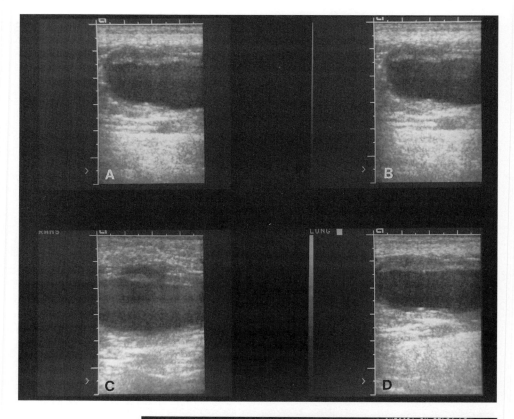

Figure 3–193. Longitudinal (A,B,&D) and transverse (C) sonograms of the urinary bladder of an 8-year-old spayed female Australian shepherd with a history of autoimmune hemolytic anemia, which had been treated with cytoxan for 3 months. The bladder wall is thickened and the contour is irregular. This is indicative of chronic cystitis. **Diagnosis:** Cytoxan cystitis.

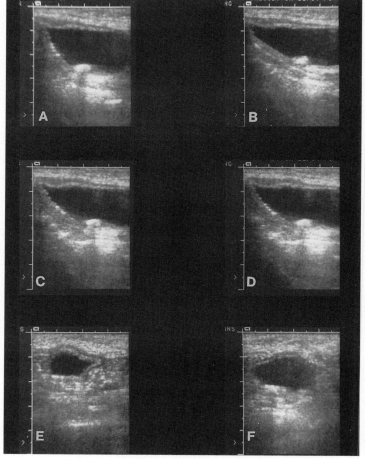

Figure 3–194. Longitudinal (A,B,C,&D) and transverse (E&F) sonograms of the urinary bladder of a 9-year-old spayed female schnauzer with a history of vomiting and diarrhea of 1 week's duration. There is a hyperechoic structure within the urinary bladder. The bladder wall is slightly thickened. This is indicative of cystitis with a cystic calculus. **Diagnosis:** Cystitis and cystic calculus.

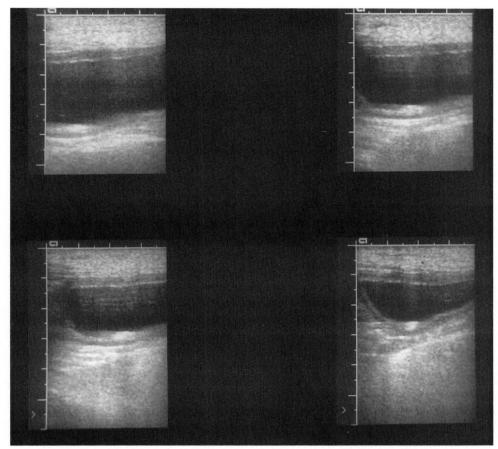

Figure 3–195. Longitudinal sonograms of the urinary bladder of a 5-year-old female mixed breed dog with a history of hematuria and dysuria of 3 weeks' duration. The bladder wall is thickened. Mineral material is present in the dependent portion of the bladder. The findings are indicative of cystitis with fine sand or calculi. **Diagnosis:** Cystitis with multiple small cystic calculi.

Usually, tumors can be detected easily as heteroechoic structures protruding into the bladder lumen (Figs. 3–196 and 3–197). The attachment of the mass to the bladder wall is often abrupt and thickening of the bladder wall at the site of attachment can usually be recognized.[210] Differentiating between an attached blood clot and a bladder tumor may be impossible.

A focal area of bladder wall thickening may be observed at the trigone of the bladder. This is the ureteral papillae and should not be mistaken for a focal mass or polyp. Careful examination using high frequency transducers permits identification of the ureter within the bladder wall or allows detection of the jet of urine that enters the bladder from the ureter.

Intraluminal objects, such as crystals, cells, calculi, blood clots, and air bubbles, may be observed during the ultrasound examination. Crystalline material, cells, air bubbles, and fat globules can be observed floating within the usually anechoic urine. Agitation of the bladder will increase the movement of these structures. Air bubbles may produce reverberation artifacts (comet tails) that help to distinguish them from other floating objects. They will eventually float to the top of the urinary bladder. A large amount of air present within the urinary bladder, either from catheterization or from emphysematous cystitis, can interfere with the ultrasound examination. The air is recognized easily because it is highly echogenic and produces reverberation artifacts. Moving the patient will help to discriminate between air in the lumen (which moves) versus air in the bladder wall (which is fixed). Crystals and cells eventually

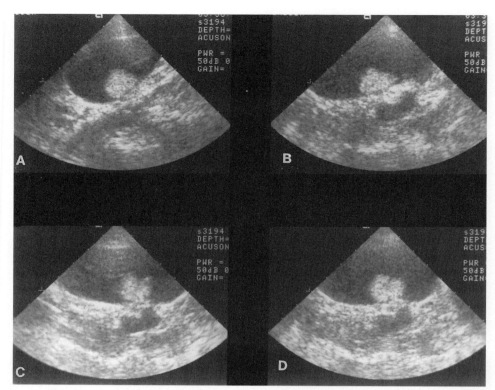

Figure 3–196.   Longitudinal (A,B,&C) and transverse (D) sonograms of the urinary bladder of a 12-year-old spayed female mixed breed dog who presented for evaluation of a cutaneous hemangiosarcoma. The dog was otherwise asymptomatic and the ultrasound examination was performed to investigate the possibility of abdominal neoplasia. There is a hyperechoic well-defined mass attached to the dorsal bladder wall. This mass appears to be pedunculated and remained fixed in position despite movement of the patient. This is indicative of a bladder mass. **Diagnosis:** Hemangioma.

Figure   3–197.   Transverse (A&B) and longitudinal (C&D) sonograms of the urinary bladder of a 10-year-old male mixed breed dog with a history of stranguria, hematuria, and incontinence of 3 months' duration. There is a heteroechoic mass associated with the right dorsal bladder wall. This mass is fixed in position and represents a tumor. **Diagnosis:** Transitional cell carcinoma.

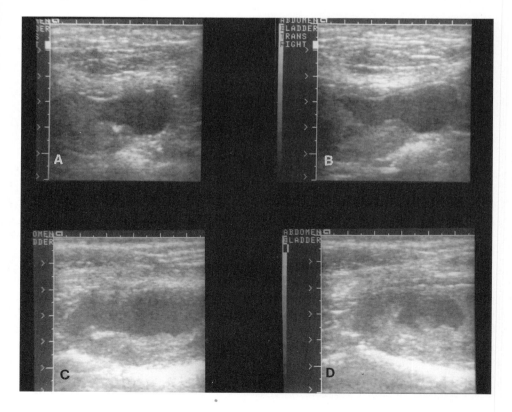

settle to the dependent part of the urinary bladder and can form a thick layer if present in large numbers. Although crystals tend to produce brighter echoes than cells, an exact diagnosis is difficult.

Urinary catheters produce paired parallel hyperechoic lines within the urinary bladder (Fig. 3–198). When a Foley catheter is in place, the balloon is also easily recognized because of its shape.

Blood clots settle to the dependent portion of the urinary bladder and will move with changes in the patient's position. Blood clots are heteroechoic and may be confused with bladder tumors. Movement of the patient and the resulting change in position of the heteroechoic mass helps determine that the lesion is a blood clot rather than a neoplasm (Fig. 3–199).

Urinary calculi are hyperechoic and often shadow (Figs. 3–194, 3–195, 3–200, and

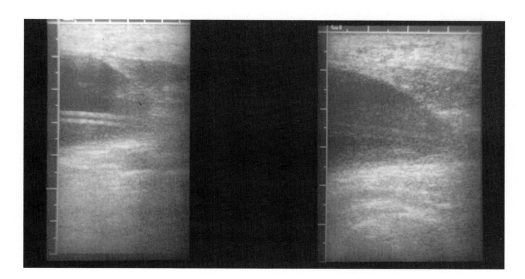

Figure 3–198. Longitudinal sonograms of the urinary bladder of a 13-year-old spayed female pit bull with a history of hematuria which was secondary to a transitional cell carcinoma of the bladder. The dog was undergoing chemotherapy. There is an echogenic structure composed of two parallel lines located within the urinary bladder. This represents a urinary catheter. **Diagnosis:** Catheter within the urinary bladder.

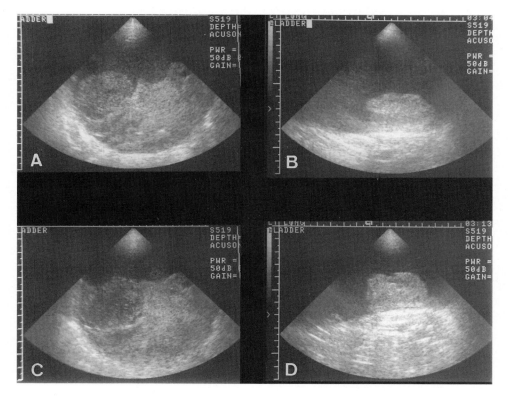

Figure 3–199. Transverse (A&C) and longitudinal (B&D) sonograms of the urinary bladder of a 4-year-old male Great Dane with a history of hematuria of four months' duration. There is an echogenic mass within the urinary bladder. The mass changes position and shape with changes in the dog's position and always remains in the dorsal (dependent) portion of the urinary bladder. This indicates that the mass is not arising from or attached to the bladder wall and therefore represents a blood clot rather than a bladder wall mass. **Diagnosis:** Blood clot in the urinary bladder.

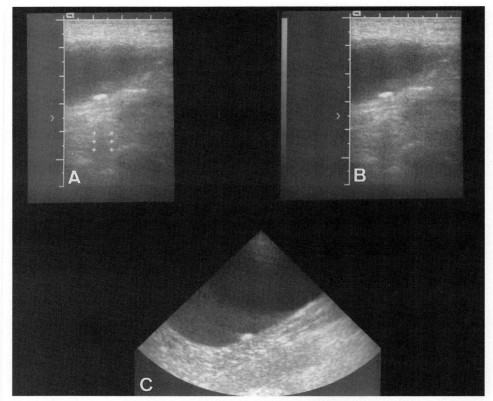

Figure 3–200. Longitudinal sonograms of the urinary bladder of an 11-year-old female dachshund with a history of abdominal distension and polycythemia. There is a highly echogenic cystic calculus visible in all three images. Shadowing is present deep to the cystic calculus. It is most obvious in the first image (*white arrows*), is less evident in "B," and there is no shadowing observed in "C." **Diagnosis:** Cystic calculus.

3–201). Although shadowing is not always present, when identified it indicates the presence of calculi. Calculi settle to the dependent portion of the bladder and move with agitation of the bladder or changes in patient position.(Fig. 3–202) The colon can produce a hyperechoic shadow adjacent to the urinary bladder and can appear to be within the bladder. Examination of the bladder from several different angles will prevent this mistake.[211]

Bladder wall mineralization can be identified as a hyperechoic area within the bladder, which also shadows. The lesion will be fixed in location when the patient is moved or the bladder is agitated, and this helps to determine that the lesion is within the bladder wall rather than within the lumen.

Air within the urinary bladder produces a hyperechoic lesion that can be recognized as air rather than mineral, because it floats to the top (non-dependent surface) of the urinary bladder and produces a reverberation artifact (comet tail) (see Fig. 3–202). If the air is trapped within the bladder wall, such as in emphysematous cystitis, the reverberation artifact will still occur and the lesion can be recognized as air despite the fact that it does not change position in response to gravity.

URETHRA

In the male and female dog the urethra differs greatly in length, while in cats its length is similar in both sexes.[146,159,160,161] The urethra in both species and sexes is a smooth tube of nearly constant diameter connecting the bladder neck to the urethral orifice. Abnormalities detectable on survey radiographs are limited. Radiopaque calculi may be seen anywhere along the length of the urethra but are most commonly lodged at the ischial arch, at the base of the os penis in the male dog, or

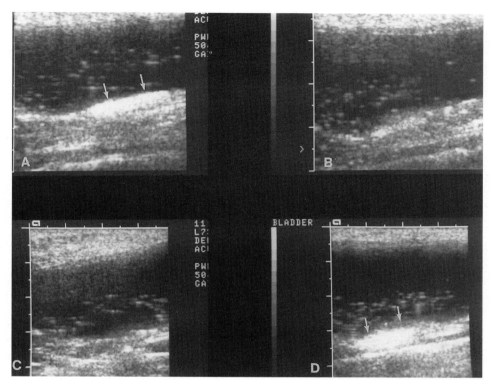

Figure 3–201. Longitudinal sonograms (A,B,C,&D) of the urinary bladder of a 4-year-old spayed female English cocker spaniel who presented with a history of lumbosacral pain. There is echogenic material in the dependent portion of the urinary bladder. In scans A and D the material is predominantly layered on the dorsal (dependent) surface (*arrows*). In scans B, C, and D the bladder has been agitated and the material is evident floating within the urine. **Diagnosis:** Sand or fine calculi within the urinary bladder.

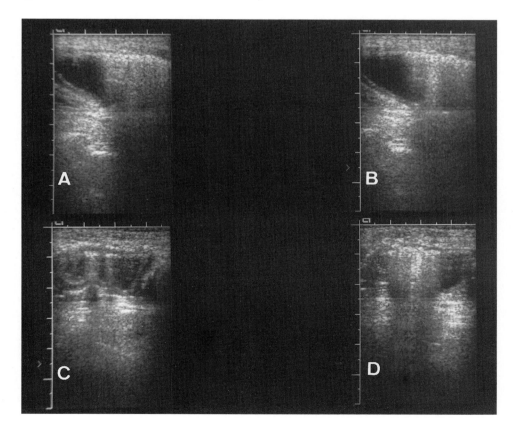

Figure 3–202. Longitudinal (A&B) and transverse (C&D) sonograms of the urinary bladder of a 14-year-old spayed female mixed breed dog with a history of polyuria and polydipsia. There is a hyperechoic region within the urinary bladder with a reverberation artifact indicating the presence of air. This region was consistent in position despite changes in the dog's position. It is indicative of air within the bladder wall. **Diagnosis:** Emphysematous cystitis.

at the urethral papilla in the female dog (Fig. 3–203). Urethral calculi are rarely seen in the cat but may lodge within the penile urethra. Occasionally, fractures of the os penis may be seen, and if significant callus has formed this may interfere with urination.

A urethrogram is required in many urethral diseases to characterize the lesions.[144,157] The normal urethrogram should outline a smooth, regular tube throughout the entire urethral length with slight narrowing at the ischial arch and pelvic brim in the male dog. The colliculus seminalis may be noticeable as a dorsal filling defect in the prostatic urethra (Fig. 3–204).[168] In some normal male dogs, the prostatic urethra may appear narrow but the borders will be smooth and regular.

Density and Shape Changes

Radiolucent urethral calculi may be seen on the urethrogram (Fig. 3–205). These will appear as irregularly shaped radiolucencies, usually small in size, within the column of contrast media. It is important that proper urethrographic technique is followed so that air bubbles are not introduced during contrast injection and mistaken for calculi. Air bubbles are usually smooth and round or oval in shape. They may fill the urethra but do not distend it, and when they are large they become more oval or elongated rather than distorting the urethral lumen. Calculi are often more irregular in shape with uneven margins. When they are large they will distort the urethral contour.[144,157] Although not a totally reliable differentiating feature, air bubbles are often easily displaced during successive contrast injections while calculi tend to remain in a fixed position. Radiolucent calculi can be detected during urethral catheterization, and the contrast urethrogram is performed to document or determine the number and location of the calculi that are present.

Rupture of the urethra may occur as a result of trauma or tearing by urethral calculi. In urethral rupture, the urethrogram will reveal extravasation of contrast media from the lumen (Fig. 3–206). If the rupture involves the distal urethra in males, the

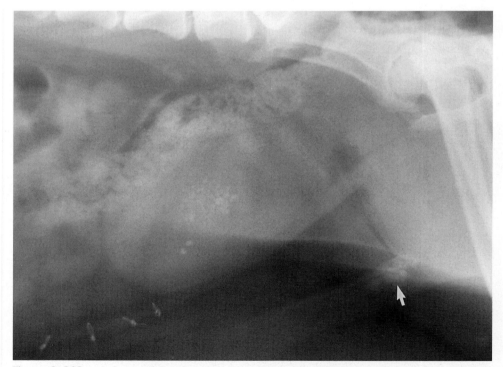

Figure 3–203. A 6-year-old male miniature schnauzer with chronic hematuria and acute stranguria. There are radiodense calculi visible in the bladder. There are also calculi seen in the urethra at the level of the os penis (*white arrow*). Healed pelvic fractures are noted as an incidental finding. **Diagnosis:** Cystic and urethral calculi.

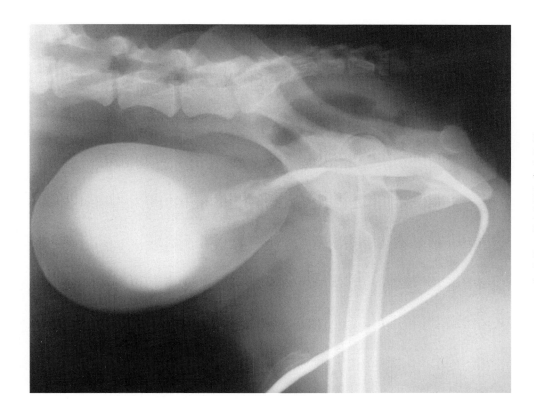

Figure 3–204. A 4-year-old male Weimaraner with hematuria. The urethrogram was within normal limits. The apparent narrowing through the prostatic urethra is normal. Differential diagnoses include normal or prostatic disease (the urethrogram may be normal in the face of early prostatic pathology). **Diagnosis:** Normal urethrogram.

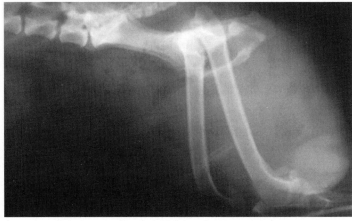

A

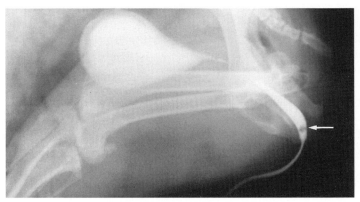

B

Figure 3–205. A 12-year-old male mixed breed dog with pollakiuria and hematuria for 3 weeks and tenesmus for 1 week. (A) The survey radiograph revealed no gross abnormalities. (B) The urethrogram revealed an irregularly bordered filling defect (*white arrow*) in the urethra in the area of the ischial arch. Differential diagnoses include radiolucent urethral calculus or urethral polyp. **Diagnosis:** Radiolucent urethral calculus.

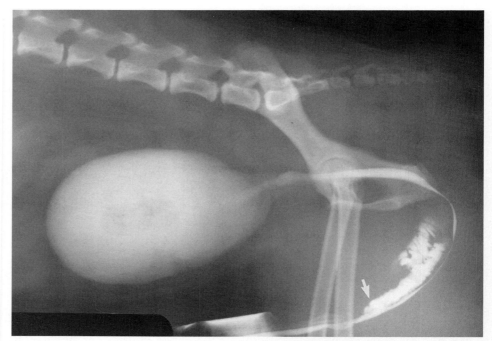

Figure 3–206. A 10-year-old male poodle with urinary obstruction, pyrexia, and swelling of the inguinal and perineal areas. There were three radiopaque calculi located approximately 2 cm proximal to the base of the os penis as well as several cystic calculi seen on the survey radiograph. The urethrogram revealed extravasation of contrast media into the corpus cavernosum urethra (*white arrow*) at the site of the urethral calculi. The urethra proximal to this is narrowed, which may be the result of urethral spasm or periurethral edema or fibrosis. **Diagnosis:** Ruptured urethra secondary to urethral calculi, urethral spasm, and cystic calculi.

contrast media may be seen entering the corpus cavernosum urethra where it will appear as if in multiple small contiguous compartments. It may be possible to see the contrast media being carried through the vascular system into the veins of the pelvic area. If the tear occurs proximal to the level where the corpus cavernosum joins the urethra, the contrast will be seen in the periurethral tissues dissecting along fascial planes or accumulating within the pelvic canal.

Urethral carcinoma and granulomatous urethritis are most commonly seen in the female dog.[212–214] These usually are manifested by focal or diffuse irregularity of the urethral lumen (Fig. 3–207). They are nearly impossible to differentiate radiographically and exfoliative cytology may be necessary to reach a diagnosis.[212] In some cases of neoplasia, the lesion is predominately in the periurethral area. This produces displacement of the normal urethral position, but a normal smooth mucosal surface persists. Urethral neoplasia is seen occasionally in the male dog (Fig. 3–208).[144,157,213,214]

In the male, periurethral fibrosis (presumably due to trauma or previous urethral rupture, surgery, or inflammation) may be seen as an area of decreased urethral lumen size with a normal urethral mucosal pattern (Fig. 3–209). Because the contrast injection is made retrograde, the urethra will be dilated distal to the site of urethral stricture or narrowing. Usually, the point of narrowing must be documented on two views or two contrast injections so that urethral spasm is not mistaken for a stricture. The urethra is normally narrower at the pelvic brim and at the ischial arch. These should not be confused with strictures. If a questionable area is detected, the catheter should be positioned as close as possible to the suspicious area and a contrast injection performed at that location.

Congenital anomalies, such as urethrorectal fistulae, urethral diverticulae, and duplicate urethra, have also been demonstrated by urethrography (Fig. 3–210). The

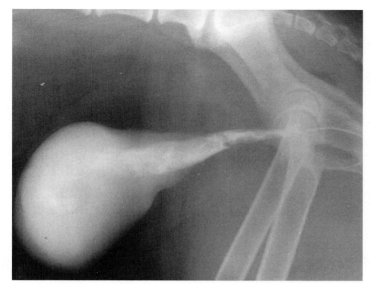

A

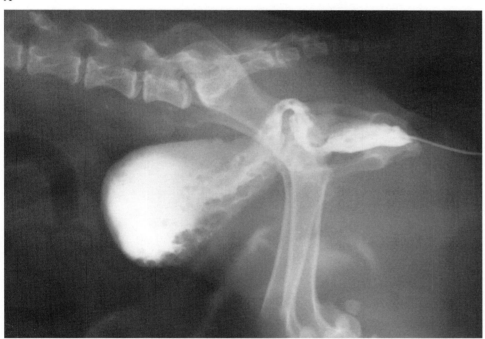
B

Figure 3–207. (A) A 12-year-old female mixed breed dog with chronic stranguria. There was marked irregularity of the urethra with multiple filling defects in both views. Differential diagnoses include urethritis or urethral neoplasia. **Diagnosis:** Chronic urethritis. (B) An 11-year-old neutered female German shepherd with stranguria for 2 months. There was marked tortuosity of the urethra with marked mucosal irregularity which extended into the bladder. Differential diagnoses include urethral neoplasia, inflammation, or periurethral fibrosis. **Diagnosis:** Transitional cell carcinoma involving the bladder and urethra.

contrast will be observed entering the rectum if a fistula is present.[215] Urethral diverticulae are easily identified as outpouchings of the urethra that contain contrast material. These outpouchings should be consistent on two views or on the same view after two separate contrast injections.

Urethral Ultrasound

The urethra does not lend itself to ultrasound examination because it is contained within the pelvic canal. The prostatic urethra may be observed as an anechoic linear or oval area within the prostate if the prostate is enlarged and displaced out of the pelvic canal. In most cases, the prostatic urethra is not identified. Calculi may be identified within the urethra as hyperechoic focal lesions that shadow; however, this is rarely observed and is not necessary for the diagnosis or evaluation of urinary calculi. Urethral carcinoma may extend onto the bladder neck, and this lesion may be

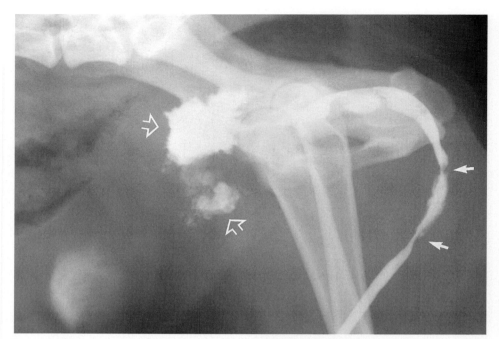

Figure 3–208. A 9-year-old male Samoyed with stranguria for 3 weeks. The urethrogram revealed irregularity to the urethral mucosa immediately distal to the ischial arch (*solid white arrows*) as well as cavitation of the prostate (*open white arrows*) and prostatic enlargement. Differential diagnoses include prostatic neoplasia with extension to the urethra or cavitating prostatitis and urethritis. **Diagnosis:** Prostatic carcinoma with extension down the urethra.

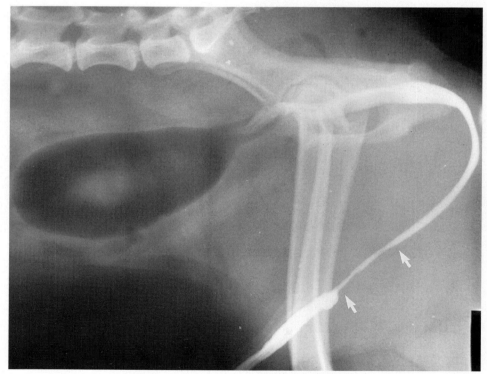

Figure 3–209. A 7-year-old male cocker spaniel with chronic stranguria. The urethrogram revealed narrowing of the urethra proximal to the os penis (*white arrows*), which was present on multiple views. The differential diagnoses include urethral neoplasia or periurethral fibrosis. **Diagnosis:** Periurethral fibrosis.

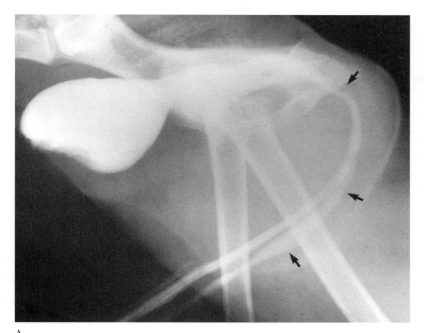

A

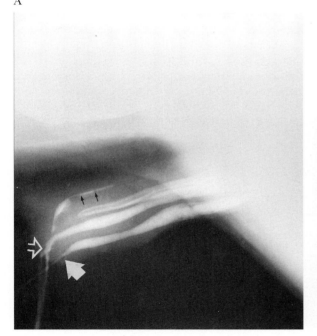

B

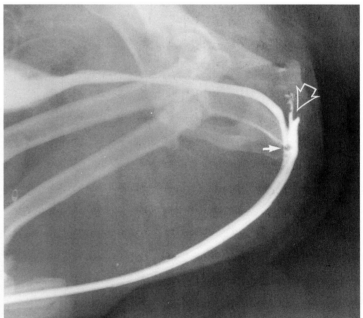

C

Figure 3–210. (A) A 1-year-old male Siberian husky with chronic hematuria. The retrograde urethrogram revealed filling of a second tubular structure (*black arrows*) which arises near the prostate and extends to the area of the distal urethra. There are no septations, which would indicate leakage of contrast media into the corpus cavernosum urethra present. (B) A voiding urethrogram of the distal penis revealed the normal urethral orifice (*open white arrow*), contrast media in the space between the penis and prepuce (*black arrows*), and the termination of the second tubular structure on the distal prepuce (*solid white arrow*). **Diagnosis:** Incomplete duplicate urethra. (C) A 5-year-old male Lhasa apso that had a cystotomy for cystic calculi 1 year prior to examination. The dog had been pollakiuric and passing sand for 1 day. The survey radiographs were normal. A retrograde urethrogram revealed a small radiolucent calculus (*solid white arrow*) at the ischial arch and a blind ended extension of the urethra into the soft tissues (*open white arrow*). **Diagnosis:** Radiolucent urethral calculus and urethral diverticulum.

identified using ultrasound. An increase in the urethral diameter producing a heteroechoic round or oval structure without an increase in the size of the urethral lumen is usually observed in these cases.

GENITAL SYSTEM

Contrast techniques such as vaginography and hysterosalpingography to visualize portions of the female genital system have been described but are not used routinely.[35,36,216,217] Vaginography has been used to demonstrate ectopic ureter. Contrast is injected into the vagina allowing for the demonstration of flow into the urethra and into the ectopic ureter.

ABNORMAL FINDINGS

OVARIES

Although normally not visible, the ovaries, which are located just caudal to the kidneys, may enlarge. Cysts are the most common cause of enlargement; however, neoplasia and hemorrhage must also be considered as causes of ovarian enlargement (Fig. 3–211). The position of the adjacent kidney is an important clue to the presence of an ovarian mass, because the kidney may be cranially and laterally displaced. Ovarian tumors are often accompanied by a large amount of peritoneal fluid and this masks their presence.

UTERUS AND VAGINA

The uterus is not readily visualized unless it becomes enlarged.[34,218] In a fat dog, the uterine body may be visible dorsal to or superimposed upon the bladder and ventral to the colon on the lateral radiograph. When enlarged, the uterus becomes visible as a tubular-shaped soft tissue structure that displaces the small intestine cranially, dorsally, and toward the midline. The uterus folds upon itself and appears oval or sausage shaped. Although fluid-filled distended loops of intestine may create a similar appearance, the presence of gas within the intestines is an important feature that helps to distinguish between an enlarged uterus and distended small intestines. Enlargement of the uterus may be due to pregnancy, postpartum, hemorrhage, infection (pyometra or endometritis), accumulation of secretions (such as mucometra or

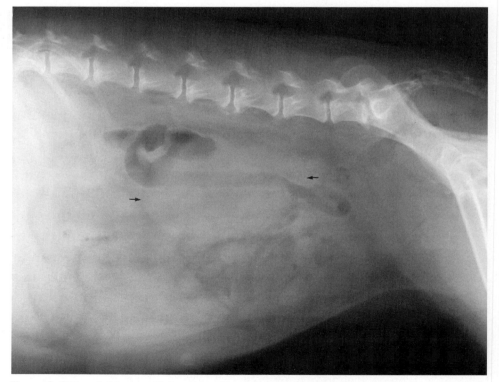

Figure 3–211. A 14-year-old female collie with polyuria and polydipsia for 3 months and a palpably enlarged spleen. There is a soft tissue-dense mass (*black arrows*) caudal to the left kidney. Differential diagnoses include enlarged left ovary, intestinal mass, or mesenteric lymph node. **Diagnosis:** Left ovarian papillary adenocarcinoma.

hydrometra), or neoplasia (Fig. 3–212). In both the dog and the cat the differentiation of these conditions may be difficult based solely on radiographic signs. If the cervix is open, allowing the uterus to drain, or if it is early on in the process, the uterus may not be readily apparent. In these instances, the use of abdominal compression may aid in defining the uterus (Fig. 3–213). Displacing the intestines cranially away from the urinary bladder often allows the uterine body to become visible

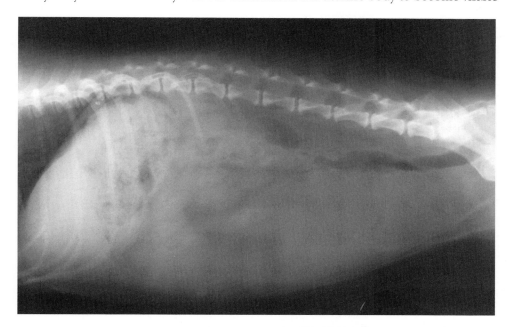

Figure 3–212. A 7-year-old female domestic short-haired cat with anorexia for 2 days. The lateral radiograph revealed massive uterine enlargement which displaced the abdominal organs cranially and slightly dorsally. Differential diagnoses include uterine enlargement (pregnancy, pyometra, or mucometra), distension of the urinary bladder, or mass arising from the caudal abdominal organs. **Diagnosis:** Pyometra.

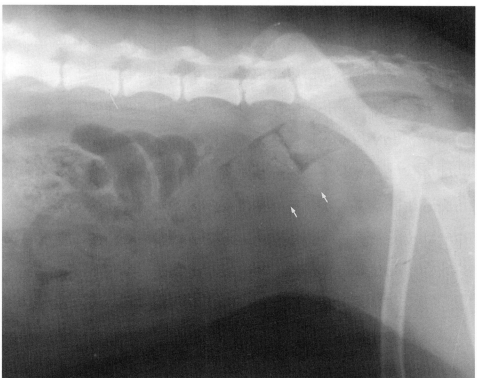

Figure 3–213. A 7-year-old female Brittany spaniel with polyuria and polydipsia for 1 week. The survey radiographs were within normal limits. Because pyometra was a strong clinical suspicion, a lateral compression ("spoon") view was performed. This revealed a visible uterus that was larger than normal (normally the uterus is not seen). Differential diagnoses include pyometra, endometritis, or mucometra. **Diagnosis:** Pyometra.

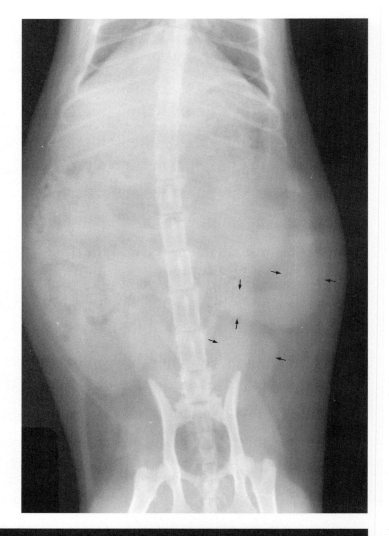

Figure 3–214. A 7-year-old female domestic short-haired cat with anorexia and depression for 3 days. The ventrodorsal radiograph revealed segmented tubular densities (*black arrows*) in the lateral portions of the caudal abdomen. Differential diagnoses include pyometra or pregnancy. **Diagnosis:** Pyometra.

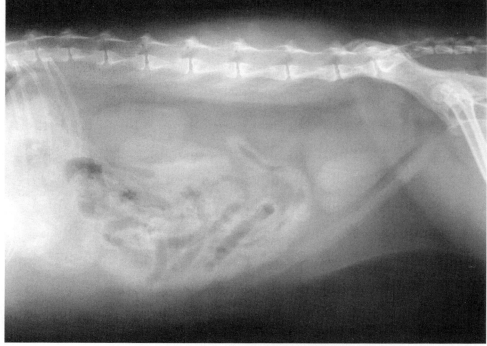

Figure 3–215. A 12-year-old neutered female domestic short-haired cat with anorexia for 5 days. The lateral radiograph revealed a mass between the bladder and colon. Differential diagnoses include uterine stump infection or neoplasm. **Diagnosis:** Abscess of the uterine stump.

because it cannot be displaced. While pyometra usually involves the entire uterus, only one horn or only one portion of one horn may be affected. In cats, uterine infection may present as a series of segmental enlargements which mimic pregnancy (Fig. 3–214). Infection of the uterine stump in spayed dogs and cats may be recognized as a mass between the colon and urinary bladder (Fig. 3–215). Tumors of the uterus may present as focal masses, a segmental horn, or diffuse enlargements (Fig. 3–216).

Unless they are quite large, lesions affecting the vagina are readily apparent radiographically only if contrast is used. In most cases, the vagina lends itself to thorough physical or endoscopic examination and radiography is rarely needed. Pneumo- or positive-contrast vaginography may be helpful in outlining the cranial extent of a vaginal mass when an endoscope cannot be passed beyond the mass. Differentiation between inflammatory and neoplastic lesions is not possible radiographically.

A linear mineralized structure may be seen within the labia or perineal soft tissues. This represents an os clitoris. (Fig. 3–217). It is usually an incidental finding; however, it may be observed in conjunction with anomalies of the genital tract such as pseudohermaphroditism.

PREGNANCY

The definitive determination of pregnancy by radiography is not possible until approximately the 42nd day of pregnancy, when the fetal skeletons calcify sufficiently to be visualized (Fig. 3–218). Before this fetal calcification, the visible uterine enlargement is nonspecific. A symmetrical segmentation of the pregnant uterus may be observed at 25 to 30 days of gestation. The mammary glands may become prominent as pregnancy develops, but this may also be seen with uterine infections or may

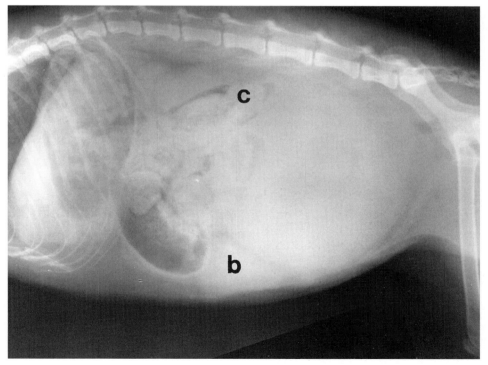

Figure 3–216. A 5-year-old female domestic short-haired cat with anorexia for 5 days. The cat was in heat 1 week prior to the onset of signs. There is a large soft tissue density mass between the bladder (*black b*) and colon (*black c*). Differential diagnoses include segmental pyometra, uterine tumor, or focal pregnancy. **Diagnosis:** Leiomyosarcoma.

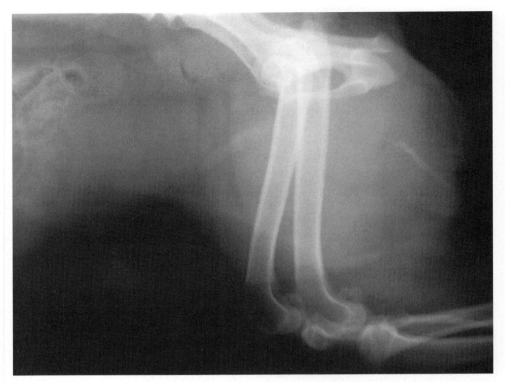

Figure 3–217. Close-up view of pelvic region of a 2-year-old spayed female Weimaraner with a history of chronic hematuria. There is a linear bone density visible in the perineal soft tissues in the region of the vulva. This represents an os clitoris. It is usually without clinical signs. **Diagnosis:** Os clitoris

be the result of a previous pregnancy. The uterus involutes by 21 days postpartum. It can be detected radiographically up to 12 days postpartum.[219]

Radiography is superior to ultrasound for determination of litter size in the bitch.[220] Pregnant females are rarely radiographed because of difficult deliveries. Radiographs are helpful in eliminating pelvic malformation as a cause of dystocia. The fetuses may be examined radiographically to determine their viability. The signs of fetal death include gas in the fetal GI tract and/or perifetal area, overlap of the frontal and parietal bones over the fontanelle, loss of fetal flexion, uneven bone density, or mummification (Fig. 3–219).[221,222]

ULTRASOUND OF THE ABNORMAL OVARY AND UTERUS

The normal anestrus ovary is small and hard to identify, but it becomes larger and more easily identified during proestrus and estrus.[29] The ovary is normally smooth but may become irregularly shaped prior to ovulation. At the time of ovulation, the anechoic follicles become hypoechoic. These hypoechoic structures are replace by the corpora lutea, which are anechoic centrally with a hypoechoic margin.[29] The anechoic central portion of the corpora lutea gradually becomes obliterated. If the ovary is easily found it may be enlarged. Size comparison with the opposite ovary is helpful. Ovarian cysts are anechoic, vary in size, and may be solitary or multiple (Fig. 3–220). Tumors are heteroechoic and may contain anechoic cystic areas.[223,224] Follicles may be identified before ovulation as anechoic structures within the ovary, and the enlargement, rupture, and regression of the follicles can be followed.

Differentiating the pregnant from the non-pregnant uterus using ultrasound is easy; however, endometritis, hydrometra, mucometra, hematometra, and pyometra have similar appearances.[225,226]

Pyometra can be recognized when the uterus is enlarged, thin-walled, and filled with echogenic fluid (Fig. 3–221). When the uterus is only slightly enlarged with

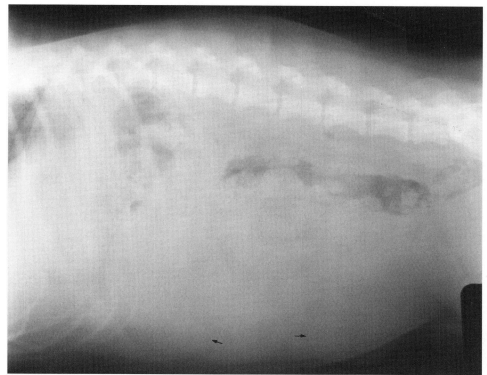

Figure 3–218. A 4-year-old female golden retriever that had been bred 6 weeks prior to examination. The lateral radiograph revealed an enlarged uterus which displaced the small intestines dorsally and cranially. Close scrutiny revealed early calcification of the fetal skeletons (*black arrows*). The presence of skeletons limits the differential diagnoses to pregnancy. **Diagnosis:** Forty-two day pregnancy.

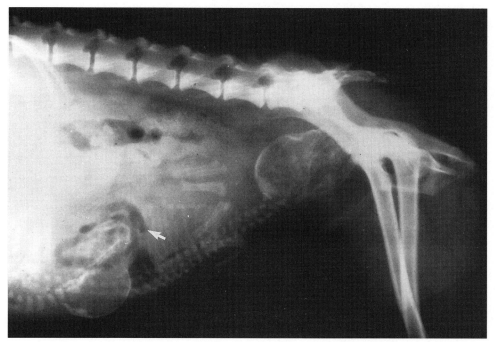

Figure 3–219. A 5-year-old female beagle that had been bred 65 days prior to the examination and had been in labor for 18 hours. The radiograph revealed the presence of two puppies. The pup nearest the birth canal has gas within its small intestine (*white arrow*) and overlap of the bones of the calvarium at the fontanelle. These are signs of fetal death. The pup more proximal in the uterus shows no signs of fetal death. **Diagnosis:** Dystocia with one fetus confirmed dead and the other fetus possibly alive (a cesarean section was performed and the puppy in the birth canal was dead but the other was alive).

Figure 3–220. Transverse sonograms of the caudal abdomen (A,B,&C) and longitudinal sonogram of the midabdomen (D) of a 14-month-old female cat with a history of weight loss, anorexia, depression, and recurrent estrus for 2 to 4 months. There is a round heteroechoic structure (*small arrows*) located dorsal and to the right of the urinary bladder. The lumen of this structure contains echogenic material (A&C) and a small amount of fluid (B). This represents an enlarged uterus. There is a heteroechoic structure in the midabdomen (*arrows*) which represents an enlarged ovary (D). The aorta can be seen deep to the ovary. There are multiple hypoechoic structures within the ovary. This is indicative of a cystic ovary. **Diagnosis:** Uterine enlargement with cystic ovary.

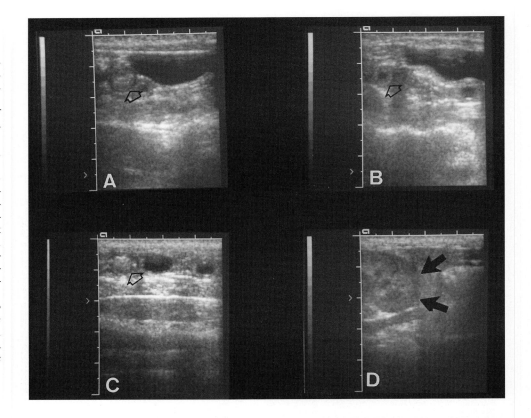

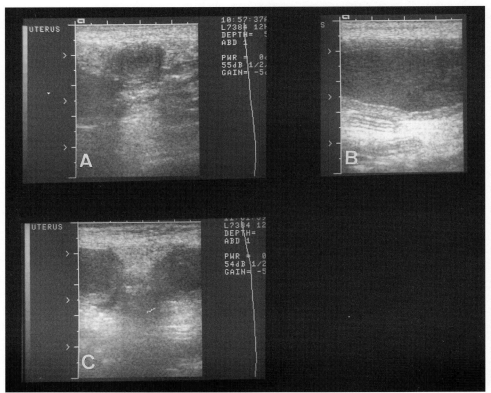

Figure 3–221. Transverse (A&C) and longitudinal (B) sonograms of the caudal abdomen of a 10-year-old female mixed breed dog with a history of leucocytosis, abdominal pain, and hypothermia. There is an elongated oval structure in the caudal abdomen that has a thick echogenic wall and echogenic material within the lumen. The structure divides into two tubes in the transverse view (C). This is indicative of an enlarged uterus which contains echogenic fluid and is therefore most likely a pyometra. **Diagnosis:** Pyometra.

a thick wall, a specific diagnosis is not possible and endometritis, endometrial hyperplasia, hydrometra, mucometra, hematometra, or pyometra may be present (Figs. 3–220 and 3–222).

Uterine stump pyometra may appear as a heteroechoic or hypoechoic oval or elongated mass located between the colon and the bladder. Hyperechoic areas that may represent fibrous tissue or anechoic areas that represent fluid accumulation may be seen (Figs. 3–223 and 3–224). The location of the mass rather than its echo intensity is usually diagnostic. Uterine body, vaginal, or cervical tumors are usually more uniform in architecture. They can range from hypoechoic to hyperechoic.

The anestrus uterus may be identified as a tubular structure with hypoechoic walls

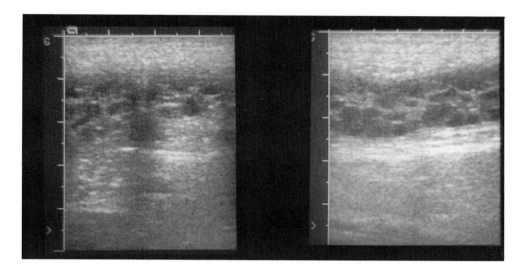

Figure 3–222. Longitudinal sonograms of the uterus of a 13-year-old female cocker spaniel that presented with a history of a mucoid vaginal discharge of 1 month's duration. There is uterine enlargement with multiple hypoechoic, irregularly shaped lesions within the wall of the uterus. This is indicative of inflammatory or infiltrative disease of the uterine wall. **Diagnosis:** Cystic endometrial hyperplasia.

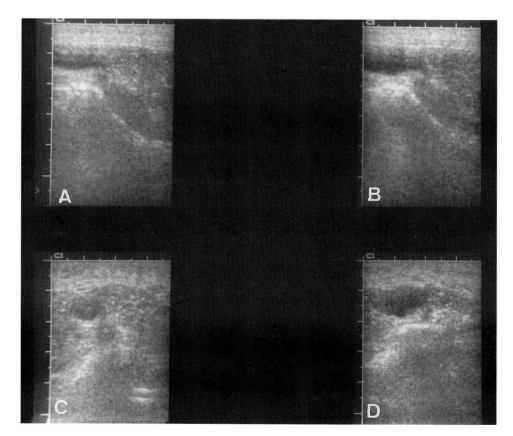

Figure 3–223. Longitudinal (A&B) and transverse (C&D) sonograms of the caudal abdomen of a 4-year-old spayed female Samoyed with a history of chronic urinary incontinence and acute onset of vomiting and icterus. There is a heteroechoic mass located caudal to the urinary bladder (A&B) and on the left lateral aspect of the bladder (C&D). This represents a uterine stump. **Diagnosis:** Stump pyometra.

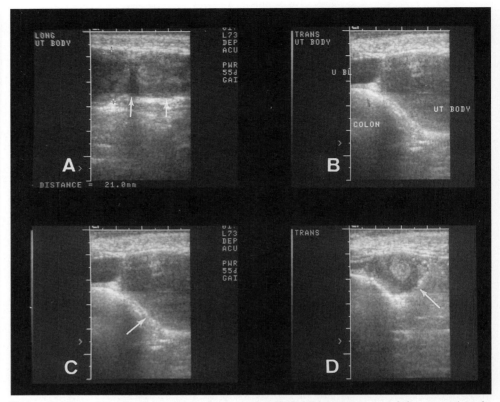

Figure 3–224. Longitudinal (A) and transverse (B,C,&D) sonograms of the posterior abdomen of a 5-year-old spayed female mixed breed dog who presented with a history of recurrent estrus and a purulent vaginal discharge which persisted despite a second ovariohysterectomy with removal of residual ovarian tissue. There is a heteroechoic elongated somewhat oval-shaped mass (*arrows*) evident caudal and to the left of the urinary bladder. In the region of the cervix there is a centrally located hyperechoic region. This represents a uterine stump. **Diagnosis:** Stump pyometra.

and a hyperechoic lumen. It may be identified dorsal to the urinary bladder but can rarely be traced cranially because it will be obscured by overlying small intestines.

Using high frequency transducers, pregnancy can be detected as early as 10 days in dogs and 4 days in cats.[227–232] In most cases, a pregnancy can be confirmed by 17 days. The accuracy with which a diagnosis of pregnancy can be made is 99% by 28 days. The blastocyst appears as a focal, slightly hyperechoic area in the uterine horn. A small central hyperechoic area may be observed within the blastocyst. As the blastocyst enlarges, the uterus becomes less tubular and segmentation can be observed. The diameter of the gestational sac varies even among fetuses in the same litter. In the dog, fetal cardiac activity can be identified at 20 days, and in the cat heart motion is visible at 17 days (Figs. 3–225 and 3–226). Mineralization of the mandible, ribs, spine, and skull occur at approximately 30 to 33 days of gestation. These are evident as hyperechoic symmetrical structures. By 37 days cardiac chambers can be identified. The lung and liver have equal echo intensity at 40 days, but the echo intensity of the lung increases by day 43 (Figs. 3–227 and 3–228). By day 46 long bones and facial features are evident. Intestinal motility may be observed by day 58 to 63.[227–233]

In cats, fetal heart rates remain stable during pregnancy and average 228 beats per minute (bpm). In dogs, fetal heart rates increase during pregnancy from an average of 214 bpm initially to an average of 238 bpm by day 40. The heart rate slows slightly around the time of parturition.[233]

By means of fetal head and/or body diameter measurements, ultrasound was used

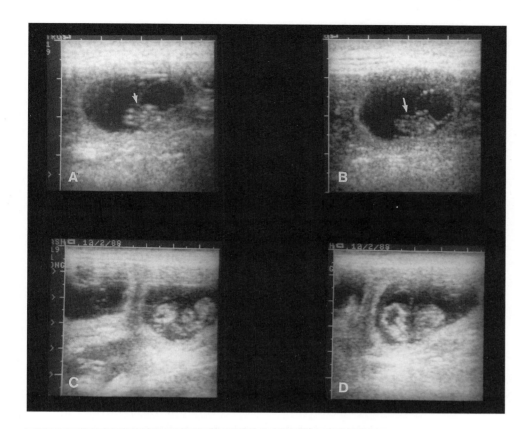

Figure 3–225. Transverse sonograms of the uterus of a 5-year-old female basset hound. The dog was being evaluated for pregnancy and was clinically normal. Sonograms were obtained at 23 days (A&B) and at 30 days (C&D) post-breeding. Fluid is evident within the uterus at 23 days and the fetus can also be identified (*arrows*). A heart beat could be detected at this stage. At 30 days, the size of the fetus has increased and the head and limb buds are visible. **Diagnosis:** Normal pregnancy.

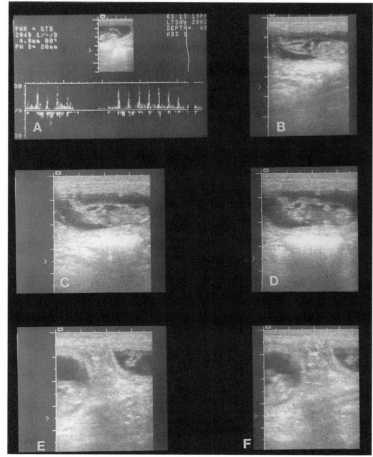

Figure 3–226. Doppler (A), longitudinal (B, C,&D), and transverse (E&F) sonograms of the uterus of a 2-year-old female Pomeranian. The dog was clinically normal and the examination was performed as a routine pregnancy evaluation 30 days after breeding. The fetal heart beat can be identified in the Doppler sonogram. The fetus and fetal membranes can be identified in the other views. **Diagnosis:** Normal 30 day pregnancy.

Figure 3–227. Doppler sonogram and longitudinal sonograms of the uterus of a 3-year-old female German shepherd dog. The examination was part of a routine pregnancy check 50 days post breeding. The dog was clinically normal. The Doppler examination identifies the heart and establishes the heart rate. In the longitudinal sonograms the head of the fetus can be identified. **Diagnosis:** Normal pregnancy.

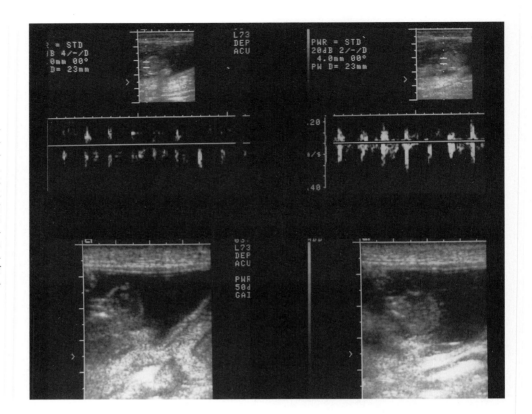

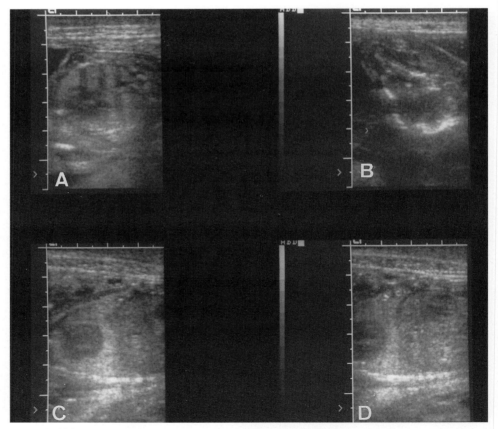

Figure 3–228. Longitudinal (A,C,&D) and transverse sonograms of the uterus of a 3-year-old German shepherd dog 57 days post-breeding. The dog was clinically normal. The heart, lung, liver, and stomach can be identified. Note that the lung is hyperechoic relative to the liver. Shadowing is evident due to calcification of the ribs (A). **Diagnosis:** Normal pregnancy.

to predict parturition dates in queens. The formula used was 61.2 minus (24.6 multiplied by the head diameter in centimeters) or 43.5 minus (10.9 multiplied by the body diameter in centimeters).[234]

The uterus is still evident on ultrasound 24 days postpartum. Variability in the appearance of the uterus was observed. In the first 1 to 4 days postpartum, the uterus is large and its contents are heteroechoic. Placentation sites may be visible as ovoid heteroechoic areas. Both hypoechoic and hyperechoic uterine contents are visible, and the uterine wall is thick. As uterine involution progresses, the wall becomes thinner and placentation sites become more uniform.[118]

PROSTATE

The prostate is normally a bilobed ovoid or round tissue-dense structure with a smooth, regular margin located almost entirely within the pelvic canal. A triangular-shaped fat density usually is observed between the bladder neck and the cranial-most aspect of the prostate and this helps to identify these two structures. Extension of the prostate cranial to the pelvic brim usually indicates enlargement (Fig. 3–229). In some chondrodystrophic breeds (e.g., Scottish terriers), the normal prostate may be located cranial to the pelvic brim. In some animals, the prostate may be normal to small in size but is displaced cranial to the pelvic brim due to urinary bladder or colonic distention. The most common cause of prostatic enlargement is benign prostatic hyperplasia. Other considerations for prostatomegaly are neoplasia, metaplasia, intraprostatic cyst, paraprostatic cyst, or inflammatory disease.[235–243] Abrupt changes in prostatic outline suggest prostatic abnormality (cyst, abscess, or tumor). Density changes within the prostate are uncommon. Punctate calcifications may be present with benign prostatic concretions (calculi), prostatic abscess, or prostatic

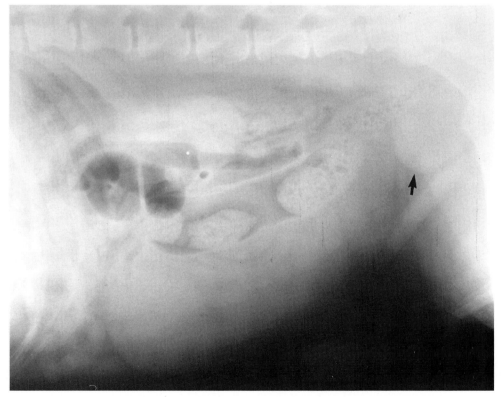

Figure 3–229. An 8-year-old male miniature poodle with a small amount of blood dripping from the penis for 3 days. The lateral radiograph reveals a moderately enlarged prostate which is clearly cranial to the brim of the pelvis (*black arrow*). Differential diagnoses include benign hyperplasia, prostatitis, or prostatic neoplasia. **Diagnosis:** Prostatitis.

carcinoma. Prostatic neoplasia may be accompanied by enlarged sublumbar lymph nodes and/or the formation of periosteal new bone on the ilial wings and/or ventral aspects of the caudal lumbar vertebrae secondary to hematogenous metastases (Fig. 3–230).[242,243] In some cases of prostatitis, inflammatory elements will penetrate the prostatic capsule and there will be hazy, streaky tissue densities in the fat between the bladder and the prostate (Fig. 3–231). In some male dogs, the persistence of

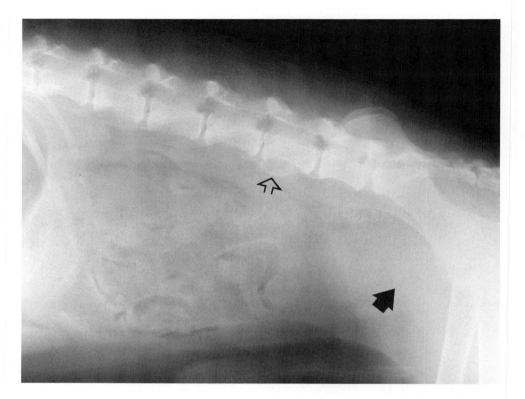

Figure 3–230. A 9-year-old male Norwegian elkhound with stranguria for 2 weeks. The lateral radiograph revealed mild prostatomegaly (*solid black arrow*). The sublumbar lymph nodes show no enlargement but there is a marked periosteal response involving the ventral aspect of L6 (*open black arrow*). **Diagnosis:** Prostatic adenocarcinoma with spinal metastasis.

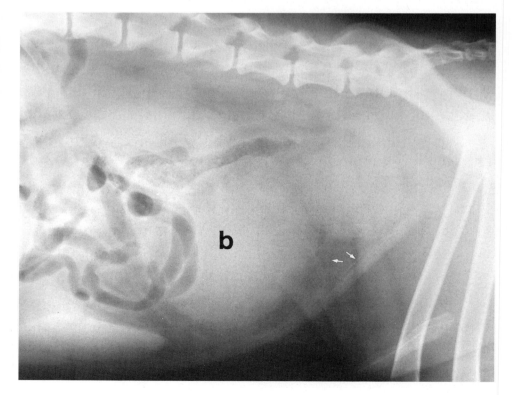

Figure 3–231. An 8-year-old male Brittany spaniel with blood dripping from the penis for 1 week and vomiting and anorexia of 3 days. The lateral radiograph revealed marked prostatomegaly which displaced the bladder (*black b*) cranially. Close scrutiny revealed streaks of tissue density in the normally homogenous fat density between the prostate and bladder (*white arrows*). This is usually indicative of the spread of inflammatory cells through the capsule of an inflamed prostate. Differential diagnoses include prostatitis, prostatic neoplasia, or benign prostatic hyperplasia. **Diagnosis:** Prostatitis.

Muellerian ducts will result in the development of paraprostatic cysts. These may be visible as round, oval, or tubular soft tissue-dense structures in the caudal ventral abdomen. These masses may be present between the colon and bladder, may be cranial or lateral to the bladder, or may even be in perineal hernia sacs. They are always attached by a stalk to the prostate gland and may have a calcified wall (Figs. 3–232 and 3-233).[241]

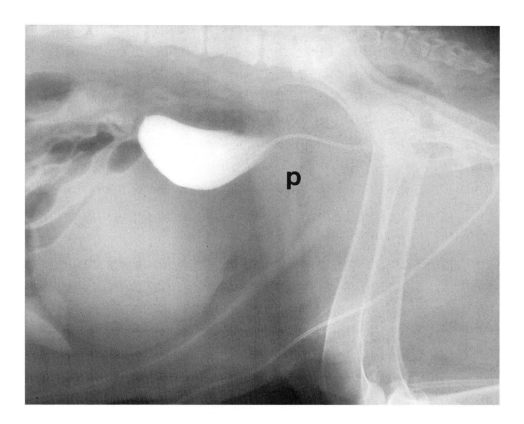

Figure 3–232. A 6-year-old male cocker spaniel with a palpable caudal abdominal mass detected on routine physical examination. The survey radiograph revealed three distinguishable caudal abdominal tissue densities. The cystogram was performed to determine the position of the urinary bladder. The mass caudal to it was presumed to be the prostate (*black p*). Differential diagnoses for the mass cranial and ventral to the opacified urinary bladder include paraprostatic cyst, neoplasm of the cranial bladder wall, splenic mass, or other forms of neoplasia. **Diagnosis:** Paraprostatic cyst.

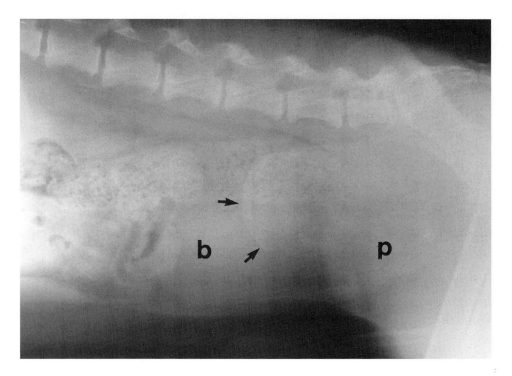

Figure 3–233. A 5-year-old male Doberman pinscher with a palpable caudal abdominal mass detected on routine physical examination. The lateral radiograph revealed the colon filled with fecal material, the bladder (*black b*) displaced cranially, moderate prostatomegaly (*black p*), and a mass (*black arrows*) with a calcified rim ("egg shell" calcification) between the bladder and colon. Differential diagnoses include paraprostatic cyst or neoplasm arising from the margin of the colon, prostate, or bladder. **Diagnosis:** Paraprostatic cyst.

Urinary tract contrast studies offer little specific information regarding the etiology of prostatic disease. When there is doubt as to the identity of a caudal abdominal mass, radiographs with a radiopaque urinary catheter in the bladder, cystograms, or urethrograms may be helpful. Although retrograde urethrography may identify a large cystic prostatic structure which communicates with the urethra, the more common situation is either a normal study or a false-negative (i.e., one in which a cystic prostatic structure does not communicate with the urethra).[241] Prostatic abscess, cyst, and necrotic tumor may produce cavitation within the prostate, which can be filled with contrast during a contrast urethrogram. A small amount of contrast may reflux into a normal prostate. The finding of contrast within the prostate is therefore non-specific.[154,162]

ULTRASOUND OF PROSTATIC ABNORMALITIES

Ultrasound is well suited for evaluation of the prostate.[38,244,245] Provided the prostate is not too deeply positioned within the pelvic canal, it can be examined easily. A specific diagnosis can be made in only a few cases; however, the number of possible diagnoses can be reduced based on the ultrasound features. Ultrasound may also be used for guidance during aspiration or biopsy of the prostate or for abscess or cyst drainage.[39]

Prostatic hyperplasia usually produces a uniformly textured enlarged prostate.[39] The echo intensity of the prostate is normal. Small hypoechoic or anechoic cysts may be identified (Fig. 3–234).

Prostatitis and prostatic carcinoma can create single or multiple foci of increased echo intensity (Fig. 3–235).[245] Differentiation of these two conditions is difficult when based solely on the ultrasound examination. Prostatitis may produce multifocal anechoic and or hypoechoic areas with smooth or irregular margins. These lesions result from focal inflammation or abscessation. Hyperechoic areas that shadow

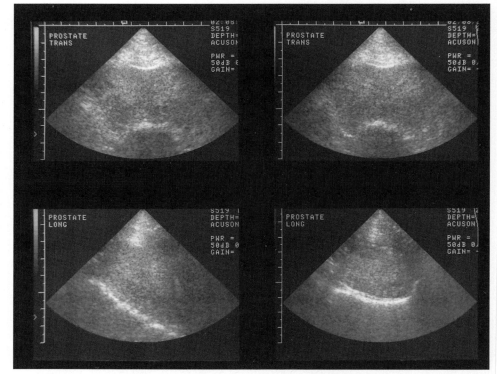

Figure 3–234. Transverse and longitudinal sonograms of the prostate of 6-year-old male rottweiler who presented with a history of stranguria and chronic urolithiasis. The prostate is enlarged but normally shaped. The architecture is uniform with multiple small hypoechoic and hyperechoic regions. This is indicative of hyperplasia. **Diagnosis:** Prostatic hyperplasia.

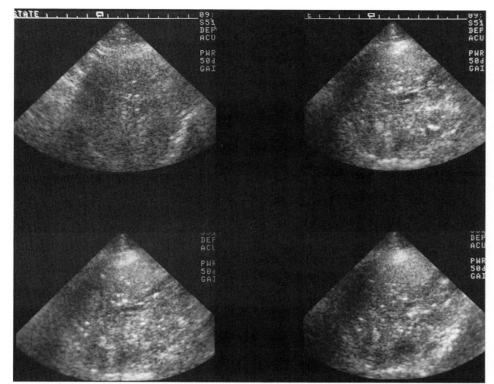

Figure 3–235. Transverse sonograms of the prostate of an 11-year-old male standard poodle with a history of chronic hematuria and prostatomegaly. The prostate is enlarged and contains multiple small hyperechoic foci. These do not shadow and therefore may not represent mineral. This is most likely due to prostatic neoplasia. **Diagnosis:** Prostatic carcinoma.

may indicate prostatic mineralization, which may occur in either prostatitis or carcinoma. Asymmetric enlargement may be seen more often with prostatic tumor. Prostatic carcinoma may be characterized by multifocal hyperechoic areas that have a tendency to coalesce. Round or oval hypoechoic masses, which represent sublumbar lymph node enlargement, may be identified. Ultrasound is more sensitive than radiography in detecting sublumbar (iliac) lymph node enlargement. Identification of enlarged lymph nodes during an ultrasound examination is a less specific finding and may occur in association with either tumor or infection. If enlarged lymph nodes are recognized on radiographs it is almost always a sign of tumor.

Prostatic abscess and intraprostatic cysts produce solitary or multiple hypoechoic or anechoic lesions (Figs. 3–236, 3–237, and 3–238). Posterior enhancement and through transmission may be identified in cysts. Cellular echoes within the cavity may be present in either cysts or abscesses. Cysts may be more smoothly marginated, however either lesion may have irregular margins. Tumor necrosis may produce hypoechoic areas within prostatic neoplasms, and this decreases the specificity of the ultrasound findings.

Paraprostatic cysts are anechoic or hypoechoic structures that may be tubular or septated (Fig. 3–239). Mineralization within the wall of the cyst may produce hyperechoic areas which shadow. Infection or hemorrhage within the cyst may produce small echoes that move with manipulation of the transducer or the patient. Communication of the paraprostatic cyst with the prostate may be identified. Criteria that could separate infected from noninfected paraprostatic cysts were not identified.[244] Distinguishing a large paraprostatic cyst from the urinary bladder may be difficult, but with careful examination from all sides the distinction can be made. If necessary, the bladder can be catheterized and saline can be injected through the urinary catheter. The air bubbles within the fluid will be identified easily.

Prostatic biopsy or aspiration can be performed easily, but the patient should be

Figure 3–236. Transverse (A,B,&C) and longitudinal (D) sonograms of the prostate of a 9-year-old male mixed breed dog with a history of stranguria and incontinence of 3 months' duration. The prostate is hyperechoic with multiple hypoechoic to anechoic irregularly shaped lesions within the prostatic tissue. These are indicative of prostatic cysts or abscesses. **Diagnosis:** Prostatic abscesses.

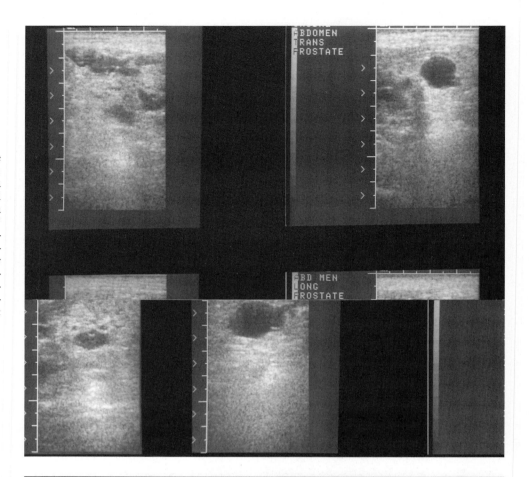

Figure 3–237. Longitudinal sonograms of the prostate of a 13-year-old male West Highland white terrier with a history of stranguria, dysuria, and hematuria of 1 month's duration. The prostate is enlarged and the architecture is abnormal with multiple irregularly shaped hypoechoic and anechoic areas throughout the prostate. This is indicative of either prostatitis with abscess formation or multiple prostatic cysts. **Diagnosis:** Prostatitis with multiple abscesses.

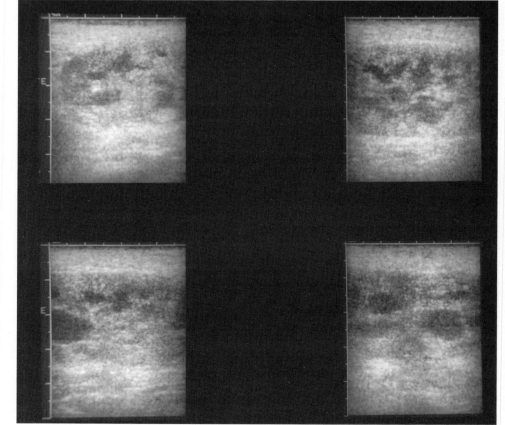

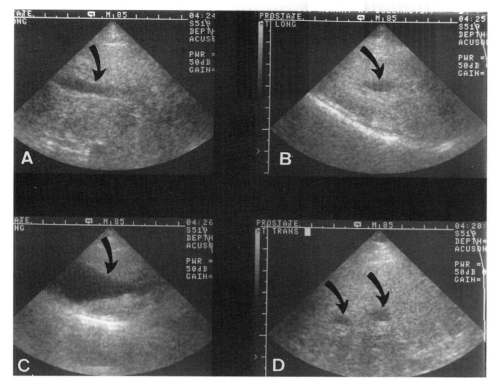

Figure 3–238. Longitudinal (A,B,&C) and transverse (D) sonograms of the prostate of a 6-year-old male bullmastiff with a history of abnormal ejaculate and low sperm counts. There are several anechoic lesions visible within the prostate (*arrows*). These represent intraprostatic cysts. The remainder of the prostate appears normal. **Diagnosis:** Prostatic cysts.

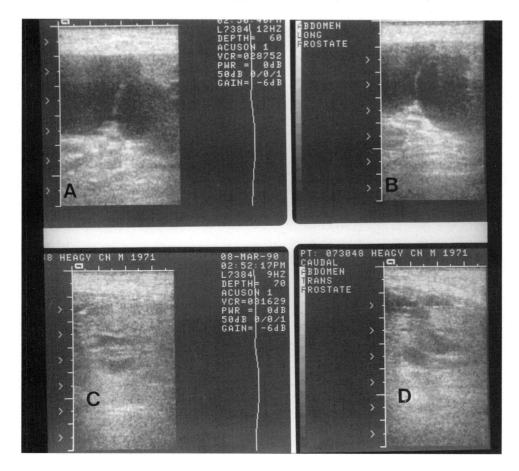

Figure 3–239. Longitudinal (A&B) and transverse (C&D) sonograms of the prostate of a 9-year-old male mixed breed dog with a history of stranguria for 4 months. There is an anechoic septated structure which was located cranial to the prostate and lateral to the urinary bladder. The anechoic lesion can be identified lateral, ventral, and to the right of the prostate in the transverse sonograms. This is indicative of a paraprostatic cyst. **Diagnosis:** Paraprostatic cyst.

anesthetized or heavily sedated. Biopsy guides may be used, however directing the needle without the guide is accomplished easily. Cyst or abscess drainage may be performed using ultrasound guidance and may eliminate the need for surgery.[39]

TESTICLES

Unless they are enlarged, undescended testicles are rarely radiographically apparent. They may be found anywhere from just caudal to the kidneys to the inguinal ring (Fig. 3–240). Intra-abdominal testicles are prone to neoplastic changes, especially Sertoli cell tumor. In these cases, a large abdominal mass may be accompanied by prominent nipples. Another, less common cause of enlargement of a retained testicle is torsion.[246] Although most scrotal testicular tumors are benign, extension of a tumor along the epididymis may be recognized radiographically as an irregular enlargement extending through the inguinal ring into the sublumbar area.

ULTRASOUND OF THE ABNORMAL TESTICLE

Usually, testicular tumors are hypoechoic, but may also be heteroechoic or hyperechoic relative to the surrounding normal testicle. Most are well circumscribed and round or oval in shape. The size of the tumor and the sharpness of the interface between the tumor and the normal testicular tissue determine the echogenicity of the tumor. Smaller tumors tend to be hypoechoic, while larger tumors are often heteroechoic. Only a few hyperechoic tumors have been reported. Smaller tumors also tend to have sharper margins while larger tumors are often poorly demarcated from

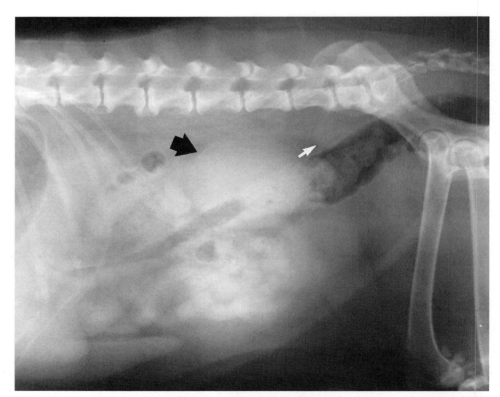

Figure 3–240. A 5-year-old male beagle with a retained testicle, ventral alopecia, and enlarged nipples. There is a tissue-dense mass in the caudal abdomen (*black arrow*) and enlarged sublumbar lymph nodes (*white arrow*). Differential diagnoses include testicular tumor (Sertoli cell tumor, seminoma), nonobstructing small intestinal mass (leiomyosarcoma), or tumor or granuloma arising from the mesentery. **Diagnosis:** Sertoli cell tumor with metastasis to the sublumbar lymph nodes.

the surrounding normal tissue.[247] Small masses that cannot be palpated can be detected using ultrasound. A consistent sonographic pattern has not been associated with tumor type (Figs. 3–241 and 3–242). Intra-abdominal retained testicles can also be identified accurately using ultrasound. They can be recognized because of their normal hyperechoic appearance despite their abnormal location.[248] The testicle may appear hypoechoic when it is atrophied.

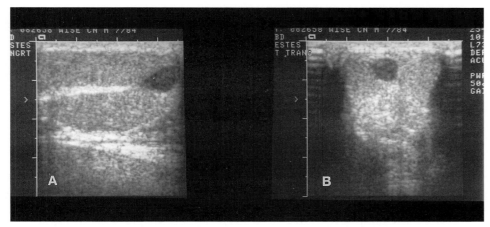

Figure 3–241. Longitudinal (A) and transverse (B) sonograms of the left testicle of an 8-year-old male Labrador retriever with a history of fecal incontinence, hematuria, and pyrexia. There is a well-defined hypoechoic lesion in the caudal portion of the testes. This is indicative of a testicular tumor. **Diagnosis:** Sertoli cell tumor.

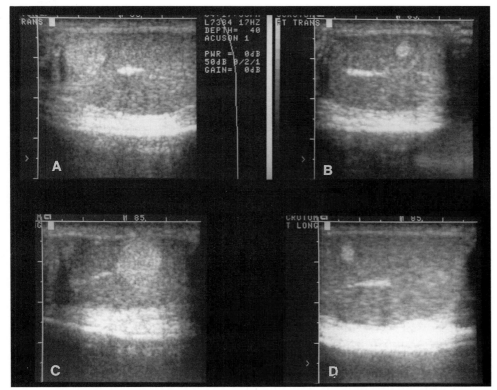

Figure 3–242. Transverse (A&B) and longitudinal (C&D) sonograms of the right testicle of a 6-year-old male bullmastiff with a history of abnormal ejaculate and low sperm counts. There are two hyperechoic foci visible within the testicle. These represent testicular tumors. **Diagnosis:** Sertoli cell tumor.

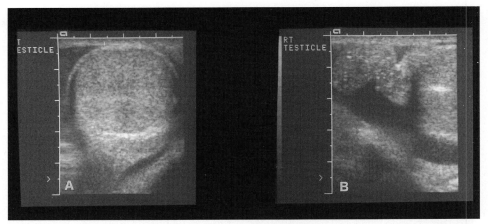

Figure 3–243. Transverse (A) and longitudinal (B) sonograms of the right testicle of a 9-year-old male Labrador retriever with a history of abdominal distension and scrotal swelling for 1 month. The testicle is normal. There is a large amount of scrotal fluid surrounding the testicle. **Diagnosis:** Scrotal fluid secondary to splenic mass and ascites.

Doppler examination has been used in humans to distinguish testicular torsion from testicular neoplasia. Since testicular torsion is rare and most neoplasms are small this may not be necessary in dogs. Orchitis and torsion may produce fluid within the scrotum. Ultrasound can be used to identify and evaluate the testicle within the fluid distended scrotum when it cannot be palpated. Ultrasound can distinguish the testicular from the nontesticular causes for scrotal swelling and can differentiate unilateral from bilateral disease (Fig. 3–243).[248]

A diffuse, patchy hypoechoic pattern has been identified with orchitis in dogs. Enlargement of the epididymis was also observed.[248]

HEMOLYMPHATIC SYSTEM

ABNORMAL FINDINGS

SPLEEN

The major abdominal organ of this system is the spleen. There are no practical special procedures to evaluate the spleen; however, there are a number of changes that may be identified on survey radiographs. Evaluation of splenic size is completely subjective. The most common finding in the dog is a generalized enlargement. Determining the significance of generalized enlargement may be difficult, because the spleen is a very dynamic organ and its size can change dramatically as a normal response to various physiologic states. Excessive enlargement may be due administration of various drugs (phenothiazines or barbiturates), passive congestion, torsion, splenitis, extramedullary hematopoiesis, immune mediated diseases, or diffuse infiltration (Fig. 3–244). Except for the response to pharmaceuticals, changes in splenic size in the cat are much less common. In cats, generalized splenic enlargement most often indicates infiltrative disease (lymphosarcoma or mast cell tumor) (Fig. 3–245).

Changes in the shape of the spleen are almost always due to healed fractures or focal masses. These may be multiple and small, as is frequently seen with nodular hyperplasia, or may be large and solitary, as those seen in hematoma, hemangioma, leiomyosarcoma, or hemangiosarcoma (Fig. 3–246). Splenic hemangiosarcoma in dogs may rupture resulting in hemorrhage or metastasis into the adjacent peritoneum (Fig. 3–247). This will appear as a vaguely definable mass in an area of poor visceral detail.

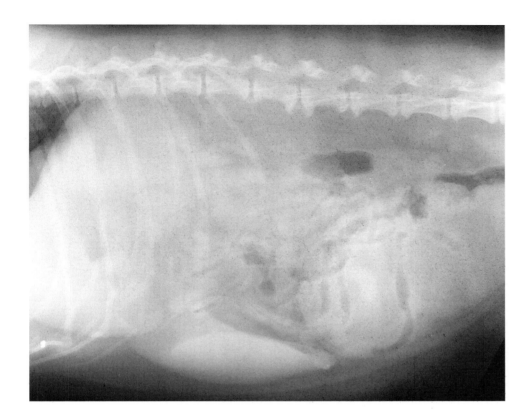

Figure 3–244. An 8-year-old male standard poodle with anemia. The lateral radiograph revealed marked splenomegaly. Differential diagnoses include splenic dilation secondary to tranquilization or anesthesia, lymphosarcoma, hypersplenism, autoimmune hemolytic anemia, or mast cell tumor. **Diagnosis:** Hypersplenism.

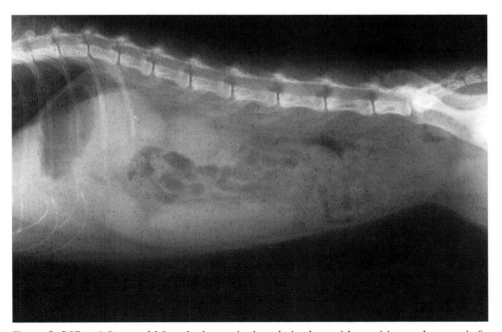

Figure 3–245. A 5-year-old female domestic short-haired cat with vomiting and anorexia for 2 weeks. The lateral radiograph revealed diffuse splenomegaly. Differential diagnoses include lymphosarcoma or mast cell tumor. **Diagnosis:** Mass tumor.

The spleen of the dog is fairly mobile within the abdominal cavity. Occasionally, it will rotate around its mesenteric axis. This results in splenic torsion, as indicated by a generally enlarged spleen that is displaced from its normal position and with a poorly-defined margin. The gastric shape may be distorted as the pylorus is pulled closer to the cardia due to traction on the gastrosplenic ligament. This exaggerates

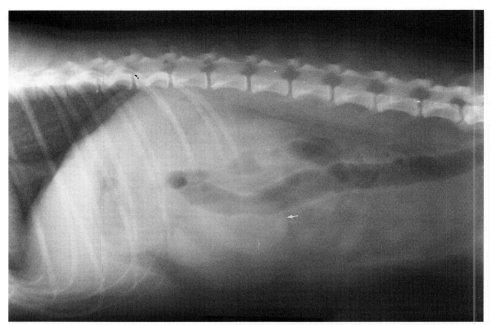

Figure 3–246. A 6-year-old male poodle with anorexia for 2 days. The lateral radiograph revealed a ventral tissue-dense mass with clearly discrete margins just caudal to the stomach and liver (*white arrow*). Differential diagnoses include masses involving the spleen (hematoma, leiomyosarcoma, or hemangiosarcoma) or caudal borders of a lateral liver lobe (cyst or neoplasia). **Diagnosis:** Splenic hematoma.

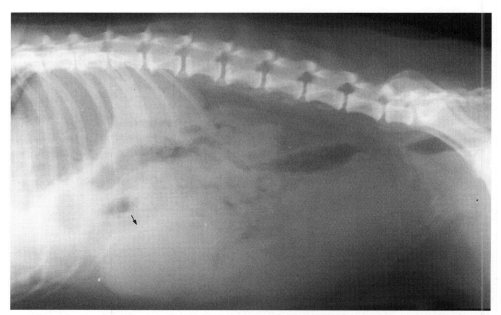

Figure 3–247. An 8-year-old female German shepherd dog with acute collapse. The lateral radiograph revealed a mass (*black arrow*) caudal and ventral to the stomach which displaces the small bowel dorsally. The borders of the mass are indistinct indicating local hydroperitoneum. Differential diagnoses include splenic mass or lateral lobe hepatic mass. The hydroperitoneum suggests an active process. **Diagnosis:** Ruptured hemangiosarcoma of the spleen.

the normal "C" shape of the stomach. Peritoneal fluid may be present, especially around the area of the spleen.[249–251]

Mineralization of the spleen is rare. Granulomas, hematomas, and tumors may become mineralized. Gas may be seen within the spleen secondary to splenic infarct.[252]

Ultrasound of the Abnormal Spleen

Splenic size can vary greatly and still be normal. Identification of normal splenic architecture during the ultrasound examination despite splenic enlargement may reflect splenomegaly associated with drugs, extramedullary hematopoiesis, or immune mediated anemia. Infiltrative diseases of the spleen, such as lymphosarcoma, can also cause splenic enlargement without altering the echo intensity or architecture of the spleen. Diffuse alterations in echo intensity of the spleen may be seen in association with disseminated mast cell tumors and lymphosarcoma, which may cause a diffuse increase in echo intensity and in splenic torsion, which, in turn, may cause a diffuse decrease in echo intensity (Fig. 3–248).[251,253] Lymphosarcoma most often produces multifocal hypoechoic lesions that do not alter the splenic contour.[79,253] Focal splenic lesions are more common. Splenic tumor, nodular hyperplasia, hematoma, or abscess may produce solitary or multifocal lesions (Fig. 3–249).[83] These may be hyperechoic or hypoechoic relative to the normal spleen. Splenic hemangiosarcoma may produce a mixed or heteroechoic mass with areas ranging from hyperechoic to hypoechoic when compared to the normal spleen. The hypoechoic regions most likely represented blood-filled cavernous regions, chronic hematomas, or cysts, while the hyperechoic areas may represent fibrosis or more recent hemorrhage.[253–256] Myelolipoma may produce large hyperechoic areas within the spleen. Hyperechoic areas that shadow may be observed if mineralization of the lesion has occurred. Hematomas may have a similar appearance with heteroechoic lesions representing the hematoma in varying states of organization. Biopsy or aspirate usually is required for a specific diagnosis. The presence of other lesions, such as peritoneal or pericardial fluid, or additional lesions in the liver are indicators of neoplasia. Lymphosarcoma may be diffuse, causing a general increase in splenic echo intensity or may produce multiple, poorly marginated hypoechoic nodules. These nodules do not often alter the splenic contour (i.e., bulge from the margin of

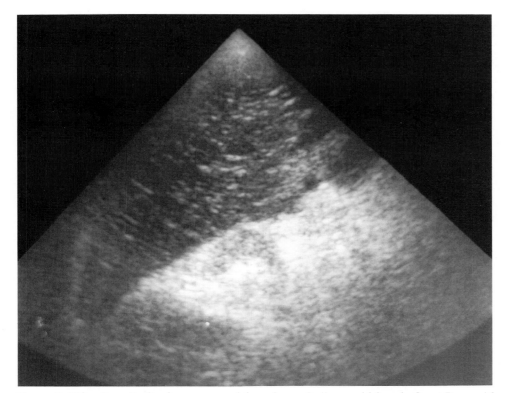

Figure 3–248. Longitudinal sonogram of the spleen of a 5-year-old female Great Dane with a history of vomiting, anorexia, and fever of 8 days' duration. The spleen is enlarged and uniformly hypoechoic. This is indicative of splenic torsion or infarct. **Diagnosis:** Splenic torsion.

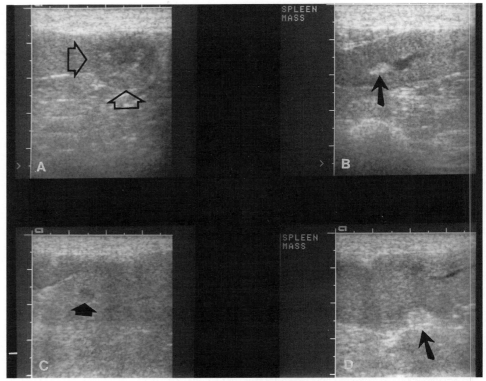

Figure 3–249. Transverse sonograms of the spleen of a 9-year-old female Vizsla with a history of acute collapse associated with thrombocytopenia and mild anemia. There is a hypoechoic round mass associated with the tail of the spleen (*open arrows*, A). There is a hyperechoic lesion adjacent to the splenic vein (*arrows*, B&D). An additional small hypoechoic mass can be identified (*closed arrow*, C). These hypoechoic lesions could be tumors or areas of nodular hyperplasia. The position of the hyperechoic lesion adjacent to the splenic vein identifies it as an area of infolding of fat at the splenic hilus. **Diagnosis:** Nodular hyperplasia.

the spleen).[253] Splenic masses may be very large and at times localization of the mass to a portion of the spleen can be difficult. Invasion of the gastrosplenic ligament may occur (Fig. 3–250).

In humans, acute splenic infarct may be hypoechoic or anechoic, wedge shaped or round, irregularly delineated or smooth. In dogs, the appearance of splenic infarct (diffuse hypoechoic) is similar to that of splenic torsion.[252] Splenic necrosis and infarct may produce focal hypoechoic or isoechoic, circular, well-defined nodular masses with alteration of the splenic contour, or a diffuse hypoechoic or heteroechoic coarse pattern without marginal deformity (Fig. 3–251).[252]

ABDOMINAL LYMPH NODES

The remainder of the intra-abdominal hemolymphatic system is composed of various lymphatics and lymph nodes. One group is clustered around the mesenteric root ventral to L2. These are rarely seen unless they are severely enlarged (Fig. 3–252). The other major group constitutes the sublumbar lymph nodes: the external iliac, internal iliac, and coccygeal lymph nodes. These lymph nodes are located ventral to the caudal lumbar vertebrae and extend into the pelvic canal. Enlargement of these lymph nodes produces an increased density dorsal to the colon, which alters the normal smooth contour of the sublumbar muscles. There may be ventral colonic displacement, and in extreme cases the nodes may impinge upon the colon and cause constipation or dyschezia. Reactive lymphadenitis from infection of organs drained (uterus or prostate), primary neoplasia (lymphosarcoma), or metastatic neoplasia (prostate, testicle, uterine, or urinary bladder) may enlarge these nodes.

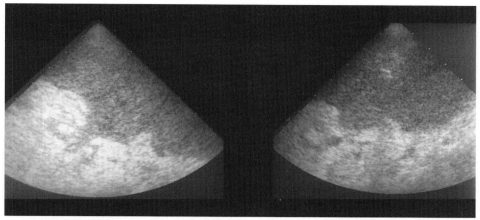

Figure 3–250. Longitudinal sonograms of the spleen of a 7-year-old male Doberman pinscher with a 3/6 systolic murmur, weight loss, and lethargy of 5 weeks' duration. The spleen is enlarged and the contour is irregular, especially at the interface between the spleen and the adjacent fat. This is indicative of a splenic tumor. **Diagnosis:** Sarcoma of the spleen with invasion of the gastrosplenic ligament.

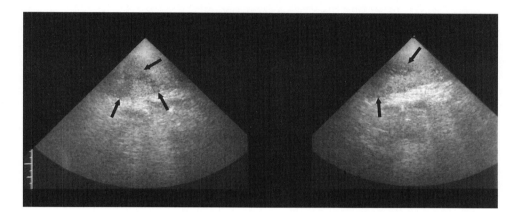

Figure 3–251. Transverse sonograms of the spleen of a 7-year-old male old English sheepdog with a history of vomiting and icterus. There are multiple poorly marginated hypoechoic lesions within the spleen (*arrows*). These may represent abscesses, infarcts or tumors. **Diagnosis:** Splenic infarcts.

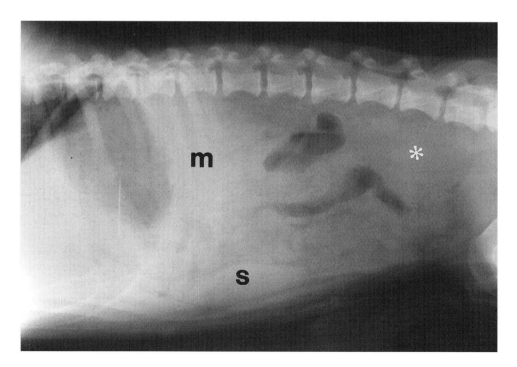

Figure 3–252. A 10-year-old male dachshund with polyuria and polydipsia for 2 weeks. The lateral radiograph revealed a large spleen (*black s*), enlarged mesenteric lymph nodes (*black m*), and enlarged sublumbar lymph nodes (*white* *). A needle foreign body is noted in the stomach. **Diagnosis:** Lymphosarcoma.

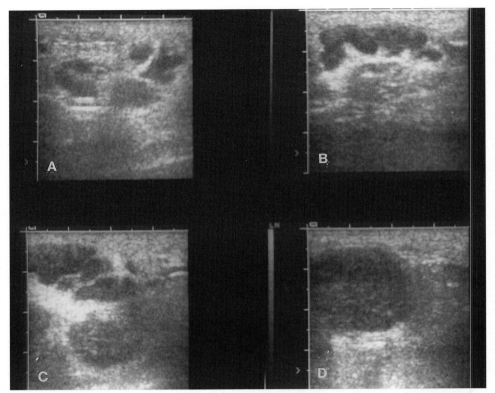

Figure 3-253. Longitudinal (A,B,&C) and transverse (D) sonograms of the midabdomen of a 1-year-old castrated male cat with a history of anorexia, hepatomegaly, and a palpable abdominal mass. There are multiple hypoechoic irregularly shaped abdominal masses. The hyperechoic area along the margin of the mass represents mesenteric fat. These masses represent enlarged abdominal lymph nodes. **Diagnosis:** Lymphosarcoma.

Ultrasound of Lymphadenopathy

Enlarged lymph nodes can be readily detected during an ultrasound examination. Most lymph nodes are hypoechoic and may be round, oval or irregularly shaped (Figs. 3–35, 3–253, and 3–254).[5] They can be found at the root of the mesentery, along the mesentery adjacent to the intestines, caudal to the stomach, adjacent to the ileocecocolic junction, and in the sublumbar region. The ultrasound appearance of the lymph nodes is not particularly helpful in distinguishing neoplastic from infectious or reactive lymphadenopathy. Lymph node masses may become large and can be misinterpreted as splenic, hepatic, or intestinal masses.

ENDOCRINE SYSTEM

ABNORMAL FINDINGS

ADRENAL GLANDS

The major abdominal endocrine organs are the adrenal glands and the pancreas (discussed previously in this chapter under the GI system). In the normal animal, the adrenal glands are not seen radiographically. In some cases of neoplasia, the adrenal enlargement may be calcified and apparent on the survey radiograph (Fig. 3–255). In cats, dense calcification has been noted without evidence of adrenal enlargement, neoplasia, or other disease (Fig. 3–256). The significance of this calcification is unknown. One special procedure that may be helpful in evaluating the adrenal gland is the pneumoperitoneum utilizing a dorsoventral or standing lateral

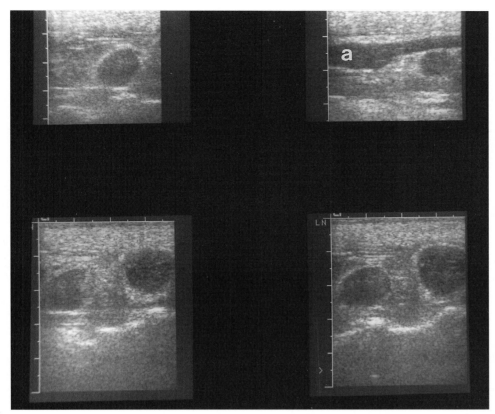

Figure 3-254. Longitudinal sonograms of the sublumbar region of a 13-year-old spayed female mixed breed dog with a history of generalized lymphadenopathy and anorexia. There are multiple oval hypoechoic masses noted in the sublumbar region. The aorta is visible as a linear hypoechoic structure ventral to these masses (a). These findings are indicative of sublumbar (external iliac) lymphadenopathy. **Diagnosis:** Lymphosarcoma.

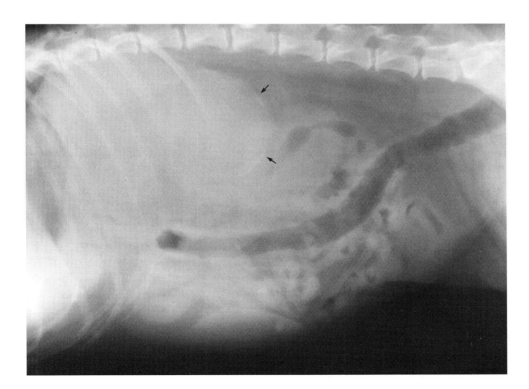

Figure 3-255. A 10-year-old female miniature poodle with hematuria and polydipsia for 2 weeks. The lateral radiograph revealed a tissue density mass that has a calcified rim just cranial to the left kidney (*black arrows*). Differential diagnoses include adrenal adenoma or adenocarcinoma. **Diagnosis:** Adrenal adenocarcinoma.

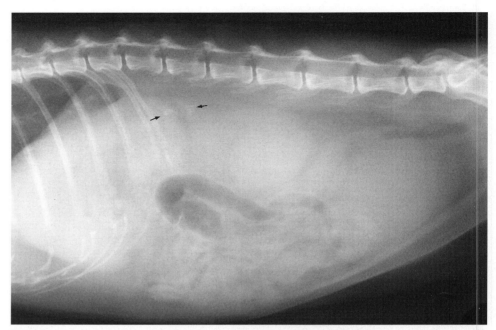

Figure 3-256. A 9-year-old female domestic short-haired cat with vomiting for 1 day. The lateral radiograph revealed two focal areas of calcification cranial to the kidneys (*black arrows*). **Diagnosis:** Calcification within the adrenal glands.

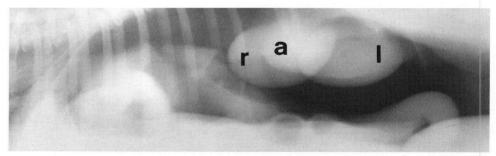

Figure 3-257. A 10-year-old female cocker spaniel with polyuria and polydipsia for 2 months. There was a pendulous abdomen and mild alopecia. Survey radiographs were within normal limits. A pneumoperitoneum was performed. The horizontal beam lateral radiograph shows the abdominal gas surrounding the retroperitoneal structures. The left kidney (*black l*) and right kidney (*black r*) are clearly demonstrated. A third tissue-dense structure (*black a*) is seen superimposing the area where the two renal shadows overlap. **Diagnosis:** Left adrenal adenocarcinoma.

view with a horizontal x-ray beam (Fig. 3–257). Some adrenal tumors extend into the caudal vena cava. A contrast venogram may show the obstruction or abnormal venous blood flow patterns.

Ultrasound of Adrenal Abnormalities

The adrenal glands can be measured directly from the ultrasound image. Changes in size can be detected provided care is exercised in obtaining a true sagittal and transverse image so that the dimension of the adrenal gland is not altered due to obliquity. Most abnormalities result in an adrenal gland that is enlarged and hypoechoic, although large masses may be heteroechoic (Figs. 3–258 and 3–259). The echo intensity of adrenal masses often is similar to that of the renal cortex, although adrenocortical tumors range from hypoechoic to hyperechoic. The hypoechoic regions may represent hemorrhage or necrosis.[30,257] Distortion of the shape of the

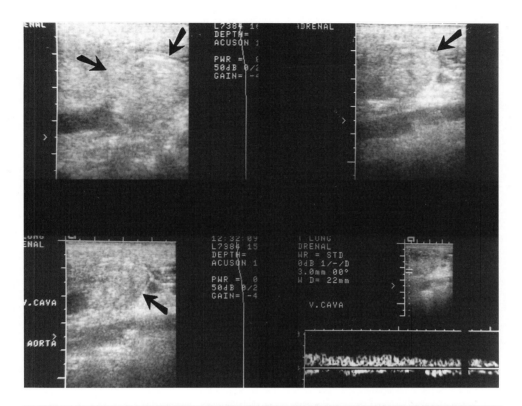

Figure 3-258. Longitudinal sonograms of the cranial abdomen of a 15-year-old spayed female dachshund who presented for acute rear limb paralysis which occurred secondary to a fall from the owner's arms. The dog was pot-bellied and had a long standing history of polyuria and polydipsia. There is an oval heteroechoic mass noted (*arrows*) compressing or invading the cuadal vena cava. The aorta is evident deep to this mass. This represents an adrenal tumor. **Diagnosis:** Adrenal adenoma.

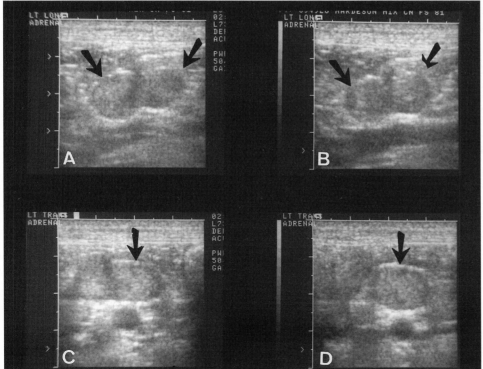

Figure 3-259. Longitudinal (A&B) and transverse (C&D) sonograms of the left adrenal gland of a 12-year-old spayed female mixed breed dog with a history of panting and gagging. There was a palpable mass in the laryngeal region. The adrenal gland is enlarged and abnormally shaped (*arrows*). This may be secondary to adrenal tumor or hyperplasia. The cervical mass was determined to be a thyroid adenocarcinoma. **Diagnosis:** Adrenal adenocarcinoma.

gland may be evident, with rounded nodules causing the gland to be asymmetrically shaped. Cavitation of the adrenal mass may produce hypoechoic areas within a heteroechoic mass. Pheochromocytomas were heteroechoic with ultrasound characteristics ranging from hypoechoic to hyperechoic. These characteristics correlated with their histological architecture.[257] Mineralization of the adrenal gland may produce hyperechoic areas that shadow.[24] These may be associated with adrenal tumors or may be seen in normal-aged animals. Adrenal tumors may invade into the caudal vena cava, and this may be observed during the ultrasound examination.[257] It may be difficult to distinguish between compression and invasion of the vena cava. Alteration of the normal blood flow may be detected using Doppler.

REFERENCES

1. Love NE. The appearance of the canine pyloric region in right versus left lateral recumbent radiographs. Vet Radiol Ultrasound 1993;34:169.
2. Carrig CB, Mostosky UV. The use of compression in abdominal radiography of the dog and cat. JAVRS 1976;17:178.
3. Farrow CS. Abdominal compression radiography in the dog and cat. JAAHA 1978;14:337.
4. Aronson MG, Fagella AM. Surgical techniques for neutering 6- to 14-week-old kittens. JAVMA 1993;202:53.
5. Pugh CR. Ultrasonographic examination of abdominal lymph nodes in the dog. Vet Radiol Ultrasound 1994;35:110.
6. Nyland TG, Park RD. Hepatic ultrasonography in the dog. Vet Radiol 1983;24:74.
7. Nyland TG, Hager DA. Sonography of the liver, gallbladder and spleen. VCNA 1985;15:1123.
8. Kleine LJ, Lamb CR. Comparative organ imaging: The gastrointestinal tract. Vet Radiol 1989;30:133.
9. Spaulding KA. Ultrasound corner. Gallbladder wall thickness. Vet Radiol Ultrasound 1993;34:270.
10. Moentk J, Biller DS. Bilobed gallbladder in a cat: Ultrasonographic appearance. Vet Radiol Ultrasound 1993;34:354.
11. Weber WJ, Spaulding KA. Ultrasound corner hepatic pseudomasses caused by normal anatomic structures in the dog. Vet Radiol Ultrasound 1994;35:307.
12. Jakovljevic S, Gibbs C. Radiographic assessment of gastric mucosal fold thickness in dogs. AJVR 1993;54:1827.
13. Penninck DG, Nyland TG, Fischer PE, Kerr LY. Ultrasonography of the normal canine gastrointestinal tract. Vet Radiol 1989;30:272.
14. Miles KG, Lattimer JC, Krause GF, Knapp DW, Sayles CE. The use of intraperitoneal fluid as a simple technique for enhancing the sonographic visualization of the canine pancreas. Vet Radiol 1988;29:258.
15. Saunders HM. Ultrasonography of the pancreas. Prob Vet Med 1991;3:583.
16. Wood AKW, McCarthy PH, Angles JM. Ultrasonographic-anatomic correlation and imaging protocol for the spleen in anesthetized dogs. AJVR 1990;51:1433.
17. Grandage J. Some efects of posture on the radiographic appearance of the kidneys of the dog. JAVMA 1975;166:165.
18. Lee R, Leowijuk C. Normal parameters in abdominal radiology of the dog and cat. JSAP 1982;23:251.
19. Barr FJ, Holt PE, Gibbs C. Ultrasound measurement of normal renal parameters. JSAP 1990;31:180.
20. Nyland TG, Kantrowitz BM, Fisher P, Olander HJ, Hornof WJ. Ultrasonic determination of kidney volume in the dog. Vet Radiol 1989;30:174.
21. Felkai CS, Voros K, Vrabely T, Karsai F. Ultrasonographic determination of renal volume in the dog. Vet Radiol Ultrasound 1992;33:292.
22. Konde LJ, Wrigley RH, Park RD, Lebel JL. Ultrasound anatomy of the normal canine kidney. Vet Radiol 1984;25:173.
23. Konde LJ. Sonography of the kidney. VCNA 1985;15:1149.
24. Wood AKW, McCarthy PH. Ultrasonographic-anatomic correlation and an imaging protocol of the normal canine kidney. AJVR 1990;51:103.
25. Walter PA, Feeney DA, Johnston GR, Fletcher TF. The normal feline renal ultrasonogram: Quantitative analysis of imaged anatomy. AJVR 1987;48:596.
26. Walter PA, Johnston GR, Feeney DA, O'Brien TD. Renal ultrasonography in healthy cats. AJVR 1987;48:600.
27. Yaeger AE, Anderson WI. Study of association between histologic features and echogenicity of architecturally normal cat kidneys. AJVR 1989;50:860.
28. Pugh CR, Schelling CG, Moreau RE, Golden D. Ultrasound corner iatrogenic renal pyelectasia in the dog. Vet Radiol Ultrasound 1994;35:50.
29. England GCW, Yeager AW. Ultrasonographic appearance of the ovary and uterus of the bitch during oestrus, ovulation and early pregnancy. J Reprod Fertil Suppl 1993;47:107.
30. Kantrowitz BM, Nyland TG, Feldman EC. Adrenal ultrasonography in the dog: Detection of tumors and hyperplasia in hyperadrenocorticism. Vet Radiol 1986;27:91.
31. Voorhut G. X-ray computed tomography, nephrotomography and ultrasonography of the adrenal glands of healthy dogs. AJVR 1990;51:625.
32. Biller DS, Kantrowitz B, Partington B, Miyabayashi T. Diagnostic ultrasound of the urinary bladder. JAAHA 1990;26:397.

33. Douglass JP. Ultrasound corner: Bladder wall mass effect caused by the intrmural portion of the canine ureter. Vet Radiol Ultrasound 1993;34:107.
34. Ackerman N. Radiographic evaluation of the uterus: A review. Vet Radiol 1981;22:252.
35. Collery L. Contrast hysterography in the bitch. Irish Vet J 1956;10:99.
36. Funkquist B, Lagerstedt A-S, Linde C, Obel N. Hysterography in the bitch. Vet Radiol 1985;26:12.
37. Stone EA, Thrall DE, Barber DL. Radiographic interpretation of prostatic disease in the dog. JAAHA 1978;14:115.
38. Cartee RE, Rowles T. Transabdominal sonographic evaluation of the canine prostate. Vet Radiol 1983;24:156.
39. Finn ST, Wrigley RH. Ultrasonography and ultrasound-guided biopsy of the canine prostate. In: Kirk RW, ed. Current veterinary therapy X. Philadelphia: WB Saunders, 1989.
40. Pugh CR, Konde LJ, Park RD. Testicular ultrasound in the normal dog. Vet Radiol 1990;31:194.
41. Spaulding KA. Ultrasound corner—helpful hints in identifying the caudal abdominal aorta and caudal vena cava. Vet Radiol Ultrasound 1992;33:90.
42. Kantrowitz BM, Nyland TG, Fisher P. Estimation of portal blood flow using duplex realtime and pulsed doppler ultrasound imaging in the dog. Vet Radiol 1989;30:222.
43. Rendano VT. Positive contrast peritoneography: An aid in the radiographic diagnosis of diaphragmatic hernia. JAVRS 1979;20:67.
44. Schmidt S, Suter PF. Angiography of the hepatic and portal venous system in the dog and cat: An investigative method. Vet Radiol 1980;21:57.
45. Suter PF. Portal vein anomalies in the dog: Their angiographic diagnosis. JAVRS 1975;16:84.
46. Hornof WJ, Suter PF. The use of prostaglandin El and tolazoline to improve cranial mesenteric portography in the dog. JAVRS 1979;20:15.
47. Allan GS, Dixon RT. Cholecystography in the dog: Choice of contrast media and optimum dose rates. Vet Radiol 1975;16:98.
48. Allan GS, Dixon RT. Cholecystography in the dog: Assessment of radiographic positioning and the use of a double contrast examination by visual and densitometric methods. JAVRS 1977;18:177.
49. Carlisle CH. A comparison of techniques for cholecystography in the cat. JAVRS 1977;18:173.
50. Wrigley RH, Reuter RE. Percutaneous cholecystography in normal dogs. Vet Radiol 1982;23:239.
51. Finn ST, Park RD, Twedt DC, Curtis CR. Ultrasonographic assessment of sincalide-induced canine gallbladder emptying: An aid to the diagnosis of biliary obstruction. Vet Radiol 1991;32:269.
52. Zontine WJ. Effect of chemical restraint drugs on the passage of barium sulfate through the stomach and duodenum of dogs. JAVMA 1973;162:878.
53. Hogan PM, Aronson EA. Effect of sedation on transit time of feline gastrointestinal contrast studies. Vet Radiol 1988;29:85.
54. O'Brien TR. Radiographic diagnosis of abdominal disorders in the dog and cat. Davis, CA: Covell Park Vet Co, 1981.
55. Agut A, Sanchez-Valverde MA, Lasaosa JM, Murciano J, Molina F. Use of iohexol as a gastrointestinal contrast medium in the dog. Vet Radiol Ultrasound 1993;34:171.
56. Allan GS, Rendano VT, Quick CB, Meunier PC. Gastrografin as a gastrointestinal contrast medium in the cat. Vet Radiol 1979;20:110.
57. Williams J, Biller DS, Miyabayashi T, Leveille R. Evaluation of iohexol as a gastroinestinal contrast medium in normal cats. Vet Radiol Ultrasound 1993;34:310.
58. Morgan JP. The upper gastrointestinal tract in the cat: A protocol for contrast radiography. JAVRS 1977;18:134.
59. Miyabayashi T, Morgan JP. Gastric emptying in the normal dog: A contrast radiographic technique. Vet Radiol 1984;25:187.
60. Miyabayashi T, Morgan JP, Atilola MAO, Muhumuza L. Small intestinal emptying time in normal beagle dogs. Vet Radiol 1986;27:164.
61. Burns J, Fox SM. The use of a barium meal to evaluate total gastric emptying time in the dog. Vet Radiol 1986;27:169.
62. Evans SM, Laufer I. Double contrast radiography in the normal dog. Vet Radiol 1981;22:2.
63. Evans SM, Biery DL. Double contrast radiography in the cat: Technique and normal radiographic appearance. Vet Radiol 1983;24:3.
64. Evans SM. Double versus single contrast radiography in the dog and cat. Vet Radiol 1983;24:6.
65. Nyland TG, Ackerman N. Pneumocolon: A diagnostic aid in abdominal radiography. JAVRS 1978;19:203.
66. Root CR. Contrast radiography of the alimentary tract. In: Ticer JW, ed. Radiographic technique in veterinary practice. 2nd ed. Philadelphia: WB Saunders, 1984;364.
67. Probst CW, Stickle RL, Bartlett PC. Duration of pneumoperitoneum in the dog. AJVR 1986;47:176.
68. Probst CW, Bright RM, Ackerman N, Goring RL, Waldron DR. Spontaneous pneumoperitoneum subsequent to gastric volvulus in two dogs. Vet Radiol 1984;25:37.
69. Henley RK, Hager DA, Ackerman N. A comparison of two-dimensional ultrsonography and radiography for the detection of small amounts of free peritoneal fluid in the dog. Vet Radiol 1989;30:121.
70. Konde LJ, Lebel JL, Park RD, Wrigley RH. Sonographic application in the diagnosis of intrabdominal abscess in the dog. Vet Radiol 1986;27:151.
71. Kirpensteijn J, Fingland RB, Ulrich T, Sikkema D, Allen SW. Cholelithiasis in dogs: 29 cases (1980–1990). JAVMA 1993;202:1137.
72. Lord PF, Wilkins RJ. Emphysema of the gall bladder in a diabetic dog. JAVRS 1972;13:49.
73. vanBree H, Jacobs V, Vandekerkhove P. Radiographic assessment of liver volume in dogs. AJVR 1989;50:1613.
74. Owens JM. Radiographic interpretation for the small animal clinician. St. Louis: Ralston Purina Co, 1982.
75. Godshalk CP, Badertscher RR II, Rippy MK, Ghent AW. Quantatative ultrasonic assessment of liver size in the dog. Vet Radiol 1988;29:162.

76. Barr F. Ultrasonographic assessment of liver size in the dog. JSAP 1992;33:359.
77. Barr F. Normal hepatic measurements in mature dogs. JSAP. 1992;33:367.
78. Biller DS, Kantrowitz B, Miyabayashi T. Ultrasonography of diffuse liver disease. JVIM 1992;6:71.
79. Lamb CR, Hartzband LE, Tidwell AS, Pearson SH. Ultrasonographic findings in hepatic and splenic lymphosarcoma in dogs and cats. Vet Radiol 1991;32:117.
80. Voros K, Vrabely T, Papp L, Hovarth L, Karsai F. Correlation of ultrasonographic and pathomophological findings in canine hepatic diseases. JSAP 1991;32:627.
81. Yaeger AE, Mohammed H. Accuracy of ultrasonography in the detection of severe hepatic lipidosis in cats. AJVR 1992;53:597.
82. Stowater JL, Lamb CR, Schelling SH. Ultrasonographic features of canine nodular hyperplasia. Vet Radiol 1990;31:268.
83. Feeney DA, Johnston GR, Hardy RM. Two-dimensional ultrasonography for assessment of hepatic and splenic neoplasia in the dog and cat. JAVMA 1984;184:68.
84. Nyland TG, Gillett NA. Sonographic evaluation of experimental bile duct ligation in the dog. Vet Radiol 1982;23:252.
85. Berry CR, Ackerman N, Charach M, Lawrence D. Iatrogenic biloma (biliary pseudocyst) in a cat with hepatic lipidosis. Vet Radiol Ultrasound 1992;33:145.
86. Neer TM. A review of disorders of the gallbladder and extrahepatic biliary tract in the dog and cat. JVIM 1992;6:186.
87. Wrigley RH, Konde LJ, Park RD, Lebel JL. Ultrasonographic diagnosis of portacaval shunts in young dogs. JAVMA 1987;191:421.
88. Payne JT, Martin RA, Constantinescu GM. The anatomy and embryology of portosystemic shunts in dogs and cats. Semin Vet Med Surg (Small Animal) Portovascular Anomalies 1990;5:76.
89. Bailey MQ, Willard MD, McLoughlin MA, Gaber C, Hauptman J. Ultrasonographic findings associated with congenital hepatic arteriovenous fistula in three dogs. JAVMA 1988;192:1099.
90. Nyland TG, Fisher PE. Evaluation of experimentally induced canine hepatic cirrhosis using duplex doppler ultrasound. Vet Radiol 1990;31:189.
91. Lattgen PJ, Whitney MS, Wolf AM, Scruggs DW. Heinz body hemolytic anemia associated with high plasma zinc concentration in a dog. JAVMA 1990;197:1347.
92. Huml RA, Konde LJ, Sellon RK, Forrest LJ. Gastrogastric intussusception in a dog. Vet Radiol Ultrasound 1992;33:150.
93. Miller RI. Gastrointestinal phycomycosis in 63 dogs. JAVMA 1985;186:473.
94. Van Der Gaag II, Happe RD, Wolvekamp WTC. A boxer dog with chronic hypertrophic gastritis resembling Menetrier's disease in man. Vet Pathol 1976;13:172.
95. Happe RP, Van Der Gaag II, Wolvekamp WTC. Pyloric stenosis caused by hypertrophic gastritis in three dogs. JSAP 1981;22:7.
96. Huxtable CR, Mills JN, Clark WT, Thompson R. Chronic hypertrophic gastritis in a dog: Successful treatment by partial gastrectomy. JSAP 1982;23:639.
97. Walter MC, Goldschmidt MH, Stone EA, et al. Chronic hypertrophic pyloric gastropathy as a cause of pyloric obstruction in the dog. JAVMA 1985;186:157.
98. Penninck DG, Nyland TG, Kerr LY, Fisher PE. Ultrasonographic evaluation of gastrointestinal diseases in small animals. Vet Radiol 1990;31:134.
99. Lamb CR, Hijfte MF. Ultrasound corner beware the gastric pseudomass. Vet Radiol Ultrasound 1994;35(5):398.
100. Penninck DG, Moore AS, Tidwell AS, Matz ME, Freden GO. Ultrasonography of alimentary lymphosarcoma in the cat. Vet Radiol Ultrasound 1994;35:200.
101. Grooters AM, Biller DS, Ward H, Miyabayashi T, Couto G. Ultrasonographic appearance of feline alimentary lymphoma. Vet Radiol Ultrasound 1994;35:468.
102. Biller DS, Partington BP, Miyabayashi T, Leveille R. Ultrasonographic appearance of chronic hypertrophic pyloric gastropathy in the dog. Vet Radiol Ultrasound 1994;35:30.
103. Grooters AM, Miyabayashi T, Biller DS. Sonographic appearance of uremic gastropathy in four dogs. Vet Radiol Ultrasound 1994;35:35.
104. Tidwell AS, Penninck DG. Ultrasonography of gastrointestinal foreign bodies. Vet Radiol Ultrasound 1992;33:160.
105. Kleine LJ, Hornbuckle WE. Acute pancreatitis: The radiographic findings in 182 dogs. JAVRS 1978;19:102.
106. Garvey MS, Zawie DA. Feline pancreatic disease. VCNA 1984;14:1231.
107. Root CR. Abdominal masses: The radiographic differential diagnosis. JAVRS 1974;15:26.
108. Salisbury SK, Lantz GC, Nelson RW, Kazacos EA. Pancreatic abscess in dogs: Six cases (1978–1986). JAVMA 1988;193:1104.
109. Ackerman N, Silverman S. Intra-abdominal soft tissue calcifications. MVP 1977;58:619.
110. Nyland TG, Mulvaney MH, Strombeck DR. Ultrasound features of experimentally induced pancreatitis. Vet Radiol 1983;24:260.
111. Murtaugh RJ, Herring DJ, Jacobs RM, DeHoff WD. Pancreatic ultrasonography in dogs with experimentally induced acute pancreatitis. Vet Radiol 1985;26:27.
112. Simpson KW, Shiroma JT, Biller DS, Wicks J, Johnson SE, Dimski D, Chew D. Antemortem diagnosis of pancreatitis in four cats. JSAP 1994;35:93.
113. Rutgers C, Herring DS, Orton EC. Pancreatic pseudocyst asssociated with acute pancreatitis in a dog: Ultrasonographic diagnosis. JAAHA 1985;21:411.
114. Parker WM, Presnell KR. Mesenteric torsion in the dog: Two cases. Can Vet J 1972;13:283.
115. Felts JF, Fox PR, Burk RL. Thread and sewing needles as gastrointestinal foreign bodies in the cat: A review of 64 cases. JAVMA 1984;184:56.
116. Weichselbaum RC, Feeney DA, Hayden DW. Comparison of upper gastrointestinal radiographic findings to histopatholgic observations: A retrospective study of dogs and cats with suspected small bowel infiltrative disease (1985–1990). Vet Radiol Ultrasound 1994;35:418.

117. Thrall DE, Leininger JR. Irregular intestinal mucosal margination in the dog. JAVMA 1969; 155:713.
118. O'Brien TR, Morgan JP, Lebel JL. Pseudoulcers in the duodenum of the dog. JAVMA 1969; 155:713.
119. Myers NC, Penninck DG. Ultrasonographic diagnosis of gastrointestinal smooth muscle tumors in the dog. Vet Radiol Ultrasound 1994;35:391.
120. Watson DE, Mahaffey MB, Neuwirth LA. Ultrasonographic detection of duodenojejunal intussuception in a dog. JAAHA 1991;27:367.
121. Spaulding KA, Cohn LA, Miller RT, Hardie EM. Enteric duplication in two dogs. Vet Radiol 1990;31:83.
122. Fluke MH, Hawkins EC, Elliott GS, Blevins WE. Short colon in two cats and a dog. JAVMA 1989;195:87.
123. Anderson GR, Geary JC. Canine pneumatosis coli. JAAHA 1973;9:354.
124. Morris EL. Pneumatosis coli in a dog. Vet Radiol Ultrasound 1992;33:154.
125. Ewing GO, Gomez JA. Canine ulcerative colitis. JAAHA 1973;9:392.
126. Miller WW, Hathcock JT, Dillon AR. Cecal inversion in eight dogs. JAAHA 1984;20:1009.
127. Ackerman N. Intravenous pyelography. JAAHA 1974;10:277.
128. Ackerman N. Intravenous pyelography—interpretation of the study. JAAHA 1974;10:281.
129. Bartels JE. Feline intravenous urography. JAAHA 1973;9:349.
130. Biery DN. Chapter 11, upper urinary tract. In: O'Brien TR, ed. Radiographic diagnosis of adominal disorders of the dog and cat. Davis CA: Covell Park Vet Co, 1981.
131. Kneller SK. Role of the excretory urogram in the diagnosis of renal and ureteral disease. VCNA 1974;4:843.
132. Lord PF, Scott RC, Chan KF. Intravenous urography for evaluation of renal disease in small animals. JAAHA 1974;10:139.
133. Feeney DA. Effect of dose on quality of excretory urography. JAVRS 1977;18:34.
134. Feeney DA, Thrall DE, Barber DL, Culver DH, Lewis RE. Normal canine excretory urogram: Effects of dose, time, and individual dog variation. AJVR 1979;40:1596.
135. Byrd L, Sherman RL. Radiocontrast-induced acute renal failure: A clinical and pathophysiologic review. Medicine 1979;58:270.
136. Davidson AJ. Diagnosis of renal parenchymal disease. Philadelphia: WB Saunders, 1984.
137. Walter PA, Feeney DA, Johnston GA. Diagnosis and treatment of adverse reactions to radiopaque contrast agents. In: Kirk RW, ed. Current veterinary therapy IX. Philadelphia: WB Saunders, 1986.
138. Carr AP, Reed AL, Pope ER. Persistant nephrogram in a cat after intravenous urography. Vet Radiol Ultrasound 1994;35:350.
139. Root CR. Contrast radiography of the urinary system. In: Ticer JW, ed. Radiographic technique in veterinary practice. 2nd ed. Philadelphia: WB Saunders, 1984;374.
140. Thrall DE, Finco DR. Canine excretory urography: Is quality a function of BUN? JAAHA 1976; 12:446.
141. Feeney DA, Osborne CA, Jessen CR. Effects of radiographic contrast media on results of urinalysis, with emphasis on alteration in specific gravity. JAVMA 1980;176:1378.
142. Feeney DA, Walter PA, Johnston GR. The effect of radiographic contrast media on the urinalysis. In: Kirk RW, ed. Current veterinary therapy IX. Philadelphia: WB Saunders, 1986.
143. Ruby AL, Ling GV, Ackerman N. Effect of sodium diatrizoate on the *in vitro* growth of three common canine urinary bacterial species. Vet Radiol 1983;24:222.
144. Park RD. Chapter 12, radiology of the urinary bladder and urethra. In: O'Brien TR, ed. Radiographic diagnosis of abdominal disorders of the dog and cat. Davis, CA: Covell Park Vet Co, 1981.
145. Johnston GR, Feeney DA. Comparative organ imaging: Lower urinary tract. Vet Radiol 1984; 25:146.
146. Johnston GR, Feeney DA, Osborne CA. Urethrography and cystography in cats, part 1. Techniques, normal radiographic anatomy and artifacts. Comp Cont Ed 1982;4:823.
147. Mahaffey MB, Barber DL, Barsanti JA, Crowell WA. Simultaneous double-contrast cystography and cystometry in dogs. Vet Radiol 1984;25:254.
148. Mahaffey MB, Barsanti JA, Crowell WA, Shotts E, Barber DL. Cystography: Effect of technique on diagnosis of cystitis in dogs, Vet Radiol 1989;30:261.
149. Ackerman N, Wingfield WE, Corley EA. Fatal air embolism associated with pneumourethrography and pneumocystography in a dog. JAVMA 1972;160:1616.
150. Zontine WJ, Andrews LK. Fatal air embolism as a complication of pneumocystography in two cats. JAVRS 1978;19:8.
151. Christie BA. Vesicoureteral reflux in dogs. JAVMA 1973;162:772.
152. Kipnis RM. Vesicoureteral reflux in a cat. JAVMA 1975;167:288.
153. Newman L, Bucy JG, McAlister WH. Incidence of naturally occurring vesicoureteral reflux in mongrel dogs. Invest Radiol 1973;8:354.
154. Ackerman N. Prostatic reflux during positive retrograde urethrography in the dog. Vet Radiol 1983;24:251.
155. Ackerman N. Use of the pediatric Foley catheter for positive-contrast retrograde urethrography. MVP 1980;684.
156. Johnston GR, Feeney DA, Osborne CA, Johnston SD, Smith FO, Jessen CR. Effects of intravesical hydrostatic pressure and volume on the distensibility of the canine prostatic portion of the urethra. AJVR 1985;46:748.
157. Johnston GR, Jessen CR, Osborne CA. Retrograde contrast urethrography. In: Kirk RW, ed. Current veterinary therapy VI. Phliadelphia: WB Saunders, 1977.
158. Johnston GR, Jessen CR, Osborne CA. Effects of bladder distention on canine and feline retrograde urethrography. Vet Radiol 1983;24:271.
159. Johnston GR, Osborne CA, Jessen CR. Effects of urinary bladder distention on the length of the dog and cat urethra. AJVR 1985;46:509.

160. Johnston GR, Osborne CA, Jessen CR, Feeney DA. Effects of urinary bladder distention on location of the urinary bladder and urethra of healthy dogs and cats. AJVR 1986;47:404.
161. Feeney DA, Johnson GR, Osborne CA, Tomlinson MJ. Dimensions of the prostatic and membranous urethra in normal male dogs during maximum distention retrograde urethrocystography. Vet Radiol 1984;25:249.
162. Feeney DA, Johnston GR, Osborne CA, Tomlinson MJ. Maximum-distention retrograde urethrocystography in healthy male dogs: Occurrence and radiographic appearance of urethroprostatic reflux. AJVR 1984;45:948.
163. Barsanti JA, Crowell W, Losonsky J, Talkington FD. Complications of bladder distention during retrograde urethrography. AJVR 1981;42:819.
164. Poogird W, Wood AKW. Radiologic study of the canine urethra. AJVR 1986;47:2491.
165. Ticer JW, Spencer CP, Ackerman N. Positive contrast retrograde urethrography: A useful procedure for evaluating urethral disorders in the dog. Vet Radiol 1980;21:2.
166. Johnston GR, Stevens JB, Jessen CR, Osborne CA. Effects of prolonged distention of retention catheters on the urethra of dogs and cats. AJVR 1983;44:223.
167. Johnston GR, Stevens JB, Jessen CR, Osborne CA. Complications of retrograde contrast urethrography in dogs and cats. AJVR 1983;44:1248.
168. Jacobs G, Barsanti J, Prasse K, Selcer B. Colliculus seminalis as a cause of a urethral filling defect in two dogs with Sertoli cell testicular neoplasms. JAVMA 1988;192:1748.
169. Miller JB, Sande R. Osseous metaplasia in the renal pelvis of a dog with hydronephrosis. JAVRS 1980;21:146.
170. Kaufmann ML, Osborne CA, Johnston GR, O'Brien TD, Levine SH, Hartmann WL. Renal ectopia in a dog and a cat. JAVMA 1987;190:73.
171. Barber DL, Finco DR. Radiographic findings in induced bacterial pyelo-nephritis in dogs. JAVMA 1979;175:1183.
172. Biery DN. Radiographic evaluation of the kidneys. In: Bovee KC, ed. Canine nephrology. Philadelphia: Harwell Publishing Co, 1984;275.
173. Ettinger SJ, Feldman EC. Ethylene glycol poisoning in a dog. Mod Vet Pract 1977;58:237.
174. Kneller SK. Role of the excretory urogram in the diagnosis of renal and ureteral disease. VCNA 1974;4:843.
175. Lord PF, Scott RC, Chan KF. Intravenous urography for evaluation of renal disease in small animals. JAAHA 1974;10:139.
176. Watson ADJ. The nephrotic syndrome due to renal amyloidosis in a dog. Aust Vet J 1971;47:398.
177. Feeney DA, Barber DL, Osborne CA. The functional aspects of the nephrogram in excretory urography: A review. Vet Radiol 1982;23:42.
178. Biller DS, Chew DJ, DiBartola SP. Polycystic kidney disease in a family of Persian cat. JAVMA 1990;196:1288.
179. Johnson ME, Denhart JD, Graber ER. Renal cortical hypoplasia in a litter of cocker spaniels. JAAHA 1972;8:268.
180. Cartee RE, Selcer BA, Patton CS. Ultrasonographic diagnosis of renal disease in small animals. JAVMA 1980;176:426.
181. Ackerman N, Hager DA, Kaude JV. Ultrasound appearance and early detection of VX 2 carcinoma in the rabbit kidney; comparison with renal angiography and excretory urography. Vet Radiol 1989;30:88.
182. Walter PA, Johnston GR, Feeney DA, O'Leary TP. Ultrasonographic evaluation of renal parenchymal disease in dogs: 32 cases (1981–9186). JAVMA 1987;191:999.
183. Konde LJ, Wrigley RH, Park RD, Lebel JL. Sonographic appearance of renal neoplasia in the dog. Vet Radiol 1985;26:74.
184. Konde LJ, Park RD, Wrigley RH, Lebel JL. Comparison of radiography and ultrasonography in the evaluation of renal lesions in the dog. JAVMA 1986;188:1420.
185. Walter PA, Johnston GR, Feeney DA, O'Brien TD. Applications of ultrasonography in the diagnosis of parenchymal kidney disease in cats: 24 cases (1981–1986). JAVMA 1988;192:92.
186. Biller DS, Schenkman DI, Bortnowski H. Ultrasonographic appearance of renal infarction in a dog. JAAHA 1991;27:370.
187. Neuwirth L, Mahaffey M, Crowell W, Selcer B, Barsanti J, Cooper R, Brown J. Comparison of excretory urography and ultrasonography for detection of experimentally induced pyelonephritis in dogs. AJVR 1993;54:660.
188. Kaude JV, Kekomoki M, Walker D, Fitzsimmons JR. Imaging of unilateral hydronephrosis in an experimental animal. Acta Radiol Diag 1985;25:501.
189. Barr FJ, Patteson MW, Lucke VM, Gibbs C. Hypercalcemic nephropathy in three dogs: Sonographic appearance. Vet Radiol 1989;30:169.
190. Biller DS, Bradley GA, Partington BP. Renal medullary rim sign: Ultrasonographic evidence of renal disease. Vet Radiol Ultrasound 1992;33:286.
191. Adams WH, Toal RL, Walker MA, Breider MA. Early renal ultrasonographic findings in experimentally induced ethylene glycol nephrosis. AJVR 1989;50:1370.
192. King W, Kimme-Smith C, Winter J. Renal stone shadowing: An investigation of contributing factors. Radiology 1985;154:191.
193. Ackerman N. Canine ureteral ectopia. Cal Vet 1978;32:9.
194. Johnston GR, Osborne CA, Wilson JW, Yano BL. Familial ureteral ectopia in the dog. JAAHA 1977;13:168.
195. Lennox JS. A case report of unilateral ectopic ureter in a male siberian husky. JAAHA 1978;14:331.
196. Osborne CA, Dieterich HF, Hanlon GF, Anderson LD. Urinary incontinence due to ectopic ureter in a male dog. JAVMA 1975;166:911.
197. Owen R, Ap R. Canine ureteral ectopia—A review. JSAP 1973;14:407.
198. Smith CW, Stowater JL, Kneller SK. Ectopic ureter in the dog. A review of cases. JAAHA 1981;17:245.

199. Tidwell AS, Ullman SL, Schelling SH. Urinoma (para-ureteral pseudocyst) in a dog. Vet Radiol 1990;31:203.

200. Root CR, Scott RC. Emphysematous cystitis and other radiographic manifestations of diabetes mellitus in dogs and cats. JAVMA 1971;158:721.

201. Scherding RG, Chew DJ. Nondiabetic emphysematous cystitis in two dogs. JAVMA 1979;174:1105.

202. Adams WM, DiBartola SP. Radiographic and clinical features of pelvic bladder in the dog. JAVMA 1983;182:1212.

203. Mahaffey MB, Barsanti JA, Barber DL, Crowell WA. Pelvic bladder in dogs without urinary incontinence. JAVMA 1984;184:1477.

204. Johnston GR, Osborne CA, Jessen CR, Feeney DA. Effects of urinary bladder distention on location of the urinary bladder and urethra of healthy dogs and cats. AJVR 1986;47:404.

205. Crow SE, Theilen GH, Madewell BR, et al. Cyclophosphamide-induced cystitis in the dog and cat. JAVMA 1977;171:259.

206. Stanton ME, Legendre AM. Effects of cyclophosphamide in dogs and cats. JAVMA 1986;188:1319.

207. Laing EJ, Miller CW, Cochrane SM. Treatment of cyclophosphamide-induced hemorrhagic cystitis in five dogs. JAVMA 1988;193:233.

208. Halliwell WH, Ackerman N. Botryoid rhabdomyosarcoma of the urinary bladder and hypertrophic osteoarthropathy in a young dog. JAVMA 1974;165:911.

209. Johnston SD, Osborne CA, Stevens JB. Canine polypoid cystitis. JAVMA 1975;166:1155.

210. Leveille R, Biller DS, Partington BP, Miyabayashi T. Sonographic investigation of transitional cell carcinoma of the urinary bladder in small animals. Vet Radiol Ultrasound 1992;33:103.

211. Berry CR. Ultrasound corner—differentiating cystic calculi from the colon. Vet Radiol Ultrasound 1992;33:283.

212. Moroff SD, Brown BA, Matthiesen DT, Scott RC. Infiltrative urethral disease in female dogs: 41 cases (1980–1987). JAVMA 1991;199:247.

213. Ticer TW, Spencer CP, Ackerman N. Transitional cell carcinoma of the urethra in four female dogs: Its urethrographic appearance. Vet Radiol 1980;21:12.

214. Burk RL, Schaubhut CW. Obstructive urethritis in the female dog. VMSAC 1976;71:898.

215. Osborne CA, Engen MH, Yano BL, Brasmer TH, Jessen CR, Blevins WE. Congenital urethrorectal fistula in two dogs. JAVMA 1975;166:999.

216. Adams WM, Biery DN, Millar HC. Pneumovaginography in the dog: A case report. JAVRS 1978;19:80.

217. Holt PE, Gibbs C, Latham J. An evaluation of positive contrast vagino-urethrography as a diagnostic aid in the bitch. JSAP 1984;25:531.

218. Cobb LM, Archibald J. The radiographic appearance of certain pathological conditions of the canine uterus. JAVMA 1959;134:393.

219. Pharr JW, Post K. Ultrasonography and radiography of the canine post partum uterus. Vet Radiol Ultrasound 1992;33:35.

220. Toal RL, Walker MA, Henry GA. A comparison of real-time ultrasound, palpation and radiography in pregnancy detection and litter size determination in the bitch. Vet Radiol 1986;27:102.

221. Bartels JE. Radiology of the genital tract. In: O'Brien TR, ed. Radiographic diagnosis of abdominal disorders in the dog and cat. Davis, CA: Covell Park Vet Co, 1981;615.

222. Farrow CS, Morgan JP, Story EC. Late term fetal death in the dog: Early radiographic diagnosis. JAVRS 1976;17:11.

223. Goodwin JK, Hager DA, Philips L, Lyman R. Bilateral ovarian adenocarcinoma in a dog: Ultrasonographic-aided diagnosis. Vet Radiol 1990;31:265.

224. Wrigley RH, Finn ST. Ultrasonography of the canine uterus and ovary. In: Kirk RW, ed. Current veterinary therapy X. Philadelphia: WB Saunders, 1989.

225. Poffenbarger EM, Feeney DA. Use of gray-scale ultrasonography in the diagnosis of reproductive disease in the bitch: 18 cases (1981–1984). JAVMA 1986;189:90.

226. Fayrer-Hoskin RA, Mahaffey M, Miller-Liebl D, Caudle AB. Early diagnosis of canine pyometra using ultrasonography. Vet Radiol 1991;32:287.

227. Davidson AP, Nyland TG, Tsutsui T. Pregnancy diagnosis with ultrasound in the domestic cat. Vet Radiol 1986;27:109.

228. Schille VM, Gontarek J. The use of ultrasound for pregnancy diagnosis in the bitch. JAVMA 1985;187:1021.

229. Concannon P, Rendano V. Radiographic diagnosis of canine pregnancy: Onset of fetal skeletal radiopacity in relation to times breeding, preovulatory luteinizing hormone release, and parturition. AJVR 1983;44:1506.

230. Cartee RE, Rowles T. Preliminary study of the ultrasonographic diagnosis of pregnancy and fetal development in the dog. AJVR 1984;45:1259.

231. Rivers B, Johnston GR. Diagnostic imaging of the reproductive organs of the bitch—methods and limitations. VCNA 1991;21:437.

232. Johnston SD, Smith FO, Bailie NC, Johnston GR, Feeney DA. Prenatal indicators of puppy viability at term. Comp Cont Ed Pract Vet 1983;5:1013.

233. Verstegen JP, Silva LDM, Onchin K, Donnay I. Echocardiographic study of heart rate in dog and cat fetuses in utero. J Reprod Fertil 1993;47(Suppl):175.

234. Beck KA, Baldwin CJ, Bosu WTK. Ultrasound prediction of parturition in queens. Vet Radiol 1990;31:32.

235. O'Shea JD. Studies on the canine prostate gland. I. Factors influencing its size and weight. J Comp Pathol 1962;72:321.

236. O'Shea JD. Studies on the canine prostate gland. II. Prostatic neoplasms. J Comp Pathol 1963;73:244.

237. O'Shea JD. Squamous metaplasia of the canine prostate gland. Res Vet Sci 1963;4:431.

238. Berg OA. The normal prostate gland of the dog. Acta Endocrinol 1958;27:129.

239. Berg OA. Parenchymatous hypertrophy of the canine prostate gland. Acta Endocrinol 1958;27:140.

240. Berg OA. Effect of stilbestrol on the prostate gland in normal puppies and adult dogs. Acta Endocrinol 1958;27:155.

241. Atilola MAO, Pennock PW. Cystic uterus masculinus in the dog: Six case history reports. Vet Radiol 1986;27:8.

242. Leav I, Ling GV. Adenocarcinoma of the canine prostate. Cancer 1968;22:1329.

243. Stone EA, Thrall DE, Barber DL. Radiographic interpretation of prostatic disease in the dog. JAAHA 1978;14:115.

244. Stowater JL, Lamb CR. Ultrasonographic features of paraprostatic cysts in nine dogs. Vet Radiol 1989;30:232.

245. Feeney DA, Johnson GR, Klausner JS, et al. Canine prostatic disease-comparison of ultrasonographic appearance with morphological and microbiological findings: 30 cases (1981–1985). JAVMA 1987;190:1027.

246. Naylor RW, Thompson SMR. Intra-abdominal testicular torsion: A report of two cases. JAAHA 1979;15:763.

247. Johnston GR, Feeney DA, Johnston SD, O'Brien TD. Ultrasonographic features of testicular neoplasms in dogs: 16 cases (1980–1988). JAVMA 1991;198:1770.

248. Pugh CR, Konde LJ. Sonographic evaluation of canine testicular and scrotal abnormalities: A review of 26 case histories. Vet Radiol Ultrasound 1991;32:243.

249. Stevenson S, Chew DJ, Kociba GJ. Torsion of the splenic pedicle in the dog: A review. JAAHA 1981;17:239.

250. Stickle R. Radiographic signs of isolated splenic torsion in dogs: Eight cases (1980–1987). JAVMA 1989;194:103.

251. Konde LJ, Wrigley RH, Lebel JL, Park RD, Pugh C, Finn S. Sonographic and radiographic changes associated with splenic torsion in the dog. Vet Radiol 1989;30:41.

252. Schelling CG, Wortman JA, Saunders HM. Ultrasonic detection of splenic necrosis in the dog. Three case reports of splenic necrosis secondary to infarction. Vet Radiol 1988;29:277.

253. Wrigley RH, Konde LJ, Park RD, Lebel JL. Ultrasonographic features of splenic lymphosarcoma in dogs: 12 cases (1980–1986). JAVMA 1988;193:1565.

254. Wrigley RH, Konde LJ, Park RD, Lebel JL. Clinical features and diagnosis of splenic hematoma in dogs: 10 cases (1980–1987). JAAHA 1989;25:371.

255. Hanson JA, Penninck DG. Ultrasonographic evaluation of a traumatic splenic hematoma and literature review. Vet Radiol Ultrasound 1994;35:463.

256. Wrigley RH, Park RD, Konde LJ, Lebel JL. Ultrasonographic features of splenic hemangiosarcoma in dogs: 18 cases (1980–1986). JAVMA 1988;192:1113.

257. Poffenbarger EM, Feeney DA, Hayden DW. Gray-scale ultrasonography in the diagnosis of adrenal neoplasia in dogs: Six cases (1981–1986). JAVMA 1988;192:228.

Chapter Four

THE APPENDICULAR SKELETON

INTRODUCTION

The radiographic diagnosis of bone and joint disease is composed of two processes: description and interpretation of the lesion. Description of a lesion usually requires at least two radiographs that are centered on the region of interest, carefully positioned, properly exposed, and at right angles to each other. The radiographs should include the joints that are proximal and distal to the lesion. For joint lesions, the radiograph should be centered on the joint.

Radiographs generally are described by the path that the x-ray beam traverses. Commonly used views include ventrodorsal, dorsoventral, dorsopalmer, dorsoplantar, mediolateral, and lateromedial.[1] Several other views to evaluate specific areas of patient anatomy have been described.[2-9]

Knowledge of normal musculoskeletal anatomy, especially with regard to the immature animal, is essential for lesion recognition. The location and dates of closure for the growth plates can be very important in evaluating the radiograph (Table 4–1).[10] Comparison radiographs of the opposite limb can be extremely valuable (Fig. 4–1).

Radiographs must be evaluated systematically. One approach involves sequentially examining the soft tissues surrounding the bone, the periosteal and endosteal surfaces, the cortical thickness and density, the medullary density and trabecular pattern, the articular surfaces, the subchondral bone density and thickness, and the joint space width.

Interpretation of a bone lesion requires knowledge of the age, breed, and species involved, the usual site or sites of involvement (i.e., specific joint, bone, or location within the bone), the number of bones or joints involved, (i.e. mono- or polyostotic, mono- or polyarticular), and whether a disease usually is localized or generalized.

Bone can respond to stress or injury only by removal of existing bone (destruction or osteolysis) or by adding new bone (bony proliferation or sclerosis). A loss of 30% to 50% of the bone density is required before the loss can be detected radiographically. (1) Alteration of the trabecular pattern or loss of the normal bone density within the medullary canal or subchondral bone, or (2) a decrease in cortical thickness or break in cortical continuity may be seen when bony destruction is present. Bone loss within the cortex may be detected more easily than bone loss within the medullary canal. Bony proliferation may originate from the periosteum (outer cortical margins) or endosteum (inner cortical margin) or within the medullary canal.

The aggressiveness, activity, or rate of change of a bony lesion can be estimated by evaluating the amount and nature of the bony destruction and/or proliferation that is present and the margin between the normal and abnormal bone. Slowly progressive or inactive (non-aggressive or benign) bone or joint lesions are characterized by a well-defined, smooth, well-mineralized, uniformly dense margin on periosteal and

TABLE 4-1. Age at Appearance of Ossification Centers and of Bony Fusion in the Immature Canine

ANATOMICAL SITE	AGE AT APPEARANCE OF OSSIFICATION CENTER	AGE WHEN FUSION OCCURS	ANATOMICAL SITE	AGE AT APPEARANCE OF OSSIFICATION CENTER	AGE WHEN FUSION OCCURS
Scapula			Ilium	Birth	4–6 mo
Body	Birth		Ischium	Birth	4–6 mo
Tuber scapulae	7 wk	4–7 mo	Os acetabulum	7 wk	5 mo
Humerus			Iliac crest	4 mo	1–2 yr
Diaphysis	Birth		Tuber ischii	3 mo	8–10 mo
Proximal epiphysis	1–2 wk	10-13 wk	Ischial arch	6 mo	12 mo
Distal epiphysis		6–8 mo to shaft	Caudal symphysis pubis	7 mo	5 yr
			Symphysis pubis		5 yr
Medial condyle	2–3 wk	6 wk to lateral condyle	*Femur*		
			Diaphysis	Birth	
			Proximal epiphysis (head)	2 wk	7–11mo
Lateral condyle	2–3 wk		Trochanter major	8 wk	6–10 mo
Medial epicondyle	6–8 wk	6 mo to condyles	Trochanter minor	8 wk	8–13 mo
Radius			Distal epiphysis		8–11 mo to shaft
Diaphysis	Birth		Trochlea	2 wk	3 mo condyle to trochlea
Proximal epiphysis	3–5 wk	6–11 mo			
Distal epiphysis	2–4 wk	8–12 wk	Medial condyle	3 wk	
			Lateral condyle	3 wk	
Ulna					
Diaphysis	Birth		*Patella*	9 wk	
Olecranon	8 wk	6–10 mo	Tibia		
Distal epiphysis	8 wk	8–12 mo	Diaphysis	Birth	
Anconeal process	12 wk	4–5 mo	Condyles		
Carpus					
Ulnar	4 wk		Medial	3 wk	6 wk to lateral
Radial	3–4 wk				
Central	4–5 wk		Lateral	3 wk	6–12 mo to shaft
Intermediate	3–4 wk				
Accessory			Tuberosity	8 wk	6–8 mo to condyles
Body	2 wk				
Epiphysis	7 wk	4 mo			6–12 mo to shaft
First	3 wk				
Second	4 wk		Distal epiphysis	3 wk	8–11 mo
Third	4 wk		Medial malleolus	3 mo	5 mo
Fourth	3 wk		*Fibula*		
Sesamoid bone	4 mo		Diaphysis	Birth	
Metacarpus			Proximal epiphysis	9 wk	8–12 mo
Diaphysis	Birth		Distal epiphysis	2–7 wk	7–11 mo
Distal epiphysis (2–5)ᵃ	4 wk	6 mo	*Tarsus*		
Proximal epiphysis (1)ᵃ	5 wk	6 mo	Tibial	Birth-1 wk	
Phalanges			Fibular	Birth-1 wk	
First phalanx			Tuber calcis	6 wk	3–8 mo
Diaphysis (1–5)ᵃ	Birth		Central	3 wk	
Distal epiphysis (2–5)ᵃ	4 wk	6 mo	First	4 wk	
Distal epiphysis (1)ᵃ	6 wk	6 mo	Second	4 wk	
Second phalanx			Third	3 wk	
Diaphysis (2–5)ᵃ	Birth		Fourth	2 wk	
Proximal epiphysis(2–5)ᵃ	5 wk	6 mo			
Second phalanx absent or fused with first in first digit.			Metatarsus and pelvic limb phalanges are approximately the same as the metacarpus and pectoral limb phalanges.		
Third phalanx			*Sesamoids*		
Diaphysis	Birth		Fabellar	3 mo	
Volar sesamoids	2 mo		Popliteal	3 mo	
Dorsal sesamoids	4 mo		Plantar phalangeal	2 mo	
Pelvis			Dorsal phalangeal	5 mo	
Pubis	Birth	4–6 mo			

ᵃDigit numbers.

From: Ticer JW. Radiographic technique in small animal practice. Philadelphia: WB Saunders Co, 1975;101. Reproduced courtesy of publisher.

endosteal surfaces and the presence of an organized trabecular pattern in the medullary canal (Fig. 4–2). Rapidly progressive, active (aggressive or malignant) bone lesions have poorly defined, irregular, unevenly mineralized margins and gradual transition between the normal, uninvolved bone and the lesion (Fig. 4–3).

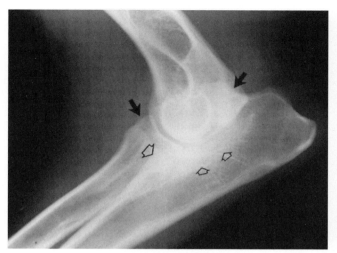 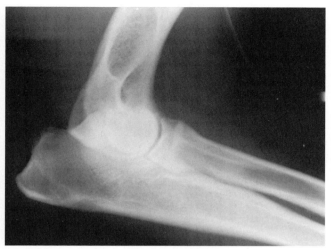

A   B

Figure 4–1. A 9-month-old male German shepherd dog that has been lame in the right fore-limb for 2 months. The dog resented manipulation of the elbow. (A) A lateral radiograph of the right elbow and (B) a comparison lateral radiograph of the left elbow were obtained. (A) There is increased density involving the subchondral bone of the proximal right ulna (*small open arrows*). The coronoid process is flattened and indistinct (*large open arrow*). There is a slight amount of bony proliferation with remodeling of the proximal aspect of the anconeal process and irregularity involving the proximal aspect of the radius (*solid arrows*). These changes in this elbow are more apparent when compared with the normal left elbow. **Diagnosis:** Fragmented coronoid process.

Other imaging methods of evaluating bones and joints include scintigraphy, computed tomography (CT) and magnetic resonance imaging (MRI). Ultrasound studies can be useful in selected situations. Each methodology has unique strengths and weaknesses. Scintigraphy is particularly useful in identifying the location of a lesion because increased uptake of radionuclide frequently occurs in lesions that may not be radiographically apparent.[11,12] CT is useful because it is more sensitive than standard radiographs in detecting decalcification and evaluating a cross sectional image.[13] MRI provides superior soft tissue resolution and may be particularly useful in evaluating cartilage and other soft tissue structures. Ultrasound can be used when skeletal structures are not calcified (e.g., neonates) or to evaluate associated soft tissue structures (e.g., tendons, ligaments).[14]

Bone and joint lesions may be classified as traumatic, neoplastic, infectious, nutritional, metabolic, toxic, anatomic, developmental congenital, and idiopathic. Each time a bone lesion is identified these disease categories should be reviewed.

FRACTURE, FRACTURE HEALING, COMPLICATIONS

DEFINITION AND CLASSIFICATION

A fracture is a complete or incomplete discontinuity or break in a bone. Two radiographs exposed at right angles, which include the joints proximal and distal to the fracture site, must be obtained to define the fracture appropriately. Fractures are classified according to the bone involved, the location within the bone, the path of discontinuity, the position of the distal (relative to the proximal) fragment (including any rotational distraction), involvement of the joint and/or physis, evidence of underlying or pre-existing disease, and damage to surrounding soft tissues.[15]

Various reference points have been designated to describe fracture location. These reference points include anatomic sites (i.e., epiphyseal, metaphyseal, diaphyseal) or arbitrary points (i.e., proximal, middle, distal thirds of the bone, or the junctions between these points). The path or direction of the fracture must also be

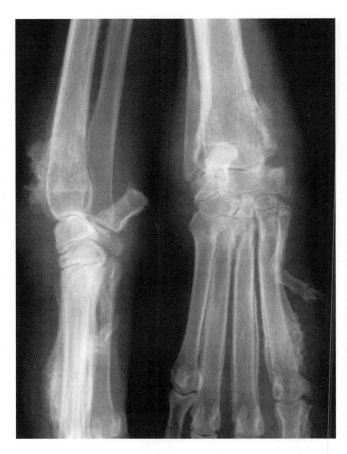

Figure 4–2. A 6-year-old spayed Great Dane with a chronic soft tissue infection of the right front foot. There is extensive bony proliferation involving the cranial medial aspect of the distal radius; radial carpal bone; 1st, 2nd, and 3rd metacarpal bones; and 1st and 2nd phalanges of the 2nd digit. The bony proliferation is smooth, well-mineralized, and possesses an organized trabecular pattern. **Diagnosis:** Benign or chronic inflammation. In this case, the reaction is secondary to chronic soft tissue infection.

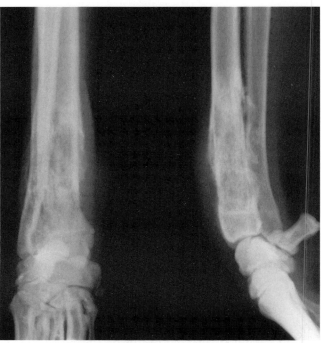

Figure 4–3. A 9-year-old female Great Dane presented with a 5-week history of swelling and lameness in the left front leg. There is localized soft tissue swelling around the distal radius and ulna, and poorly mineralized, poorly defined bony proliferation on the cranial and medial surfaces of the distal radius. There is extensive bony destruction present. The irregular poorly mineralized bony proliferation indicates an aggressive process. The location of the lesion and its destructive nature as well as the localized soft tissue swelling are indicative of a primary bone neoplasm. **Diagnosis:** Osteosarcoma.

described according to the fracture's relation to the bone's long axis or cortical margins. The proper description of many fractures will require the use of more than one descriptor from the following list:

1. Transverse: The fracture line is perpendicular to the long axis or both cortices of the bone (Fig. 4–4).

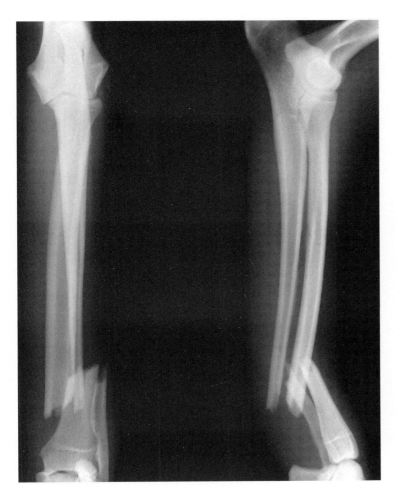

Figure 4–4. A 2-year-old female greyhound presented with a non-weight-bearing left foreleg. There is marked soft tissue swelling of the left foreleg. There are transverse fractures of the radius and ulna involving the middle and distal thirds. There is lateral and cranial displacement of the distal fragments with overriding. **Diagnosis:** Transverse fracture.

2. Oblique: The fracture line strikes the long axis or cortex at an angle other than 90° (Fig. 4–5).

3. Spiral: The fracture line encircles the shaft and forms a spiral relative to the long axis of the bone (Fig. 4–6).

4. Comminuted (butterfly fragment, segmental): Multiple fracture lines within the same bony segment dividing the fracture into more than two fragments (Fig. 4–7).

5. Impaction (depression, compression): Displacement of one fragment forcibly into another.

6. Incomplete (greenstick, torus): The fracture line does not completely separate the cortex on one side (Fig. 4–8).

7. Multiple (segmental): Two or more separate fractures within the same bone with no communication of fracture lines (Fig. 4–9).

8. Fissure (incomplete fracture): A crack in the cortex (Fig. 4–10).

9. Avulsion: Displacement of fragment at the site of muscle or tendinous insertion (Fig. 4–11).

10. Pathologic: Fracture that results from underlying disease, which decreases bone strength (Fig. 4–12).

11. Fatigue (stress): Discontinuity due to repetitive stress with gradual interruption of the bone structure at a greater rate than can be offset by the reparative process.

The position of the major distal fragment relative to the major proximal fragment must be described according to its location on both views (i.e., displacement may be

text continued on p. 437

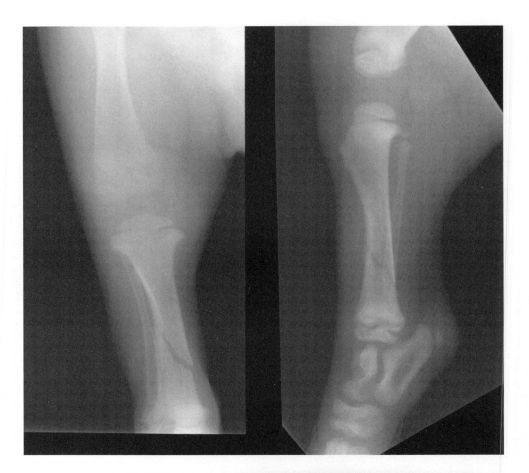

Figure 4–5. A 3-month-old male Australian shepherd that became acutely lame in the right rear leg after playing with a big dog. There is an oblique fracture of the middle portion of the right tibia. The fibula is intact. There is only slight displacement of the fracture fragments and slight soft tissue swelling. **Diagnosis:** Oblique fracture.

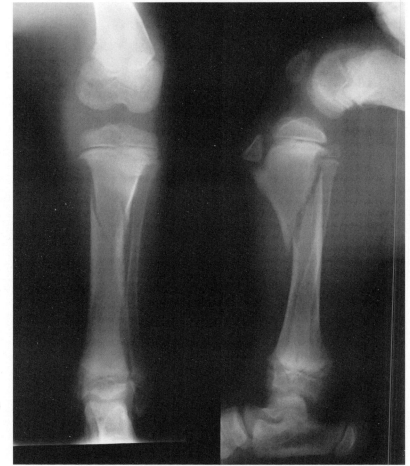

Figure 4–6. A 2-month-old male Rhodesian ridgeback that fell off the porch and presented with a non-weight-bearing left rear leg. There is a spiral fracture of the left tibia involving the proximal and middle third. There is caudal medial displacement of the distal fragment with overriding. The fibula is intact and this most likely explains the minimal displacement that has occurred. **Diagnosis:** Spiral fracture. The widened joint spaces both proximal and distal to the fracture are due to the dog's young age.

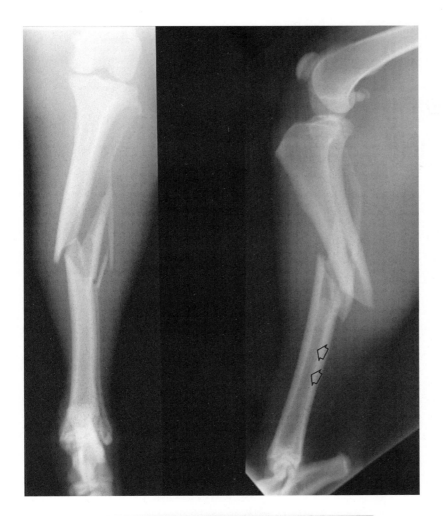

Figure 4–7. A 2-year-old female Australian shepherd was hit by a car and presented non-weight-bearing on the right rear limb. There is a comminuted fracture involving the midportion of the right tibia. There is a large butterfly fragment separated from the lateral cortex of the tibia. There is cranial and lateral displacement of the distal tibia fragment with slight overriding of the fracture fragments. There is a thin fissure fracture extending distally in the distal tibia (*arrows*). Fractures of this sort should be carefully noted on pre-operative radiographs. There are a multiple fractures of the fibula with fracture lines at three sites. **Diagnosis:** Comminuted tibial fracture and multiple fibular fractures.

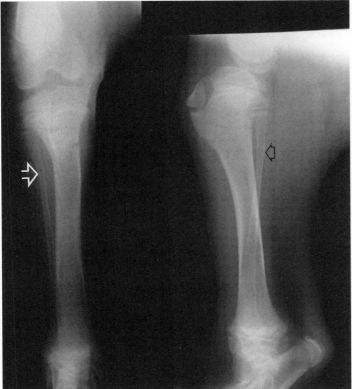

Figure 4–8. A 3-month-old female mixed breed dog was stepped on by the owner and has been non-weight-bearing on the left hindlimb since that time. There is an incomplete fracture involving the proximal third of the left tibia. There is also a folding fracture involving the proximal fibula (*arrows*). The overall bone density appears decreased and the cortices are thin. The thin cortices, poor bone density, and folding-type fracture are indicative of pathologic fractures due to secondary hyperparathyroidism. This dog's diet was predominantly meat and therefore a diagnosis of nutritional secondary hyperparathyroidism was made. **Diagnosis:** Green stick and folding fractures. The dog had an additional green stick fracture of the left femur.

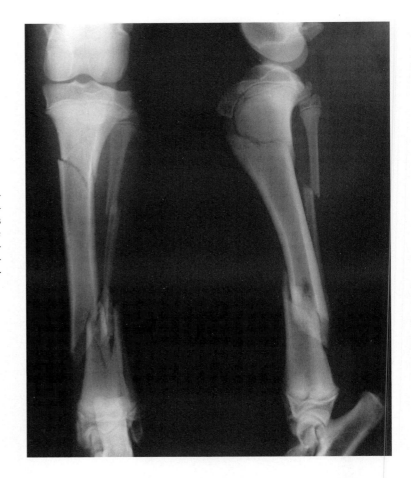

Figure 4–9. A 7-month-old male Doberman pinscher that was hit by a car and was non-weight-bearing on the right rear leg. There are multiple fractures of the right tibia and fibula. The distal tibial fracture is comminuted. There is cranial and lateral displacement of the distal fragment and cranial medial displacement of the middle fragment of the tibia. **Diagnosis:** Multiple fractures.

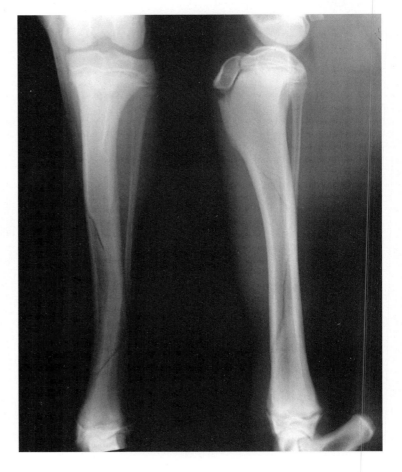

Figure 4–10. A 7-month-old male Labrador retriever presented with an acute lameness in the right rear leg. There was no history of trauma; however, the dog had been running free. There is soft tissue swelling involving the midshaft right tibia. There is an incomplete fracture involving the middle and distal thirds of the right tibia. The fibula is intact and displacement is minimal. **Diagnosis:** Fissure fracture.

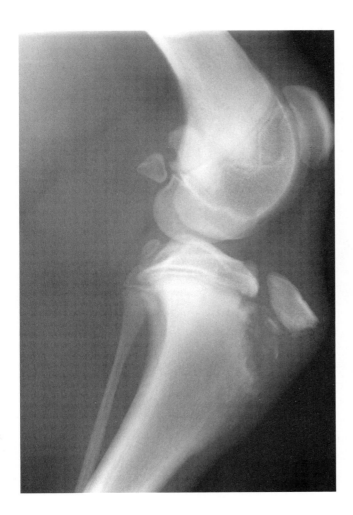

Figure 4–11. A 5-month-old male greyhound presented with a left rear lameness of 10 day's duration. There is an avulsion fracture involving the tibial tuberosity. There are multiple fragments of bone noted at the fracture site. There is proximal displacement of the tibial tuberosity. **Diagnosis:** Avulsion fracture.

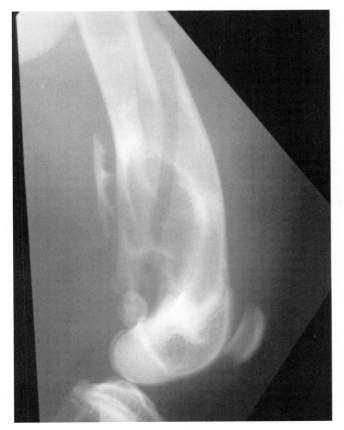

Figure 4–12. A 9-month-old male Doberman pinscher presented with an acute onset of left rear leg lameness. There was no evidence of trauma. There is a large radiolucent lesion in the middle and distal portions of the left femur. The lesion's margins are smooth, the cortex is thin, and there is no evidence of periosteal proliferation. There is a comminuted fracture through this area with cranial displacement of the distal fragment. **Diagnosis:** Pathologic fracture. This fracture has occurred through a primary bone cyst.

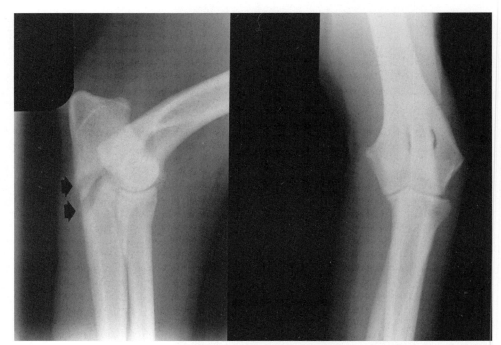

Figure 4–13. A 16-month-old female Irish setter that was hit by a car and presented with left front leg lameness. There is a fracture involving the proximal ulna that extends into the joint. There is only slight displacement of the fracture fragments. The margins of the fracture are smooth and there is a faint periosteal response on the caudal aspect of the ulna (*arrows*). This is because the fracture was 12-days-old. **Diagnosis:** Intra-articular transverse fracture.

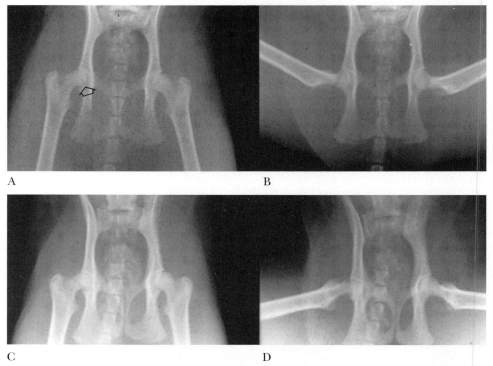

A

B

C

D

Figure 4–14. A 3-month-old domestic short-haired cat presented with a right rear limb lameness, which occurred after a tape recorder fell on the cat. Pain was elicited on palpation of the right hip. On (A&B) the initial radiograph obtained at the time of presentation, there is slight malalignment of the right femoral capital epiphysis (*arrow*). Radiographs were obtained 3 days later (C&D). The fracture line and fracture displacement are obvious. **Diagnosis:** Femoral capital epiphyseal fracture (Salter type I).

cranial and lateral, caudal and medial, etc.). In addition, the degree of proximal displacement (overriding) of fragments, displacement of one fragment into another (impaction), axial alignment (e.g., varus or valgus), and joint or physeal involvement should be noted (Fig. 4–13).

Physeal lines, secondary ossification centers, and irregular ossification patterns may be mistaken for fractures. Comparison radiographs of the uninjured opposite extremity may be extremely helpful in evaluating immature patients.

Fractures in immature patients frequently involve the growth plate (physis). The common patterns of physeal fractures are classified according to the direction and extent of the fracture line as described in the following list:

Classification of physeal fractures

Type I—Fracture extending through the physis with epiphyseal displacement (Fig. 4–14).

Type II—Fracture extending through the physis into the metaphysis with a triangular segment of metaphysis accompanying the displaced epiphysis (Fig. 4–15).

Type III—Fracture extending from the joint through the epiphysis, to the physis, and then along the physis with displacement of a portion of the epiphysis.

Type IV—Fracture extending from the joint through the epiphysis, physis, and adjacent metaphysis (Fig. 4–16).

Type V—Impaction (crushing) injury to physis without displacement (Fig. 4–17).

Any fracture that involves a physis may result in a growth disturbance. The probability of a growth disturbance increases from Type I to Type V fractures.[16,17]

The growth disturbance that results from physeal trauma varies depending upon the trauma site, severity of the injury, and the animal's remaining growth potential

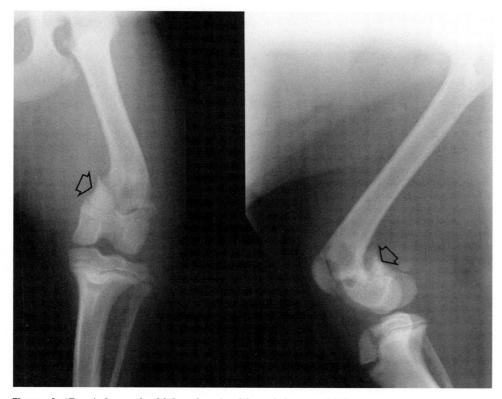

Figure 4–15. A 6-month-old female mixed breed that was hit by a car and presented non-weight-bearing on the right rear leg. There is a Salter II fracture of the distal femur. A medial metaphyseal fragment can be seen (*arrows*). There is caudal and medial displacement of the distal fragment with overriding. **Diagnosis:** Salter II fracture.

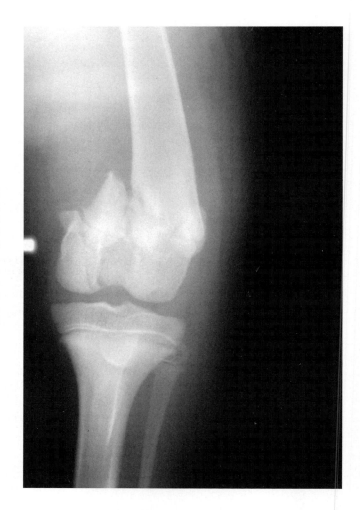

Figure 4–16. A 6-month-old male Great Dane was presented after falling from a moving truck and was non-weight-bearing on the left rear leg. Lateral and postero-anterior radiographs were obtained: only the postero-anterior is illustrated. There is a Salter IV fracture of the distal left femur. The fracture line extends through the distal femoral metaphysis and epiphysis. The articular surface is involved. The medial condyle and medial portion of the distal femoral metaphysis are displaced medially. The fracture line also extends through the physeal plate to the lateral side of the distal femur. This has resulted in medial displacement of the lateral femoral condyle. **Diagnosis:** Salter IV fracture.

at the time of the injury. Lateral deviation of the foot is most often observed in association with altered distal ulnar and radial growth (Fig. 4–17A and 4–17B). Subluxation of the humeroradial (humeroulnar) articulation or anconeal fracture may also occur (Fig. 4–18 and 4–19). Because the angular deformity may be more easily corrected if diagnosed early, all animals with known or suspected physeal trauma (especially radial or ulnar) should be examined frequently, and radiographs of the affected and non-affected limb should be compared.

Growth disturbances may also result from metaphyseal infection or alterations in normal endochondral ossification (i.e., hypertrophic osteodystrophy, retained endochondral cartilage). Infection may cause retarded growth if growth cartilage is damaged; however, accelerated growth in response to local inflammation has also been observed.

Non-displaced physeal or incomplete (fissure) fractures may not be visible on radiographs that are obtained immediately after an injury. If a suspected fracture is not obvious on initial radiographs, a repeat exam 3 to 7 days afterward usually will demonstrate the fracture, because the resorption of bone along the fracture edges and early periosteal reaction will make the discontinuity more apparent (see Fig. 4–14).

A closed fracture has the overlying skin intact. An open fracture has a break in the overlying skin and soft tissues allowing communication between the bone and the

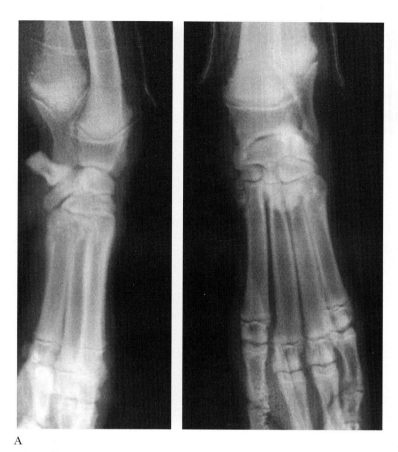

A

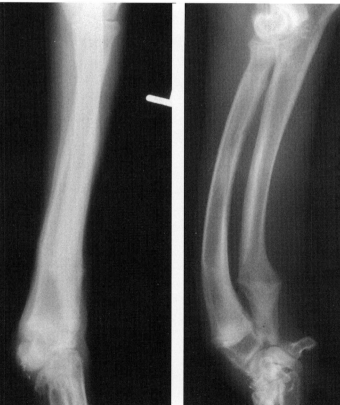

B

Figure 4–17. A 6-month-old female Labrador retriever was presented after being hit by a car. The dog was lame in the left front leg and pain was elicited upon palpation of the carpus. (A) In the initial radiograph there is minimal lateral displacement of the distal radial epiphysis. Close scrutiny of the distal ulna reveals that the cranial and medial aspects of the physis (growth cartilage) are narrower than the caudal and lateral aspects. This represents a Salter V fracture. The limb was immobilized in a cast at the owners request. Later, the owner removed the splint and did not return with the dog for 6 months. At that time, there was (B) marked cranial bowing and lateral angulation of the distal limb. **Diagnosis:** Salter V fracture of the distal ulnar physis with resultant premature closure of the distal ulnar physis with angulation deformity.

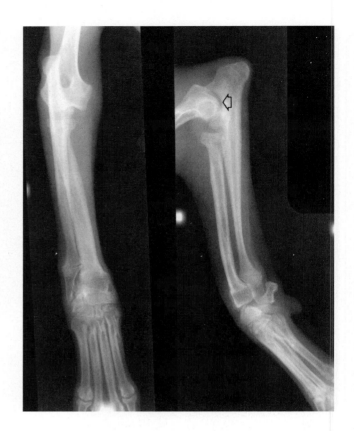

Figure 4–18. A 7-month-old male miniature poodle that had been dropped by the owners at 2 months of age and experienced pain for 2 weeks following the injury. The dog was lame and the right elbow was painful on palpation. There is subluxation of the radial humeral articulation with a large gap between the radial head and the distal humeral condyle. The coronoid process of the ulna is irregular and there is sclerosis of the subchondral bone of the ulna. The humeral ulnar articulation is widened (*arrow*). The cranial cortex of the radius and the ulna are thickened. There is a slight bowing deformity of the radius. The proximal radial and distal ulnar growth plates remain open while the distal radial growth plate appears to be closed. **Diagnosis:** Premature closure of the distal radial physis. The resultant lack of radial growth has produced the elbow subluxation with remodeling and secondary degenerative joint disease.

Figure 4–19. A 6-month-old female bassett hound was injured at 4 months of age. The injury was mild and was not treated at that time. The right foreleg became deviated laterally. There is subluxation of the humeral ulnar articulation (*open arrow*). The radius and ulna are curved. The proximal and distal radial growth plates remain open. The distal ulnar growth plate is closed except for a small remnant, which remains open on the caudal and lateral aspects (*closed arrows*). **Diagnosis:** Premature closure of the distal ulnar physis. This has resulted in growth deformity with the upward pressure of the radius on the distal humerus causing the elbow subluxation. If this continues, fracture of the anconeal process could result. Although some degree of limb curvature is considered normal in a dog of this breed, the changes noted here were more severe than in the opposite limb.

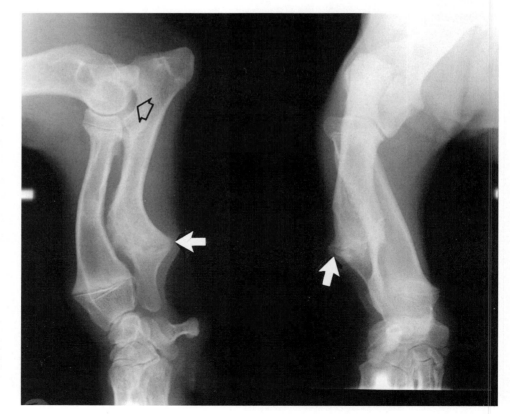

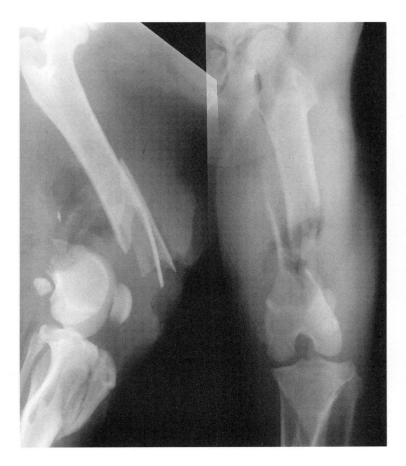

Figure 4–20. A 9-month-old female Labrador retriever was hit by a car. There is a comminuted fracture involving the distal third of the left femur. There is caudal and medial displacement of the distal fragment. There are multiple butterfly fragments at the fracture site. There is gas present in the soft tissues both at the fracture site and on the cranial surface of the limb. These indicate that the fracture is open. There is a comminuted fracture involving the proximal tibia. The fibula is intact. The tibial articular surface is involved and the fracture fragments are impacted. **Diagnosis:** Open comminuted femoral and tibial fractures.

ambient environment. The presence of air within the surrounding soft tissue suggests an open fracture (Fig. 4–20). This may be the first indication of an open wound that is hidden by the animal's coat of hair.

Bone density and trabecular pattern should be examined carefully in all fractures, particularly those fractures that occur with minimal trauma. A loss of bone density, evidence of periosteal proliferation, or disturbance of the normal trabecular pattern at the time of the initial injury indicates an underlying pathologic process. A pathologic fracture is due in part to the weakness caused by the underlying disease.[18] The bone may bend, producing an incomplete (torus or greenstick) rather than complete fracture. Tumors, infections, and primary and secondary hyperparathyroidism may be associated with pathologic fractures.

Involvement of joints should also be described. Joint derangements can include dislocation (complete loss of contact between the usual articular surface components), subluxation (partial loss of contact between the usual articular surface components), or diastasis (frank separation of a slightly moveable joint—e.g., pubic symphysis or distal tibiofibular syndesmosis).[15]

POSTOPERATIVE EVALUATION

Postoperative radiographs are mandatory after attempted reduction (either open or closed) of fracture fragments. Alignment and apposition of the fracture fragments and position of any surgical apparatus (i.e., pins, plates, etc.) should be evaluated (Fig. 4–21). Specific attention should be paid to the number and types of appliances as well as their relationship to the fracture and to each other. Postoperative radiographs also serve as a basis for comparison in evaluating the course of fracture healing.

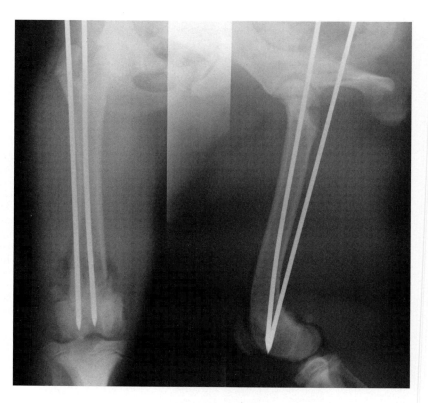

Figure 4–21. Post-operative radiographs of the same dog as in Figure 4–15. The fracture has been repaired by means of two intramedullary pins. The caudal lateral pin does not engage the proximal fragment. This illustrates the importance of post-operative radiographs to check not only for alignment and apposition of fracture fragments, but also for stability of the repair.

The rate at which a fracture heals depends upon the animal's age, general health and nutrition, the blood supply to the bone, and the stability of fragments. Fractures in young, growing animals, in areas with a rich blood supply, and those that are rigidly immobilized heal more rapidly. Clinical union usually precedes radiographic healing.

Fracture fragments should have distinct margins at the time of initial injury. Typically, endochondral healing leads to fracture repair. In this method of healing, the fracture margins will become less distinct due to absorption of bone within 2 to 3 days (inflammatory phase). Periosteal proliferation usually becomes evident within 10 to 14 days after the injury; however, in growing animals, periosteal proliferation may be evident as early as 3 to 5 days (Fig. 4–22). Callus (an unorganized meshwork of loosely woven bone developed on the pattern of the original fibrin clot that is formed immediately following the fracture) may develop from the stem cells from the periosteum, endosteum, or haversian canal lining (reparative phase).[19] The amount of callus varies considerably depending upon the animal's age, the fracture site, and the method of fixation (Figs. 4–23, 4–24, 4–25, and 4–26). As time passes, the callus will mature (remodeling phase) by laying down new bone along the lines of stress and resorbing trabeculae that are poorly aligned to the stresses.[15,19,20]

Membranous healing may occur if the fracture fragments are rigidly affixed in intimate contact. With this method of healing, callus is kept to a minimum and the fracture gap is filled with periosteal and endosteal new bone.

The nature of the fracture, the type of repair and its adherence to proper fixation principles, and the patient's clinical signs determine the frequency with which follow-up radiographs should be obtained. A change in the patient's status (i.e., reluctance to use the limb, sudden onset of swelling, pain, or discharge) is an indication for immediate reevaluation. Follow-up radiographs should be examined carefully for the progression of healing or for the presence of complications.

COMPLICATIONS OF FRACTURE HEALING

Complications that may be detected radiographically include the following:

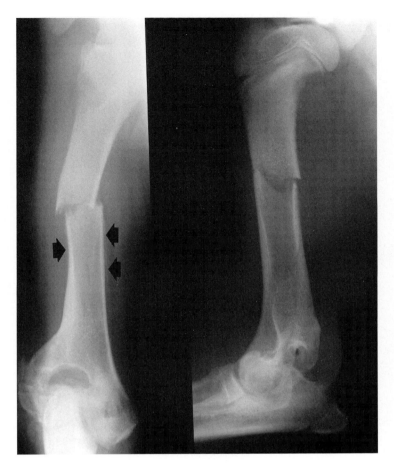

Figure 4–22. A 4-month-old female mixed breed dog that was hit by a car and had a fracture of the right elbow repaired 6 weeks previously. The dog was again presented non-weight-bearing on the right front leg. There is a transverse fracture of the right humerus. The fracture fragment margins are indistinct. There is a faint periosteal response on the medial and lateral aspects of the distal fragment (*arrows*). There is medial displacement of the distal fragment. There is an old malunion fracture of the distal right humerus. The lateral condyle is displaced proximally. This fracture has healed with callus bridging the old fracture site and considerable elbow deformity. There is sclerosis of the ulnar articular surface indicating the presence of degenerative joint disease. The indistinct margins and bony proliferation in the midshaft humerus are compatible with a 1-week-old fracture. There is no evidence of underlying bone disease. The cortical thickness and medullary density are normal. This represents early healing and not a pathologic fracture. **Diagnosis:** Healing transverse humeral fracture.

1. Infection.[21]
2. Fracture fragment movement.
3. Orthopedic device movement or failure.
4. New injury.
5. Joint disease.
6. Soft tissue abnormality, such as swelling, contracture, subcutaneous emphysema, atrophy, or calcification.[22]
7. Premature physeal closure.
8. Fracture induced sarcoma.[23]

Identifying osteomyelitis at the site of a healing fracture can be difficult because the radiographic changes indicative of osteomyelitis are similar to those observed with normal fracture healing (i.e., periosteal proliferation and bone lysis).[24] The presence of excessive periosteal proliferation or bone lysis, especially when located away from the actual fracture site, suggests osteomyelitis (Figs. 4–27 and 4–28).[25] Exuberant periosteal proliferation may also occur in young dogs when multiple intramedullary pins (stack pinning) are used or extensive periosteal stripping occurs. This may resemble infection; however, the absence of bony destruction is helpful in recognizing this reaction.

Motion and/or infection will result in absorption of bone around orthopedic devices (Fig. 4–29).[26,27] Motion usually results in a smoothly marginated, uniform loss of bony density around the device—when infection is present, a more uneven pattern of bone density loss occurs. Soft tissue swelling also is frequently present with infection. The presence of metallic fixation devices complicates the treatment of infection.[28,29] Because radiographic changes lag behind clinical signs, it is best to treat

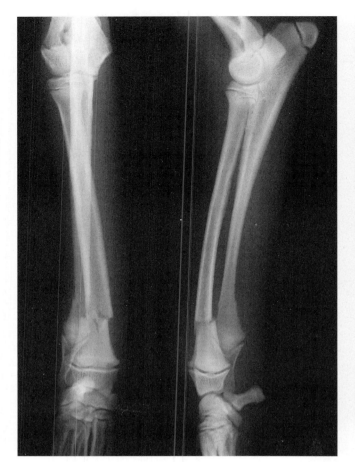

A

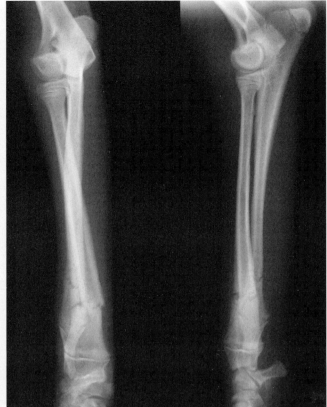

B

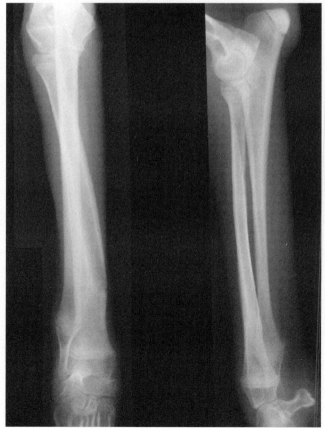

C

Figure 4–23. A 6-month-old male mixed breed dog was hit by a car and presented with a non-weight-bearing lameness of the right front leg. (A) There are transverse fractures of the radius and ulna involving the junction of the middle and distal thirds. There is slight lateral and caudal displacement of the distal fragments. There is mild soft tissue swelling of the area. (B) Follow-up radiographs were obtained 2 weeks following the initial injury. The leg had been placed in a cast. There is no change in position of the fracture fragments when compared with the initial radiographs. The fracture lines appear slightly wider with indistinct margins due to resorption at the fracture edges. There is a minimal amount of periosteal proliferation. The physes appear normal without evidence of growth plate trauma. (C) Follow-up radiographs were obtained 1 month after the initial injury. The fracture has healed completely and the fracture lines are no longer visible. There is slight malalignment at the fracture site. The distal radial and ulnar physes remain open without evidence of growth deformity. There is demineralization of the bones distal to the fracture site. This is due to disuse from immobilization of the limb in a cast. **Diagnosis:** Healed transverse fracture.

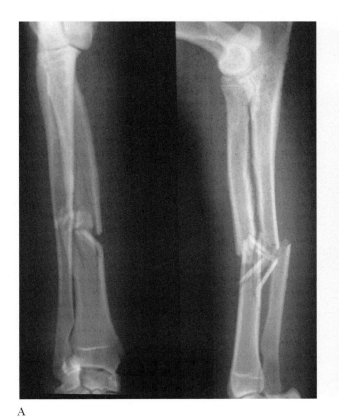

A

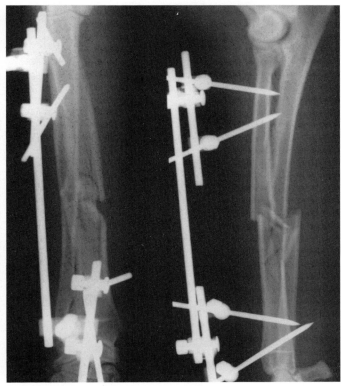

B

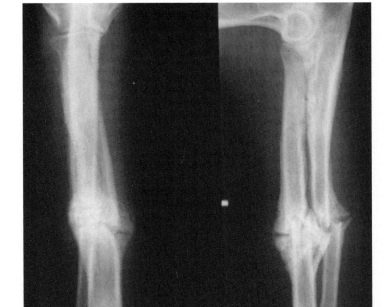

C

Figure 4–24. An 18-month-old male mixed breed dog was hit by a car. (A) There are midshaft comminuted fractures of the radius and ulna. There are linear fissure fractures extending both proximal and distal to the major fracture. There is caudal displacement of the distal fragment. The slight irregularity between the radius and ulna in their proximal thirds is the site of normal interosseous muscle attachment. The longitudinal fissure fractures both proximal and distal to the fracture site are of great importance and should be carefully evaluated in a fracture of this type. (B) Postoperative radiographs of the right radius and ulna reveal that the fracture has been repaired by means of a Kirschner Ehmer device. Alignment and apposition are good. The pins are well placed in the proximal and distal fragments. (C) Radiographs were obtained 5 weeks after surgical repair. The Kirschner Ehmer device has been removed. There is extensive callus, which bridges the fracture completely. A radiolucent line is still evident at the fracture site. There is an increase in bony density within the proximal radius and ulna. A similar area is in the distal radius at the site from which the pins were removed. **Diagnosis:** Healing fracture with slight malalignment of the fracture fragments. The bony response seen at the site of pin placement is normal and there is no evidence of infection.

for infection based on clinical signs rather than waiting for the radiographic diagnosis to become evident.

Loss of a bone fragment's blood supply due to the original trauma or subsequent

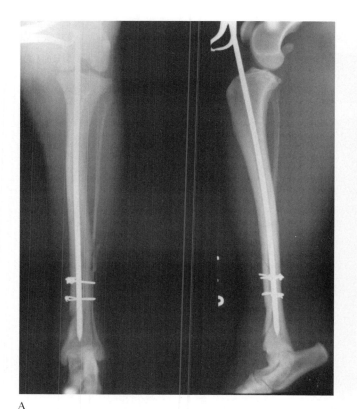

A

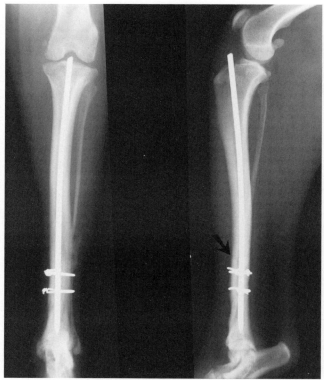

B

Figure 4–25. A 2-year-old male mixed breed dog was hit by a car. (A) Post-operative radiographs of the right tibia reveal the presence of an oblique fracture of the distal right tibia and a comminuted fracture of the right fibula at the junction of the middle and distal third. The fracture has been repaired by the means of an intramedullary pin and two cerclage wires. The intramedullary pin does not extend fully into the distal fragment (i.e., it is within 0.5 cm of the distal articular surface and only approximately 1 cm into the distal fracture fragment). Alignment and apposition of the fracture fragments are excellent. There is marked soft tissue swelling. (B) On radiographs obtained 5 weeks following the repair, there is no change in position of the orthopedic devices. The fracture line is no longer visible except for a small linear radiolucency proximal to the most proximal cerclage wire (*black arrow*). There is little periosteal callus with only a small amount on the lateral aspect of the middle third of the tibia. **Diagnosis:** Healing fracture. The minimal callus formation and rapid healing are the result of the solid fixation and fracture stability.

infection may result in sequestrum formation. A sequestrum cannot be identified radiographically at the time of the initial injury; however, as the fracture heals, the sequestrum will remain dense and its edges will remain distinct. An area of relative radiolucency (involucrum) will form around the sequestrum while other fracture fragments show evidence of bony proliferation or absorption (Fig. 4–30). A large sequestrum will interfere with fracture healing while smaller sequestra may be revascularized eventually. A persistent sequestrum will interfere with or prevent complete fracture healing.[30] Therefore, sequestrum recognition is important because its removal usually is necessary.

Delayed union, which is the failure of a fracture to heal in the normally expected time, is difficult to define precisely because of the many factors that normally affect the rate of healing. However, this diagnosis may be apparent in some situations. A non-union occurs when the fracture remains and there is cessation of bone healing. The diagnosis of non-union should not be tendered as long as there is continued evidence of healing progress (i.e., additional callus present at the fracture site when sequential radiographs are compared). A non-union is identified by a persistent fracture line and smooth, rounded, and dense fracture fragment margins with obliteration of the marrow cavity by callus (Figs. 4–31 and 4–32).[22] With time, a non-union may develop a pseudoarthrosis. This is characterized by the development of a joint

text continued on p. 451

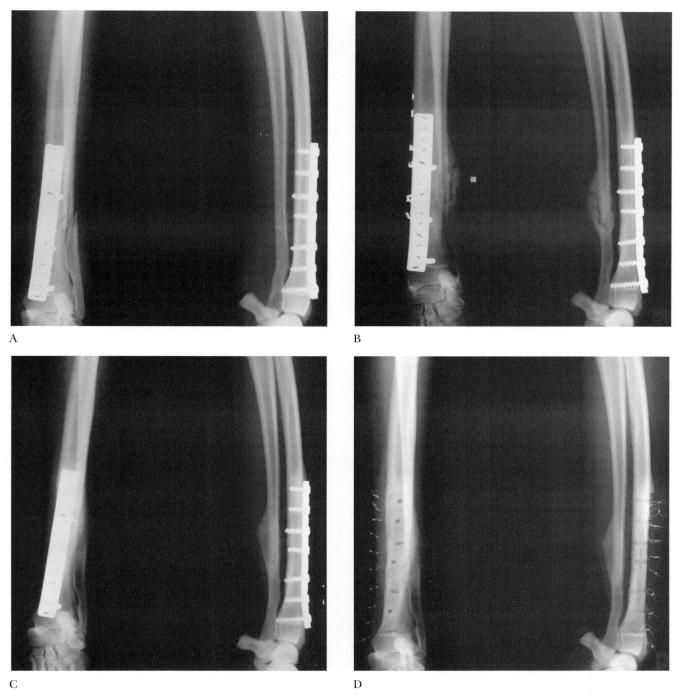

A

B

C

D

Figure 4–26. (A) Postoperative radiographs of the left radius and ulna of a 2-year-old female greyhound. The previously illustrated fracture (see Fig. 4–4) has been repaired by the means of a 7-hole dynamic compression bone plate. There is excellent alignment and apposition of the radial fracture fragments. There is slight malalignment of the distal ulna. All screws except the most proximal one appear to engage the caudal radial cortex. (B) Follow-up radiographs obtained 6 weeks after the surgical repair. There is exuberant callus formation around the distal ulna. There is minimal callus formation around the radius. Increased bony density is present between the screws. This represents normal healing. Note that the radius, which is rigidly stabilized, has a minimal amount of callus with disappearance of the fracture line while the ulna, which was less well-stabilized, exhibits a greater amount of callus. The absence of soft tissue swelling and bony destruction indicate that the ulna is healing normally without infection. (C) Post-operative radiographs 10 weeks after initial surgical repair. The fractures have healed and the fracture lines are not visible. The bony callus is smooth and contains a normal trabecular pattern. The margins of the ulnar fragments are smooth and a dense cortical shadow is forming. There is a small amount of bony callus around the proximal end of the bone plate. The bone plate and screws are intact. (D) The bone plate has been removed and the healing of the fracture is apparent. There is some loss of bone density beneath the bone plate; however, this is minimal. The radius has healed without deformation and with minimal callus due to the rigid immobilization provided by the bone plate. The ulna has also healed; however, with a larger amount of callus. The changes in the radius represent the usual pattern of bone healing associated with rigid fixation. **Diagnosis:** Healed fracture.

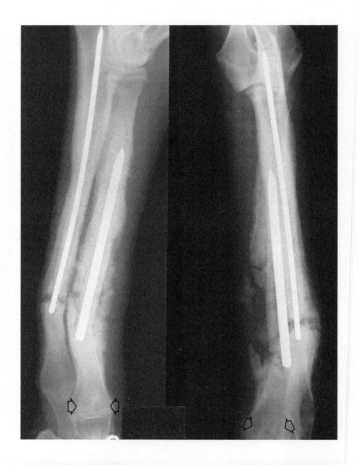

Figure 4–27. An 8-month-old female collie had transverse fractures of the radius and ulna repaired 5 weeks previously. There are two intramedullary pins in the radius and ulna, which extend into the distal fragments for a short distance. There is cranial and medial angulation of the distal fragments and diffuse mild soft tissue swelling. There is marked, active, irregular periosteal reaction both proximal and distal to the fracture site. There is increased density within the medullary canal of both the radius and ulna. Areas of irregular bony reabsorption are present around the distal aspect of the radial intramedullary pin and areas of radiolucency with slightly increased density are visible within the proximal and distal radial metaphyses (*arrows*). There is extensive bony destruction at the fracture site. **Diagnosis:** Osteomyelitis at the site of fracture repair. The extensive bony proliferation distant to the fracture site and the areas of bony destruction within the radial metaphysis and the fracture site suggest the diagnosis of infection. The irregular, mottled periosteal response should be contrasted with the more uniform and evenly mineralized callus usually associated with a healing fracture.

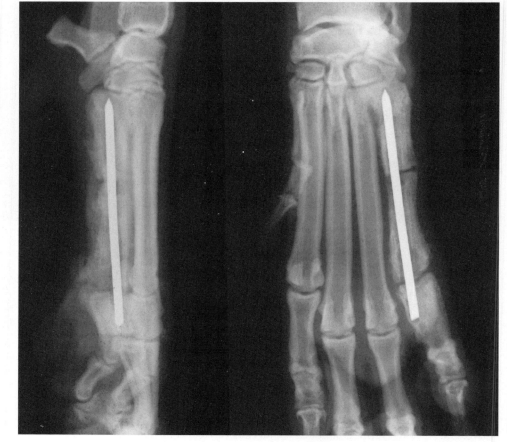

Figure 4–28. A 4-year-old male Siberian husky whose left front foot was traumatized 4 months previously. A fractured 5th metacarpal bone was pinned at that time. The fracture is still visible and an intramedullary pin is present within the 5th metacarpal bone. There is no evidence of callus at the fracture site. There is an irregular radiolucency around the intramedullary pin and extensive bony proliferation around both the proximal and distal fragments as well as on the 1st phalanx of the 5th digit. **Diagnosis:** Non-union fracture secondary to infection and instability.

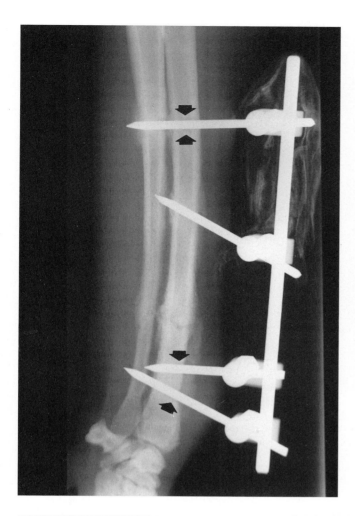

Figure 4–29. A 13-month-old male golden retriever that had transverse fractures of the distal third of the radius and ulna, which were repaired by the means of a Kirschner Ehmer device 1 month previously. Callus is present bridging the fracture. There are areas of radiolucency around the Kirschner Ehmer pins (*arrows*). There is bony proliferation on the caudal aspect of the ulna at the site of proximal pin penetration and on the cranial surface of the radius in association with the Kirschner Ehmer pins. **Diagnosis:** Infection. The irregular nature of the radiolucencies indicates that infection rather than motion is responsible for the loss of bone.

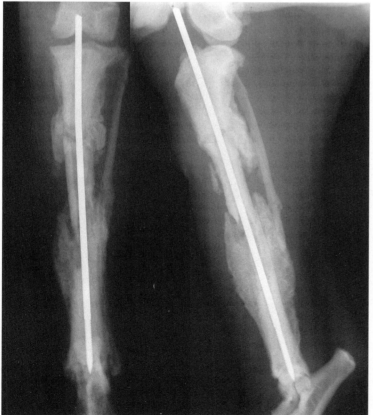

Figure 4–30. A 14-month-old male mixed breed dog had an open comminuted fracture of the right tibia repaired one month previously. An intramedullary pin is present and extensive bony proliferation involves the proximal and distal fragments. There is a very dense, sharply marginated fragment in the midportion of the tibia. The bony proliferation surrounds but does not contact or involve this bony fragment. There is irregular reabsorption of bone surrounding the intramedullary pin and diffuse extensive soft tissue swelling. **Diagnosis:** Osteomyelitis and lack of bone healing (delayed union) due to the presence of infection and a sequestrum. This fracture was successfully treated by removal of the sequestrum and intramedullary pin and administration of systemic antibiotics.

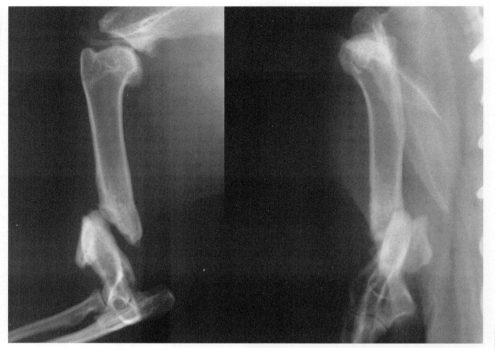

Figure 4–31. A 2-year-old spayed domestic short-haired cat was hit by a car 9 months previously and a fracture of the right humerus was immobilized in a coaptation splint. There is a fracture of the right humerus at the junction of the middle and distal thirds. The fracture fragments are smooth: their margins and medullary canals are sclerotic. There is no callus crossing the fracture site. **Diagnosis:** Non-union humeral fracture. There is remodeling of the distal scapular glenoid and proximal humeral head, which most likely resulted from previous trauma with malarticulation and degenerative joint disease.

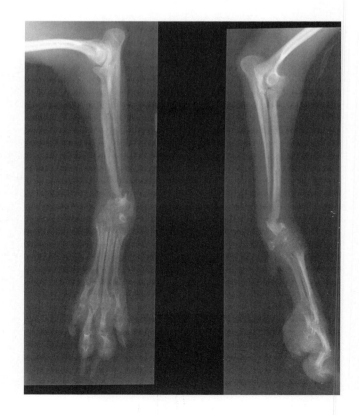

Figure 4–32. An 18-month-old male toy poodle suffered a fractured left radius and ulna 8 months previously. The leg has been immobilized in an external splint since that time. There is little evidence of callus. The fracture margins are smooth and sclerotic. There is a marked loss of bone, especially, at the distal ulna. The distal ulna has become thin and there is sclerosis of the radial cortex. There is marked demineralization of the carpal bones as well as the proximal and distal aspects of the metacarpal bones and phalanges. These changes are due to disuse from immobilization in a cast. **Diagnosis:** Non-union fracture with marked bone atrophy. This type of disuse atrophy frequently occurs in small breed dogs with fractures that are immobilized.

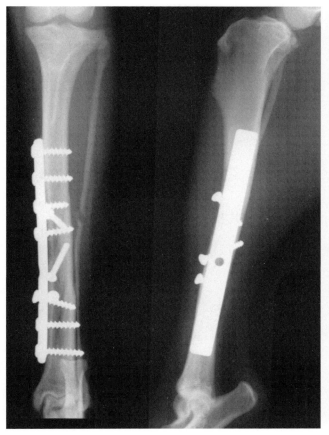
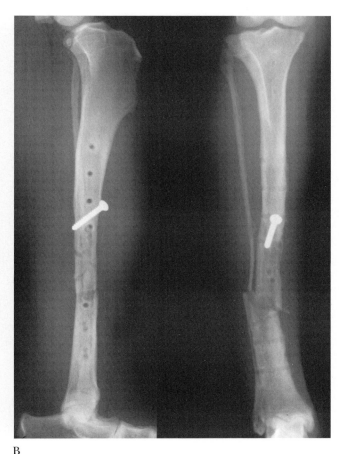

A   B

Figure 4–33.   A 1-year-old female English pointer was hit by a car 8 weeks previously. A comminuted fracture was repaired with a bone plate and interfragmentary screws. (A) In the radiographs obtained 8 weeks after fracture repair, the fracture has apparently healed with minimal callus and the fracture lines are barely visible in the distal and middle portions of the tibia. The findings are indicative of a healing fracture. There is a slight loss of bony density beneath the distal portion of the bone plate. The fibula has not healed. The plate was removed and the dog kept in a cage. The dog became acutely lame the following day. (B) Additional radiographs were obtained. One interfragmentary bone screw remains. There is a fracture involving the tibia at the junction of the middle and distal thirds. There is lateral displacement of the distal fragment with medial angulation and slight overriding. The fracture has occurred through an area of decreased bone density. This decreased density was the result of stress protection provided by the bone plate. **Diagnosis:** Pathologic fracture.

space and joint capsule, which is lined by synovium, between the two bone fragments. Radiographically, a pseudoarthrosis may appear as two adjacent fragments with smooth, sclerotic ends that have remodeled to form congruent surfaces, which resemble a false ball and socket joint between the bone fragments. Osteomedullography (injection of contrast media into the medullary canal of the distal fragment) can be performed in fractures that are older than 4 weeks to confirm the suspicion of a delayed union or non-union. Failure of the contrast to cross the fracture line confirms the diagnosis.[31] Fractures may heal with malaligned fragments. This is described as a malunion.[32]

Stress protection may result in osteopenia beneath the bone plate after a fracture has healed (Fig. 4–33).[33,34] This weakness can then result in a pathologic fracture. Thin cortices and coarse trabeculation beneath or around the bone plate are radiographic evidence of stress protection-induced osteopenia.

Disuse osteopenia (a more generalized form of stress protection induced osteopenia) can result from immobilization of a limb. The loss of bone density usually is more apparent distal to the fracture (Fig. 4–34). Severe disuse osteopenia predisposes to a pathologic fracture. This usually occurs if the animal exercises vigorously

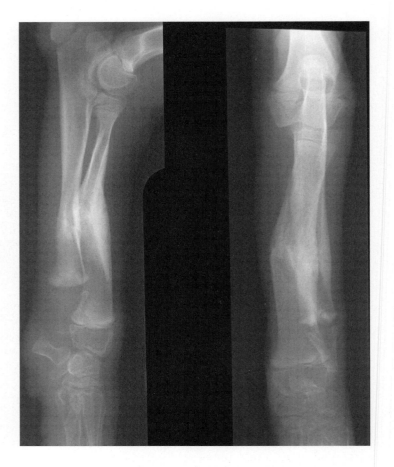

Figure 4–34. A 6-month-old male mixed breed dog had a transverse, midshaft radius and ulna fracture immobilized in a cast 4 weeks previously. The fractures have healed with moderate malalignment. There is a loss of bone density distal to the fracture. This is due to immobilization of the limb. **Diagnosis:** Healed fracture (malunion) with bone atrophy. The malalignment and bone atrophy did not affect this dog's return to normal limb usage.

soon after the immobilization device is removed. A gradual return to normal weight bearing should be prescribed when disuse osteopenia is evident.

TUMORS

PRIMARY BONE TUMORS

Most neoplasms of the appendicular skeleton are malignant and may be categorized as primary bone tumors, tumors metastatic to bone, or primary soft tissue tumors with bone invasion. A definitive diagnosis requires both radiographic and histologic evaluation of the neoplasm. The age, breed, and clinical history must also be considered. The following lists several specific radiographic features to be considered when evaluating the radiograph:

1. The soft tissue around the bone lesion.
2. The anatomic location of the lesion within the bone (i.e., metaphyseal, diaphyseal, etc.).
3. The number of bones involved.
4. The density of the bone in and around the lesion.
5. The margination of the lesion.
6. Any change since previous radiographs.
7. The presence of lesions in other parts of the animal.

Osteosarcoma is the most frequent primary bone tumor in dogs.[35–40] It accounts for approximately 85% of the primary bone tumors. Chondrosarcomas account for about 10%. Hemangiosarcoma, fibrosarcoma, malignant fibrous histiocytoma, lymphoma, liposarcoma, myeloma, giant cell tumor, and chondroma together account for the remaining 5%. Large and giant breed dogs (e.g., great Dane, Irish setter, German shepherd, St. Bernard, etc.) account for 90% of the osteosarcoma occurrences. Two peak occurrence rates are seen in dogs at approximately 18 months of age and again in older individuals (greater than 6 years of age); the incidence is decreased between these times.[37]

Primary bone tumors are uncommon in cats. The radiographic features of feline primary bone tumors are similar to those of the dog.[35,36] The incidence of metastasis is lower in the cat than it is in the dog.

Primary bone tumors are frequently osteolytic; however, both osteoblastic and mixed lesions are also common. The cortex may be destroyed at several points, and the normal trabecular pattern destroyed or distorted. There is irregular, poorly defined, and mineralized periosteal and endosteal proliferation. The affected area will blend gradually with the normal bone, resulting in what has been termed "a long transition zone." As a general rule, they do not cross joint spaces or involve adjacent bones. Most primary bone tumors are highly aggressive, and rapid expansion of the lesion will be evident if the tumor is reevaluated after 1 to 2 weeks.

The presence of a suspected primary bone tumor raises the question about metastasis to other sites. Scintigraphic and radiographic surveillance of other bony structures have been discussed and may be appropriate in selected situations; however, because bone metastasis with osteosarcoma is relatively infrequent, neither routine scintigraphy nor radiographic bone surveys are recommended.[12,41,42] Thoracic radiographs should always be obtained when a bone tumor is suspected. The presence of pulmonary metastasis may aid in establishing the diagnosis of tumor.

Osteosarcoma

Osteosarcoma usually produces a localized soft tissue swelling, which may contain mineralized foci. The bony changes can vary from almost completely osteolytic to totally osteoblastic,[23,35,37,43–51] although a mixed (predominately osteolytic) pattern is seen most often. Osteosarcomas are observed most frequently in the metaphyseal portion of the proximal humerus, distal radius and ulna, distal femur, and proximal tibia (Figs. 4–3, 4–35, 4–36, 4–37). When they become large they can expand into an

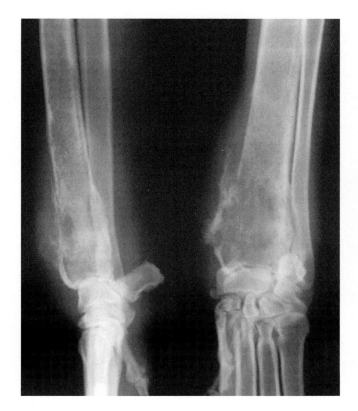

Figure 4–35. A 6-year-old female Great Dane presented with a right foreleg lameness with an acute onset. The carpus was swollen. There is soft tissue swelling surrounding the radial metaphysis. There is extensive bony destruction with the cortex eroded at several sites. Mild periosteal reaction is present. There is poor demarcation between the involved and normal bone. **Diagnosis:** Osteosarcoma.

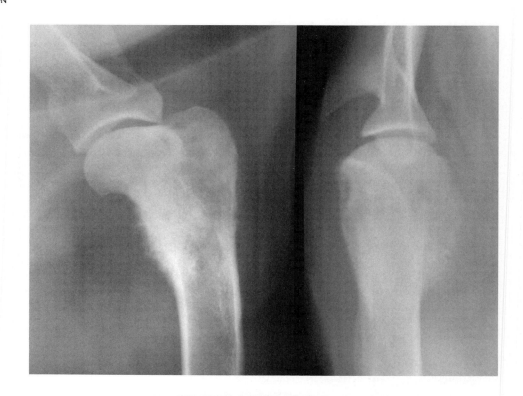

Figure 4–36. A 5-year-old female Irish setter presented with an acute onset of left foreleg lameness which had become more severe and painful over 3 days. Left shoulder muscle atrophy was present. There is bony proliferation noted involving the proximal humeral metaphysis with bony destruction involving the medullary canal and cortex in this area. There is increased density within the medullary canal with poor demarcation between the involved metaphysis and normal-appearing diaphyseal areas. **Diagnosis:** Osteosarcoma.

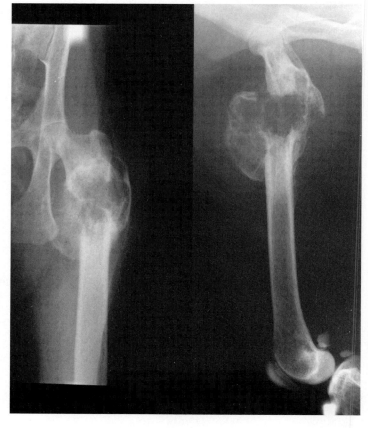

Figure 4–37. A 7-year-old female domestic short-haired cat was presented with a 1-month lameness of the left rear leg. There is focal bony destruction involving the proximal third of the left femur. There is extensive soft tissue calcification present. The margins of the bony lesion are poorly defined. The radiographic findings are indicative of an expansile neoplasm arising within the medullary cavity and extending into the soft tissues. **Diagnosis:** Osteosarcoma.

adjacent bone. This occurs most often in the distal radius and ulna and in the tibia and fibula. It is evident radiographically as periosteal proliferation or destruction of the adjacent bone (Fig. 4–38). Osteosarcoma has been reported as a late sequela to complicated fracture repair and the long-term presence of metallic orthopedic

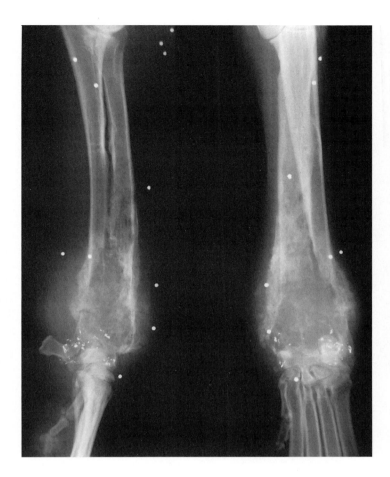

Figure 4–38. An 8-year-old male mixed breed dog was lame on the left foreleg for 3 weeks. The swelling had increased gradually and the dog was non-weight-bearing. There is a localized soft tissue swelling centered over the distal radius and ulna. There is massive bony destruction involving the middle and distal portions of the radius and the medial and cranial aspects of the distal ulna. There is irregular, amorphous soft tissue mineralization surrounding these bones with poorly defined areas of periosteal proliferation. There are multiple metallic shotgun pellets throughout the soft tissues with fragmentation of these metallic fragments in the carpal joint area. **Diagnosis:** Osteosarcoma. The spread of this lesion to the ulna is unusual; however, the size of this lesion and close relationship between the radius and ulna at this point contributed to the extension of the tumor into the ulna.

implants.[36,52,53] In these cases, the tumor has occurred at the previous fracture site (Fig. 4–39).

Multicentric and metastatic osteosarcomas have been reported.[54,55] Simultaneous involvement of several bones indicates a multicentric tumor, while multiple bone involvement, after some time delay, indicates metastasis (Figs. 4–40 and 4–41).

Other primary bone neoplasms occur infrequently; therefore, it is difficult to characterize their features. Some general comments may be made regarding their radiographic features.

Parosteal Osteosarcoma

Parosteal osteosarcoma has been reported, but its incidence is low.[35,56] The described radiographic features are similar to those of osteosarcoma; however, the lesion is centered on the periosteum rather than the medullary canal and extends into the soft tissue of the limb. Extensive, poorly organized, and poorly mineralized patterns of bone density occur within the soft tissue mass (Fig. 4–42). Bony destruction is present within the medullary canal. Discrimination between osteosarcoma and parosteal osteosarcoma may be important. In humans, parosteal osteosarcoma metastasizes less frequently than does osteosarcoma.

Chondrosarcoma

Although chondrosarcomas may affect long bones, they most frequently arise from flat bones such as the pelvic bones, scapulae, or ribs (Figs. 4–43 and 4–44).[35,57–59] This tumor occurs more often in older, medium and large breed dogs and rarely affects giant breeds. Chondrosarcomas usually are highly destructive masses. Calcifications in the soft tissue mass frequently appear as multilobulated globules ("popcorn calcification") but they may also appear less organized. Chondrosarcoma may arise at the site of an osteochondroma or cartilaginous exostosis.[60]

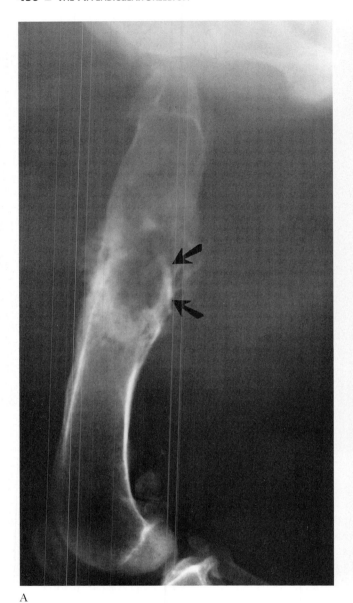
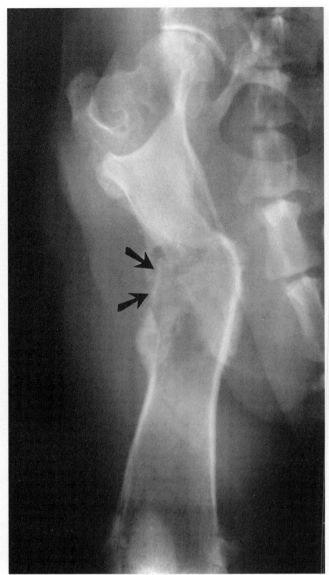

A   B

Figure 4–39. (A&B) An 8-year-old female Weimeraner had been hit by a car 6 years previously and had a fractured right femur repaired surgically. A draining tract had persisted. The dog had become acutely lame during the last 2 weeks. There is a destructive lesion involving the middle portion of the right femur. There is poorly organized and mineralized periosteal proliferation surrounding this area of bony destruction. The area of bony destruction is poorly defined within the medullary canal. There is a thin, somewhat linear bone density on the caudal lateral aspect of the midshaft femur (*arrows*). This represents a sequestrum. **Diagnosis:** Osteosarcoma at the site of previous surgical repair and chronic osteomyelitis. The site of this lesion within the femoral diaphysis is unusual for primary bone tumors: the presence of a chronic infection may have contributed to its occurrence at this site.

Fibrosarcoma

Fibrosarcoma has been reported in young and old dogs and cats.[35,61–64] It typically produces an osteolytic lesion in the metaphysis of the long bones (Fig. 4–45). A large soft tissue mass without calcification may be present. Periosteal new bone formation is rare.

Malignant Fibrous Histiocytoma

Malignant fibrous histiocytoma is thought to be a tumor of histiocytic origin. Radiographically, the lesion is similar to that seen with fibrosarcoma. Bony changes are

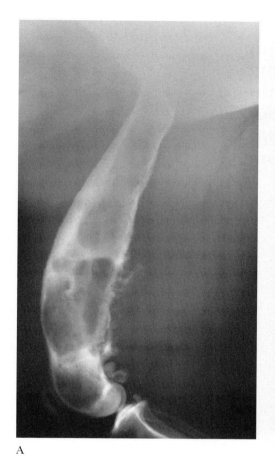

A

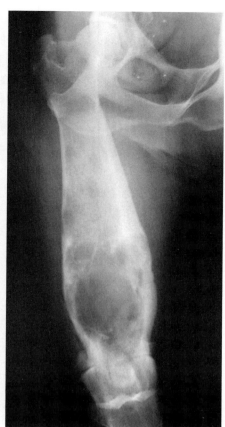

B

Figure 4–40. (A&B) A 7-year-old female rottweiler had a right rear leg lameness for 6 weeks. Swelling was noted in the area of the right stifle. There is an expansile bony lesion involving the entire femoral diaphysis extending into the proximal and distal metaphyses. Endosteal scalloping is present. There is smooth periosteal proliferation on the medial and cranial aspect of the right femur. There is irregular, poorly mineralized bony proliferation present on the caudal aspect of the distal femur. **Diagnosis:** Osteosarcoma.

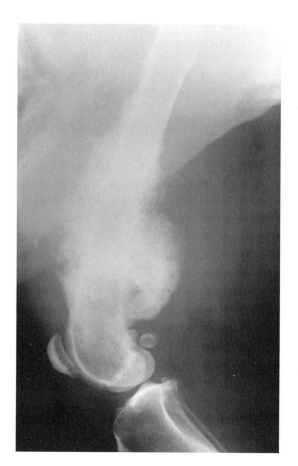

Figure 4–41. An 8-year-old female rottweiler whose right rear leg was amputated 1 year previously because an osteosarcoma was present in the right femur at that time (see Fig. 4–40). The dog was then presented with a mass on the left rear leg. There is a marked amount of bony proliferation noted involving the middle and distal portions of the left femur. The periosteal proliferation is poorly defined and irregularly mineralized. Several areas of bony destruction are present within the medullary canal. There is a large soft tissue swelling associated with this bony lesion. **Diagnosis:** Osteosarcoma. This may represent a metastatic lesion of the previous right femoral osteosarcoma. While multicentric osteosarcoma can occur, the diagnosis requires simultaneous occurrence of the bone tumors. There was no evidence of pulmonary metastasis in this dog. The difference in appearance of the right femoral and left femoral lesions reflects the wide variation observed in osteosarcomas.

457

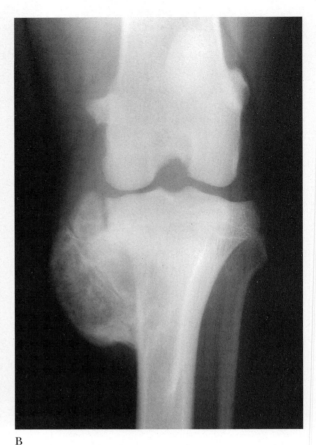

A   B

Figure 4–42. (A&B) A 9-year-old male golden retriever was presented with a right rear limb lameness. There was pain on manipulation of the stifle and a palpable mass. There is a bony mass on the medial aspect of the proximal tibia. The margins of the mass are well-defined with a thick cortical shadow. The bony lesion appears to be contiguous with the medullary canal. **Diagnosis:** Parosteal osteosarcoma.

predominately lytic. Minimal periosteal reaction may be present. The lesions tend to be poorly defined and may have associated soft tissue swelling.[65]

Hemangiosarcoma

Hemangiosarcoma is a highly destructive lesion that usually involves the metaphysis or diaphysis of a long bone (Fig. 4–46). The pattern of destruction typically presents as an overall osteopenia with a superimposed pattern of numerous, small, well-defined lytic foci.[35,66,67] Minimal amounts of periosteal proliferation may be present.[68,69] Soft tissue calcification has been observed occasionally. The tumor has a tendency to remain confined to the medullary cavity, while expanding proximally and distally. Pathologic fractures may occur.

Myeloma

Plasma cell myeloma occasionally presents as a solitary lesion but is more commonly present with multiple lesions.[70,71] The lesions may involve any long or flat bones. The bony changes usually are well-defined, discrete areas of cortical lysis that lack sclerotic margins (Fig. 4–47). Occasionally, these may show some proliferative change.[71,72] Rarely, a generalized loss of bone density may be all that is observed (see Fig 6-34).

Liposarcoma

A few liposarcomas of bone have been reported.[40] Multiple areas of metaphyseal bony lysis and reactive periosteal proliferation were described.

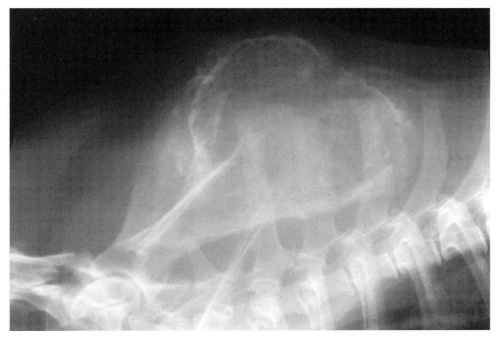

A

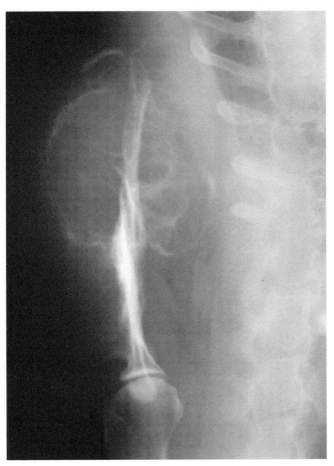

B

Figure 4–43. (A&B) A 12-year-old female Labrador retriever that had a 6-month history of left forelimb lameness. A firm mass was detected in the area of the proximal left scapula 1 month previously. There is an expansile bony lesion involving the proximal two-thirds of the left scapula. There are irregular, amorphous areas of calcification within this mass. **Diagnosis:** Chondrosarcoma.

Giant Cell Tumor

The giant cell tumor is an unusual tumor of bone.[73–75] It is characterized by a lytic, expansile lesion of the metaphysis and epiphysis. The appearance can be very similar to a bone cyst, but the zone of transition usually is longer and less distinct with giant cell tumor.

459

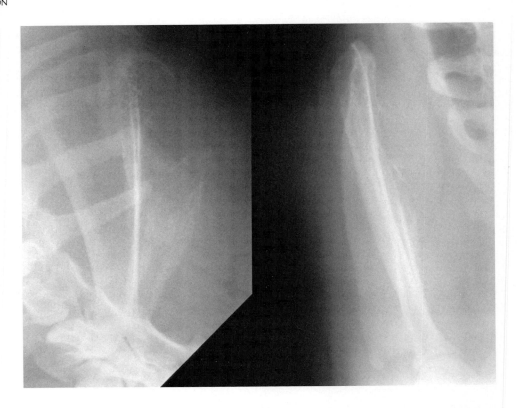

Figure 4–44. A 6-year-old male wire-haired fox terrier presented with a firm swelling over the left scapula. There was no pain or lameness. There is soft tissue swelling medial, proximal, and cranial to the left scapula. There is bony destruction involving the cranial medial aspect of the scapula with irregular bony densities within the area of bony destruction. There is no evidence of bony proliferation. **Diagnosis:** Chondrosarcoma.

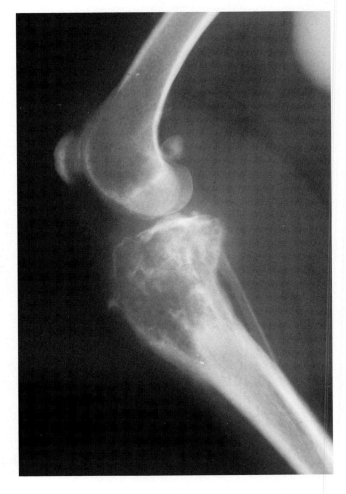

Figure 4–45. A 12-year-old male Labrador retriever with left hindlimb lameness for 6 weeks. There was a mild degree of swelling in the area of the proximal tibia, which was painful. The lateral radiograph reveals a lytic lesion of the proximal tibia. The margins of the lesion are not clearly demarcated. No periosteal reaction is noted. The cortex has been breached and mild soft tissue swelling is present. **Diagnosis:** Fibrosarcoma.

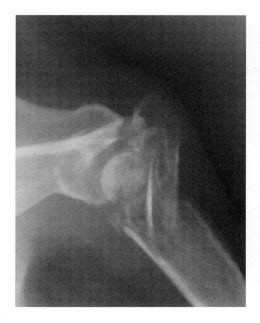

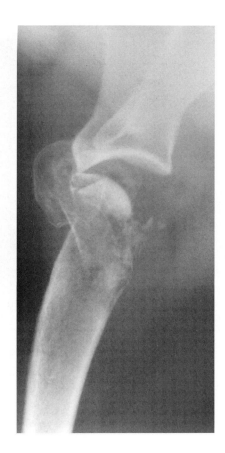

Figure 4–46. A 6-year-old male golden retriever presented with an acute onset of left foreleg lameness. The dog was painful when the leg was manipulated. There is a pathological fracture involving the proximal humerus. The bone density is decreased with a pattern of radiolucency extending into the mid-diaphysis. There is no evidence of bony proliferation or soft tissue calcification. The scapula is not involved despite the extensive humeral destruction. **Diagnosis:** Hemangiosarcoma. The radiographic changes indicate a pathologic fracture secondary to a primary bone tumor. The final diagnosis was based on the histology of the lesion.

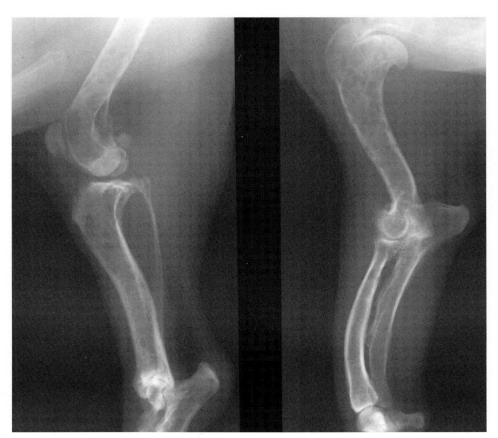

Figure 4–47. A 12-year-old male Welsh corgi presented with anorexia, depression and weight loss of 1 month duration. Radiographs of the long bones were obtained after abnormalities were noted on the thoracic and abdominal radiographs. There are multiple semicircular lytic lesions within the femur and humerus that do not have sclerotic margins. There is no evidence of periosteal proliferation. **Diagnosis:** Multiple myeloma.

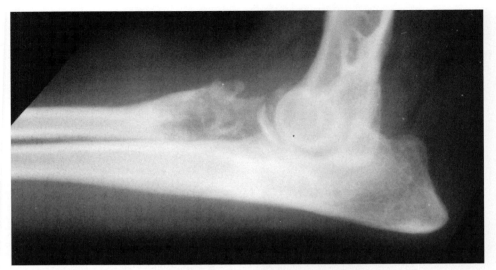

Figure 4–48. A 5-year-old male golden retriever presented with an ill-defined lameness and weight loss. The lateral view of the right elbow reveals an ill-defined, lytic lesion that lacks clearly defined margins that involves the proximal radius. No periosteal reaction is present. Similar lesions were present in the pelvis and left tibia. **Diagnosis:** Lymphoma.

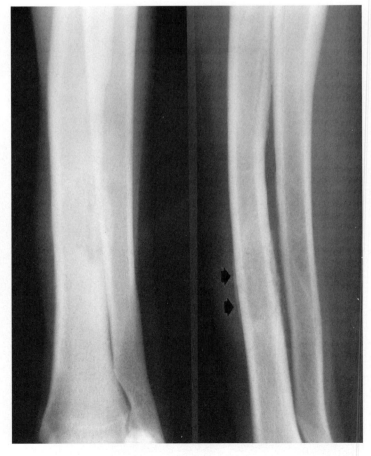

Figure 4–49. A 10-year-old male German shepherd dog presented with lameness in the left foreleg of 1 month's duration. A periprostatic cyst had been removed 5 months previously. There is a destructive lesion involving the central portion of the radial diaphysis. There is a faint periosteal proliferation cranial to this area of bony destruction (*arrows*). There is poor demarcation of the lesion from the surrounding normal bone. There is increased density surrounding this area of bony destruction especially on the caudal proximal aspect of the ulna. **Diagnosis:** Metastatic neoplasm. This was a metastatic prostatic adenocarcinoma.

Lymphoma of Bone

Primary lymphoma of bone is an unusual manifestation of lymphoma.[35,76–79] It is characterized radiographically by multiple focal to confluent areas of osteolysis, which do not have sclerotic margins (Fig. 4–48). Multiple bones usually are involved. Periosteal reaction is rare except in cases with concomitant pathological fractures.

METASTATIC TUMORS

Tumor metastases to bone are more commonly metaphyseal but occasionally may be diaphyseal. The commonly reported sites include the femur, humerus, and tibia, although any bone may be involved and the lesion is frequently polyostotic. The radiographic appearance of metastatic lesions varies.[35,39,80–87] They may be osteolytic, osteoblastic, or mixed (Figs. 4–49, 4–50, and 4–51). Soft tissue swelling usually is minimal unless cortical penetration has occurred. Soft tissue calcification and marked periosteal responses are rare. The margins of the lesion usually are poorly defined. If a metastatic tumor is suspected, the patient should be evaluated for a primary soft tissue neoplasm, which often is carcinoma of the lung, mammary gland, or prostate. Bony metastasis may be present with or without pulmonary metastasis.

SOFT TISSUE TUMORS

Soft tissue tumors arise from the soft tissues adjacent to bones and joints and affect them by direct extension. These tumors may involve adjacent bones. The pattern of destruction usually is centered on one aspect of the cortex (Fig. 4–52).

Synovial Cell Sarcoma

Synovial sarcoma (arising from the secretory lining of the joint capsule or tendon sheath) frequently involves more than one bone in a joint. Although any joint may be involved, it is observed most often in the elbow and stifle (Fig. 4–53).

This tumor usually crosses the joint space to involve the adjacent epiphyseal and metaphyseal areas. The lesion is predominantly osteolytic, periosteal proliferation is minimal, and soft tissue mineralization is rare.[88–91]

Fibrosarcoma

Fibrosarcoma arising from the fibrous connective tissue capsule of a joint usually has an appearance similar to synovial cell sarcoma. However, fibrosarcoma of the joint

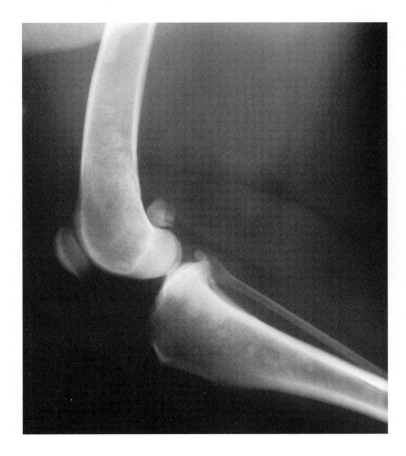

Figure 4–50. A 10-year-old female Doberman pinscher presented with a right limb lameness and generalized stiffness with difficulty getting up and down. Multiple cutaneous nodules were present. Both right and left rear limbs were radiographed. The right stifle is illustrated. There are multiple areas of increased medullary density involving the distal right femur and proximal and middle portions of the right tibia. Similar densities were noted within the diaphysis and metaphysis of the left femur and tibia. These intermedullary densities with no evidence of periosteal proliferation are suggestive of disseminated bony metastasis. **Diagnosis:** Metastatic carcinoma.

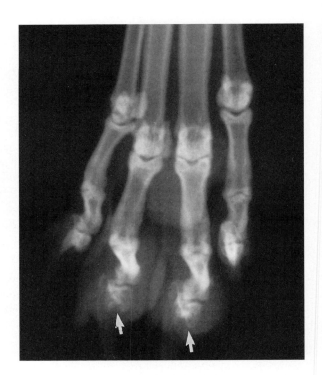

Figure 4–51. A 9-year-old female Russian blue cat presented with a right hindlimb lameness of 4 day's duration. Examination reveals swelling of the digits. The dorsoplantar radiograph reveals osteolysis of the ungual process of the 3rd phalanx of the 3rd and 4th digits (*arrows*). Soft tissue swelling of the area is also present. Radiographs of the thorax revealed a large, solitary mass in the right caudal lung lobe. **Diagnosis:** Metastatic bronchogenic adenocarcinoma.

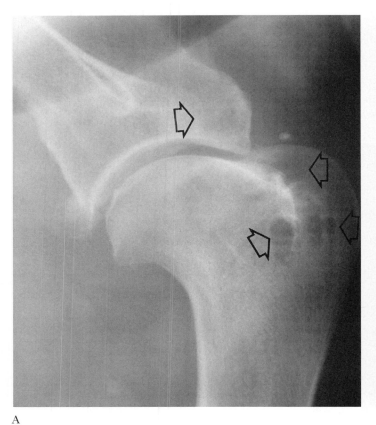

A

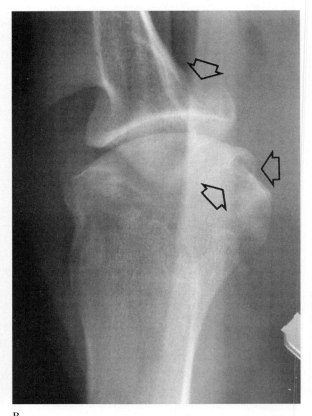

B

Figure 4–52. (A&B) A 7-year-old male Great Dane presented with a right front leg lameness of 2½ weeks' duration. There was pain on flexion and deep palpation of the shoulder. There are periarticular osteophytes on the caudal aspect of the scapular glenoid and the caudal aspect of the proximal humeral head. The articular surface of the humerus is uneven. There is a small bone density proximal to the greater tubercle. There are areas of bony lysis within the bicipital groove and within the metaphysis of the proximal humerus. These are most severe on the cranial and medial aspect of the humerus (*arrows*). Similar bony destructive lesions are present in the cranial medial aspect of the scapula (*arrows*). **Diagnosis:** Soft tissue neoplasm which is invading the proximal humerus and distal scapula. This lesion is superimposed upon degenerative joint disease. The lesion was a leiomyosarcoma.

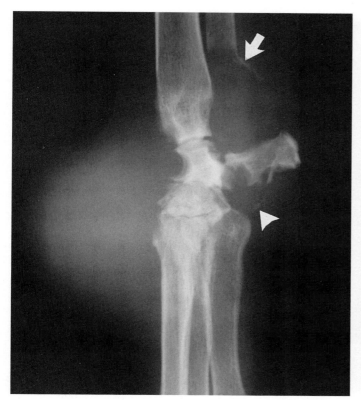

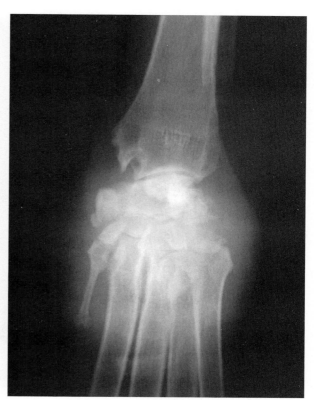

A   B

Figure 4–53. (A&B) A 7-year-old male standard poodle that was presented with a 1-month history of a mass on the left carpus. The size of the mass appeared to increase rapidly. There is marked local soft tissue swelling centered over the carpal-metacarpal joint. There is marked bony destruction involving the distal ulna, distal radius, accessory carpal bone, radial carpal bone, and metacarpal bones. There is a small amount of bony proliferation caudal to the ulna (*arrow*). There is a small amount of soft tissue mineralization on the caudal aspect of the carpus (*arrowhead*). **Diagnosis:** Soft tissue neoplasm invading the carpal joint. This neoplasm was identified as a synovial cell sarcoma.

occurs less frequently than synovial cell tumor. Histology is required to distinguish between these two possibilities.

Squamous Cell Carcinoma of the Nail Bed

Squamous cell carcinoma of the nail bed (nail bed carcinoma) is highly malignant and often locally invasive. Squamous cell carcinoma produces a localized soft tissue swelling, which may involve the adjacent bones producing an osteolytic lesion with minimal bony proliferation (Fig. 4–54).[35,86,92,93] Disorganized or punctate areas of mineralization may be present within this soft tissue mass. Local recurrence with tumor extension to adjacent bones after amputation is frequent. Metastasis to the lung or other bones rarely occurs. The tumors may be multicentric, involving multiple digits on one or several limbs.

BENIGN BONE TUMORS

Osteochondroma (Cartilaginous Exostosis)

Multiple or solitary osteochondroma (cartilaginous exostosis) typically affects young animals by producing lesions at the metaphysis of long bones, the dorsal spinous processes of the vertebrae, or the costochondral junctions.[40,94–98] Growth of the lesions usually stops at the time of physeal plate closure. Radiographically, osteochondromas are typified in dogs by one of two radiographic appearances. One form

Figure 4–54. An adult female Doberman pinscher presented with a growth on her left rear foot that had been present for 2 months. There is a local soft tissue swelling involving the 5th digit of the left rear foot. There is marked destruction of the 3rd phalanx of this digit. There is a small amount of soft tissue calcification cranially and laterally. There is no evidence of periosteal proliferation. **Diagnosis:** Squamous cell carcinoma of the digit.

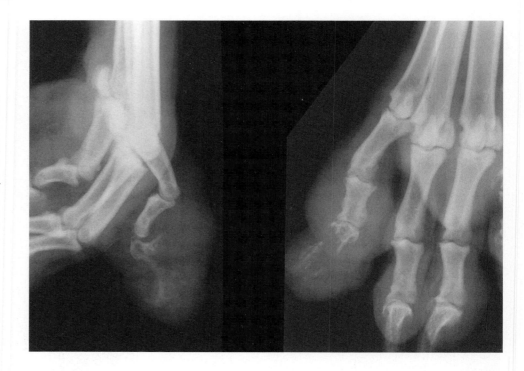

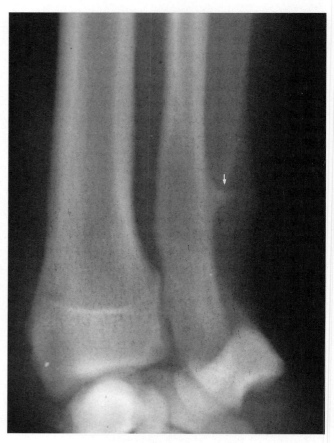

Figure 4–55. A 2-year-old male English pointer was presented with an acute lameness of the left forelimb that developed during a field trial. The lateral radiograph of the distal left radius and ulna reveals a small, broad-based bony projection extending from the distal ulnar metaphysis (*arrow*). The projection tapers to a small tip and is oriented at a 90° angle to the long axis of the ulna. **Diagnosis:** Osteochondroma. This was not apparently significant as the dog completely recovered with 48 hours of rest.

has a wide base attached to the metaphysis of a long bone, which projects to a narrower tip. The osteochondroma usually is at right angles to the axis of the host bone (Fig. 4–55). The other form has an eccentric expansile lesion of the bone (usually metaphyseal) with smooth cortex, a trabecular pattern, and no periosteal reaction.

These usually are asymptomatic unless they cause a mechanical interference with locomotion. In dogs, this is thought to be a hereditary disease.

A viral etiology has been suggested in some cats.[95] The radiographic appearance of the viral associated disease in the cat is that of polyostotic, poorly defined, variably sized and irregularly mineralized lesions with large, radiolucent areas interspersed within mature trabecular bone. These occur in both diaphyseal and metaphyseal regions. In the cat, the lesions usually appear after skeletal maturity, grow progressively, and often increase in number.

Some osteochondromas may undergo transformation to chondrosarcoma at a later time. Malignant transformation is reportedly more frequent in multiple osteochondroma than solitary osteochondroma. Rapid growth of the lesion after physeal closure and the presence of an irregularly mineralized mass suggests malignant transformation.

Enchondroma

Enchondroma is an extremely rare, benign neoplasm that may produce radiolucent defects with cortical thinning in the metaphysis or diaphysis of a long bone.[99] These lesions may be the result of a failure of normal endochondral ossification with retention of physeal growth cartilage.[100] In humans, the lesion may grow slowly, thinning and expanding the cortex, and resulting in a pathologic fracture.

CYSTIC BONE LESIONS

Primary Bone Cysts

Bone cysts may be monostotic or polyostotic and usually are located in the metaphysis and diaphysis (Figs. 4–12 and 4–56).[101,102] The condition is seen most often in

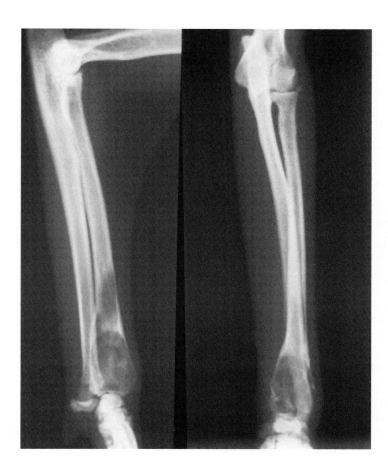

Figure 4–56. A 7-year-old male domestic short-haired cat presented with a right forelimb lameness. A swelling was noted in the distal radial area. The distal radius is widened. The cortex is smooth. The lucent lesion is well-demarcated from the normal bone. There are no fractures identified. **Diagnosis:** Bone cyst.

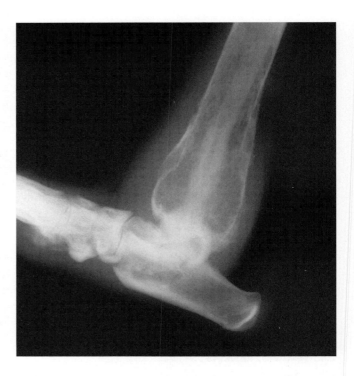

Figure 4–57. An 11-year-old spayed dalmatian was presented with a 6-week history of non-weight-bearing lameness of the right hindlimb. The right hock was swollen. The lateral radiograph of the right tibia reveals a septated, mildly expansile, lytic lesion involving the distal third of the tibia. Minimal periosteal reaction is present. **Diagnosis:** Aneurysmal bone cyst.

young dogs, 5 to 24 months old; however, bone cysts may be asymptomatic and, therefore, any age may be affected. Bone cysts also occur in cats. Radiographically, the bone is expanded with thin cortical margins. In multicameral cysts, thin bony partitions within the medullary canal divide the lesion into compartments. If a pathologic fracture occurs, periosteal proliferation and callus may be observed. Recurrence or malignant transformation has not been observed after curettage.

Aneurysmal Bone Cyst

Aneurysmal bone cyst is a rare lesion. It usually is eccentrically located within the metaphysis and produces bony lysis with minimal cortical or periosteal reaction (Fig. 4–57).[35,103–105]

Epidermoid Cyst

Epidermoid cysts of bone are rare neoplasms. They consist of an island of squamous cells embedded in a bone.[65] Reported cases involved vertebral bodies and terminal phalanges.[106,107] All were characterized by localized radiolucent areas with sclerotic margins.[106,107]

Subperiosteal Cortical Defect

Subperiosteal cortical defect (fibrous cortical defect) is a symptom-less rarefaction of cortical bone.[108,109] These defects are predominately metaphyseal lesions arising close to the growth plate (Fig. 4–58). In humans, they usually arise from the posterior wall of a tubular bone and affect the medial osseous surface producing focal, shallow radiolucent areas in the cortex with normal or sclerotic adjacent bone.[109] Their exact cause is unknown.

OSTEOMYELITIS (INFECTION)

Osteomyelitis (infection of bone) can be caused by bacterial, fungal, or protozoal organisms. Viral organisms have also been rarely reported.[110] Pathogens may gain access to bone by direct inoculation, extension from an adjacent soft tissue infection, or hematogenous spread. The most common cause of osteomyelitis is complication of fracture healing or repair.

THE APPENDICULAR SKELETON ■ 469

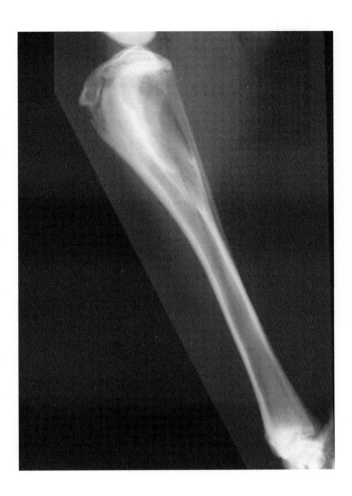

Figure 4–58. A 9-month-old male Doberman pinscher that had a pathologic fracture of the left femur (see Fig. 4–12). The right tibia was radiographed as part of a bone survey. An eccentric lytic lesion is noted in the proximal tibial metaphysis with a sclerotic cortex deep to it. The lesion is clearly demarcated from the normal bone and is eccentrically placed. **Diagnosis:** Subperiosteal cortical defect.

The radiographic changes caused by infection share many characteristics with those caused by neoplasia.[24] Typically, soft tissue swelling, bone lysis, and periosteal reaction are seen. In some specific infections, one or more of these signs tend to predominate.

BACTERIAL OSTEOMYELITIS

Bacterial osteomyelitis may occur anywhere within a bone.[111,112] One (monostotic) or multiple (polyostotic) bones may be affected.[113] Monostotic lesions usually are due to direct inoculation or extension of infections, whereas polyostotic disease usually is due to hematogenous spread.[114] Both aerobic and anaerobic bacteria may be involved.[115–119] Anaerobes may be involved in up to 70% of osteomyelitis cases.[110]

Radiographic findings center on bone destruction associated with extensive periosteal and endosteal proliferation. Soft tissue swelling usually is diffuse.[120] These findings may mimic those seen with neoplasia.[24]

Bacterial osteomyelitis associated with a fracture can lead to other complications. It may cause the formation of a sequestrum, which is an avascular piece of bone that appears abnormally radiodense and has distinct margins. If the sequestrum is within the bone, a radiolucent area (involucrum) may be seen surrounding it. If the process breaches the cortex, a defect (cloaca) may be seen, which may extend to the skin with a draining fistulous tract (Figs. 4–59, 4–60, and 4–61).

Hematogenous osteomyelitis in young dogs may involve the metaphyses (Fig. 4–59). Irregular bony lysis and periosteal proliferation will be seen. This lesion may mimic hypertrophic osteodystrophy (HOD); however, unlike HOD, the involvement is asymmetric involving different areas to a greater or lesser extent. This type of infection may be seen in weimeraners with immune deficiency states.

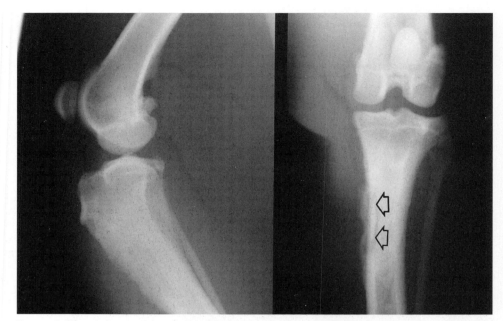

Figure 4–59. A 1-year-old male English bulldog was in a dog fight 3 weeks previously and has had intermittent lameness since that time. Soft tissue swelling extended from the stifle to the hock. There is bony proliferation with increased density within the medullary canal involving the proximal third of the right tibia. A dense bony fragment is present in the medial cortex of the proximal tibia (*arrows*). This is surrounded by an area of radiolucency. There is extensive periosteal proliferation medial to this dense fragment. This fragment represents a sequestrum. **Diagnosis:** Osteomyelitis.

Figure 4–60. A 5-year-old male German shepherd dog was in a fight with another dog 3 weeks ago. Clinically, there is swelling involving the left forelimb. Diffuse soft tissue swelling is evident radiographically. There is periosteal proliferation involving the middle portions of the radius and ulna. The endosteal surfaces of both the radius and ulna are sclerotic. **Diagnosis:** Osteomyelitis.

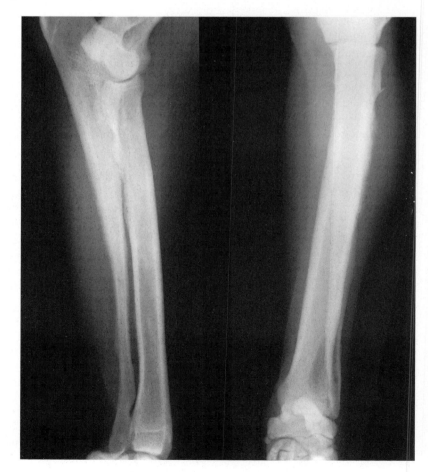

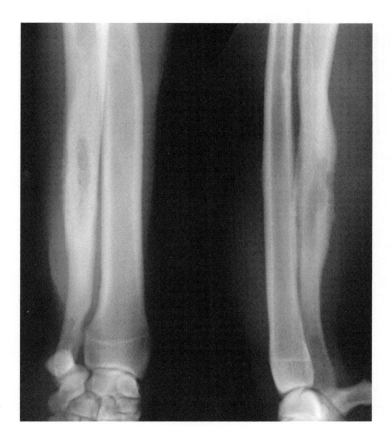

Figure 4–61. A 2-year-old male rottweiler had a bite wound on his right foreleg 5 months ago. The wound had been treated with antibiotics but the swelling recurred. On physical exam the limb was swollen at the carpus and forearm and a draining tract was present. There is diffuse soft tissue swelling involving the right forelimb. There is bony proliferation involving the distal third of the ulna. There is a central area of radiolucency which extends through the caudal ulnar cortex (cloaca). The bone proximal and distal to the area of radiolucency is dense. **Diagnosis:** Chronic osteomyelitis. A sequestrum is not observed in this case. This lesion responded to surgical curettage.

In young dogs, the entire diaphyseal cortex may develop into a large sequestrum. Extensive, reactive periosteal proliferation will surround the dense cortical sequestrum. Fortunately, this lesion will respond to antibiotics since removal of the sequestrum is not possible.

An unusual sequestrum may be seen when a bone is penetrated by a pin used as a fixator. The radiographic appearance of concentric zones of osteosclerosis and osteolucency surrounding the bone defect caused by a pin has been called a "ring sequestrum."[121] Although infection is a likely cause in this situation, bone necrosis from the heat related to drilling the pin must also be considered.

An unusual outcome of bacterial osteomyelitis is the formation of a chronic bone (Brodie's) abscess. This is a chronic abscess of bone that is incarcerated by a wall of granulation tissue and a fibrous capsule. The abscess becomes static and sterile. Radiographically, a chronic bone abscess appears as a focal lucency surrounded by a zone of mild to moderate sclerosis.[122]

MYCOTIC AND HIGHER BACTERIAL OSTEOMYELITIS

Coccidioidomycosis and blastomycosis account for the majority of cases of mycotic osteomyelitis; however, infections due to histoplasmosis, aspergillosis, cryptococcosis, paeciliomycosis, nocardiosis, actinomycosis, and sporotrichosis have been reported (Figs. 4–62, 4–63, 4–64, 4–65, and 4–66).[30,123–133] Mycotic osteomyelitis is most frequently polyostotic. The periosteal and endosteal bony proliferation in mycotic infection usually is denser and more extensive than that seen with bacterial osteomyelitis. However, some lesions associated with histoplasmosis and other systemic mycoses have been predominately lytic (Fig. 4–67).[124,133] Sequestrum formation is uncommon. The differentiation between mycotic osteomyelitis and neoplasia is aided by knowing the geographic distribution of mycotic diseases and the fact that young animals are affected more often than older animals.

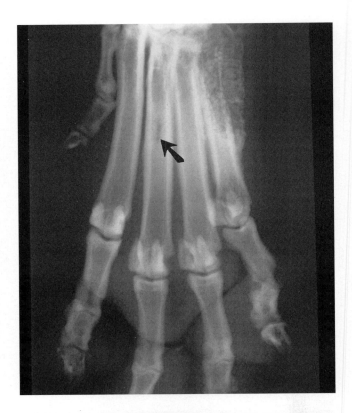

Figure 4–62. A 2-year-old female Saint Bernard presented with lameness of the left forelimb. There is swelling involving the carpal and metacarpal area as well as the 4th and 5th digits. There is extensive bony destruction and proliferation involving the 5th metacarpal bone. The changes are more severe proximally; however, the entire shaft of this metacarpal bone is involved. There is a radiolucent area within the midportion of the 3rd metacarpal bone (*arrow*). There is destruction involving the distal end of the 2nd phalanx of the 4th digit and areas of bony destruction involving the distal end of the 1st phalanx of the 5th digit. The multi-focal nature of this lesion and proliferative response are suggestive of mycotic infection. **Diagnosis:** Blastomycosis.

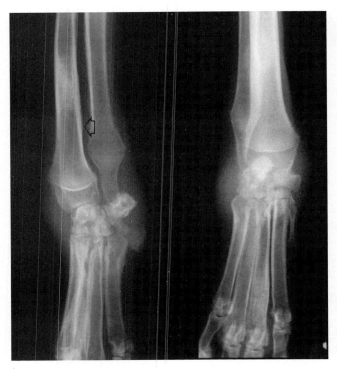

A

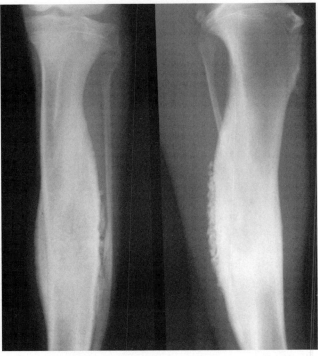

B

Figure 4–63. An 8-month-old female Doberman pinscher presented with an elevated temperature and reluctance to walk. There was swelling noted around both carpi and the right tibia. (A) On radiographs of the right carpus a swelling is evident in the area of the carpal joint. There is an increase in bony density within the mid- and distal portions of the right radius. There is a laminar periosteal response on the caudal cortex of the radius (*arrow*). There is a small amount of bony proliferation on the ulna adjacent to this site. There is an area of increased bone density within the medullary canal of the 3rd metacarpal bone. (B) There is a marked increase in medullary density within the midshaft tibia. There is a laminar periosteal proliferation on the cranial and medial cortex of the tibia and a less regular area of periosteal proliferation on the caudal lateral aspect of the tibia. The presence of multi-focal areas of increased density with periosteal proliferation in a dog of this age is indicative of an infection. The dog lived in the lower Sonoran valley. **Diagnosis:** Coccidioidomycosis.

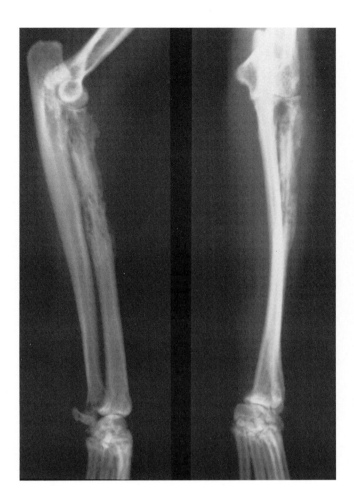

Figure 4–64. A 4-year-old female domestic short-haired cat was presented with a chronic right foreleg lameness with swelling. There is soft tissue swelling involving the right forelimb. There is an area of bony destruction involving the proximal half of the right radius. There is a small amount of bony proliferation cranially and medially. The localized nature of this lesion with the massive bony destruction with little bony proliferation suggested a primary neoplasm. A biopsy was not performed. The leg was amputated. **Diagnosis:** Cryptococcosis. A destructive pattern may occur with infections that mimic the patterns seen with a primary neoplasm. This case identifies the critical role of a bone biopsy.

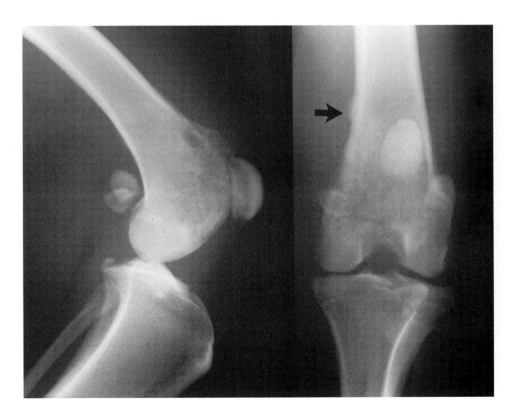

Figure 4–65. A 3-year-old male Labrador retriever presented with a left rear leg lameness, a draining tract medial to the left stifle, and a distended and painful joint. There is soft tissue swelling involving the stifle joint. There is bony destruction within the left femur in the distal metaphysis. A small amount of periosteal new bone formation is present on the medial aspect of the left femur (*arrow*). There is some loss of bone density within the patella. The diffuse soft tissue swelling and involvement of both the distal femur and patella are suggestive of infection. **Diagnosis:** Septic arthritis and osteomyelitis. This was due to *Nocardia* infection.

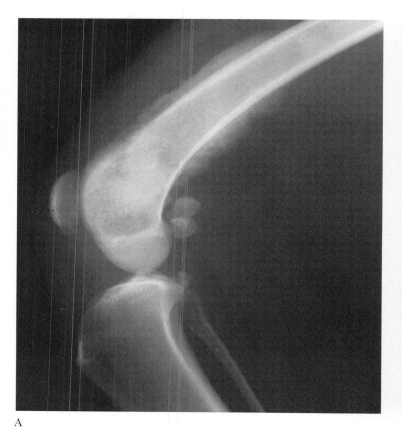

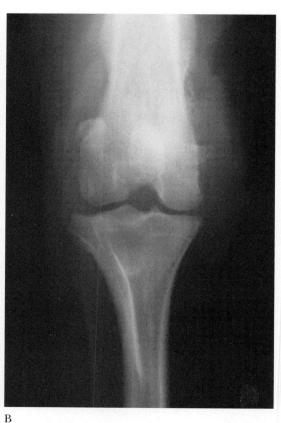

A

B

Figure 4–66. (A&B) A 4 year-old male coonhound had been lame for 1 month in the right rear leg. The dog was afebrile. There is soft tissue swelling which extends into the stifle joint. There is extensive bony proliferation involving the distal right femur. The medullary canal density is increased. There is no evidence of bony destruction. **Diagnosis:** Actinomycosis. This lesion has many features of a primary bone tumor and indicates the need for bone biopsy.

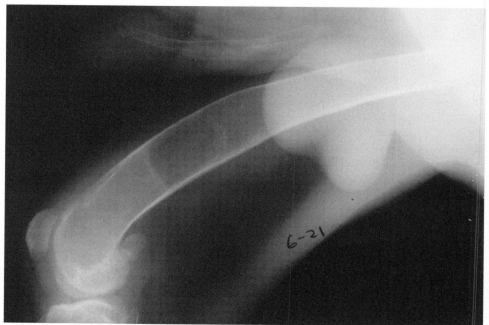

Figure 4–67. A 2-year-old mixed breed male dog was presented with diarrhea, weight loss, and intermittent right hindlimb lameness of 6 month's duration. The lateral radiograph of the right femur reveals an osteolytic, minimally expansile lesion of the midshaft. The cortex is thinned in this region. **Diagnosis:** Histoplasmosis.

PARASITIC INFESTATION

Periosteal proliferation has been observed in association with a protozoan parasite infestation (*Hepatozoan sp.*).[134,135] Protozoan-like elements have been identified in the neutrophils within the bone marrow. Smooth periosteal proliferation involved the vertebral bodies, ribs, and the diaphyses of all long bones proximal to the tarsus and carpus. The bony proliferation was reduced one year after diagnosis, despite the continued presence of protozoan parasites; therefore, the relationship between the organism and the bone lesion is not clear.

Multiple bone involvement has also been reported in dogs with visceral leishmaniasis.[136] Leishmanial organisms were observed in synovial biopsies and within the bone. Periosteal proliferation, cortical destruction, and increased medullary density were reported in the diaphysis of long bones. Osteolytic lesions were seen around the joints. The site of involvement and degree of bony response was variable, but there was a tendency for the lesions to be symmetrical.

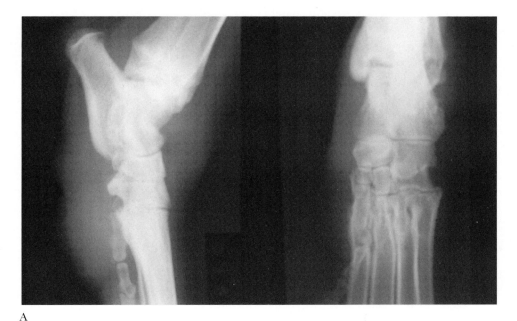

A

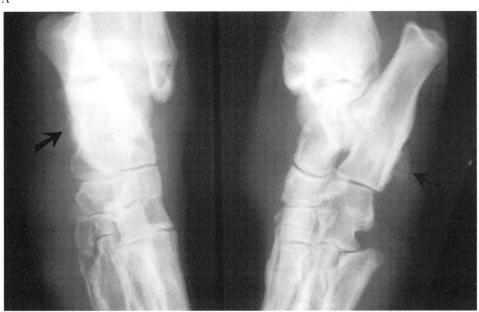

B

Figure 4–68. (A&B) A 9-month-old female Doberman pinscher presented with a swollen left hock. The swelling had been present for 3 months. There is irregular soft tissue swelling surrounding the tarsus. The swelling extends beyond the joint margins. There is minimal smooth bony proliferation on the lateral and caudolateral aspects of the joint (*arrows*). This is secondary to the chronic soft tissue infection and does not indicate bone infection. **Diagnosis:** Chronic soft tissue infection.

TABLE 4-2. Differential Diagnosis of Bone Neoplasia and Infection

	SIGNALMENT			LOCATION			SOFT TISSUE		
	AGE (YRS)	BREED	SEX (M:F)	DIA-PHYSEAL	META-PHYSEAL	DISTRI-BUTION	SWELLING	DENSITY	BONE
Tumor									
Primary[a]	1.5 6	Giant	1.2:1	+[b]	+++[c]	Monostotic	Focal	Bone	D[d] > P[e]
Metastatic	Old	Any	—	+++	++[f]	Polyostotic	Focal	Fluid	D = P
Infection									
Bacterial	Any	Any	—	++	++	Polyostotic	Diffuse	Fluid	D < P
Mycotic	Young	Any	—	++	++	Polyostotic	Diffuse	Fluid	D < P

[a]Osteosarcoma
[b]+ = Occurs rarely
[c]+++ = Most often occurs
[d]D = Bone destruction
[e]P = Bone production
[f]++ = May occur

SOFT TISSUE INFECTION

Periosteal proliferation may result from chronic soft tissue infections or inflammation (Fig. 4–68). The periosteal proliferation often is well-defined, evenly mineralized, and may extend along the diaphysis or metaphysis. Endosteal or medullary changes may occur late in the disease process if an infection progresses.

PARONYCHIA

Chronic infection or inflammation around the nail bed (paronychia) can affect the distal phalanges. Paronychia will result in lysis of the third phalanx and stimulate bony proliferation around the second or first phalanges. It may be difficult to distinguish infection from the changes caused by tumors such as squamous cell carcinoma of the nail bed. The presence of a diffuse soft tissue swelling, rather than a localized mass, and an extensive amount of periosteal proliferation along the diaphysis of the second phalanx are important clues to the diagnosis of infection.

DIFFERENTIAL DIAGNOSIS OF INFECTION AND NEOPLASIA

Both infection and neoplasia produce a wide spectrum of destructive and productive bony changes (Table 4–2). Unfortunately, there is a great deal of overlap of many of the radiographic features. This is particularly true early in the pathogenesis of the diseases. For that reason, a diagnosis based solely on the radiographic findings may be erroneous. All radiographic changes must be evaluated in light of the clinical and historical information. Biopsy, culture, and serology usually are required to reach a final diagnosis. The histology should be evaluated in conjunction with the radiographic changes and with knowledge of the site from which the biopsy was obtained.

NUTRITIONAL AND METABOLIC

GROWTH HORMONE DEFICIENCY (PITUITARY DWARFISM)

Pituitary dwarfism results from inadequate growth hormone during the growth phase of life. German shepherds appear to be the most commonly affected variety of dogs.[137] The dogs are proportionate dwarfs and have delayed closure of their growth plates, incomplete calcification of the epiphyses, and delayed appearance of some centers of ossification.

HYPERPARATHYROIDISM (PRIMARY, SECONDARY) AND PSEUDOHYPERPARATHYROIDISM

Primary hyperparathyroidism, due to a functional parathyroid tumor, occurs infrequently.[138–141] Secondary hyperparathyroidism, either renal or nutritional (due to a calcium/phosphorus imbalance, a deficiency in calcium, or vitamin D), occurs more frequently than primary hyperparathyroidism. Secondary hyperparathyroidism more frequently results in radiographic changes of bone.[142–145] Pseudohyperparathyroidism, which is associated with various neoplastic diseases such as lymphosarcoma and perianal apocrine adenocarcinoma, usually does not cause radiographically apparent bone loss.

The radiographic findings of hyperparathyroidism (any form) may include decreased bone density, subperiosteal bone resorption, cortical resorption tunnels, double cortical lines, loss of the lamina dura dentes, physeal aberrations, pathologic fractures, expansile lesions (Brown's tumor), and soft tissue calcification.

Secondary renal hyperparathyroidism may cause extensive demineralization of the skull, vertebral column, and/or long bones. The lesions usually are more severe in juvenile animals. Occasionally, renal secondary hyperparathyroidism may cause osteopetrosis rather than osteopenia.

Loss of the lamina dura dentes has been described as an early change. This loss also may occur due to periodontal disease. Generalized loss of bone from the skull accentuates the difference between the density of the teeth and that of the mandible and maxilla, which creates an appearance described as "floating teeth." Diffuse soft tissue swelling may be present around the mandible and maxilla due to replacement of bone by fibrous tissue. Pathologic (including folding, "torus") fractures may result from the extensive loss of mineral in the bones. Collapse of the pelvis with abnormal curvature of the ilium and ischium and narrowing of the pelvic canal may be present. Before physeal plate closure occurs, limb growth and physeal appearance are normal despite the generalized loss of bone density and pathologic fractures. Cortices usually are thin and may show cortical resorption tunnels and subperiosteal resorption.[144] Diaphyseal and metaphyseal trabeculation frequently is accentuated. Pathologic fractures usually heal rapidly at the expense of additional loss of cortical and medullary bone, although permanent bony deformity frequently remains.

Severe secondary nutritional hyperparathyroidism usually results in marked, generalized loss of bone density. Pathologic bowing and folding fractures are most common, but complete fractures may be present (Figs. 4–8 and 4–69). Physeal growth

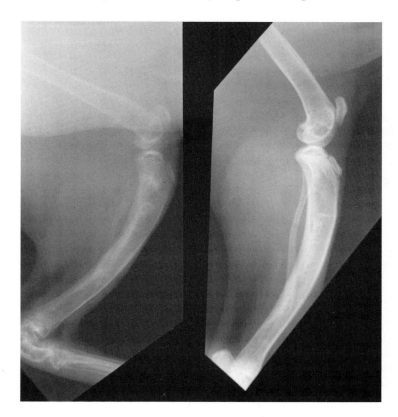

Figure 4–69. A 6-month-old female domestic short-haired cat presented with a history of generalized weakness, pain, and reluctance to walk. (A) A lateral radiograph of the tibia and (B) a follow-up radiograph 3 months later are illustrated. There is a decrease in bony density in the radiograph obtained at the time of admission. The cortices are thin and the leg is bowed. A pathological fracture is present in the distal femur, proximal tibia and fibula. On the follow-up radiograph the normal bone density has returned. The pathological fractures have healed; however, a residual bony deformity (tibial curvature) is present. **Diagnosis:** Nutritional secondary hyperparathyroidism.

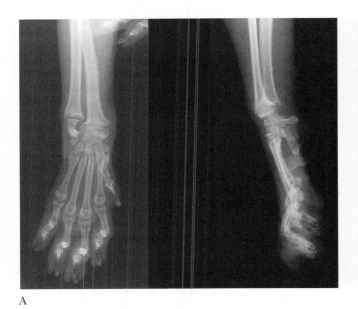

A

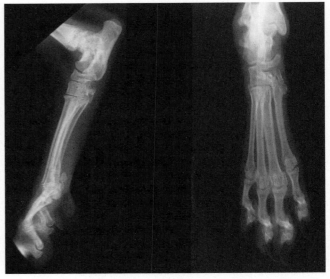

B

Figure 4–70. A 3-year-old female domestic short-haired cat was presented with a history of poor hair coat and shortened stature. The cat was reluctant to walk. Radiographs of the fore and rear limbs, the pelvis, and the spine were obtained. Radiographs of (A) the right carpus, (B) right tarsus, and (C) pelvis are illustrated. The distal radial and ulnar physes remain open despite the fact that the cat is 3 years old. Open physes are also noted in the proximal and distal femur, proximal tibia, and acetabulum. The distal ulnar epiphysis is irregularly mineralized. There is subluxation of both coxofemoral joints; however, the apparent lateral patellar dislocation is a positional artifact. The retarded epiphyseal closure and irregular mineralization of the distal ulnar epiphysis are indicative of an epiphyseal dysplasia with retarded bone growth. **Diagnosis:** Hypothyroidism. Mucopolysaccharidosis could also be considered; however, delayed epiphyseal closure would not be expected in that disease.

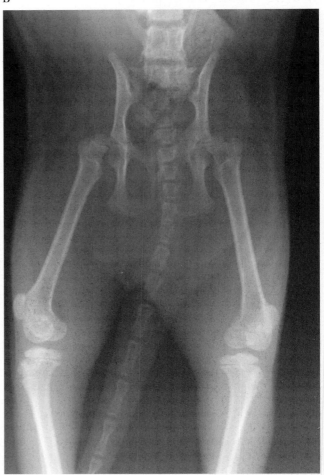

C

usually is normal, and fracture healing is at the expense of bone loss in other areas. Reversal of the bony changes is rapid once the dietary imbalance is corrected.

Soft tissue mineralization may be present with either secondary or other forms of hyperparathyroidism at many different sites. Bronchial and pulmonary, renal parenchymal, gastric mucosal, vascular calcifications, and extensive foot pad calcification may be seen.

HYPOTHYROIDISM

Hypothyroidism usually affects middle-aged or older dogs and does not produce radiographic changes. Congenital hypothyroidism may result in disproportionate dwarfism.[146-150] Radiographic findings include absence or delayed appearance and retarded development of epiphyseal growth centers (Fig. 4–70). Thickening of the radial and ulnar cortices as well as radial bowing may be seen. Facial bone and mandibular shortening combined with a full complement of deciduous and permanent teeth may result in crowding of the teeth. Cranial sutures may remain open. The bony changes may respond to early hormone replacement.

HYPERADRENOCORTICISM

Hyperadrenocorticism may result in demineralization of the skeleton. Although this is uncommon, it generally is associated with long-standing disease. The radiographic changes that may be seen include subtle loss of bone density.[151,152] This is most often observed in the vertebral bodies.

HYPERVITAMINOSIS A

Hypervitaminosis A produces fusion of cervical vertebrae due to bony proliferation along the dorsal spinous processes, vertebral bodies, and articular facets.[153,154] Bridging exostoses also may occur across articulations of the appendicular skeleton (Fig. 4–71). Coarse medullary trabeculation, decreased bony density, thin cortices, and soft tissue mineralization have been described (Fig. 4–72). In affected young growing dogs, a decrease in long bone length and width, premature physeal closure, transverse metaphyseal widening, periarticular osteophytes, metaphyseal periosteal proliferation, and spontaneous fractures have been described.[153] Permanent retardation of growth may result.

LEAD INTOXICATION

An uncommon finding in lead intoxication in the juvenile animal is metaphyseal sclerosis (lead lines). Radiographically, bands of increased density adjacent to the physeal growth plate are identified.[100]

ERYTHROCYTE PYRUVATE KINASE DEFICIENCY IN BASENJIS

An anemia associated with erythrocyte pyruvate kinase deficiency has been described in basenjis.[155] A progressive, diffuse osteosclerosis has been associated with this syndrome (Fig. 4–73).

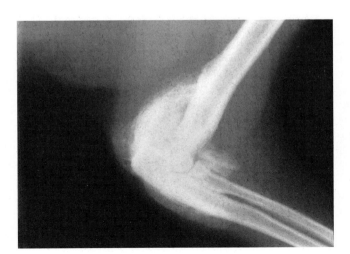

Figure 4–71. A 9-year-old female domestic short-haired cat that was presented with a 3-month history of reluctance to walk. The joints appeared stiff and the cat resented joint manipulation. There is extensive periarticular soft tissue mineralization around the elbow. Similar changes were present in the other limbs. **Diagnosis:** Hypervitaminosis A.

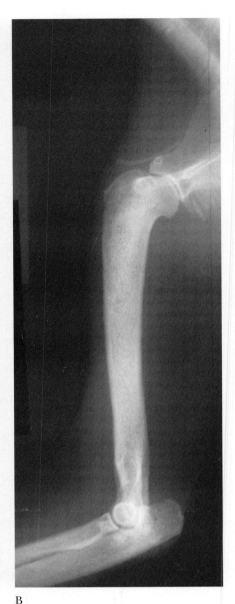

Figure 4–72. An 11-year-old male domestic short-haired cat was presented with a 9-month history of anorexia and depression. The cat was reluctant to walk. All four limbs were radiographed. (A) Radiographs of the left (B) and right forelimbs are presented. There is increased density within the diaphyses of all bones. The cortex is thickened and the medullary trabeculation is coarse. The joints were not affected. **Diagnosis:** Hypervitaminosis A.

A

B

ANATOMIC, CONGENITAL, DEVELOPMENTAL, IDIOPATHIC

CHONDRODYSPLASIA

Several inherited chondrodysplasias (conditions due to abnormal cartilage development) have been described. These include Alaskan malamute dwarfism, chondrodysplasia of great Pyrenees, endochondrodystrophy of English pointers, osteochondrodysplasia in Scottish deerhounds, skeletal and retinal dysplasia in Labrador retrievers, chondrodysplasia in a cat, pseudoachondroplasia in poodles, and congenital epiphyseal dysplasia in beagles and poodles.[156–164] In some breeds (e.g., English bulldogs and bassett hounds), the deformity resulting from chondrodysplasia is considered to be normal and desirable.

Alaskan Malamute Dwarfism

A Mendelian recessive short-limbed dwarfism has been described in Alaskan malamute dogs.[159,160] The skeletal lesion was generalized and symmetrical and best demonstrated in the carpus of 4- to 12-week-old dogs (Fig. 4–74). The distal ulnar

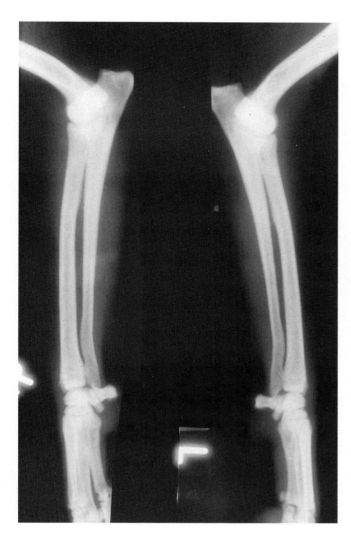

Figure 4–73. A 4-year-old male basenji was presented with a moderate anemia. The lateral radiographs of the forelimbs reveals a generalized increase in density (osteosclerosis) in all bones. Similar changes were present in the hindlimbs and ribs. **Diagnosis:** Erythrocyte pyruvate kinase deficiency of basenjis.

and radial metaphyses were widened and irregular. The time of appearance and the ossification of epiphyseal growth centers were delayed compared to normal Alaskan malamutes. Lateral deviation of the paw and stunted growth were observed.

Skeletal And Retinal Dysplasia in Labrador Retrievers

A skeletal dysplasia of Labrador retrievers has been described. The radiographic changes have included delayed epiphyseal development with retarded radial, ulnar, and tibial growth, un-united and hypoplastic anconeal processes, and coxofemoral joint deformities combined with retinal dysplasia, retinal detachment, and cataract formation (Fig. 4–75).[158,165] Abnormal skeletal development can be detected at 8 weeks of age. Radiographically, distal ulnar growth plate irregularities with retained cartilaginous cores and delayed development of the anconeus, coronoid, and medial humeral epicondyle may be seen.[165] The radius and ulna were shortened and curved. Shallow acetabuli, thickened femoral necks, and periarticular osteophytes were described. Stifle osteoarthrosis and shortened femurs also occurred.

Pseudoachondroplasia in Poodles

Pseudoachondroplastic dysplasia becomes evident at 3 weeks of age in affected miniature poodles.[162] Joint enlargement, short, bent limbs, flattened rib cages, and abnormal locomotion with hind limb abduction has been described. Retarded epiphyseal ossification results in stippled, patchy densities in the epiphyses. The skull is not affected.

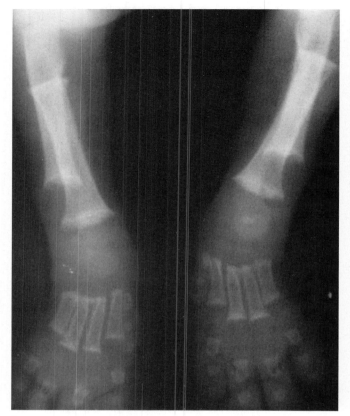

A

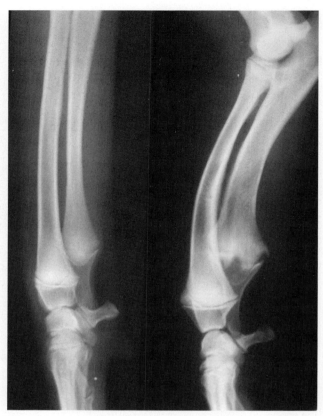

B

Figure 4–74. A 4-week-old female malamute from a litter of puppies was evaluated for dwarfism. (A) Antero-posterior radiographs of both carpi were obtained. The distal radial and ulnar metaphyses are widened and irregular. The distal ulnar metaphysis does not have the expected cone shape. (B) On radiographs obtained at 9 months of age, an angular limb deformity is apparent, especially when compared to a normal littermate. The distal ulnar metaphysis is irregular and an area of cartilage remains uncalcified. The proximal radial-ulnar joint is malaligned and the radius is bowed. **Diagnosis:** Malamute dwarfism.

Epiphyseal Dysplasia

Epiphyseal dysplasia has been reported in beagles and poodles.[161] The dogs showed hind limb dysfunction at birth and osteoarthrosis as adults. Punctate calcifications with irregularly stippled epiphyses were described in the humerus, femur, metacarpals, metatarsals, carpal and tarsal bones, and vertebral bodies (Fig. 4–76). The disease may be recognized up to 4 months of age, after which the irregular calcifications become incorporated in the ossified bone. Non-specific osteoarthritic changes persist in the adult. These cannot be distinguished from other causes of secondary degenerative joint disease.

ECTRODACTYLY

Ectrodactyly, or split-hand deformity, is an abnormal limb development with separation noted between metacarpal bones, digit contracture, digit aplasia, metacarpal hypoplasia, and metacarpal fusions (Fig. 4–77).[166] Unilateral involvement is most common. In dogs, there is equal involvement of left and right limbs and no breed or sex predisposition. In the cat, ectrodactyly is caused by a dominant gene with variable expressivity.

HEMIMELIA

Hemimelia is a rare disease in which one bone in a paired set is partially or completely absent. This usually affects the radius of the radius/ulna, or occasionally af-

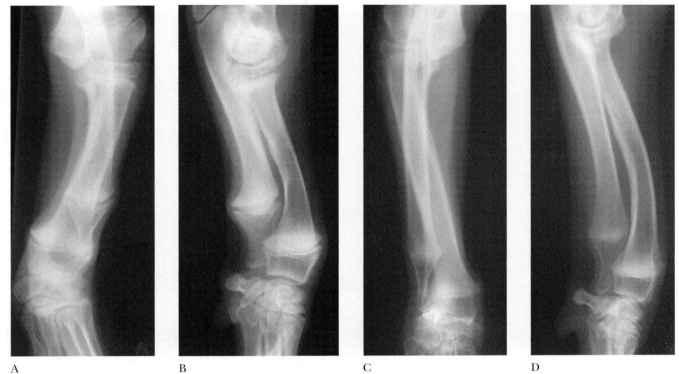

A B C D

Figure 4–75. A 4-month-old female Labrador retriever was presented with a history of apparent blindness. The dog managed well at home but seemed lost in new surroundings. The dog appeared smaller than anticipated. (A&B) There is a bowing deformity of the radius with irregularity of the distal ulnar metaphysis. The foot is slightly laterally deviated. (C&D) At 9 months of age the angular limb deformity has increased. The distal ulnar metaphysis remains irregular and the physis has partially closed. **Diagnosis:** Skeletal dysplasia of Labrador retrievers.

fects the tibia of the tibia/fibula.[167,168] The bone of the affected "pair" that is present usually is somewhat larger in diameter than normal. The joint proximal and/or distal to the bone may be subluxated or luxated.

SESAMOID BONE ABNORMALITIES IN ROTTWEILERS

Abnormalities of the sesamoid bones of rottweilers have been reported.[169,170] Lesions usually involve the medial sesamoids of the metacarpal phalangeal joints of digits 2 and 5. Lesions range from a single radiodensity separated from an otherwise normal sesamoid to replacement with multiple, small radiodense bones. This finding usually is not associated with clinical signs.

OSTEOGENESIS IMPERFECTA

Osteogenesis imperfecta is related to a defect in collagen production and is typified by fragile bone that fractures spontaneously or with minimal trauma. It has been reported in a kitten.[171] Radiographically, the bone density was normal. Multiple healing fractures with active callus formation were noted.

OSTEOPETROSIS

Osteopetrosis is a rare hereditary, familial, and congenital bone abnormality manifested by a generalized increase in bone density, especially in subchondral bone, which involves the axial and appendicular skeleton (Fig. 4–78). Cortical thickening and increased medullary densities ("marble bone") will partially or completely obliterate the medullary canal.[172–174] Pathologic fractures may occur despite the markedly

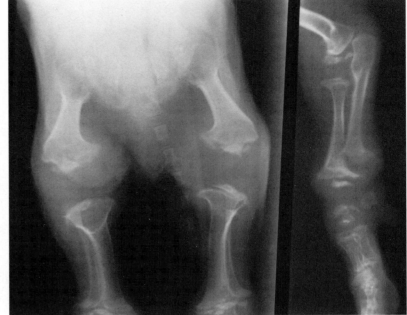

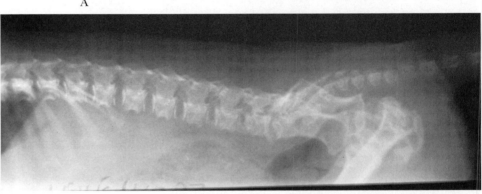

A

B

Figure 4–76. A 2-month-old male miniature poodle was presented because it was smaller and seemed to be less healthy than its littermates. (A) Forelimb and pelvic and (B) spinal radiographs are illustrated. The epiphyses are irregularly ossified and delayed in appearance for a dog of this age. **Diagnosis:** Epiphyseal dysplasia.

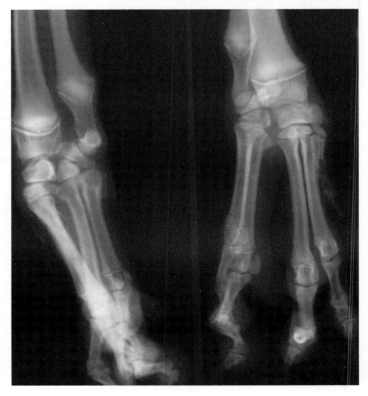

Figure 4–77. A 6-month-old male Shetland sheepdog presented with a congenital anomaly of the right front limb. There were no clinical signs associated with this deformity. There is a marked deformity of the metacarpal and carpal bones. The distal row of carpal bones are deformed. The 3rd and 4th digits are separated, with articulation of the 4th and 5th digits with the ulnar and accessory carpal bones, and articulation of the 1st, 2nd, and 3rd digits with the radial, 2nd, and 3rd carpal bones. The lateral carpal bones appear to articulate with the ulna and the medial carpal bones with the radius. **Diagnosis:** Ectrodactyly. The left forelimb was normal.

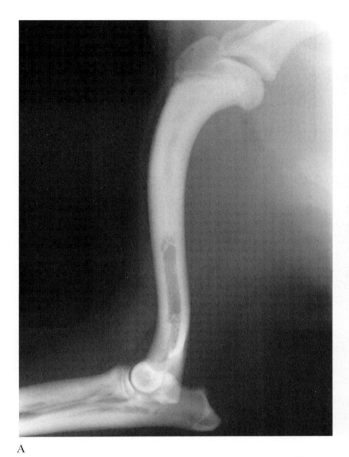

A

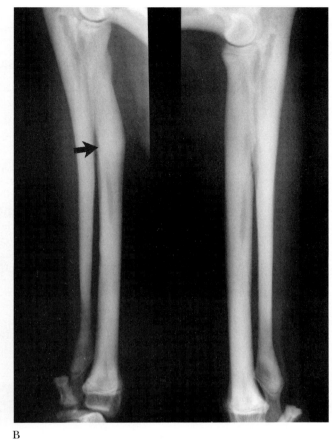

B

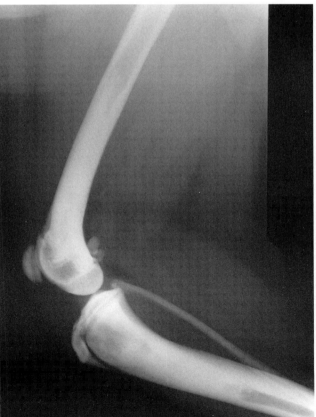

C

Figure 4–78. An 11-month-old female collie presented with a history of recurrent shifting leg lameness. (A) The density and cortical thickness of the humerus is increased. (B) There is a marked increase in medullary and cortical density involving right and left radii. The medullary canal is obliterated. There is no soft tissue swelling. A linear radiolucency is noted crossing the radius at the junction at the proximal and middle third's (*arrow*). There is slight deformity of the radial outline at this point. This is a pathologic fracture. The growth plates are open and are unaffected. The density of the metacarpal bones appears increased although the carpal bones are spared. (C) There is thickening of the right femoral and tibial cortices with an increased bony density in the medullary canal of these bones. The fibula also appears dense. There is no evidence of soft tissue swelling. **Diagnosis:** Osteopetrosis with a pathological fracture of the radius.

increased bone density. Clinical signs may be related to the fractures or to an anemia, which results from obliteration of the bone marrow.[173,175]

PANOSTEITIS (EOSINOPHILIC PANOSTEITIS, ENOSTOSIS)

Panosteitis is a self-limiting bone disorder that causes lameness due to an acute onset of long bone pain. It most frequently affects large breed dogs. While mainly a disease of the young (being reported in dogs as young as 2 months), it does occasionally affect older individuals up to 7 years of age. The acute lameness may undergo spontaneous remission, and may recur in the same limb or reappear in another limb. Evidence of pain can frequently be elicited by applying direct pressure to the affected bone.

The radiographic findings in panosteitis center on the nutrient foramina and involve the diaphysis and metaphysis of the long bones.[176,177] Four radiographically distinct phases have been described. The earliest phase reveals a zone of radiolucency at the nutrient foramen. This is rarely identified clinically and usually requires a retrospective analysis. The second phase begins with an increase in endosteal and medullary density; there is blurring of the normal trabecular pattern. Contrast between the medulla and cortex is reduced (Figs. 4–79 and 4–80). In the third phase, the radiodense areas tend to coalesce, become patchy, mottled, and expand to fill the medullary canal. The endosteal surface may become irregular and mild periosteal proliferation may be present (Fig. 4–81). These changes persist for 4 to 6 weeks and then gradually recede. During the fourth (final) phase, the medullary

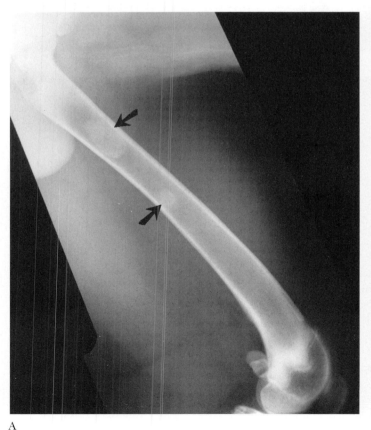

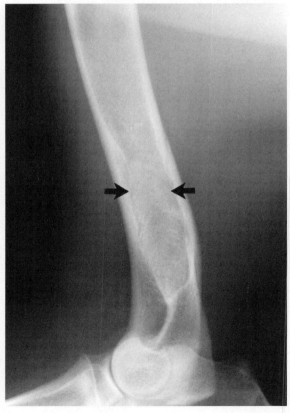

A   B

Figure 4–79. (A&B) An 8-month-old male Great Dane had a recurrent shifting leg lameness. Radiographs of both fore and rear limbs were obtained. The left femur and right humerus are illustrated. There is a localized area of increased medullary density within the proximal and mid-diaphysis of the left femur (*arrows*). There is a less well-defined area of increased medullary density involving the distal third of the right humeral diaphysis (*arrows*). **Diagnosis:** Panosteitis.

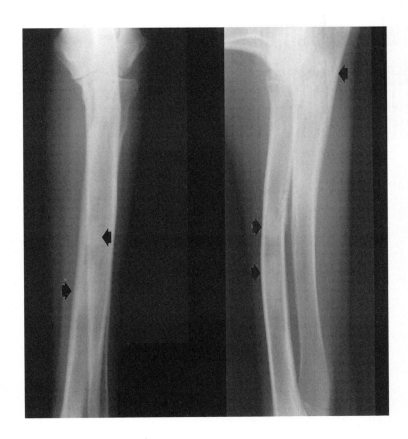

Figure 4–80. A 1-year-old male Great Dane that had been lame for 1 week and exhibited pain upon palpation of the right forelimb and elbow. There is an increase in medullary density involving the mid-diaphyseal portion of the radius. These densities appear poorly defined (*arrows*). There is increased density within the proximal ulnar diaphysis (*arrows*). **Diagnosis:** Panosteitis.

canal regains a normal or decreased density and cortical thickening may persist. Detecting very early lesions is difficult, especially if the radiograph is underexposed. Comparison radiographs of the unaffected limb may be extremely helpful. The radiographic lesion may not be visible at the time the lameness is first observed.

Differential diagnosis of these lesions should include panosteitis as well as neoplasia and hematogenous osteomyelitis. The history and clinical signs are important in determining a final diagnosis.

HYPERTROPHIC OSTEODYSTROPHY

Hypertrophic osteodystrophy usually is seen in rapidly growing large breed dogs between 3 and 8 months of age.[178,179] The cause is unknown, although infectious and nutritional etiologies have been proposed.[180–183] The affected dog may be intermittently depressed, anorectic, febrile, and reluctant to walk or stand. Often, there are obvious distal metaphyseal swellings, which may feel warm on palpation. Spontaneous remission may occur; however, recurrent episodes are common. Severe disease may result in angular limb deformity and retarded growth.

Initial radiographic changes include the presence of transverse radiolucent bands within the metaphysis adjacent to the physeal plate and soft tissue swelling. All long bones may be affected, and lesions may also be seen at the costochondral junctions. The abnormalities are most obvious in the distal radius, ulna, and tibia due to the rapid rate of bone growth in these areas. With time, the metaphyses will appear widened and their opacity will increase. A cuff of periosteal proliferation may be seen that is separated from the metaphysis by a thin linear radiolucency but gradually blending with the diaphyseal cortex. The bony changes appear to progress toward the diaphysis as the dog grows. The physis and epiphysis usually are not involved (Figs. 4–82 and 4–83). Although the condition disappears with maturity, a residual bowing deformity of the forelimbs may result and mild thickening of the metaphysis may remain. Some deaths have been reported in dogs with hypertrophic osteodystrophy.

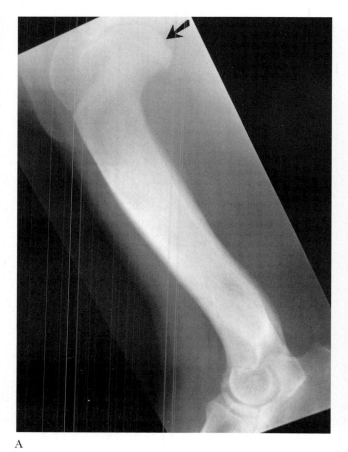

A

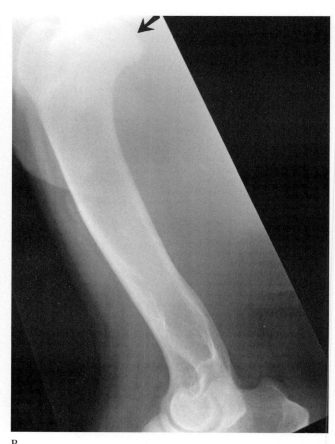

B

Figure 4–81. A 9-month-old male German shepherd dog presented with a right foreleg lameness and pain on palpation of the right humerus. Pain was also noted on extension and flexion of the right shoulder. (A) Initial and (B) 4-month follow-up radiographs of the right humerus are illustrated. There is an increase in medullary density within the entire diaphysis of the right humerus with mild periosteal proliferation on the cranial and caudal surfaces of the humeral diaphysis. There is flattening of the proximal humeral head (*arrow*) with sclerosis in the subchondral bone. This is indicative of panosteitis and osteochondrosis. (B) In the follow-up radiograph, the increased right humeral diaphyseal density has resolved. Several fine linear densities are present in the middle and distal portions of the humeral diaphysis. The cortical density and thickness is normal. There is a slight residual flattening in the proximal humeral head (*arrows*). **Diagnosis:** Panosteitis and osteochondrosis.

Many normal, rapidly growing, young, large breed dogs have mild irregularities of the distal ulnar and radial metaphysis. This must be considered when evaluating a dog suspected of having hypertrophic osteodystrophy. The line of demarcation between normal and mild disease is indistinct.

Hypertrophic osteodystrophy and craniomandibular osteopathy have been reported simultaneously in a few large breed dogs, and some terriers affected with craniomandibular osteopathy have had long bone changes resembling hypertrophic osteodystrophy.

HYPERTROPHIC OSTEOPATHY

Hypertrophic osteopathy produces a generalized, symmetrical, palisading periosteal proliferation, which involves the diaphyses of the long bones (Figs. 4–84 and 4–85). The condition most often is associated with either infectious or neoplastic intrathoracic lesions (i.e., pleural, pulmonary, cardiac, and mediastinal); however, hypertrophic osteopathy has been reported in association with bladder, liver, and ovarian tumors without thoracic disease.[184–191]

The periosteal proliferation becomes more extensive as the disease progresses. The bony proliferation usually affects the distal portions of the limbs more severely;

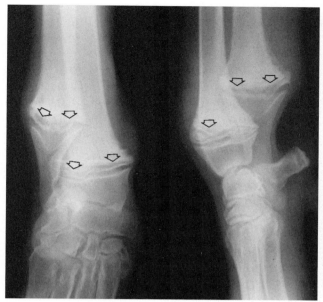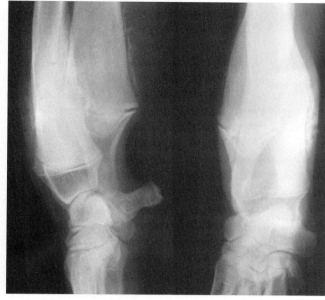

A   B

Figure 4–82. A 5-month-old female Great Dane had been non-ambulatory for 3 days at the time of presentation. Swelling was present in the distal metaphyseal area of the radius and ulna and in the distal tibial metaphyses bilaterally. Radiographs of these areas were obtained. (A) Radiographs of the right carpus and (B) follow-up radiographs obtained 2 months later are illustrated. There is soft tissue swelling in the area proximal to the carpal joint. The metaphyseal regions of the distal radius and ulna are widened and the periosteal margins are irregular. A radiolucent line is present in the distal radial and ulnar metaphyses immediately proximal to the physeal growth plate (*arrows*). There is a zone of sclerosis proximal to this radiolucent line. The distal ulnar metaphysis has lost its normal conical shape. (B) In the radiographs obtained 2 months after the first presentation, the distal radial and ulnar metaphyses remained widened. The ossification pattern within the medullary canal is irregular. The distal ulnar metaphysis has regained its conical shape. There is periosteal proliferation surrounding the distal radial and ulnar metaphyses. The distal radial and ulnar physes appear normal; however, a mild bowing and valgus deformity had resulted from the altered growth of the limb. **Diagnosis:** Hypertrophic osteodystrophy.

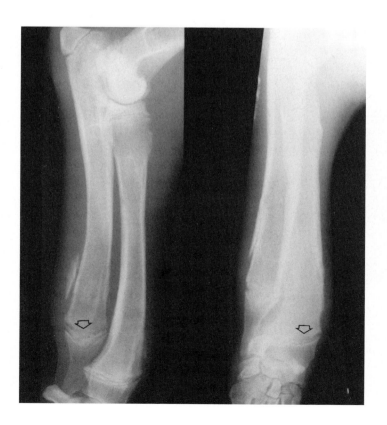

Figure 4–83. A 5-month-old female Weimeraner that had been lame, reluctant to walk, and had an intermittent fever for 5 weeks. Radiographs of both forelimbs were obtained. The left forelimb radiographs are illustrated. There are areas of increased density within the proximal and distal radial and ulnar metaphyses. An area of radiolucency is noted within the distal radial and ulnar metaphyses (*arrows*). Periosteal proliferation is noted along the medial surface of the distal radius and caudal aspect of the distal ulna. Similar periosteal proliferation is present on the cranial surface of the proximal radius and on the medial aspect of the distal humeral metaphysis. **Diagnosis:** Hypertrophic osteodystrophy. The radiolucent band has been referred to as a double epiphyseal line. Similar lesions were present in the right forelimb.

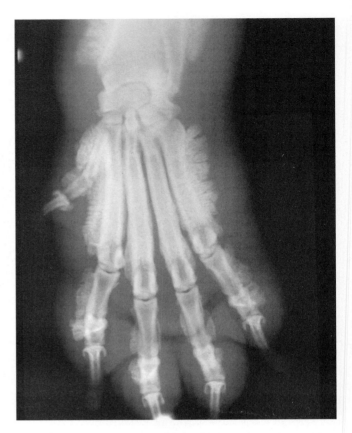

Figure 4–84. A 10-year-old male mixed breed dog that had a renal carcinoma removed 2 months previously presented with limb swelling and lethargy. Radiographs of all four extremities were obtained. The antero-posterior radiograph of the left forelimb is illustrated. There is soft tissue swelling diffusely involving the left forelimb. There is periosteal proliferation involving the radius, ulna, and both axial and abaxial surfaces of the metacarpal bones and phalanges. The bony proliferation is more severe on the lateral and medial surfaces of the foot, however all surfaces are involved. The periosteal proliferation appears to be perpendicular to the long axis of the limb. **Diagnosis:** Hypertrophic osteopathy. Similar findings were present in the other limbs. Pulmonary metastases were present.

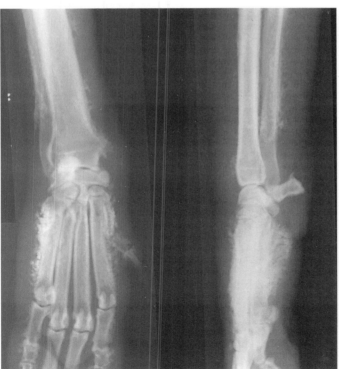

A

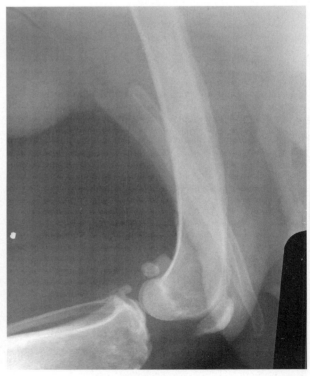

B

Figure 4–85. (A&B) A 7-year-old male pit bull presented with progressive rear limb ataxia and weakness with muscle atrophy and swollen distal extremities. Radiographs of all four limbs were obtained. Lateral radiographs of the left femur and right radius are illustrated. There is a smooth bony proliferation on the cranial and caudal surfaces of the left femur. Irregular periosteal proliferation is present along the radial and ulnar diaphyses and along the metacarpal bones. **Diagnosis:** Hypertrophic osteopathy secondary to a primary lung tumor. Note that the pattern of bony proliferation along the femur is smoother than that occurring along the radius and ulna.

however, involvement of the proximal portion also may be observed. The tarsal and carpal bones and abaxial surfaces of the 2nd and 5th metatarsal and metacarpal bones are involved most often. The periosteal proliferation usually is irregular and oriented perpendicular to the cortex, but it may also be smooth and/or oriented parallel to the cortex.

The limb swelling and periosteal proliferation may be the earliest sign of an asymptomatic thoracic lesion. Regression of the bony proliferation occurs after treatment of the primary disease, but the bones remain abnormal for a long time.

BONE INFARCTS

Bone infarcts are areas of necrosis within the medulla. Radiographically, bone infarcts appear as multiple, irregularly demarcated, distinct intramedullary densities in one or several bones (Fig. 4–86). Usually, there are no clinical signs directly associated with the infarcts. Bone infarcts may be seen in conjunction with sarcomas; however, whether or not they represent a cause or effect is unclear.[49,50,192–195]

JOINT DISEASE

Radiography aids in diagnosis, prognosis, and monitoring the response to therapy in the evaluation of patients with joint disease. The radiographic findings usually indicate a general category of joint disease (e.g., degenerative, infectious, neoplastic, immune) and not a specific entity.

The following classification scheme is suggested for use when considering joint disease in small animals.

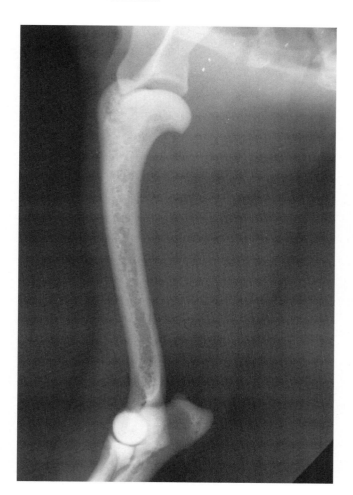

Figure 4–86. A 10-year-old mixed breed female dog was presented for treatment of mammary gland tumors. Bone lesions were noted on the thoracic radiographs and survey radiographs of the limbs obtained. A lateral radiograph of the left humerus is illustrated; however, similar lesions were present in the fore and rear limbs. There are multiple punctate densities present through the humeral diaphysis and metaphysis. **Diagnosis:** Bone infarcts. Although these are often associated with sarcomas of bone, none were identified in this dog.

CLASSIFICATION OF JOINT DISEASE

Degenerative Joint Disease (Osteoarthritis, Osteoarthrosis)

Primary. Joint disease that results from apparently normal wear and tear. No specific or predisposing cause can be identified.

Secondary. Joint disease that results from a specific or predisposing condition or event such as those listed below.

Causes of degenerative joint disease include:

Trauma

Injury to adjacent bone, ligament, tendon, articular cartilage, joint capsule.

Conformational or Developmental Abnormality

Abnormal stress or use of the limb which results from congenital, inherited or acquired limb deformities.

Metabolic, Nutritional, and Idiopathic Disorders

Disorders such as hemophilia, mucopolysaccharidosis, hypervitaminosis A, hyperparathyroidism, or congenital hypothyroidism.

Neoplastic Arthropathy

This includes tumors arising from the periarticular soft tissues.

Infectious Arthritis

Includes bacterial, mycotic, viral and mycoplasmal arthritis.

Immune-Mediated Arthritis

Erosive

Nonerosive

Crystal Induced Arthritis

Includes gout and pseudogout.

Villonodular Synovitis

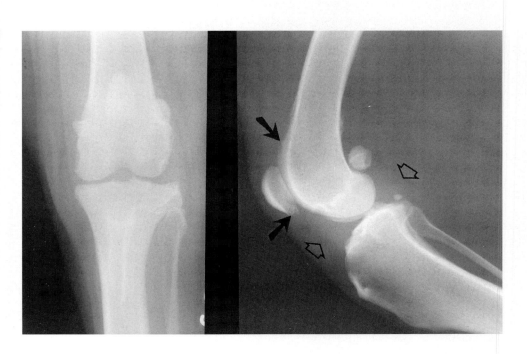

Figure 4–87. A 4-year-old male mixed breed dog had a right rear limb lameness for 5 months. There is soft tissue swelling noted in the stifle joint (*open arrows*). There are areas of irregular bony proliferation on the proximal and distal margins of the patella and on the proximal aspect of the distal femoral articular surface (*closed arrows*). **Diagnosis:** Mild degenerative joint disease. This was proved to be secondary to rupture of the cranial cruciate ligament.

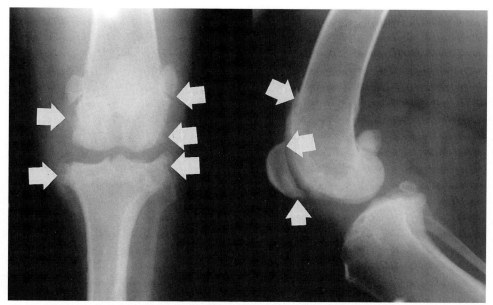

Figure 4–88. A 3-year-old male Doberman pinscher exhibited pain in both rear limbs. The lameness had been present in the right rear limb for 1 year and was present for 3 months in the left rear limb. There is soft tissue swelling involving the right stifle. There are areas of bony proliferation involving the distal femoral articular surface, both femoral epicondyles, fabellae, and the proximal and distal margins of the patella (*arrows*). There are areas of bony proliferation on the medial and lateral aspects of the proximal tibia (*arrows*). There is irregularity of the distal femoral articular surface. **Diagnosis:** Severe degenerative joint disease. This dog was found to have bilateral cranial cruciate ligament ruptures.

DEGENERATIVE JOINT DISEASE

Degenerative joint disease (DJD), also known as osteoarthritis and osteoarthrosis, is a common arthropathy with many diverse causes. The radiographic features of DJD are similar regardless of the underlying etiology (Figs. 4–87 and 4–88).[196–199] Soft tissue swelling usually is minimal. Periarticular periosteal proliferation occurs at the sites of joint capsule and ligamentous attachment and at the margins of the articular cartilage. This proliferation usually is smooth and uniformly mineralized with well-defined margins. The subchondral bone may become thinned, thickened, dense, or irregular. Intra- or periarticular bony densities may be seen. These densities may be due to avulsion fractures, joint capsule or tendinous calcifications, or calcification of detached articular cartilage fragments (joint mice, synovial osteochondromatosis).[200] Narrowing or collapse of the joint space and subchondral bone cysts may be observed. Malalignment of articular surfaces or joint subluxation may be seen with some specific conditions; however, weight-bearing or stress radiographs may be required to demonstrate joint instability (Fig. 4–89). In most cases, the radiographic findings are less extensive than those observed at surgery or necropsy. The more severe the radiographic findings, the poorer the prognosis despite the correction of any underlying disease. With severe degenerative changes, the underlying cause may be obscured. The progression of the radiographic changes usually is slow with little difference observed over several months.

Primary degenerative joint disease (resulting from normal wear and tear on a joint) is uncommon in small animals but may be observed as an incidental finding. It typically occurs in older, large breed dogs, and is most often observed in the shoulder but may be seen in any joint.[196]

Secondary degenerative joint disease is a great deal more common. Many different conditions may cause secondary degenerative joint disease.[201–203]

Trauma

Trauma to any of the tendinous or ligamentous structures around the joint may cause minor or major joint instability and ultimately lead to secondary joint disease. Fractures involving the articular surface or that change the way that stress is loaded

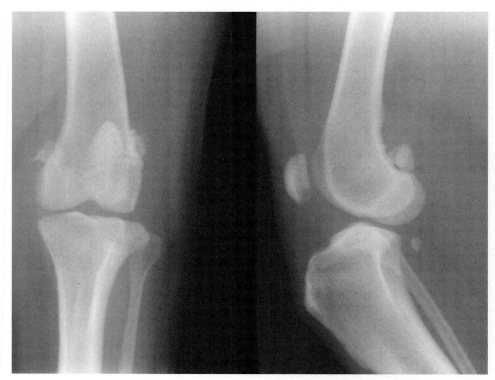

Figure 4–89. A 10-year-old female keeshound was lame in the right rear limb for 4 months. There was no history of trauma; however, palpation of the right stifle revealed ligamentous instability. There is mild soft tissue swelling of the stifle joint. There is malalignment of the proximal tibia and distal femur with the proximal tibia displaced cranially relative to the distal femur. The popliteal sesamoid bone is displaced distally. There are two small bone densities associated with the distal aspect of the medial fabellae and proximal aspect of the lateral fabellae. There is no evidence of secondary degenerative joint disease at this time. **Diagnosis:** Ruptured cranial cruciate ligament. The small bone densities associated with the fabellae may be due to trauma to the gastrocnemius muscle attachments. This degree of malalignment is very unusual in dogs with ruptured cranial cruciate ligament. The presence of obvious bony malalignment on a non-stressed lateral radiograph indicates severe ligamentous damage.

on a joint also may result in degenerative joint disease. Ligament and/or cartilage damage frequently accompanies intra-articular fractures. Soft tissue swelling; avulsion fracture fragments at the site of joint capsule, ligament, or tendon attachments; joint space collapse; or malalignment of bones are indicative of soft tissue injury. Weight-bearing or stress radiographs may be required to demonstrate the extent of the joint instability. In most cases of joint trauma, secondary degenerative joint disease will occur despite treatment.

Most joint luxations are accompanied by ligamentous injury. Small avulsion fractures may be evident. These fragments should be identified because they reflect the extent of the soft tissue injury and affect the patient's prognosis. With coxofemoral dislocations, avulsion fractures may occur at the fovea capitus due to ligamentum teres rupture. These fragments and the associated soft tissue injury can complicate reduction of the dislocation. Chip fractures of the acetabular rim also may be observed. Pre-existing joint diseases (e.g., hip dysplasia) should be recognized because they may complicate reduction of the dislocation.

Sacroiliac luxations may accompany pelvic trauma. The width of the sacroiliac joint is a poor sign of sacroiliac luxation. Alignment between the ilium and sacrum is best judged by tracing the medial aspect of the ilium from the acetabulum cranially to the point at which it joins the sacrum. The margins should be continuous (Fig. 4–90). Deviation or malalignment at the junction point indicates sacroiliac luxation. Fractures of the sacrum or ilium may be present; however, luxation without fracture is more common.

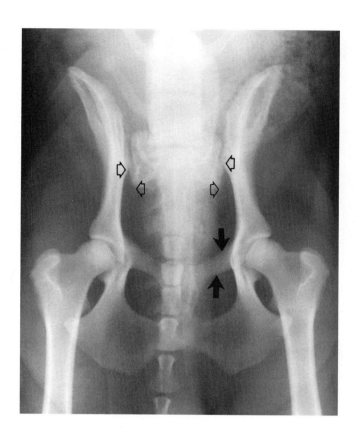

Figure 4–90. A 2-year-old male mixed breed dog presented after being hit by a car. The dog was reluctant to walk and painful in the pelvic area. There is a bilateral sacro-iliac luxation. The ilial shafts are displaced cranially from their normal junction point with the sacrum (*open arrows*). There is an incomplete, nondisplaced left pubic fracture (*closed arrows*) and a minimally displaced right acetabular fracture. **Diagnosis:** Bilateral sacro-iliac luxation with pubic fracture.

Conformational or Developmental Hip Dysplasia

Hip dysplasia is a multifactorial, clinically complex arthropathy with structural alterations of the coxofemoral joints. While dogs are most commonly afflicted, cats may also have hip dysplasia.[204,205] The anatomic alterations of hip dysplasia include shallow acetabulae, swelling or tearing of the round ligament, joint subluxation, erosion of articular cartilage, and remodeling of the acetabulum as well as the femoral head and neck surfaces.[206] One or both hips may be involved.[207–209] The causes of canine hip dysplasia are numerous and possibly are interactive.[210–213] The manner and degree in which these pathologies cause radiographic changes is not consistent. Any or all of the radiographic changes of canine hip dysplasia, including shallow acetabulae, coxofemoral subluxation, remodeling of the acetabulum, femoral head, or femoral neck, or periarticular osteophytosis, may be present (Figs. 4–91, 4–92, 4–93, 4–94 and 4–95). The degree of radiographic change does not necessarily correlate with the clinical signs.

The acetabulum is considered shallow when its depth is less than one-half the width of the femoral head. Acetabular remodeling results in a semi-elliptical (or egg-shaped) appearance rather than a normal semicircular shape. The medial bony margin of the acetabulum may become thickened. Femoral head remodeling results in the loss of the head's rounded, weight-bearing, articular surface. Instead, the femoral head appears flattened and less distinct at its junction with the femoral neck. Lateral displacement or femoral head subluxation changes the joint space from a normal, even crescent to a wedge shape. When secondary degenerative joint disease is present, the periarticular periosteal proliferation will be visible at the margin of the femoral or acetabular articular cartilage or at the sites of joint capsule attachment. Decreased or increased density or irregularity of the subchondral bone may be observed.

Although multiple radiographic techniques have been recommended, the standard ventrodorsal projection has been generally accepted since 1961.[214] This positioning standard calls for the dog to be in dorsal recumbency with its rear limbs

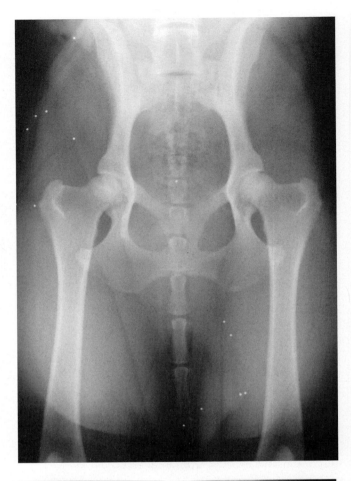

Figure 4–91. A 2-year-old female Labrador retriever which was radiographed for hip dysplasia evaluation. Both femoral heads are well-seated within their respective acetabulae. The joint spaces are thin and there is good congruity between the femoral head and acetabular rim. The conformation of this dog is excellent. The small radiopaque densities noted in the soft tissues are shotgun pellets. **Diagnosis:** Normal pelvis.

Figure 4–92. A 4-year-old male German shepherd dog presented for bilateral rear limb weakness. There is severe subluxation of both coxofemoral joints and extensive remodeling changes involving both femoral heads and necks. There is bony proliferation on the cranial and caudal surfaces of the acetabular margins bilaterally. The medial aspect of the acetabulum has been filled in with bone making it very shallow. **Diagnosis:** Severe bilateral canine hip dysplasia with extensive degenerative joint disease.

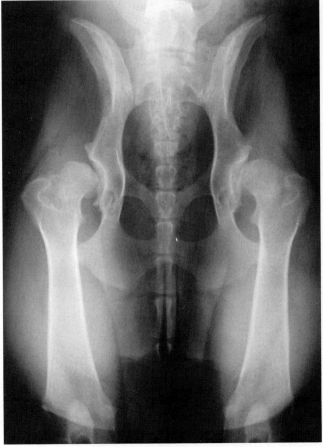

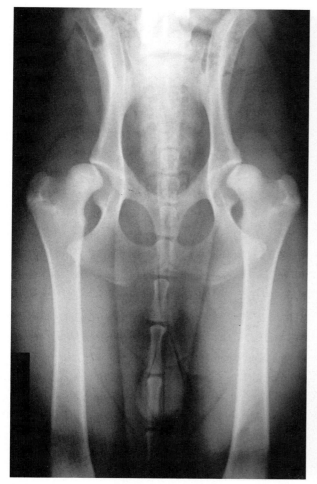
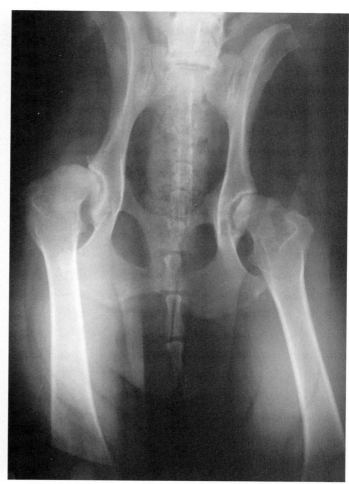

A   B

Figure 4–93. A male German shepherd dog that had pelvic radiographs taken at (A) 9 months (B) and 4 years of age. Subluxation of both coxofemoral joints is evident in the radiographs obtained at 9 months of age. Less than 50% of the femoral head is in the acetabular cavity. The density of the subchondral bone in the acetabulum is uneven—it is thinner medially. The acetabular rim is straight and does not have the normal semicircular shape. In the ventrodorsal pelvic radiographs obtained at 4 years of age, the progress of the degenerative joint disease is readily apparent. The acetabular cups have filled with bone. There are periarticular osteophytes on the acetabular margins. There is extensive remodeling of the femoral head and neck. **Diagnosis:** Severe osteoarthritis secondary to bilateral canine hip dysplasia.

pulled back until the stifle and hock are fully extended. The rear limbs are then adducted until the femurs parallel each other. The femurs also are rotated medially (inwardly) until the patellas are dorsally centered. Although not specifically stated in the standard, it is generally assumed that the femurs should be as parallel as possible with the spine, table, or film.[215] The pelvis must not be rotated. The entire pelvis and enough of the femurs to show the patellas should be included on the radiograph. Sedation or anesthesia is routinely recommended but may not be required in some cases.[215–217]

Because malpositioning can create difficulty or errors in diagnosis, especially in dogs with borderline pelvic conformation, careful positioning is mandatory for proper radiographic evaluation.[218] In a properly positioned ventrodorsal pelvic radiograph, the size and shape of the obturator foramina and iliac wings are identical and the pelvic canal is smoothly oval. The femoral shafts are parallel and the patellas are centered over the femoral trochlea.

Positioning errors can be identified by certain radiographic changes. Pelvic rotation will result in a difference in size of the obturator foramina and iliac wings—the

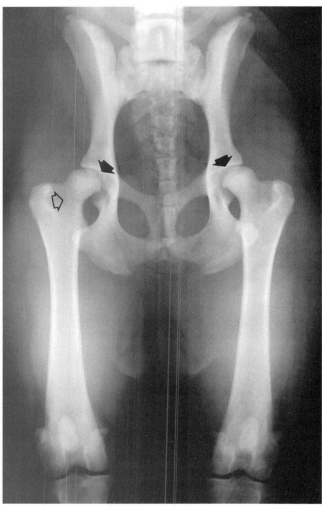

A

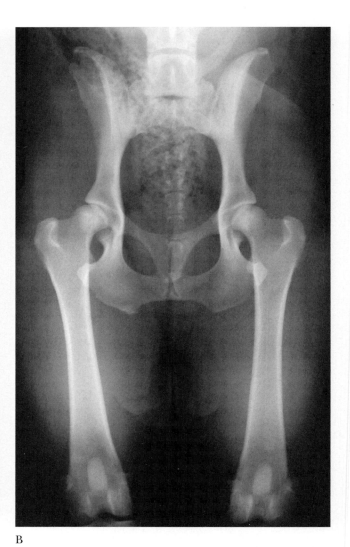

B

Figure 4–94. A 1-year-old female rottweiler presented for routine pelvic evaluation at (A) 1 year of age and again at (B) 2 years of age. (A) In the pelvic radiographs obtained at 1 year of age, there is mild subluxation of both coxofemoral joints. Less than 50% of the femoral heads are within their respective acetabulae. There is widening of the coxofemoral joint space, especially at its medial aspect (*closed arrows*). There is a faint radiodense line on the right femoral neck (*open arrow*). This is indicative of mild degenerative joint disease with bony proliferation at the site of joint capsule attachment. (B) The pelvic radiographs were repeated when the dog was 2 years of age. The degree of subluxation of the coxofemoral joint remains unchanged. There is poor congruity between the femoral heads and their respective acetabulae. The craniodorsal acetabular margins are flattened. The bony proliferation on the right femoral neck has increased. **Diagnosis:** Progressive osteoarthritis secondary to mild bilateral canine hip dysplasia.

smaller foramen and wider iliac wing will appear on the same side as the apparently shallower acetabulum. Divergence of the femoral shafts distally will increase the apparent congruity of the femoral head and acetabulum. External rotation of the stifle with the patella placed over the lateral femoral condyle will make the femoral neck appear shorter and thicker and will accentuate any subluxation that is present. Internal rotation of the stifle with the patella placed over the medial femoral condyle will minimize the degree of subluxation. Slight malpositioning does not interfere with the diagnosis in a dog that has excellent or good pelvic conformation or moderate or severe dysplastic pelvic conformation. However, in those dogs with fair or mild dysplastic conformation, a well-positioned, properly exposed radiograph is essential.

The Orthopedic Foundation for Animals (OFA) has served as a referral service for certification of the pelvic conformation of dogs since 1966.[219] OFA's minimum age

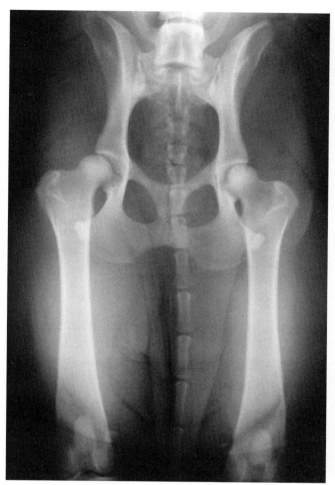 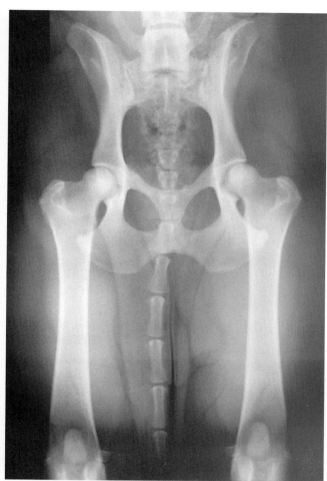

A   B

Figure 4–95. A 2-year-old female Chesapeake Bay retriever was presented for routine hip evaluation. (A) There is subluxation of the right coxofemoral joint with no remodeling changes present. (B) Follow-up radiographs were obtained 2 years later. At this time both femoral heads appear deeply seated within their respective acetabulae. Joint surfaces are smooth. There is no evidence of degenerative joint disease. The pelvic conformation appears normal at this age. Although the animal appeared to be dysplastic at 2 years of age, the follow-up radiographs indicate that the pelvis is normal. This is an unusual occurrence; however, it emphasizes the need for follow-up radiographs in animals in which the radiographic evidence of hip dysplasia is minimal. **Diagnosis:** Normal pelvis.

requirement for certification is 24 months, because examination prior to that age has a significant chance of producing false-negative results. In one study, only 10% of dysplastic dogs had radiographic signs of hip dysplasia at 4 months of age, 15% to 30% at 6 months of age, approximately 70% at 12 months of age, and approximately 95% at 24 months of age.[220] The same study showed that waiting until 36 months of age only increased the diagnostic rate to 97%. Therefore, an evaluation before 24 months of age should be considered provisional. A repeat study at 2½ or 3 years of age may be required in dogs with borderline pelvic conformation.

The OFA has defined standards of hip joint conformation ranging from excellent hip joint conformation (superior hip joint conformation as compared with other individuals of the same breed and age) to severe hip dysplasia (radiographic evidence of marked dysplastic changes of the hip joints). Radiographically, these depend upon the depth of the acetabulum, degree of subluxation, and the presence of any degenerative changes (see Figs. 4–91, 4–92, 4–93, 4–94, 4–95).[215] Repeated radiographic examinations may be necessary for an accurate diagnosis.

A new method of radiography using a distraction method (PennHip) has been reported for the purpose of diagnosing canine hip dysplasia in dogs younger than 2 years of age.[221,222] This method uses an adjustable distraction device to determine the degree of joint laxity present in the dog. The results of using this method have been reported for a limited number of Labrador retrievers measured at 4 and 8 months of age.[223] The results of this study indicated: (1) that a distraction index (DI) of >0.7 was associated with a high probability of developing dysplasia, (2) a DI of <0.4 predicted normal hips with a high degree of probability (88%), and (3) a DI within the range of 0.4 to 0.7 was not clinically reliable in predicting whether an individual was likely to be normal or dysplastic. Further research in the application of this technique is ongoing.

OSTEOCHONDROSIS

Osteochondrosis is a failure of normal endochondral ossification, which results in thickening of the articular epiphyseal complex.[224] This may lead to a dissecting intracartilaginous separation between the calcified and non-calcified layers, which may occur at articulations, epiphyses, or apophyses.[225] When this occurs at articular surfaces, the separation may result in the formation of a flap of articular cartilage or a complete fracture with a free, separate piece of cartilage. This is referred to as osteochondritis dissecans (OCD). If the process occurs at an apophyses (e.g., the coronoid or anconeal processes of the ulna), it may result in an apophyseal separation from the body of the parent bone.

Osteochondrosis most commonly is seen in large breed dogs that are less than 1-year-old. It may affect the shoulder, elbow, stifle, or hock, and may be unilateral or

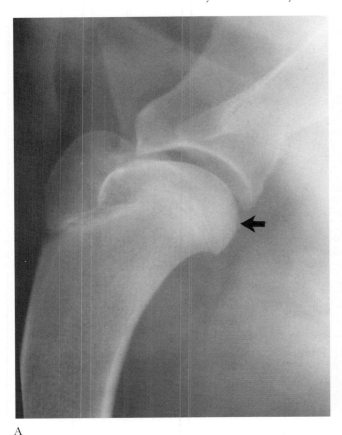

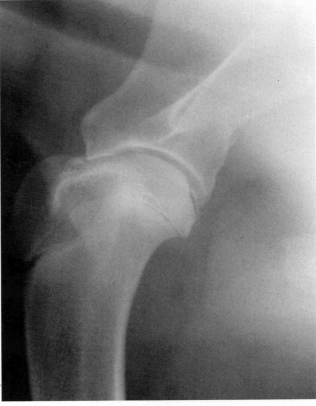

A
B

Figure 4–96. (A&B) A 15-month-old male Chesapeake Bay retriever presented with an 8-month history of lameness in the right front leg. (A) A lateral view of the shoulder reveals an area of flattening which involves the caudal aspect of the right humeral head (*arrow*). There is slight sclerosis surrounding this area of radiolucency. The limb was supinated and (B) an additional radiograph was obtained. A large calcified cartilaginous flap is readily identified. The osteochondral defect and flattening of the humeral head are also more readily observed with this positioning. **Diagnosis:** Osteochondritis dissecans. A similar lesion was present in the left shoulder.

bilateral. It usually involves the caudal aspect of the proximal humeral head, the medial humeral condyle, coronoid or anconeal process of the ulna, the lateral or medial femoral condyle, and/or the medial or the lateral trochlear ridge of the talus.

Osteochondritis Dissecans (OCD) of Articular Surfaces. The radiographic changes associated with OCD of articular surfaces are similar whether in the humeral head, humeral condyles, femoral head, femoral condyles, or the trochlear ridges of the talus.[226–235] Bilateral disease is common.[230,236,237] Radiographic findings include an area of radiolucency or a flattening within the subchondral bone immediately beneath an articular surface. Subchondral bone sclerosis may be present adjacent to the lucency or flattening, although it is difficult to identify this condition in many cases (Figs. 4–96, 4–97, 4–98, 4–99, 4–100, 4–101). Osteophytes usually are seen at the margins of the articular cartilage.[238] A joint mouse (i.e., a piece of cartilage that is loose within the joint space) or calcified cartilage fragment may be identified. In the shoulder, a cartilage fragment may migrate into the joint space under the bicipital tendon producing lameness.[239] Secondary degenerative joint disease (especially in the elbow and hock) may be the only radiographic sign of OCD. A CT scan, MRI scan, arthrotomy, arthroscopy, or arthrogram may be required to confirm the diagnosis.[236,240,241] Eventually, degenerative joint disease will result. Small lesions may heal spontaneously.

Osteochondrosis of Apophyses (Un-united Anconeal Process, Fragmented Coronoid Process). Osteochondrosis of apophyses may result in un-united anconeal process and/or fragmented (or un-united) coronoid process. In this manifestation

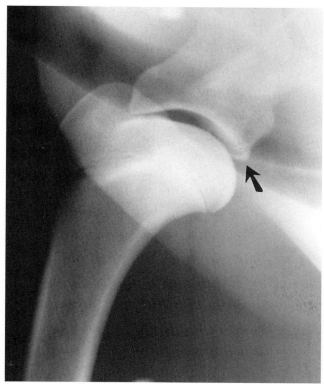

Figure 4–97. An 8-month-old male greyhound presented with a left foreleg lameness of 3 months' duration. A radiograph of the shoulder revealed (not shown) an osteochondritis dissecans lesion. A radiograph of the right shoulder was obtained for comparison and to rule out the possibility of bilateral disease. There is irregular mineralization of the caudal aspect of the glenoid (*arrow*). This appears to be a separate fragment; however, it is a normal pattern of ossification. **Diagnosis:** Normal right shoulder.

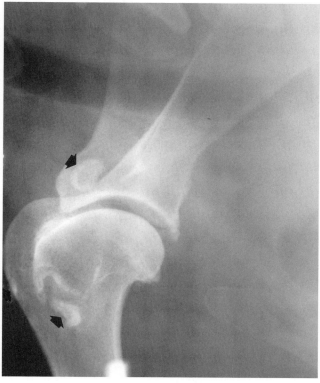

Figure 4–98. A 10-year-old male English setter presented with a 3-month lameness of the right forelimb. There are multiple calcified densities within the right shoulder. These can be seen cranial to the scapular spine and in the bicipital bursa area (*arrows*). Periarticular osteophytes are present on the caudal distal margin of the humeral articular surface and on the caudal margin of the scapular glenoid. **Diagnosis:** Severe degenerative joint disease secondary to osteochondritis dissecans.

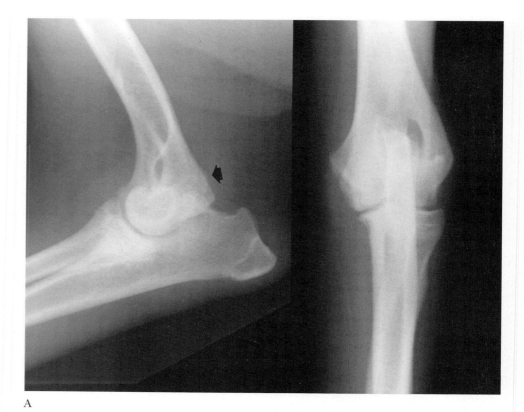

A

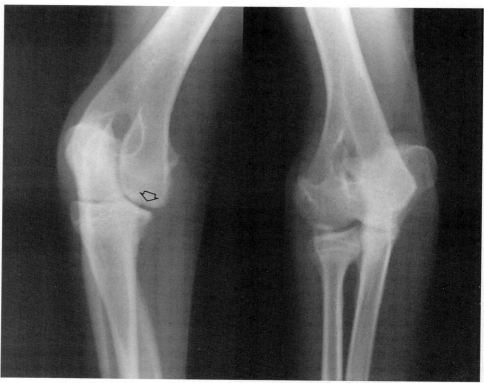

B

Figure 4–99. A 6-month-old female golden retriever presented with a right foreleg lameness of three months' duration. Muscle atrophy and some limitation of flexion and extension of both elbows were noted. Both elbows were radiographed. (A) Lateral and antero-posterior and (B) oblique radiographs of the left elbow are illustrated. There is a lucent defect in the medial humeral condyle (*open arrow*) and slight irregularity of the coronoid process. There is bony proliferation on the caudal aspect of the humeral epicondyle (*closed arrow*). **Diagnosis:** Osteochondritis dissecans of the left elbow. Similar changes were present in the right elbow.

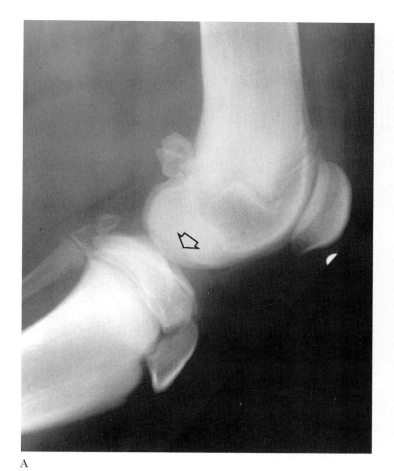
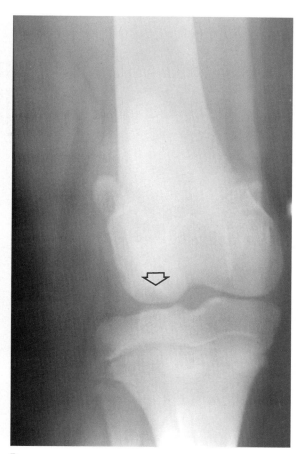

A   B

Figure 4–100. (A&B) A 6-month-old male bullmastiff presented with forelimb lameness and muscle atrophy of all four limbs. On physical examination some pain was noted with manipulation of the stifles. Both shoulders and stifles were radiographed. The left stifle is illustrated. There is soft tissue swelling of the left stifle joint and an area of flattening involving the lateral condyle of the distal left femur (*arrows*). There is no evidence of a free fragment. **Diagnosis:** Osteochondritis dissecans of the left femur. A similar lesion was present in the right stifle.

of osteochondrosis, the apophysis either fails to unite or fractures while it is still in the cartilage state.

An un-united anconeal process is identified as a bone fragment with a clear line of separation between the anconeal process and the ulna. The un-united anconeal process is best demonstrated in a flexed lateral radiograph that avoids the overlapping density of the medial humeral epicondyle (Figs. 4–1 and 4–102). The anconeal apophysis usually fuses with the remainder of the ulna around 4 months of age. A definitive diagnosis should not be made until 4½ to 5 months of age, because there is a certain amount of normal variation in the time of fusion between the anconeal process and the ulna. The prognosis is poor when secondary degenerative joint disease is present. Regardless of therapy attempted, affected joints usually will develop to significant degenerative joint disease. Both elbows should be evaluated routinely despite the absence of clinical signs in one of the elbows, because the condition frequently is bilateral.

Fracture or dislocation of the anconeal process may occur due to elbow trauma or secondary to distal ulnar physeal injury with altered growth of the radius and ulna (Fig. 4–103). Subluxation of the humeral ulnar articulation will be evident in these cases and radiographs of the entire radius and ulna will confirm the diagnosis and distinguish fracture from un-united anconeal process.

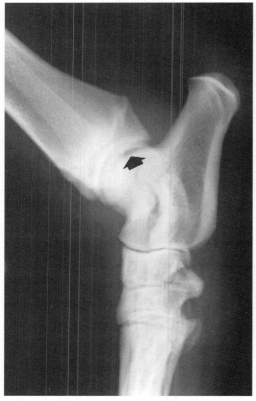

A

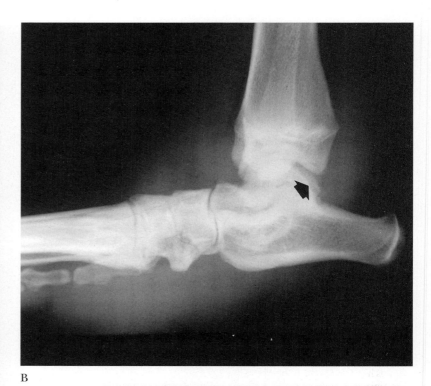

B

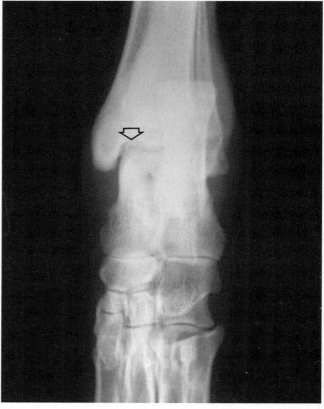

C

Figure 4–101. An 8-month-old male Saint Bernard presented with intermittent left rear leg lameness. (A) Lateral, (B) flexed lateral, and (C) antero-posterior radiographs of the right tarsus were obtained. There is a slight amount of swelling around the hock. The medial aspect of the tibiotarsal articulation is widened and a small bone density is noted within that joint space (*open arrow*). The medial trochlea of the talus appears small and the proximal aspect is flattened. Although this is evident on both (A&B) the lateral and flexed lateral views (*arrows*), flexion of the leg demonstrates the lesion more clearly. Small calcified fragments can be seen caudal to the trochlea of the talus in the flexed lateral view. **Diagnosis:** Osteochondritis dissecans of the hock.

Fragmented (Un-united) Coronoid Process. Un-united (or fragmented) coronoid process (involving either the medial and/or the lateral process) is difficult to diagnose definitively on survey radiographs.[242–252] Fragmented coronoid process usually affects both ulnas, although clinical signs may be unilateral. A flexed lateral view

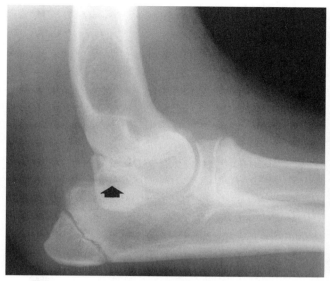
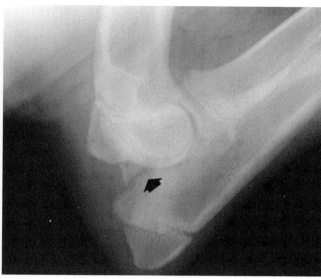

A   B

Figure 4–102. A 5-month-old female German shepherd dog presented with a left foreleg lameness of 2 weeks' duration. (A) Lateral and (B) flexed lateral radiographs of the left foreleg were obtained. There is a radiolucent line that separates the anconeal process from the proximal ulna (*arrows*). This is most obvious in the flexed lateral radiograph. The radiolucent line is hidden by the medial epicondyle of the humerus in the straight lateral view. **Diagnosis:** Un-united anconeal process. Flexion of the elbow is extremely important in evaluating an animal for un-united anconeal process since the lesion is more apparent when the joint is flexed. The un-united anconeal process is visible on the straight lateral projection.

usually is the most helpful in making the diagnosis, although other views may also be helpful. Compared to other radiographic techniques, CT has shown the highest accuracy, sensitivity, and negative-predictive values in making the diagnosis.[253]

Among the earliest radiographic signs that will be seen is mild osteophytosis on the horizontal (proximal) aspect of the anconeal process. As the condition progresses, endosteal sclerosis of the ulna immediately deep to the coronoid processes (just caudal and distal to the semilunar notch) and a widened humeral-ulnar joint space may be seen. Finally, signs of DJD may be seen including osteophytes on the cranial proximal radius, medial humeral epicondyle, proximal margin of the anconeal process, or coronoid process. The degenerative changes may be the only findings noted (Fig. 4–104). These will progress despite surgical intervention.[254] The separate coronoid fragment is rarely identified by radiography, because it usually occurs on the lateral aspect of the medial coronoid process (Fig. 4–105). The medial humeral condylar lesion of osteochondrosis may be observed concomitantly with fragmented coronoid process.

Retained Cartilage Core. Retention of endochondral cartilage occurs in young, large and giant breed dogs.[179] Although any long bone may be involved, the distal ulna is affected most frequently. An inverted radiolucent cone is seen extending proximally from the distal ulnar physis into the metaphysis (Fig. 4–106). Irregular metaphyseal radiolucencies and physeal widening may be observed in other bones. Although the lesion usually is without clinical significance and disappears as normal bone modeling occurs, growth retardation and angular limb deformities may result. Irregular patterns of metaphyseal bone density may persist after maturity. The condition usually affects both limbs in a similar manner.

PATELLA LUXATION

Medial patellar luxation is a congenital lesion seen most frequently in miniature and small breed dogs and rarely in cats.[255-257] The medial patella displacement is easily recognized; however, when the limb is extended during positioning for radiographs,

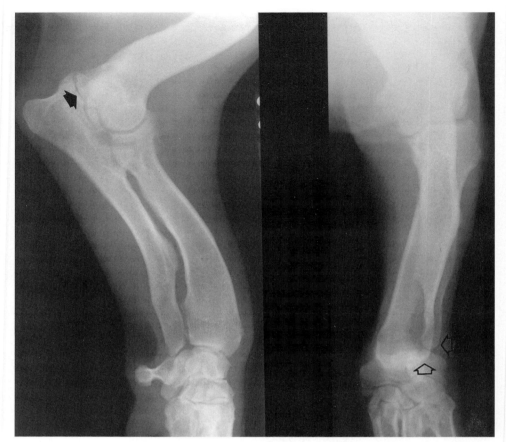

A

Figure 4–103. A 2-year-old female bassett hound presented with a 9-month history of left forelimb lameness, which had become progressively more severe. There was some restriction on extension and flexion of the left elbow. (A) There is a radiolucent line present separating the anconeal process from the proximal ulna (*closed arrows*). (B) This is most obvious in the flexed lateral radiograph. There is subluxation of the humeral ulnar articulation. The antero-posterior and lateral radiographs of the entire limb demonstrate a shortened ulna. The ulnar styloid process does not extend as far distal as the distal radius (*open arrows*). There is a bony irregularity associated with the cranial medial surface of the distal third of the ulna. This may be the site of a previous disturbance in endochondral ossification. The radius is bowed. **Diagnosis:** Un-united anconeal process. This may be secondary to the altered growth rate in the ulna and subsequent bowing deformity of the forelimb. The subluxation of the humeral ulnar articulation which is present suggests that the un-united anconeal process resulted from abnormal growth rather than being a primary un-united anconeal process.

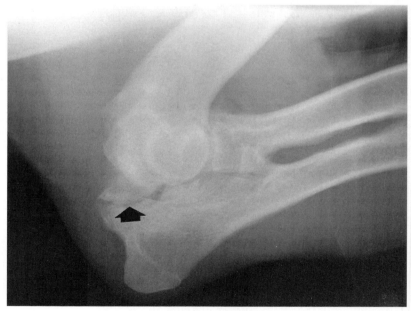

B

the patella may resume a normal position. Varying degrees of severity may be observed (Fig. 4–107). The distal femur and proximal tibia may present an "S"-shaped (sigmoid) deformity with a hypoplastic medial femoral condyle, shallow trochlear groove, and medially positioned tibial crest. Secondary degenerative joint disease may be present.

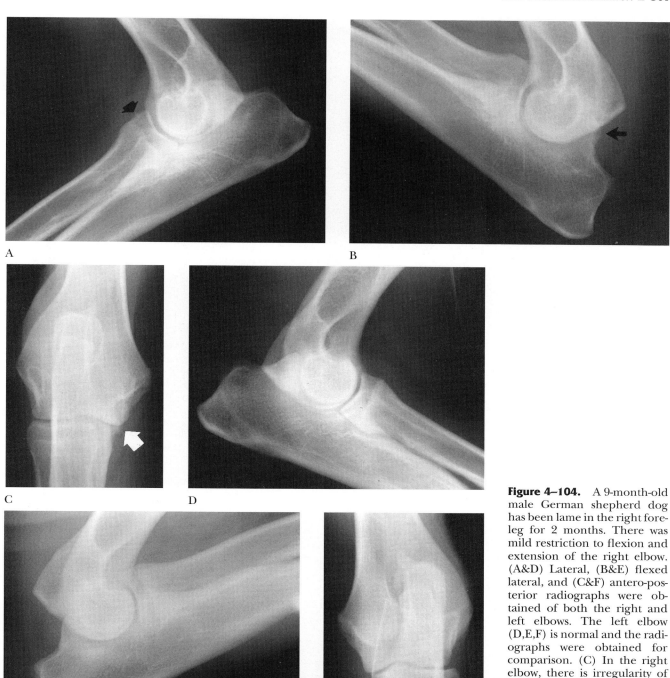

Figure 4–104. A 9-month-old male German shepherd dog has been lame in the right foreleg for 2 months. There was mild restriction to flexion and extension of the right elbow. (A&D) Lateral, (B&E) flexed lateral, and (C&F) antero-posterior radiographs were obtained of both the right and left elbows. The left elbow (D,E,F) is normal and the radiographs were obtained for comparison. (C) In the right elbow, there is irregularity of the bony margin of the medial coronoid process noted in the anterior-posterior radiograph (*arrow*). This is more obvious when compared with the normal left limb. The subchondral bone density of the ulna appears increased when the right ulna is compared to the left.

There is new bone production present on the proximal aspect of the anconeal process (*straight arrow*). This is most obvious when comparison is made between the right and left elbows in (B&E) the flexed lateral views. (A) There is bony proliferation present along the cranial proximal aspect of the proximal radius (*wide arrow*). **Diagnosis:** Fragmented coronoid process. The irregular bony margins of the coronoid process as well as the increased subchondral bone density, bony proliferation on the proximal radius, and bony proliferation on the anconeal process are the result of secondary degenerative joint disease. These bony changes may also be seen with osteochondrosis of the elbow and un-united anconeal process, and are therefore not specific for the diagnosis of fragmented coronoid process. Although the coronoid fragment cannot be identified in these radiographs, the absence of radiographic signs of osteochondrosis or un-united anconeal process permit a diagnosis of fragmented coronoid process.

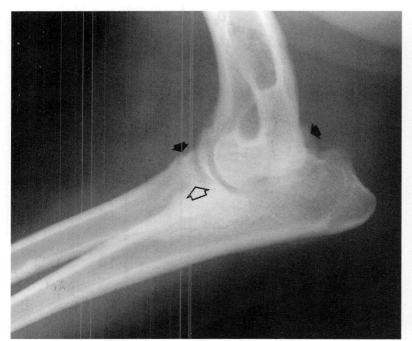
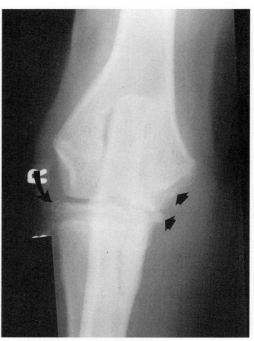

A   B

Figure 4–105. (A&B) A 10-month-old female golden retriever was lame in the right forelimb for 5 months. There was restriction to flexion and extension of the right elbow. There is mild soft tissue swelling in the area of the right elbow joint. There are areas of bony proliferation on the cranial-proximal aspect of the radius, proximal aspect of the anconeal process, medial epicondyle, and around the coronoid process (*solid arrows*). There is increased density in the subchondral bone of the proximal ulna. The area of the coronoid process on the lateral radiograph appears flattened (*open arrow*). A small, smooth, somewhat round bone density is present proximal and medial to the proximal radial articular surface (*curved arrow*). This is a normal sesamoid bone and has no clinical significance. **Diagnosis:** Fragmented coronoid process.

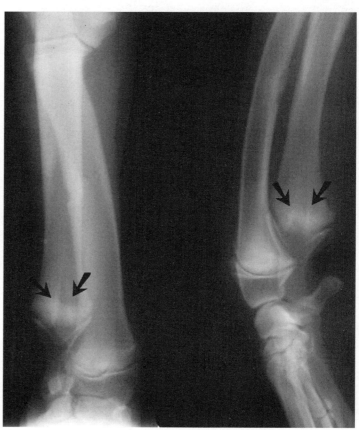

Figure 4–106. A 6-month-old male Alaskan malamute presented with mild intermittent lameness and slight lateral angulation of the foot. There is an inverted radiolucent core in the distal ulna (*arrows*). Slight lateral angulation of the foot is present. **Diagnosis:** Retained cartilage core.

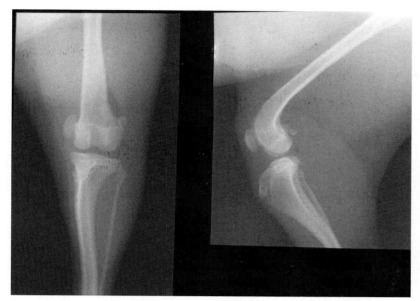

A

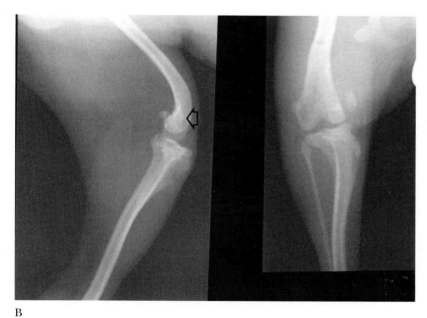

B

Figure 4–107. A 10-month-old female Chihuahua was presented with an intermittent lameness involving both rear limbs. Patella luxation was identified clinically. Both stifles were radiographed. (A) In the right stifle the patella is located medially in the posterior-anterior radiograph. It appears to be in its normal position in the lateral radiograph. The right femoral condyles appear larger than the left. The tibial crest is somewhat medially displaced; however, the degree of displacement and severity of the bowing deformity is much less than that seen in the left stifle. (B) In the left stifle the patella is medially displaced, is located medial to the femur on the posteroanterior radiograph, and is superimposed upon the distal femur in the lateral radiograph (*arrow*). The tibial crest is rotated medially, and the femoral condyles are hypoplastic. There is a bowing deformity of the proximal tibia. **Diagnosis:** Bilateral medial patella dislocation. The changes are severe on the left and moderate on the right. There is no evidence of degenerative joint disease at this time.

Lateral patellar luxation is uncommon but may be observed in large breed dogs. It is observed in some breeds as a conformational deformity but may also occur secondary to stifle trauma. Radiography is essential for evaluating the severity of the limb deformity and identifying the presence of fractures or secondary degenerative joint disease.

OSTEONECROSIS OF THE FEMORAL HEAD (LEGG-CALVE-PERTHES DISEASE)

Osteonecrosis of the femoral head may occur spontaneously in young toy and small breed dogs (4- to 11-months-old), or may be secondary to intracapsular femoral neck or capital physeal fractures.[258,259] The condition has been shown to be inherited in Yorkshire and West Highland white terriers.[260] Early radiographic signs include increased density in the femoral head and neck that usually is poorly defined. Later, joint space widening followed by a subchondral radiolucency within the femoral head is seen. Collapse of the cranial dorsal articular surface with a flattened femoral

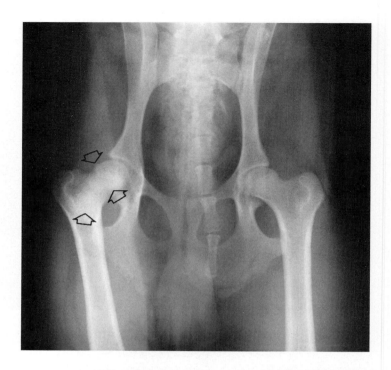

Figure 4–108. An 8-month-old male miniature pinscher presented with right rear limb muscle atrophy and weakness of 6 weeks duration. There is mild subluxation of the right coxofemoral joint. There is increased density involving the femoral neck and proximal femoral metaphysis with slight irregularity at the junction between the femoral head and neck (*arrows*). **Diagnosis:** Osteonecrosis of the right femoral head. These changes are early in the disease course. The left coxofemoral joint is normal at this time.

Figure 4–109. A 10-month-old male Yorkshire terrier had been lame since 4 months of age. It was reluctant to bear weight on the right rear limb and had muscle atrophy. There is marked collapse of the cranial dorsal aspect of the right femoral head with a decreased density in the subchondral bone beneath this flattened area. There is a loss of bone density in the right acetabulum and subluxation of the right coxofemoral joint. **Diagnosis:** Osteonecrosis of the right femoral head. The severity of the radiographic changes are indicative of a long-standing condition. The left coxofemoral joint is normal at this time.

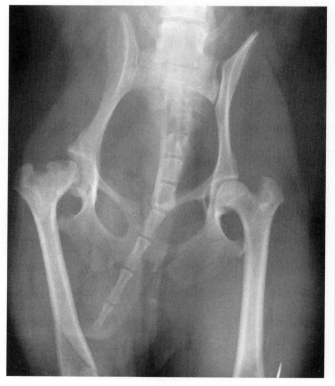

head and secondary degenerative joint disease ultimately will occur (Figs. 4–108, 4–109, and 4–110). The spontaneous disease frequently is bilateral but may not be radiographically apparent at the same time.

Intracapsular femoral neck and capital physeal fractures may result in loss of the majority or all of the blood supply to the femoral neck or head. Subsequent revascularization will result in a loss of bone from the intra- and extracapsular portions of the femoral neck. Very little bone production is evident radiographically, because the necrotic bone is gradually reabsorbed and replaced; this reestablishes the femoral architecture. If a capital epiphyseal fracture is not reduced surgically, the

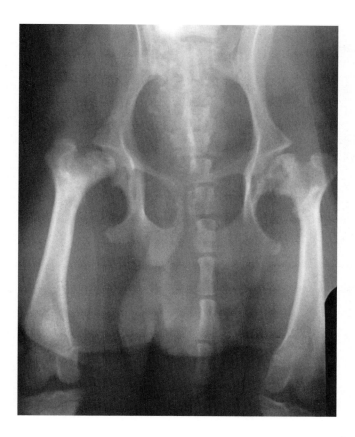

Figure 4–110. A 5-month-old male Pekingese, which was presented with a left rear leg lameness that had been present for 4 weeks. Both femoral heads are deformed and there is decreased density involving the ventrocaudal aspect of the left femoral head and neck. There is subluxation of the left coxofemoral joint with fragmentation of the left femoral head. There are areas of decreased density involving the cranial dorsal aspect of the right femoral head. Small bone densities are present in the area of the articular surface. There is subluxation of the joint. There is a slight increased density which involves the proximal metaphysis of the right femur. **Diagnosis:** Bilateral osteonecrosis. The changes in the right side appear to be more recent.

capital epiphyseal fragment may remain intact within the acetabulum with neither bony absorption nor proliferation. Bony proliferation will be observed on the femoral neck. Secondary degenerative joint disease may result in either case.

Osteonecrosis of the proximal humeral head may rarely occur in small dogs. The humeral head collapses, becomes flattened, and secondary degenerative joint disease results. The scapular glenoid remodels to conform to the altered humeral head shape.

Metabolic, Nutritional, and Idiopathic Disorders

HEMOPHILIA

Soft tissue swelling may be the only evidence of an acute hemophilic arthropathy. Chronic hemarthrosis will result in secondary degenerative joint disease. Periarticular periosteal proliferation eventually will develop along with subchondral sclerosis. The shoulders and elbows are involved more often than are the hips and stifles. In a study of a group of hemophilic dogs, a narrowed joint space and subchondral cysts were reported.[261] All dogs were affected by 1 year, with 65% showing evidence of joint disease by 6 months of age.

MUCOPOLYSACCHARIDOSIS

Bilateral subluxation of the coxofemoral joints with valgus deformity of the femoral heads and shallow acetabulae has been described in association with mucopolysaccharidosis VI in cats. Other skeletal deformities may include epiphyseal dysplasia, fusion of cervical vertebrae, flaring of the ribs at the costochondral junctions, osteoarthrosis of the vertebral articulations, and sternal deformities.[262–264] These findings are an aid in distinguishing this disease from other causes of secondary degenerative joint disease. Mucopolysaccharidosis I also has been described, and it appears similarly to mucopolysaccharidosis VI except that epiphyseal dysplasia of long bones is not seen.[265]

HYPERVITAMINOSIS A

Ankylosis of joints associated with extensive periarticular soft tissue mineralization has been associated with hypervitaminosis A in cats.[153,154,266] Lesions occur at points of ligamentous and tendinous attachment to the bone, especially in the periarticular areas (see Fig. 4–71). Periarticular osteophytes are observed most often around the elbow and shoulder, while involvement of the stifle, hip, carpal and tarsal joints is rare. The periarticular osteophytes are smooth and evenly mineralized and tend to coalesce and bridge the affected joint. The dietary history and presence of lesions in the vertebral column will help to confirm the diagnosis.

HYPOTHYROIDISM

Congenital hypothyroidism has been described in dogs and cats. Although the retarded bone development that has been observed could result in limb deformity and subsequent secondary degenerative joint disease, this has not been described.

HYPERPARATHYROIDISM

Hyperparathyroidism, either primary or secondary, may produce secondary degenerative joint disease as a result of limb deformity. Degenerative joint disease has not been reported as a direct result of hyperparathyroidism.

Neoplastic Arthropathy

Although rare, tumors may originate from the periarticular soft tissues and invade the joint. Synovial sarcoma is the most common tumor of this type, although chondrosarcoma, fibrosarcoma, lymphosarcoma, undifferentiated sarcomas, and others are observed.[88–91] The stifle or elbow are involved more frequently, although any joint may be affected. Soft tissue swelling will be identified in all cases. This frequently extends beyond the anatomic limits of the joint. Soft tissue mineralization is uncommon. A small amount of periosteal proliferation may be present at the margins of the lesion. The predominant radiographic finding usually is destruction of the bones of the affected joint. Bony destruction begins at the sites of periosteal and ligamentous attachment, but eventually the subchondral bone will also be involved.

Because joint neoplasms occur in older dogs, they may be superimposed on preexisting degenerative joint disease and some difficulty may be encountered in recognizing the presence of a tumor. The irregularly shaped localized soft tissue swelling and bony destruction should not be overlooked if the joint is evaluated carefully despite the presence of degenerative joint disease (see Figs. 4–52 and 4–53).

Infectious Arthritis

Joint infection is uncommon in dogs and cats. It may result from hematogenous spread to the synovial membrane or synovial fluid or direct joint penetration from a contiguous soft tissue or bone infection, external wound, surgical procedure, or intra-articular injection.[267–270] Bacterial infection is encountered most often, although fungal, viral, mycoplasmal, and protozoal infections have been described.[271–279]

Infectious arthritis is characterized radiographically by soft tissue swelling, subchondral bone destruction and sclerosis, and periarticular periosteal proliferation (see Figs. 4–62 and 4–65). The radiographic changes are minimal early in the disease and considerable cartilage destruction will be present by the time bony changes become evident. The earliest radiographic sign of infectious arthritis is soft tissue swelling. This often is more extensive than that seen with other joint diseases. Poorly defined or faintly mineralized bony proliferation may be observed at the points of ligamentous or joint capsule attachment. Subchondral bone destruction and sclerosis will occur later in the disease and indicates extensive destruction of articular cartilage. Although the radiographic changes observed with infectious arthritis are similar to those of secondary degenerative joint disease or some immune joint diseases, the radiographic changes generally are more severe and extensive in infectious arthritis when compared to other arthritides.

Joint space widening, described as an early radiographic change, and joint space collapse, as a late change, have been reported in infectious arthritis. Recognition of these changes is difficult because of the variation resulting from patient restraint and positioning during radiography.

Bacterial and fungal infectious arthritis produce similar radiographic changes. Only soft tissue swelling has been described in mycoplasma and viral arthritis.[278,279] In visceral leishmaniasis, the joint changes described were similar to those of degenerative joint disease.[136]

Immune-Mediated Arthritis

Numerous systemic disorders have been associated with immune-mediated arthritis in dogs and cats. These conditions may be classified radiographically into two major categories: erosive and nonerosive.

EROSIVE ARTHRITIS

Rheumatoid-like. Canine rheumatoid-like arthritis is the most frequently described erosive arthritis.[277,280–282] The carpal and tarsal joints are affected most frequently although any joint may be involved (Fig. 4–111). The condition may be monoarticular although polyarticular involvement is more common and joint involvement usually is symmetrical. Soft tissue swelling and loss of bone density around the joint is evident early in the disease. The trabecular pattern of the distal radius, ulna, tibia, fibula, and carpal and tarsal bones becomes coarse due to a loss of the finer secondary trabeculae. That portion of the distal radius and distal tibia within the joint capsule area will be affected. Round, cyst-like lucencies may develop within the subchondral bone. Progressive subchondral bone destruction occurs, especially at the articular margins. The joint space width becomes irregular and joint deformity and subluxation may occur.

Greyhound Polyarthritis. A specific erosive polyarthritis has been described in greyhound dogs 3 to 30 months of age.[197,198,283] The radiographic and pathologic changes are similar but less severe than those of canine rheumatoid arthritis.

Feline Progressive Polyarthritis. A progressive polyarthritis has been described in mature cats (predominately in males) and has been linked to feline leukemia and feline syncytial virus.[284,285] The disease is characterized radiographically by joint swelling, periarticular and subchondral erosions, and joint deformity. In most cases, bony proliferation is observed adjacent to the affected joints (Figs. 4–112 and 4–113).

NON-EROSIVE

Non-erosive immune arthritis is characterized radiographically by soft tissue swelling without erosive bony changes despite long-standing disease. Some loss of bone density may be observed; however, the subchondral bone and periarticular margins appear normal (Fig. 4–114). This form of immune arthritis has been associated with idiopathic causes; systemic lupus erythematosus; chronic inflammatory, infectious, or parasitic diseases; and some drugs.[286–292] The offending organism does not have to be present within the joint. A juvenile onset non-erosive polyarthritis has been reported in akitas. The condition is thought to be inherited.[293]

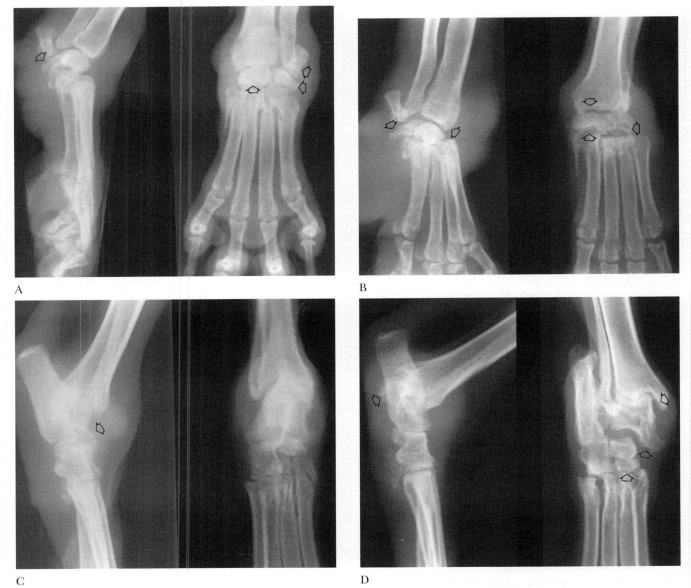

A

B

C

D

Figure 4–111. A 4-year-old male cocker spaniel had a 3-year history of lameness thought to be the result of hip dysplasia and ruptured cranial cruciate ligaments. Swelling of the carpal and tarsal joints was noted. (A&C) Left carpal and left tarsal radiographs were obtained. (A) There is soft tissue swelling of the left carpus. There is malalignment of the carpal bones especially in the carpal metacarpal joint. The accessory carpal bone is displaced proximally. There are small erosions in the carpal bones (*arrows*). There is a loss of bone density in the distal radius and in the distal metaphyseal regions of the metacarpal bones. (C) There is soft tissue swelling of the left tarsus. There is subluxation of the tibial tarsal joint with widening of the lateral aspect of this joint space. There is a generalized loss of bone density of the tarsal bones. There are bony erosions especially on the cranial surface of the talus (*arrow*). (B&D) Follow-up radiographs were obtained 7 months later. (B) In the left carpus the soft tissue swelling has increased dramatically. There is marked subluxation of the carpal metacarpal joint. There are extensive erosive changes in the radiocarpal bone and in the proximal portion of the metacarpal bones as well as in the distal radius (*arrows*). The accessory carpal bone is markedly displaced proximally. There is an overall loss of bone density especially in the periarticular regions. (D) In the left tarsus there is subluxation and malalignment of the tarsal bones especially at the proximal intertarsal joint. There are erosive changes in the distal tibia and in the talus (*arrows*). **Diagnosis:** Immune-mediated erosive arthritis.

Crystal Induced Arthritis

Crystal induced arthritis is extremely rare. Both gout urate crystal deposition in the joints and calcium pyrophosphate crystal deposition disease (CPPD, pseudogout) have been reported in dogs.[294–298]

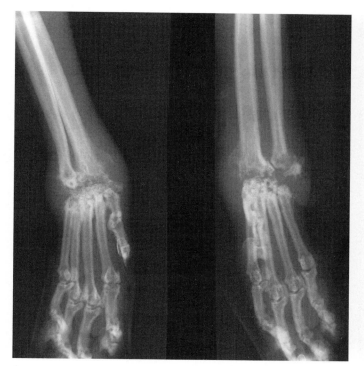 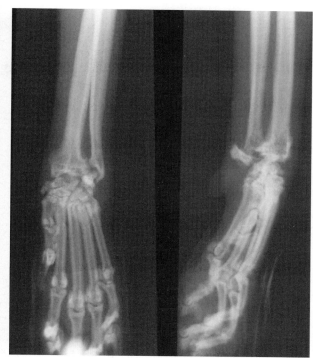

A   B

Figure 4–112. A 4-year-old female domestic short-haired cat presented with swelling of the right carpus, which had been present for 3 months. Mild swelling was also identified in the left carpus. Other joints appeared normal. Radiographs of both carpi were obtained. (A) There is soft tissue swelling in the right carpus. There is extensive bony destruction involving the distal radius and ulna and carpal bones as well as the proximal metacarpal bones. (B) There is minor soft tissue swelling of the left carpus. There is extensive demineralization of the distal radius, ulna, carpal bones, and proximal metacarpal bones. **Diagnosis:** Feline progressive polyarthritis.

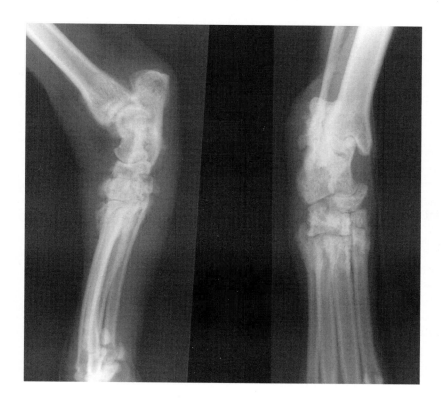

Figure 4–113. A 2-year-old female Persian cat that presented with a fever and joint swellings. There is soft tissue swelling of the right tarsus. There is bony proliferation involving the distal tibia, calcaneus, tarsal bones, and proximal metatarsal bones. There is a loss of bone density in the tarsal bones. **Diagnosis:** Feline progressive polyarthritis.

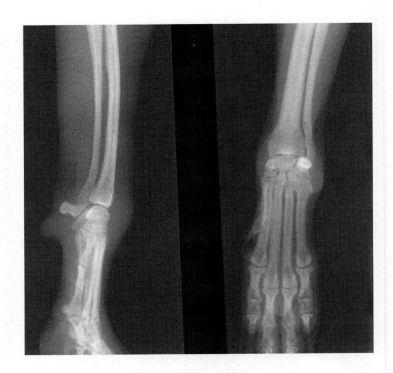

Figure 4–114. A 3-year-old female toy fox terrier had been lame for 6 months. The carpal, tarsal, and both stifle joints were swollen. There is soft tissue swelling around the left carpal joint. There is a loss of bone density involving the distal radius, distal ulna, and the carpal bones. A loss of bone density is also present in the distal metacarpal bones and in the proximal ends of the proximal phalanges. **Diagnosis:** Non-erosive immune polyarthritis.

CPPD usually is associated with the deposition of amorphous aggregates of radio-dense mineralizations in the soft tissues of the joint.[295–297] CPPD in great Danes can result in the deposition of mineral deposits in the synovial joints of the appendicular and axial skeleton.[294] Amorphous mineral opacities have been reported in the diarthrodial joints of the cervical vertebral column in puppies and in the diarthrodial joints of the cervical spine and extremities in a 1-year-old dog.[294] Abnormal bone curvature, cortical thinning, increased medullary trabeculation, and shortening of the long bones were also noted in the older dog.

Soft tissue swelling with periarticular calcification (punctate or fine linear patterns) has been described. Extensive nodular soft tissue calcification was demonstrated around one interphalangeal joint in a dog. Calcium pyrophosphate crystals were identified after the digit was removed.

Villonodular Synovitis

The etiology of villonodular synovitis is unknown. Few cases have been described in small animals.[299,300] Soft tissue swelling and cyst-like cortical erosions with marginal sclerosis have been described. The destructive bony changes were similar to, although less extensive than, those observed with joint neoplasms.

SOFT TISSUE ABNORMALITIES

SOFT TISSUE SWELLINGS/MASSES

The soft tissues should always be evaluated when the appendicular skeleton is radiographed. Swelling of the soft tissues should be categorized as local or diffuse. The location of the swelling, relative to normal anatomical structures, should be considered. Local swellings are more likely neoplastic or granulomatous, while diffuse swellings are more likely secondary to edema, hemorrhage, or inflammation (see Fig. 4–2). A localized swelling that is less dense than the surrounding soft tissues suggests a diagnosis of lipoma (Figs. 4–115 and 4–116). Local swellings that involve joints should be centered on the affected joint and should conform to the joint's

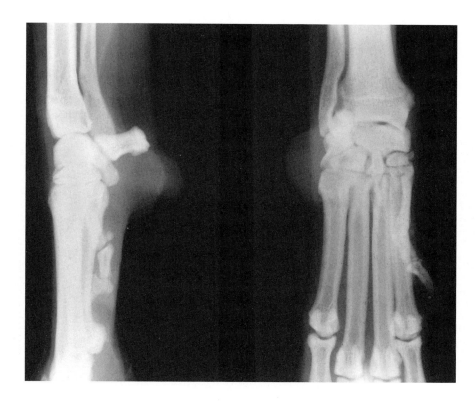

Figure 4–115. A 12-year-old female Labrador retriever was presented with a soft, somewhat fluctuant mass in the area of the right carpus. The dog was not lame. There is an area of swelling present on the caudal medial aspect of the right carpus. This swelling has a fat dense center and a tissue dense border. **Diagnosis:** Lipoma.

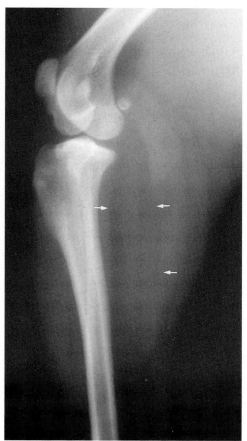

Figure 4–116. A 7-year-old neutered male miniature schnauzer presented with a swelling in the right hindlimb distal to the stifle. The lateral radiograph of the area reveals a well-marginated, fat-dense structure (*arrows*) between the gastrocnemius muscles and the deeper muscles of the tibia. **Diagnosis:** Lipoma.

anatomical limits. Identifying an area of soft tissue swelling on the radiograph indicates that a lesion may be present in the underlying bone and the bone should be examined carefully.

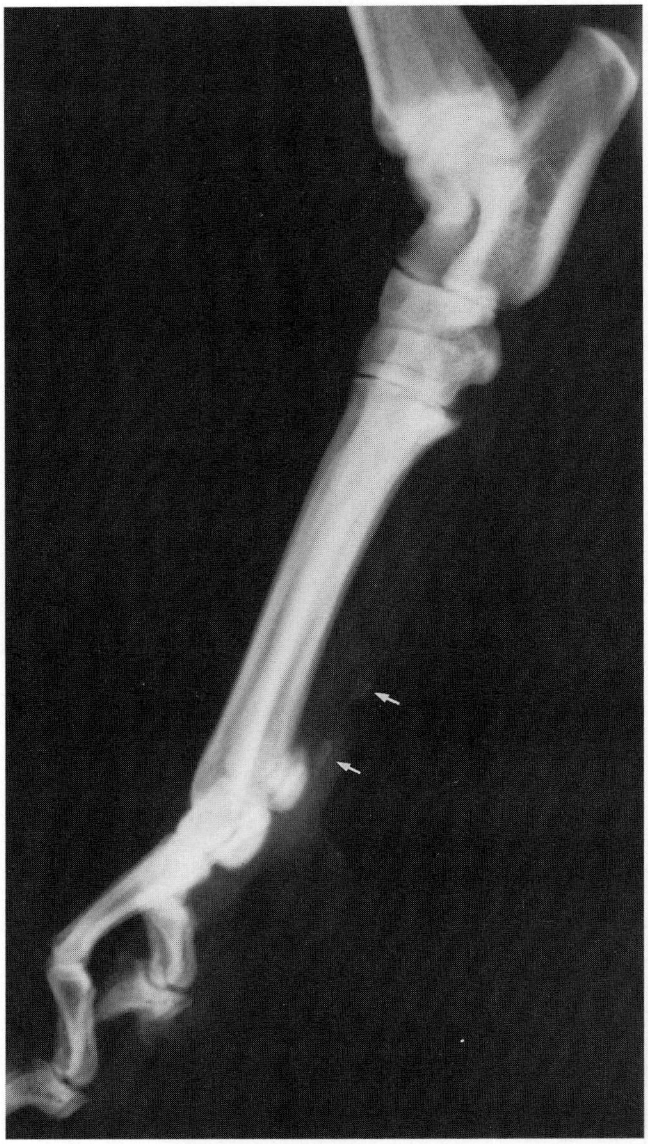

Figure 4–117. A 9-year-old neutered male Shar-Pei was presented for an acute lameness of the left hindlimb. The lateral radiograph of the tarsal region reveals multiple pairs of fine parallel calcifications caudal to the metatarsal bones (*arrows*) as well as lateral to the fibula and caudal to the tibia. Serum analysis revealed significant hypothyroidism. **Diagnosis:** Vascular calcification secondary to hypothyroidism. The lameness was due to a stifle injury.

COMPARTMENTAL SYNDROME

An unusual variant of soft tissue swelling is the compartmental syndrome. This is a post-traumatic swelling (usually due to hemorrhage) into a soft tissue area that is limited by a restrictive circumferential fascia resulting in a marked increase in pressure within the compartment and restricted perfusion. This can lead to muscle death and progressive fibrosis and contracture.[301–304]

SUBCUTANEOUS GAS

The most common cause of gas (air) accumulation within the soft tissues is the presence of an external wound. In rare cases, gas may accumulate in the subcutaneous tissues secondary to infection. Regardless of cause, gas usually accumulates or dissects along fascial planes and appears as linear radiolucencies. Large gas pockets may be seen occasionally.

SOFT TISSUE CALCIFICATIONS

Soft tissue mineralization or calcification may result from dystrophic or metastatic calcification.[305–307] Tumors, chronic infections, and hematomas may calcify and pro-

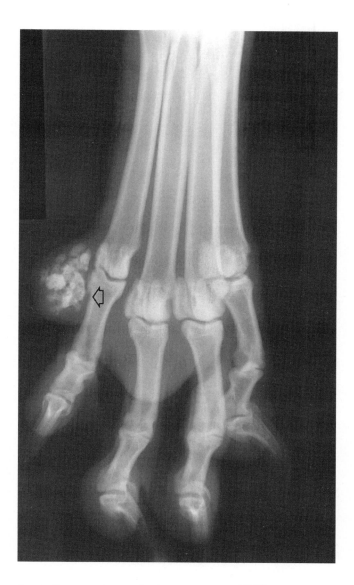

Figure 4–118. A 7-year-old male German shepherd dog presented with a 3-month history of pain when jumping. A hard mass was present on the lateral aspect of the right rear foot. There is an area of soft tissue swelling lateral to the metatarsal-phalangeal joint of the 5th digit, which contains multiple well defined mineralized densities. These densities have a poorly organized internal architecture. There is a slight erosion noted in the proximal end of the digit adjacent to the mineralized densities (*arrow*). **Diagnosis:** Calcinosis circumscripta.

duce discrete areas of mineral density.[308–310] Ossifying myositis (progressive ossification of muscle and connective tissue) may also be seen.[311,312] The pattern of calcification is not specific, and the size, shape, and location of the entire lesion (including its soft tissue component) are important in determining a radiographic diagnosis. Endocrinopathies, such as Cushing's disease or hyperparathyroidism, may result in cutaneous or subcutaneous calcification. Calcification of the foot pads and vascular calcifications have occasionally been described in association with renal failure, hyperadrenocorticism, hypothyroidism, and atherosclerosis (Fig. 4–117). Calcification in association with hypervitaminosis A has been discussed.

Ligamentous or tendon injuries may calcify.[7,313,314] These calcifications are recognized easily, because they conform to the shape and anatomic location of the ligament or tendon. However, such calcifications may be seen in asymptomatic individuals, thus other causes of lameness must be excluded before the lesion is blamed for a specific lameness.

Calcinosis circumscripta is a condition that results in localized areas of subcutaneous soft tissue calcification (Fig. 4–118).[315] These well-defined mineralized masses usually are observed in the extremities and often at pressure points.

Disseminated Idiopathic Skeletal Hyperostosis (DISH)

Disseminated idiopathic skeletal hyperostosis is an infrequently recognized problem. The majority of the lesions affect the spine and pelvis. Appendicular skeletal

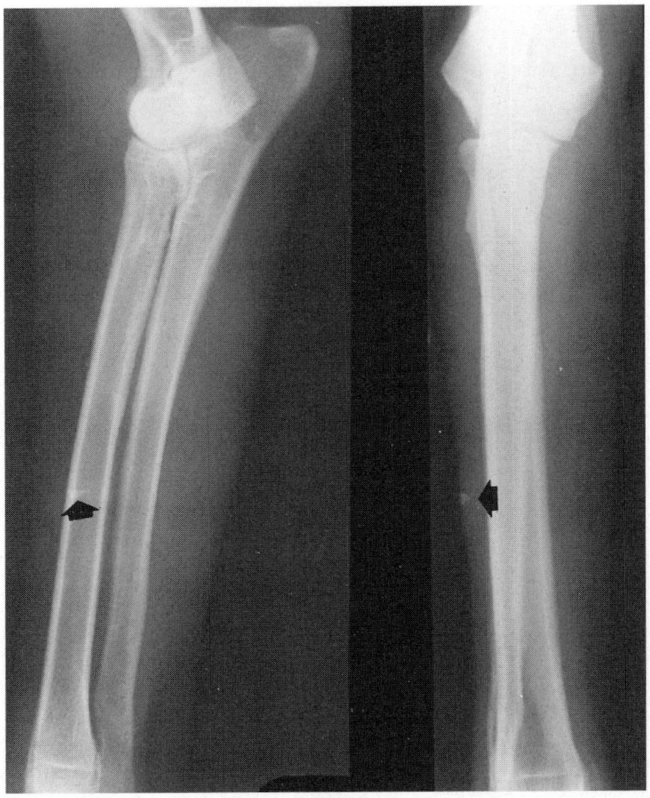

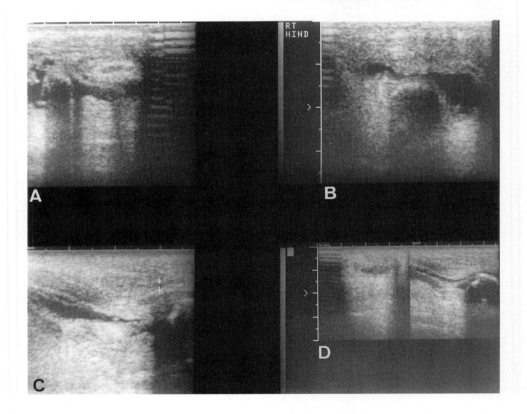

Figure 4–119. A 2-year-old female mixed breed dog presented with a swollen left forelimb. The dog roamed freely. There is diffuse soft tissue swelling along the limb. A small triangular density is visible in the soft tissues (*arrows*). There are no bony abnormalities. **Diagnosis:** Foreign body (tooth fragment) in the soft tissues.

Figure 4–120. A 1-year-old female bullmastiff presented with a right tarsal swelling of 3 weeks' duration. Transverse (A&B) and longitudinal (C) sonograms of the right common calcanean tendon and comparison transverse and longitudinal sonograms of the left (D) reveal an anechoic, peritendinous fluid that extends distally to the level of the calcaneus. (C) The tendon is disrupted at its point of attachment to the calcaneus (*arrows*). **Diagnosis:** Rupture of the right common calcanean tendon.

changes described include periarticular osteophytes and calcification and ossification of soft tissue attachments (enthesiophytes).[316]

Foreign Objects

Foreign objects may penetrate the skin and produce localized or generalized soft tissue swelling. When these foreign objects are dense, they are identified easily (Fig.

4–119). Some foreign objects are tissue-dense (radiolucent) and, therefore, will not be detected on survey radiographs. The presence of a chronic non-healing wound and periosteal proliferation in the adjacent bone suggest the presence of a radiolucent foreign body. Fistulography (i.e., injection of draining tracts with positive contrast) has been used to outline radiolucent foreign objects; however, when contrast is injected subcutaneously in dogs and cats it frequently dissects along fascial planes and does not follow the draining tract.[317]

ULTRASOUND OF APPENDICULAR SKELETON

CANINE HIP DYSPLASIA

Ultrasound has limited value in the evaluation of the appendicular skeleton. It has been used to evaluate to the coxofemoral joints of puppies. Satisfactory images of the joint were obtained in puppies up to 8 weeks of age. The coxofemoral joint space, femoral head, and acetabulum could be evaluated in longitudinal, transverse, and dorsolateral oblique planes. The predictive value of this technique for the diagnosis of canine hip dysplasia has not been determined.[14,318]

TENDON INJURY

Ultrasound also may be used for evaluation of soft tissues in the limbs. Tendinopathies may be imaged. The common calcanean tendon is the most frequently evaluated. Tendon injury, rupture, and peritendinous fluid can be observed (Fig. 4–120). Hypoechoic lesions may be observed with acute injury with hyperechoic lesions developing as the tendon heals. Dystrophic calcification of the healing tendon will reveal a hyperechoic lesion with distal shadowing. Peritendinous fluid appears as a hypoechoic or anechoic region surrounding and paralleling the tendon.

SOFT TISSUE MASSES

Ultrasound has also been use for the evaluation of soft tissue masses. Lymph node enlargement may be documented. Criteria for discriminating between reactive and neoplastic enlargement have not been established (Fig. 4–121). Hematomas vary in echogenicity, with initial hyperechoic lesions that decrease in echogenicity within 24 hours to become hypoechoic. Discrimination between hematoma and abscess is difficult because both usually are hypoechoic or anechoic with a distinct capsule. An ultrasound-guided aspirate will yield a definitive diagnosis in these cases. Tumors usually are identified as isoechoic masses in the soft tissues.

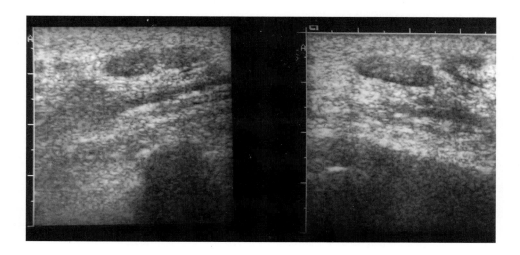

Figure 4–121. A 4-year-old male rottweiler presented with chronic, intermittent fever and swelling in the left axilla. Longitudinal sonograms reveal an oval, hypoechoic mass (lymph node) in the left axilla. This lymphadenopathy could be neoplastic or inflammatory. **Diagnosis:** Axillary lymphadenopathy secondary to chronic infection.

FOREIGN MATTER

Ultrasound has been used extensively for localization of soft tissue foreign objects in large animals. It has been used occasionally in small animals.[319] Most foreign bodies will be hyperechoic and will exhibit distal shadowing.

REFERENCES

1. Smallwood JE, Shively MJ, Rendano VT, et al. A standardized nomenclature for radiographic projections used in veterinary practice. Vet Radiol 1985;26:2.
2. Callahan TF, Ackerman N. The supinated mediolateral radiograph for detection of humeral head osteochondrosis in the dog. Vet Radiol 1985;26:144.
3. Roush JK, Lord PF. Clinical applications of a distoproximal (axial) radiographic view of the scapula. JAAHA 1990;26:129.
4. Slocum B, Devine TM. Dorsal acetabular rim radiographic view for evaluation of the canine hip. JAAHA 1990;26:289.
5. Miyabayashi T, Biller DS, Manley PA, et al. Use of a fixed dorsoplantar radiographic view of the talocrural joint to evaluate lameness in two dogs. JAVMA 1991;199:598.
6. Beck KA. Caudocranial horizontal beam radiographic projection for evaluation of femoral fracture and osteotomy repair in dogs and cats. JAVMA 1991;198:1751.
7. Flo GL, Middleton D. Mineralization of the supraspinatus tendon in dogs. JAVMA 1990;197:95.
8. Beck KA. Caudocranial horizontal beam radiographic projection for evaluation of femoral fracture and osteotomy repair in dogs and cats. JAVMA 1991;198:1751.
9. Beck KA. Caudocranial horizontal beam radiographic projection for evaluation of femoral fracture and osteotomy repair in dogs and cats. JAVMA 1991;198:1151.
10. Ticer JW. Radiographic technique in small animal practice. Philadelphia: WB Saunders Co, 1975;101.
11. Kim EE, Haynie TP. Musculoskeletal neoplasms. In: Current practice in nuclear medicine. Nuclear imaging in oncology. Norwalk: Appleton-Century Crofts, 1984;155.
12. Hahn KA, Hurd C, Cantwell HD. Single phase methylene diphosphonate bone scintigraphy in the diagnostic evaluation of dogs with osteosarcoma. JAVMA 1990;196:1483.
13. Stickle RL, Hathcock JT. Interpretation of computed tomographic images. Vet Clin North Am 1993;23:429.
14. Greshake RJ, Ackerman N. Ultrasound evaluation of the coxofemoral joints of the canine neonate. Vet Radiol Ultrasound 1993;34:99.
15. Renner RR, Mauler GG, Ambrose GL. The radiologist, the orthopedist, the lawyer and the fracture. Semin Roentgenol 1978;13:7.
16. O'Brien TR. Developmental deformities due to arrested epiphyseal growth. VCNA 1971;1:441.
17. O'Brien TR, Morgan JP, Suter PF. Epiphyseal plate injury in the dog: A radiographic study of growth disturbance in the forelimb. JSAP 1971;12:19.
18. Boulay JP, Wallace LJ, Lipowitz AJ. Pathological fracture of long bones in the dog. JAAHA 1987;23:297.
19. Vaughan LC. Limb fractures in the dog and cat: II, histological, clinical, and radiographic aspects of fracture healing. JSAP 1966;7:141.
20. Mann FA, Payne JT. Bone healing. Semin Vet Med Surg 1989;4:312.
21. Braden TD. Posttraumatic osteomyelitis. VCNA 1991;21:781.
22. Anderson GI. Fracture disease and skeletal contractures. VCNA 1991;21:845.
23. Stevenson RB, Pohler OEM, et al. Fracture associated sarcoma in a dog. JAVMA 1982;180:1189.
24. Fagin BD. Tumor or infection? Distinguishing osteomyelitis from neoplastic bone lesions. Vet Med 1988;83:1150.
25. Braden TD. Posttraumatic osteomyelitis. VCNA 1991;21:781.
26. Schrader SC. Complications associated with the use of Steinman intramedullary pins and cerclage wires for fixation of long-bone fractures. VCNA 1991;21:687.
27. Olmstead ML. Complication of fractures repaired with plates and screws. VCNA 1991;21:669.
28. Smith MM, Vasseur PB, Saunders HM. Bacterial growth associated with metallic implants in dogs. JAVMA 1989;195:765.
29. Roush JK, Kirby BM, Manley PA, et al. Chronic osteomyelitis associated with orthopedic implants and cranial cruciate repair in three dogs. JAVMA 1990;196:1123.
30. DeAngelis MP. Causes of delayed union and nonunion of fractures. VCNA 1975;5:251.
31. Sumner-Smith G. Delayed unions and nonunions. VCNA 1991;21:745.
32. Anson LW. Malunions. VCNA 1991;21:761.
33. Brinker WO, Flo GL, Braden T. Removal of bone plates in small animals. JAAHA 1975;11:577.
34. Noser GA, Brinker WO, Little RW, et al. Effect of time on strength of healing bone with bone plate fixation. JAAHA 1977;13:559.
35. Liu SK, Dorfman HD, Patnaik AK. Primary and secondary bone tumors in the cat. JSAP 1974;15:141.
36. Turrel JM, Pool RR. Primary bone tumors in the cat: A retrospective study of 15 cats and a literature review. Vet Radiol 1982;23:152.
37. Brodey RS, Riser WH. Canine osteosarcoma. A clinicopathologic study of 194 cases. Clin Orthop Rel Res 1969;62:54.
38. Ling GV, Morgan JP, Pool RR. Primary bone tumors in the dog: A combined clinical, radiographic, and histologic approach to early diagnosis. JAVMA 1974;165:55.

39. Liu SK, Dorfman HD, Hurvitz, AI et al. Primary and secondary bone tumors in the dog. JSAP 1977;18:313.
40. Theilen GH, Madewell BR. Tumors of the skeleton. In: Theilen GH, Madewell BR, eds. Veterinary cancer medicine. Philadelphia: Lea and Febiger, 1979;289.
41. Berg J, Lamb CR, O'Callaghan MW. Bone scintigraphy in the initial evaluation of dogs with primary bone tumors. JAVMA 1990;196:917.
42. LaRue SM, Withrow SJ, Wrigley RH. Radiographic bone surveys in the evaluation of primary bone tumors in dogs. JAVMA 1986;188:514.
43. Heyman SJ, Diefendorfer DL, Goldschmidt MH, et al. Canine axial skeletal osteosarcoma: A retrospective study of 116 cases (1986–1989). Vet Surg 1992;21:304.
44. Moore AS, Madewell BR, Cardinet GH, et al. Osteogenic sarcoma and myasthenia gravis in a dog. JAVMA 1990;197:226.
45. Papageorges M, Sande RD, Menard M, et al. Osteosarcoma mimicking a bone cyst in a dog. Can Vet J 1989;30:511.
46. Bradney IW, Hobson HP, Homer BL, et al. Osteosarcoma of the femoral head in a golden retriever with metastases to regional lymph nodes, lungs and heart. JAAHA 1989;25:143.
47. Thacher C, Schrader SC, Liu SK. Osteosarcoma of the patella in a dog. JAVMA 1985;187:165.
48. Phillips L, Hager D, Parker R. Osteosarcoma with a pathologic fracture in a six-month-old dog. Vet Radiol 1986;27:18.
49. Prior C, Watrous BJ, Penfold D. Radial diaphyseal osteosarcoma with associated bone infarctions in a dog. JAAHA 1986;22:43.
50. Ackerman N, Halliwell WH, Wingfield WE, et al. Bone infarction and sequestrum formation in a canine osteosarcoma. JAVRS 1975;16:3.
51. Frazier K, Herron AJ, Dee J, et al. Development of small cell osteogenic sarcoma after ulnar ostectomy in a dog. JAVMA 1991;198:432.
52. Stevenson S. Fracture-associated sarcomas. VCNA 1991;21:859.
53. Knecht CD, Priester WA. Osteosarcoma in dogs: A study of previous trauma, fracture, and fracture fixation. JAAHA 1978;14:82.
54. Owen LN. An account of multiple osteosarcomata of bone in dogs having multicentric or metastatic origin. Br J Radiol 1965;38:520.
55. Weller RE, Pool RR, Hornof WJ. Multiple skeletal metastases of osteogenic sarcoma in a dog. JAVMA 1979;56:175.
56. Banks WC. Parosteal sarcoma in a dog and a cat. JAVMA 1971;158:1412.
57. Brodey RS, Misdorp W, Riser WH, et al. Canine skeletal chondrosarcoma: A clinicopathologic study of 35 cases. JAVMA 1974;165:68.
58. Popovitch CA, Weinstein MJ, Goldschmidt MH, et al. Chondrosarcoma: A retrospective study of 97 dogs (1987–1990). JAAHA 1994;30:81.
59. Morton D. Chondrosarcoma arising in a multilobular chondroma in a cat. JAVMA 1985;186:804.
60. Doige CE, Pharr JW, Withrow S. Chondrosarcoma arising in multiple cartilaginous exostoses in a dog. JAAHA 1978;14:605.
61. Ablin LW, Berg J, Schelling SH. Fibrosarcoma of the canine appendicular skeleton. JAAHA 1991;27:303.
62. Levitt L, Doige CE. Primary intraosseous fibrosarcoma in a cat. JAVMA 1989;194:1601.
63. Gibbs C, Denny HR, Lucke VM. The radiological features of non-osteogenic malignant tumors of bone in the appendicular skeleton of the dog: A review of thirty-four cases. JSAP 1985;26:537.
64. Peiffer RL, Rebar A, Burk RL. Fibrosarcoma involving the skeleton of the dog. VMSAC 1974;69:1143.
65. Liu SK. Neoplasms of bone. In: Whittick WG, ed. Canine orthopedics. 2nd ed. Philadelphia: Lea and Febiger, 1990;873.
66. Jennings PB, Andersen GL, Mathey WS, et al. Bone haemangiosarcoma in a young Belgian Malinois. JSAP 1990;31:349.
67. Hosgood G. Canine hemangiosarcoma. Compend Cont Ed Pract Vet 1991;13:1065.
68. Barber DL, Thrall DE, Hill JR, et al. Primary osseous hemangiosarcoma in a dog. Vet Radiol 1973;14:17.
69. Bingel SA, Brodey RS, Allen H, et al. Hemangiosarcoma of bone in the dog. JSAP 1974;15:303.
70. Osborne CA, Perman V, Sautter JH, et al. Multiple myeloma in the dog. JAVMA 1968;153:1300.
71. Bartels JE, Cawley AJ, McSherry BJ, et al. Multiple myeloma (plasmacytoma) in a dog. JAVRS 1972;13:36.
72. Jergens AE, Miles KB, Moore FM. Atypical lytic proliferative skeletal lesions associated with plasma cell myeloma in a dog. Vet Radiol 1990;31:262.
73. Berg J, Gliatto JM, Wallace MK. Giant cell tumor of the accessory carpal bone in a dog. JAVMA 1990;197:883.
74. Popp JA, Simpson CF. Feline malignant giant cell tumor of bone associated with C-type particles. Cornell Vet 1976;66:528.
75. Schnelle GB. Radiology in canine practice. Evanston, IL: The North American Veterinarian, Inc, 1945;75.
76. Turnwald GH, Pechman RD, Shires PK, et al. Lymphosarcoma with osseous involvement in a dog. JAAHA 1988;24:351.
77. Olgilvie GK, Brunkow CS, Daniel GB, et al. Malignant lymphoma with cardiac and bone involvement in a dog. JAVMA 1989;194:793.
78. Rogers KS, Janovitz EB, Fooshee SK, et al. Lymphosarcoma with disseminated skeletal involvement in a pup. JAVMA 1989;195:1242.
79. Giger U, Evans SM, Hendrick MJ, et al. Orthovoltage radiotherapy of primary lymphoma of bone in a dog. JAVMA 1989;195:627.
80. Goedegebuure SA. Secondary bone tumors in the dog. Vet Pathol 1979;16:520.

81. Kas NP, van der Heul RO, Misdorp W. Metastatic bone neoplasms in dogs, cats, and a lion. Zbl Vet Med 1970;17:59.
82. Lee-Parritz DE, Lamb CR. Prostatic adenocarcinoma with osseous metastases in a dog. JAVMA 1988;192:1569.
83. Durham SK, Dietze AE. Prostatic adenocarcinoma with and without metastasis to bone in dogs. JAVMA 1986;188:1432.
84. Hahn KA, Matlock CL. Nasal adenocarcinoma metastatic to bone in two dogs. JAVMA 1990;197:491.
85. Perry RE, Weller RE, Dagle GE, et al. Transitional cell carcinoma of the bladder with skeletal metastases in a dog. JAAHA 1989;25:547.
86. Scott-Moncrief JC, Elliot GS, Radovsky A, et al. Pulmonary squamous cell carcinoma with multiple metastases in a cat. JSAP 1989;30:696.
87. May C, Newsholme SJ. Metastasis of feline pulmonary carcinoma presenting as multiple digital swelling. JSAP 1989;302:307.
88. Lipowitz AJ, Fetter AW, Walker MA. Synovial sarcoma of the dog. JAVMA 1979;174:76.
89. Mitchell M, Hurov LI. Synovial sarcoma in a dog. JAVMA 1979;175:53.
90. Silva-Krott IU, Tucker RL, Meeks JC. Synovial sarcoma in a cat. JAVMA 1993;203:1430.
91. McGlennon NJ, Houlton JEF, Gorman NT. Synovial sarcoma in the dog—a review. JSAP 1988;29:139.
92. Madewell BR, Pool RR, Theilin GH, et al. Multiple subungual squamous cell carcinomas in five dogs. JAVMA 1982;180:731.
93. Pollack M, Martin RA, Diters RW. Metastatic squamous cell carcinoma in multiple digits of a cat: Case report. JAAHA 1984;20:835.
94. Gee BR, Doige CE. Multiple cartilagenous exostoses in a litter of dogs. JAVMA 1970;156:53.
95. Brown RJ, Trevethan WP, Henry VL. Multiple osteochondroma in a Siamese cat. JAVMA 1972;160:433.
96. Gambardella PC, Osborne CA, Stevens JB. Multiple cartilaginous exostoses in the dog. JAVMA 1975;166:761.
97. Ackerman N, Halliwell WH, Renzel LG, et al. Solitary osteochondroma in a dog. JAVRS 1973;14:13.
98. Chester DK. Multiple cartilaginous exostoses in two generations of dogs. JAVMA 1971;159:895.
99. Gillette EL, Thrall DE, Lebel JL. Carlson's veterinary radiology. Philadelphia: Lea and Febiger, 1977;370.
100. Morgan JP. Radiology in veterinary orthopedics. Philadelphia: Lea and Febiger, 1972;119.
101. Schrader SC, Burk RL, Liu SK. Bone cysts in two dogs and a review of similar cystic bone lesions in the dog. JAVMA 1983;182:490.
102. Biery DN, Goldschmidt M, Riser WH, et al. Bone cysts in the dog. Vet Radiol 1976;17:202.
103. Renegar WR, Thornburg LP, Burk RL, et al. Aneurysmal bone cyst in the dog. JAAHA 1979;15:191.
104. Walker MA, Duncan JR, Shaw JW. Aneurysmal bone cyst in a cat. JAVMA 1975;167:933.
105. Pernell RT, Dunstan RW, DeCamp CE. Aneurysmal bone cyst in a six-month-old dog. JAVMA 1992;201:1897.
106. Liu SK, Dorfman HD. Intraosseous epidermoid cysts in two dogs. Vet Pathol 1974;11:230.
107. Homer BL, Ackerman N, Woody BJ, et al. Intraosseous epidermoid cysts in the distal phalanx of two dogs. Vet Radiol 1992;33:273.
108. Aegerter E, Kirkpatrick JA. Orthopedic diseases. Philadelphia: WB Saunders Co, 1975;314.
109. Resnick D, Kyriakos M, Greenway GD. Tumors and tumor-like lesions of bone: Imaging and pathology of specific lesions. In: Resnick D, ed. Bone and joint imaging. Philadelphia: WB Saunders Co, 1989;1144.
110. Johnson KA. Osteomyelitis in dogs and cats. JAVMA 1994;204:1882.
111. Dunn JK, Houlton DR. Successful treatment of two cases of metaphyseal osteomyelitis in the dog. JSAP 1992;33:85.
112. Caywood DD, Wallace LJ, Braden TD. Osteomyelitis in the dog: A review of 67 cases. JAVMA 1978;172:943.
113. Smith CW, Schiller AG, Smith AR, et al. Osteomyelitis in the dog: A retrospective study. JAAHA 1978;14:589.
114. Gilson SD, Schwarz PD. Acute hematogenous osteomyelitis in a dog. JAAHA 1989;25:684.
115. Walker, RD, Richardson, DC, Bryant, MJ, Draper, CS. Anaerobic bacteria associated with osteomyelitis in domestic animals. JAVMA 1983;182:814.
116. Muir P, Johnson KA. Anaerobic bacteria isolated from osteomyelitis in dogs and cats. Vet Surg 1992;21:463.
117. Hodgin EC, Michaelson F, Howerth EW, et al. Anaerobic bacterial infections causing osteomyelitis/arthritis in a dog. JAVMA 1992;201:886.
118. Wigney DI, Allan GS, Hay LE, et al. Osteomyelitis associated with *Penicillium verruculosum* in a German Shepherd dog. JSAP 1990;31:449.
119. Kirpenstein J, Fingland R. Cutaneous actinomycosis and nocardiosis in dogs: 48 cases (1980–1990). JAVMA 1992;201:917.
120. Walker, MA, Lewis, RE, Kneller, SK, et al. Radiographic signs of bone infection in small animals. JAVMA 1975;166:908.
121. Kantrowitz B, Smeak D, Vannini R. Radiographic appearance of ring sequestrum with pin tract osteomyelitis in the dog. JAAHA 1988;24:461.
122. Knecht CD, Slusher R, Cawley AJ. Treatment of Brodie's abscess by means of bone autograft. JAVMA 1971;158:492.
123. Iwaski M, Hagiwara M, Gandra CRP, et al. Skeletal sporotrichosis in a dog. Comp Anim Prac 1988;2:27.
124. Burk RL, Jones BD. Disseminated histoplasmosis with osseous involvement in a dog. JAVMA 1978;172:1416.

125. Lau RE, Kim SN, Piruzok RP. *Histoplasma capsulatum* infection in a metatarsal of a dog. JAVMA 1978;172:1414.
126. Wolf AM. *Histoplasma capsulatum* osteomyelitis in the cat. JVIM 1987;1:158.
127. Wolf AM. Successful treatment of disseminated histoplasmosis with osseous involvement in two cats. JAAHA 1988;24:511.
128. Millman TM, O'Brien TR, Suter PF, et al. Coccidioidomycosis in the dog: Its radiographic diagnosis. Vet Radiol 1979;20:50.
129. Ackerman N, Owens J, Ticer J. Polyostotic coccidioidomycosis in a dog. Vet Radiol 1981;22:83.
130. Roberts RE. Osteomyelitis associated with disseminated blastomycosis in nine dogs. Vet Radiol 1979;20:124.
131. Wood GL, Hirsh DC, Selcer RR, et al. Disseminated aspergillosis in a dog. JAVMA 1978;172:704.
132. Patnaik AK, Liu SK, Wilkins RJ, et al. Paecilomycosis in a dog. JAVMA 1972;161:806.
133. Clinkenbeard KD, Wold AM, Cowell RL, et al. Canine disseminated histoplasmosis. Comp Cont Ed 1989;11:1347.
134. Craig TM, Smallwood JE, Knauer KW, et al. *Hepatozoon canis* infection in dogs: Clinical, radiographic, and hematologic findings. JAVMA 1978;173:967.
135. Smallwood JE. Periosteal new bone formation associated with hepatozoon gametocytes in two dogs. Vet Radiol 1978;19:142.
136. Turrel JM, Pool RR. Bone lesions in four dogs with visceral leishmaniasis. Vet Radiol 1982;23:243.
137. Siegel ET. Endocrine disease of the dog. Philadelphia: Lea and Febiger, 1977;23.
138. Carillo JM, Burk RL, Bode C. Primary hyperparathyroidism in a dog. JAVMA 1979;174:67.
139. Legendre AM, Merkley DF, Carrig CB, et al. Primary hyperparathyroidism in a dog. JAVMA 1976;168:694.
140. Weir EC, Norrdin RW, Barthold SW, et al. Primary hyperparathyroidism in a dog: Biochemical, bone histomorphometric, and pathologic findings. JAVMA 1986;189:1471.
141. Blunden AS, Wheeler SJ, Davies JV. Hyperparathyroidism in the cat of probable primary origin. JSAP 1986;27:791.
142. Riser WH, Brodey RS, Shirer JF. Osteodystrophy in mature cats: A nutritional disease. Vet Radiol 1968;9:37.
143. Lamb CR. The double cortical line: A sign of osteopenia. JSAP 1990;31:189.
144. Burk RL, Barton CL. Renal failure and hyperparathyroidism in an Alaskan malamute pup. JAVMA 1978;172:69.
145. Campbell JR, Griffiths IR. Bone and muscles. In: Chandler EA, Sutton JB, Thompson DJ, eds. Canine medicine and therapeutics. 2nd ed. Oxford: Blackwell, 1984;138.
146. Saunders HM, Jezyk PK. The radiographic appearance of canine congenital hypothyroidism: Skeletal changes with delayed treatment. Vet Radiol 1991;32:171.
147. Peterson ME. Endocrine disorders in cats: Four emerging disorders. Comp Cont Ed 1988;10:1353.
148. Greco DS, Feldman EC, Peterson ME, et al. Congenital hypothyroid dwarfism in a family of Giant Schnauzers. JVIM 1991;5:57.
149. Arnold U, Opitz M, Grosser I, et al. Goitrous hypothyroidism and dwarfism in a kitten. JAAHA 1984;20:753.
150. Chastain CB, McNeel SV, Graham CL, et al. Congenital hypothyroidism in a dog due to an iodide organification defect. AJVR 1983;44:1257.
151. Penninck DG, Feldman EC, Nyland TG. Radiographic features of canine hyperadrenocorticism caused by autonomously functioning adrenocortical tumors; 23 cases (1978–1986). JAVMA 1988;192:1604.
152. Norrdin RW, Carpenter TR, Mailton BF, et al. Trabecular bone morphometry in Beagles with hyperadrenocorticism and adrenal adenomas. Vet Pathol 1988;25:256.
153. Cho DY, Frey RA, Guffy MM, Leipold HW. Hypervitaminosis A in the dog. AJVR 1975;36:1597.
154. Seawright AA, English PB, Gartner RJW. Hypervitaminosis A of the cat. Adv Vet Sci Comp Med 1970;14:1.
155. Giger U, Noble NA. Determination of erythrocyte pyruvate kinase deficiency in Basenjis with chronic hemolytic anemia. JAVMA 1991;198:1755.
156. Breur GJ, Zerbe CA, Slocombe RF, et al. Clinical, radiographic, pathologic, and genetic features of osteochondrodysplasia in Scottish deerhounds. JAVMA 1989;195:606.
157. Latimer KS, Rowland GN, Mahaffey MB. Homozygous Pelger-Huet anomaly and chondrodysplasia in a stillborn kitten. Vet Pathol 1988;25:325.
158. Carrig CB, MacMillan A, Brundage S, et al. Retinal dysplasia associated with skeletal abnormalities in Labrador retrievers. JAVMA 1977;170:49.
159. Sande RD, Alexander JE, Padgett GA. Dwarfism in the Alaskan malamute: Its radiographic pathogenesis. Vet Radiol 1974;15:10.
160. Fletch SM, Smart ME, Pennock PW, et al. Clinical and pathologic features of chondrodysplasia (dwarfism) in the Alaskan malamute. JAVMA 1973;162:357.
161. Rasmussen PG. Multiple epiphyseal dysplasia in a litter of beagle puppies. JSAP 1971;12:91.
162. Riser WH, Haskins ME, Jezyk PF, et al. Pseudoachondroplastic dysplasia in miniature poodles: Clinical, radiologic, and pathologic features. JAVMA 1980;176:335.
163. Bingel SA, Sande RD. Chondrodysplasia in five great Pyrenees. JAVMA 1994;205:845.
164. Whitbread TJ, Gill JJB, Lewis DG. An inherited endochondrodystrophy in the English pointer dog. A new disease. JSAP 1983;24:399.
165. Carrig CB, Schmidt GM, Tvedten HW. Growth of the radius and ulna in Labrador retriever dogs with ocular and skeletal dysplasia. Vet Radiol 1990;31:262.
166. Carrig CB, Wortman JA, Morris EL, et al. Ectrodactyly (split-hand deformity) in the dog. Vet Radiol 1981;22:123.
167. Jezyk PF. Constitutional disorders of the skeleton in dogs and cats. In: Newton CD, Nunnamaker DM, eds. Textbook of small animal orthopedics. Philadelphia: JB Lippincott, 1985;987.

168. Winterbotham EJ, Johnson KA, Francis DJ. Radial agenesis in a cat. JSAP 1985;26:393.
169. Read RA, Black AP, Armstrong SJ, et al. Incidence and clinical significance of sesamoid disease in rottweilers. Vet Rec 1992;130:533.
170. Vaughan LC, France C. Abnormalities of the volar and plantar sesamoid bones in rottweilers. JSAP 1986;27:551.
171. Cohn LA, Meuten DJ. Bone fragility in a kitten: An osteogenesis imperfecta-like syndrome. JAVMA 1990;197:98.
172. Riser WH, Frankhauser R. Osteopetrosis in the dog. JAVRS 1970;11:29.
173. Kramers P, Fluckiger MA, Rahn BA, et al. Osteopetrosis in cats. JSAP 1988;29:153.
174. O' Brien SE, Riedesel EA, Miller LD. Osteopetrosis in an adult dog. JAAHA 1987;23:213.
175. Lees GE, Sautter JH. Anemia and osteopetrosis in a dog. JAVMA 1979;175:820.
176. Barrett RB, Schall WD, Lewis RE. Clinical and radiologic features of canine eosinophilic panosteitis. JAAHA 1968;4:94.
177. Boring RH, Suter PF, Hohn RB, Marshall J. Clinical and radiologic survey of canine panosteitis. JAVMA 1970;150:870.
178. Olson SE. Radiology in veterinary pathology. Acta Radiol Suppl 1972;319:255.
179. Riser WH, Shirer JH. Normal and abnormal growth of the distal foreleg in large and giant dogs. JAVRS 1964;6:50.
180. Hedhammer A, Wu FM, Krook L, et al. Overnutrition and skeletal diseases. An experimental study in growing great Dane dogs. Cornell Vet 1974;64(Suppl 5).
181. Mee AP, Gordon MT, May C, et al. Canine distemper virus transcripts detected in the bone cells of dogs with metaphyseal osteopathy. Bone 1993;14:59.
182. Schulz KS, Payne JT, Aronson E. *Escherichia coli* bacteremia associated with hypertrophic osteodystrophy in a dog. JAVMA 1991;199:1170.
183. Woodward JC. Canine hypertrophic osteodystrophy, a study of the spontaneous disease in littermates. Vet Pathol 1982;19:337.
184. Brodey RS. Hypertrophic osteoarthropathy in the dog: A clinicopathologic survey of 60 cases. JAVMA 1971;159:1242.
185. Madewell BR, Nyland TG, Weigel JE. Regression of hypertrophic osteopathy following pneumonectomy in a dog. JAVMA 1978;172:818.
186. Caywood DD, Kramek BA, Feeney DA, et al. Hypertrophic osteopathy associated with a bronchial foreign body and lobar pneumonia in a dog. JAVMA 1985;186:698.
187. Kelly MJ. Long-term survival of a case of hypertrophic osteopathy with regression of bony changes. JAAHA 1984;20:439.
188. Hesselink JW, van den Tweel JG. Hypertrophic osteopathy in a dog with a chronic lung abscess. JAVMA 1990;196:760.
189. Gram WD, Wheaton LG, Snyder PW, et al. Feline hypertrophic osteopathy associated with pulmonary carcinoma. JAAHA 1990;26:425.
190. Brockus CW, Hathcock JT. Hypertrophic osteopathy associated with pulmonary blastomycosis in a dog. Vet Radiol 1988;29:184.
191. Wylie KB, Lewis DD, Pechman RD, et al. Hypertrophic osteopathy associated with *Mycobacterium fortuitum* pneumonia in a dog. JAVMA 1993;202:1986.
192. Ansari MM. Bone infarcts associated with malignant sarcomas. Comp Cont Ed 1991;13:367.
193. Dubielzig RR, Biery DN, Brodey RS. Bone sarcomas associated with multifocal medullary bone infarction in dogs. JAVMA 1981;179:64.
194. Riser WH, Brodey RS, Biery DN. Bone infarctions associated with malignant bone tumors in dogs. JAVMA 1972;160:411.
195. Madewell BR, Wilson DW, Hornof WJ, et al. Leukemoid blood response and bone infarcts in a dog with renal tubular adenocarcinoma. JAVMA 1990;197:1623.
196. Lunggren G, Olsson SE. Osteoarthrosis of the shoulder and elbow joints in dogs: A pathologic and radiographic study of necropsy material. Vet Radiol 1975;16:33.
197. Pedersen NC, Pool RR, Morgan JP. Joint diseases of dogs and cats. In: Ettinger SJ, ed. Textbook of veterinary internal medicine. 2nd ed. Philadelphia: WB Saunders, 1983;2187.
198. Pedersen NC, Pool RR, O'Brien TR. Naturally occurring arthropathies of animals. In: Resnick D, Niwayama G, eds. Diagnosis of bone and joint disease. Philadelphia: WB Saunders, 1981;221.
199. Morgan JP, Pool RR, Miyabayashi T. Primary degenerative joint disease in a colony of beagles. JAVMA 1987;190:531.
200. Gregory SP, Pearson GR. Synovial osteochondromatosis in a Labrador retriever bitch. JSAP 1990;31:580.
201. Vasseur PB, Berry CR. Progression of stifle osteoarthrosis following reconstruction of the cranial cruciate ligament in 21 dogs. JAAHA 1992;28:129.
202. Elkins AD, Pechman R, Kearney MT, et al. A retrospective study evaluating the degree of degenerative joint disease in the stifle joint of dogs following surgical repair of anterior cruciate ligament rupture. JAAHA 1991;27:533.
203. Bennett D, Tennant B, Lewis DG, et al. A reappraisal of anterior cruciate ligament disease in the dog. JSAP 1988;29:275.
204. Rabin KL, de Haan JJ, Ackerman N. Hip dysplasia in a litter of domestic shorthair cats. Fel Pract 1994;22:15.
205. Hayes HM, Wilson GP, Burt JK. Feline hip dysplasia. JAAHA 1979;15:447.
206. Morgan SJ. The pathology of canine hip dysplasia. VCNA 1992;22:541.
207. Keller GG, Corley EA. Canine hip dysplasia: Investigating the sex predilection and the frequency of unilateral canine hip dysplasia. Vet Med 1989;84:1162.
208. Morgan JP. Radiographic diagnosis of hip dysplasia in skeletally mature dogs. Proc Canine Hip Dysplasia Symposium, St Louis, 1972;78.
209. Riser WH. The dysplastic hip joint: Its radiographic and histologic development. Vet Radiol 1973;14:35.

210. Leighton EA, Linn JM, Wilham RL, et al. A genetic study of canine hip dysplasia. AJVR 1977;38:241.
211. Kealy RD, Olsson SE, Monti KL, et al. Effects of limited food consumption on the incidence of hip dysplasia in growing dogs. JAVMA 1992;201:857.
212. Richardson DC. The role of nutrition in canine hip dysplasia. VCNA 1992;2:529.
213. Alexander JW. The pathogenesis of canine hip dysplasia. VCNA 1992;22:503.
214. Whittington K, Banks WC, Carlson WD, et al. Report of the panel on canine hip dysplasia. JAVMA 1961;139:791.
215. Henry GA. Radiographic development of canine hip dysplasia. VCNA 1992;22:559.
216. Aronson E, Kraus KH, Smith J. The effect of anesthesia on the radiographic appearance of the cox-ofemoral joints. Vet Radiol 1991;32:2.
217. Farrow CS, Back RT. Radiographic evaluation of nonanesthetized and nonsedated dogs for canine hip dysplasia. JAVMA 1989;194:524.
218. Riser WH, Rhodes WH. Producing diagnostic pelvic radiographs for canine hip dysplasia examination. Anim Hosp 1966;2:167.
219. Corley EA. Role of the orthopedic foundation for animals in the control of canine hip dysplasia. VCNA 1992;22:579.
220. Jessen CR, Spurrell FA. Radiographic detection of canine hip dysplasia in known age groups. Proc Canine Hip Dysplasia Symposium, St Louis, 1972;93.
221. Smith GK, Gregor TP, Rhodes WH, et al. Coxofemoral joint laxity from distraction radiography and its contemporaneous and prospective correlation with laxity, subjective score, and evidence of degenerative joint disease from conventional hip-extended radiography in dogs. AJVR 1993;54:1021.
222. Smith GK, Biery DN, Gregor TP. New concepts of coxofemoral joint stability and the development of a clinical stress-radiographic method for quantitating hip joint laxity in the dog. JAVMA 1990;196:59.
223. Lust G, Williams AJ, Burton-Wurster N, et al. Joint laxity and its association with hip dysplasia in Labrador Retrievers. AJVR 1993;54:1990.
224. Paatsama SK, Rokkanen P, Jussila J, et al. A study of osteochondritis dissecans of the canine humeral head using histological, OTC bone labeling, microradiographic and microangiographic methods. JSAP 1971;12:603.
225. Cordy DR, Wind AP. Transverse fracture of the proximal humeral articular cartilage in dogs (so called osteochondritis dissecans). Pathol Vet 1969;6:424.
226. Alexander JW, Richardson DC, Selcer BA. Osteochondritis dissecans of the elbow, stifle and hock—A review. JAAHA 1981;17:51.
227. Montgomery RD, Milton JL, Henderson RA, et al. Osteochondritis dissecans of the canine stifle. Comp Cont Ed 1989;11:119.
228. Strom H, Raskov H, Arnberg J. Osteochondritis dissecans on the lateral femoral trochlear ridge in a dog. JSAP 1989;30:43.
229. Basher AW, Doige CE, Presnell KR. Subchondral bone cysts in a dog with osteochondrosis. JAAHA 1988;24:321.
230. Montgomery RD, Milton JL, Hathcock JT, et al. Osteochondritis dissecans of the canine tarsal joint. Comp Cont Ed 1994;16:835.
231. Denny HR, Gibbs C. Osteochondritis dissecans of the canine stifle joint. JSAP 1980;21:317.
232. Johnson KA, Howlett CR, Pettit GD. Osteochondrosis in the hock joints in dogs. JAAHA 1980;16:103.
233. Olson NC, Mostosky UV, Flo GL, et al. Osteochondritis dissecans of the tarsocrural joint in three canine siblings. JAVMA 1980;176:635.
234. Poulos PW. Canine osteochondrosis. VCNA 1982;12:313.
235. Rosenblum GP, Robins GM, Carlisle CH. Osteochondritis dissecans of the tibiotarsal joint in the dog. JSAP 1978;19:759.
236. van Bree H. Evaluation of the prognostic value of positive-contrast shoulder arthrography for bilateral osteochondrosis lesions in dogs. AJVR 1990;51:1121.
237. Rudd RG, Whitehair JG, Margolis JH. Results of management of osteochondritis dissecans of the humeral head in dogs: 44 cases (1982–1987). JAAHA 1990;26:173.
238. Riser WH, Woodard JC, Bloomberg MS, et al. Shoulder lesions in the greyhound with special reference to osteochondritis dissecans and chondrocalcinosis. JAAHA 1993;29:449.
239. LaHue TR, Brown SG, Roush JC, et al. Entrapment of joint mice in the bicipital tendon sheath as a sequela to osteochondritis dissecans of the proximal humerus in dogs: A report of six cases. JAAHA 1988;24:99.
240. van Bree H, Drysse H, Van Ryssen B, et al. Pathological correlations with magnetic resonance images of osteochondrosis lesions in canine shoulders. JAVMA 1993;202:1099.
241. van Bree H. Evaluation of subchondral lesion size in osteochondrosis of the scapulohumeral joint in dogs. JAVMA 1994;204:1472.
242. Voorhout G, Hazewinkel HAW. Radiographic evaluation of the canine elbow joint with special reference to the medial humeral epicondyle and the medial coronoid process. Vet Radiol 1987;28:158.
243. Studdert VP, Lavelle RB, Beilharz RG, et al. Clinical features and heritability of osteochondrosis of the elbow in Labrador retrievers. JSAP 1991;32:557.
244. Grondalen J, Lingaas F. Arthrosis in the elbow joint of young rapidly growing dogs: A genetic investigation. JSAP 1991;32:460.
245. Lewis DD, Parker RB, Hager DA. Fragmented medial coronoid process of the canine elbow. Comp Cont Ed 1989;11:703.
246. Guthrie S, Buckland-Wright JC, Vaughan LC. Microfocal radiography as an aid to the diagnosis of canine elbow osteochondrosis. JSAP 1991;32:503.
247. Berry CR. Evaluation of the canine elbow for fragmented medial coronoid process. Vet Radiol Ultrasound 1992;33:243.

248. Mason TA, Lavelle RB, Skipper SC, et al. Osteochondrosis of the elbow joint in young dogs. JSAP 1980;21:641.
249. Berzon JL, Quick CB. Fragmented coronoid process: Anatomical, clinical, and radiographic considerations with case analyses. JAAHA 1980;16:241.
250. Henry WB. Radiographic diagnosis and surgical management of fragmented medial coronoid process in dogs. JAVMA 1984;184:799.
251. Tigari M. Clinical radiographical and pathological aspects of ununited medial coronoid process of the elbow joint in dogs. JSAP 1980;21:595.
252. Read RA, Armstrong SJ, O'Keefe JD, et al. Fragmentation of the medial coronoid process of the ulna in dogs: A study of 109 cases. JSAP 1990;31:330.
253. Carpenter LG, Schwarz PD, Lowry JE, et al. Comparison of radiologic imaging techniques for diagnosis of fragmented medial coronoid process of the cubital joint in dogs. JAVMA 1993;203:78.
254. Huibregtse BA, Johnson AL, Muhlbauer MC. The effect of treatment of fragmented coronoid process on the development of osteoarthritis of the elbow. JAAHA 1994;30:190.
255. Morgan JP. Radiology in veterinary orthopedics. Philadelphia: Lea and Febiger, 1972;356.
256. Houlton EF, Meynink SE. Medial patellar luxation in the cat. JSAP 1989;30:349.
257. Roush JK. Canine patellar luxation. VCNA 1993;23:855.
258. Lee R. Legg-Perthes disease in the dog: The histological and associated radiological changes. Vet Radiol 1974;15:24.
259. Morgan JP. Radiology in veterinary orthopedics. Philadelphia: Lea and Febiger, 1972.
260. Robinson R. Legg-Calve—Perthes disease in dogs: Genetic etiology. JSAP 1992;33:275.
261. Swanton MC. Hemophilic arthropathy in dogs. Lab Invest 1959;8:1269.
262. Konde LJ, Thrall MA, Gasper P, et al. Radiographically visualized skeletal changes associated with mucopolysaccharidosis VI in cats. Vet Radiol 1987;28:223.
263. Langweiler M, Haskins ME, Jezyk PF. Mucopolysaccharidosis in a litter of cats. JAAHA 1978;14:748.
264. Jezyk PF. Feline Manoteaux-Lamy syndrome (mucopolysaccharidosis VI). In: Bojrab MJ, ed. Pathophysiology in small animal surgery. Philadelphia: Lea and Febiger, 1981;687.
265. Haskins ME, Jezyk PF, Desnick RJ, et al. Mucopolysaccharidosis in a domestic short-haired cat: A disease distinct from that seen in the Siamese cat. JAVMA 1979;175:384.
266. Goldman AL. Hypervitaminosis A in a cat. JAVMA 1992;200:1970.
267. Bennett D, Taylor DJ. Bacterial endocarditis and inflammatory joint disease in the dog. JSAP 1988;29:347.
268. Bennett D, Taylor DJ. Bacterial infective arthritis in the dog. JSAP 1988;29:207.
269. Caywood DD, Wilson JW, O'Leary TP. Septic polyarthritis associated with bacterial endocarditis in two dogs. JAVMA 1977;171:549.
270. Schrader SC. Septic arthritis and osteomyelitis of the hip in six mature dogs. JAVMA 1982;181:894.
271. Hodgin EC, Michaelson F, Howerth EW, et al. Anaerobic bacterial infections causing osteomyelitis/arthritis in a dog. JAVMA 1992;201:886.
272. Levy JK, Marsh A. Isolation of calicivirus from the joint of a kitten with arthritis. JAVMA 1992;201:753.
273. Carro T, Pedersen NC, Beaman BL, et al. Subcutaneous abscesses and arthritis caused by a probably bacterial L-form in cats. JAVMA 1989;194:1583.
274. Huss BT, Collier LL, Collins BK, et al. Polyarthropathy and chorioretinitis with retinal detachment in a dog with systemic histoplasmosis. JAAHA 1994,30:217.
275. Houlton JEF, Jeffries AR. Infective polyarthritis and multiple discospondylitis in a dog due to *Erysipelothrix rhusiopathiae*. JSAP 1989;30:35.
276. Levitt L, Fowler JD. Septic coxofemoral arthritis and osteomyelitis in a dog. Vet Radiol 1988;29:129.
277. Roush JK, Manley PA, Dueland RT. Rheumatoid arthritis subsequent to *Borrelia burgdorferi* infection in two dogs. JAVMA 1989;195:951.
278. Lissman BA, Bosler EM, Cama H, et al. Spirochete-associated arthritis (Lyme disease) in a dog. JAVMA 1984;185:219.
279. Moise NS, Crissman JW, Fairbrother JF, et al. *Mycoplasma gateae* arthritis and tenosynovitis in cats: Case report and experimental production of the disease. AJVR 1983;44:16.
280. Pedersen NC, Pool RR, Castles JJ, et al. Noninfectious canine arthritis: Rheumatoid arthritis. JAVMA 1976;169:295.
281. Biery DN, Newton CD. Radiographic appearance of rheumatoid arthritis in the dog. JAAHA 1975;11:607.
282. Schiefer B, Hurov L, Seer G. Pulmonary emphysema and fibrosis associated with polyarthritis in a dog. JAVMA 1974;164:408.
283. Woodard JC, Riser WH, Bloomberg MS, et al. Erosive polyarthritis in two greyhounds. JAVMA 1991;198:873.
284. Pedersen NC, Pool RR, O'Brien TR. Feline progressive polyarthritis. AJVR 1980;41:522.
285. Bennett D, Nash AS. Feline immune-based polyarthritis: A study of thirty-one cases. JSAP 1988;29:501.
286. Feldman DG. Glucocorticoid-responsive, idiopathic, nonerosive polyarthritis in a cat. JAAHA 1994;30:42.
287. Crawford MA, Foil CS. Vasculitis: Clinical syndromes in small animals. Comp Cont Ed 1989;11:400.
288. Cribb AE. Idiosyncratic reactions to sulfonamides. JAVMA 1989;195:1612.
289. Cowell RL, Tylker RD, Clinkenbeard KD, et al. Ehrlichiosis and polyarthritis in three dogs. JAVMA 1988;192:1093.
290. Bennett D. Immune-based non-erosive inflammatory joint disease of the dog. 3. Canine idiopathic polyarthritis. JSAP 1987;28:909.
291. Appel MJG. Lyme disease in dogs and cats. Comp Cont Ed 1990;12:617.
292. Drazner FH. Systemic lupus erythematosus in the dog. Comp Cont Ed 1980;2:243.
293. Dougherty SA, Center SA, Shae EE, et al. Juvenile-onset polyarthritic syndrome in akitas. JAVMA 1991;198:849.

294. Woodard JC, Shields RP, Aldrich HC, et al. Calcium phosphate deposition disease in great Danes. Vet Pathol 1982;19:464.
295. Gibson JP, Roenigk WJ. Pseudogout in a dog. JAVMA 1972;161:912.
296. de Haan JJ, Andreasen CB. Calcium crystal-associated arthropathy (pseudogout) in a dog. JAVMA 1992;200:943.
297. Heiman M, Carpenter L, Halverson PB. Calcium pyrophosphate deposition (chondrocalcinosis) in a dog. Vet Pathol 1990;27:122.
298. Miller RM, Kind RE. A gout-like syndrome in a dog. VMSAC 1966;61:236.
299. Kusba JK, Lipowitz AJ, Wise M, et al. Suspected villonodular synovitis in a dog. JAVMA 1983;182:390.
300. Somer T, Sittnikow K, Henriksson K, et al. Pigmented villonodular synovitis and plasmacytoid lymphoma in a dog. JAVMA 1990;197:877.
301. Olivieri M, Suter PF. Compartmental syndrome of the front leg of a dog due to rupture of the median artery. JAAHA 1978;14:210.
302. de Haan JJ, Beale BS. Compartment syndrome in the dog: Case report and literature review. JAAHA 1993;29:133.
303. Basinger RR, Aron DN, Crowe DT, et al. Osteofascial compartment syndrome in the dog. Vet Surg 1987;16:427.
304. Williams J, Bailey MQ, Schertel ER, et al. Compartment syndrome in a Labrador retriever. Vet Radiol Ultrasound 1993;34:244.
305. Barber DL, Rowland GN. Radiographically detectable soft tissue calcification in chronic renal failure. Vet Radiol 1979;20:117.
306. Barrett RB. Radiology in trauma of the musculoskeletal soft tissues of dogs and cats. Vet Radiol 1971;12:5.
307. Norris AM, Pallet L, Wilcock B. Generalized myositis ossificans in a cat. JAAHA 1980;16:659.
308. Aron DN, Rowland GN, Barber DL. Report of an unusual case of ectopic ossification and review of the literature. JAAHA 1985;21:819.
309. Dueland RT, Wagner SD, Sooy TE. von Willebrand heterotopic osteochondrofibrosis of Dobermans. Vet Surg 1989;18:78.
310. Watt PR. Posttraumatic myositis ossificans and fibrotic myopathy in the rectus femoris muscle in a dog: A case report and literature review. JAAHA 1992;28:560.
311. Waldron D, Pettigrew V, Turk M, et al. Progressive ossifying myositis in a cat. JAVMA 1985;187:64.
312. Valentine BA, George C, Randolph JF, et al. Fibrodysplasia ossificans progressiva in the cat. J Vet Intern Med 1992;6:335.
313. Muir P, Johnson KA. Supraspinatus and biceps brachii tendinopathy in dogs. JSAP 1994;35:239.
314. Muir P, Goldsmid SE, Rothwell TL, et al. Calcifying tendinopathy of the biceps brachii in a dog. JAVMA 1992;201:1747.
315. Roudebush P, Maslin WR, Cooper RC. Canine tumoral calcinosis. Comp Cont Ed 1988;10:1162.
316. Morgan JP, Stavenborn M. Disseminated idiopathic skeletal hyperostosis (DISH) in a dog. Vet Radiol 1991;32:65.
317. Lamb CR, White RN, McEvoy FJ. Sinography in the investigation of draining tracts in small animals: Retrospective review of 25 cases. Vet Surg 1994;23:129.
318. Kresken JG, Kostlin RG. The ultrasonic examination of the hip joint in young dogs. Vet Radiol Ultrasound 1993;34:99.
319. Fornage BD, Nasca S, Durville A. Sonographic detection and three-dimensional localization of a metallic foreign body in the soft-tissues in a dog. Br Vet J 1987;143:278.

Chapter Five

THE SKULL

RADIOLOGY AND ULTRASOUND OF THE SKULL

Skull or head radiographs are indicated for the evaluation of patients with clinical signs that suggest involvement of the bones, sinuses, nasal passages, teeth, eyes and orbit, brain, oral cavity, and external soft tissues. The skull is a complex structure with many overlapping shadows, and this can be intimidating when it becomes necessary to evaluate radiographs of this area. Fortunately, the skull is a relatively symmetrical structure and the right and left halves can be compared directly provided the radiograph is positioned carefully and symmetrically. Artifacts created by off-axis radiographs can mimic or obscure abnormalities. Special radiographic projections have been described for evaluation of specific areas. These are extremely valuable and should be used when clinical signs suggest an abnormality in that portion of the head.

Ultrasound has limited value in evaluation of the head. It is frequently used for evaluation of the eye and orbit, for evaluation of soft tissue masses or swelling, and for evaluation of the brain either through an open fontanelle or through a traumatic bony defect in the calvarium.

RADIOGRAPHIC POSITIONING

Multiple projections of the skull are necessary for full evaluation of pathologic change. The commonly used radiographic views are the lateral, ventrodorsal, and dorsoventral. Other views that may be helpful in evaluating specific structures include the open-mouth lateral, lateral oblique, intraoral ventrodorsal, open-mouth ventrodorsal, intraoral dorsoventral, frontal, open-mouth frontal, and modified occipital. To obtain the precise positioning required to evaluate the views of the skull, the radiographs must be taken with the patient anesthetized and the skull given the necessary support.

LATERAL VIEW

The standard lateral view of the skull is obtained by positioning the skull in true lateral recumbency; this results in superimposition of the paired structures (mandibles, osseous bullae, etc.) (Fig. 5–1). Positioning is accomplished by elevating the nose rostrally and rotating the head dorsally using radiolucent supporting material, such as a wedge-shaped piece of radiolucent foam placed under the mandibles. Failure to do this will result in an oblique view. The true lateral position is particularly useful in evaluating the nasal area and calvarium.

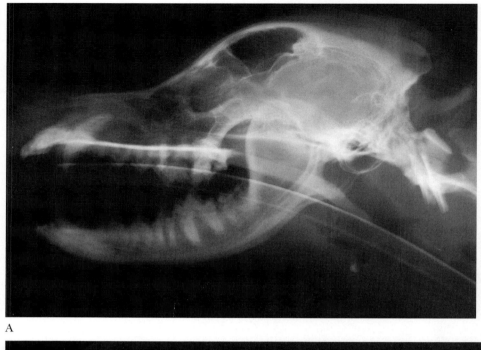

A

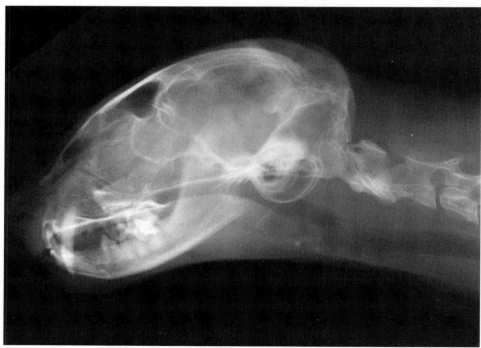

B

Figure 5–1. (A) Normal lateral canine skull radiograph. (B) Normal lateral feline skull radiograph.

VENTRODORSAL VIEW

When making the ventrodorsal view of the skull, the animal is positioned in dorsal recumbency with its head and cervical spine in a straight line and the palate parallel to the film (Fig. 5–2). There should be no obliquity to either the left or right. Radiographically, the position of both mandibles and the shape of the frontal sinuses should be symmetrical. This view is useful for evaluating the mandibles, calvarium, zygomatic arches, and temporomandibular joints.

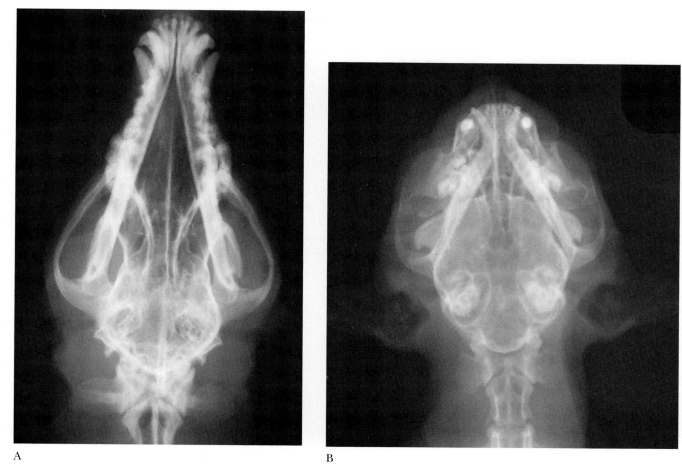

A   B

Figure 5–2. (A) Normal ventrodorsal canine skull radiograph. (B) Normal ventrodorsal feline skull radiograph.

DORSOVENTRAL VIEW

The dorsoventral view is obtained by placing the animal in sternal recumbency and extending the neck and skull in a straight line and with the plane of the hard palate parallel to that of the x-ray film (Fig. 5–3). There must be no rotation along the linear axis of the patient. The evaluation of the positioning is the same as for the ventrodorsal view. This view is useful when evaluating the mandibles, temporomandibular joints, zygomatic arches, and lateral walls of the calvarium.

OPEN-MOUTH LATERAL VIEW

The open-mouth lateral view is positioned like the standard lateral view except that the mouth is restrained in an open position (Fig. 5–4). This view aids in evaluating the rostral portion of the calvarium, because the coronoid processes of the mandibles move ventrally and do not superimpose upon the frontal and parietal regions and the upper and lower dental arcades are not superimposed.

LATERAL OBLIQUE VIEW

The lateral oblique view is obtained by placing the animal in lateral recumbency without external support to the body or skull (Fig. 5–5). This obliquity causes the structures closest to the x-ray tube (farthest from the film) to appear as the more ventral of the pair on the radiograph. In some breeds in which the head is nearly round (Boston bulldogs, pugs, etc.), it may be necessary to elevate the dorsal part of the skull slightly from the table to create adequate obliquity. This view is particularly

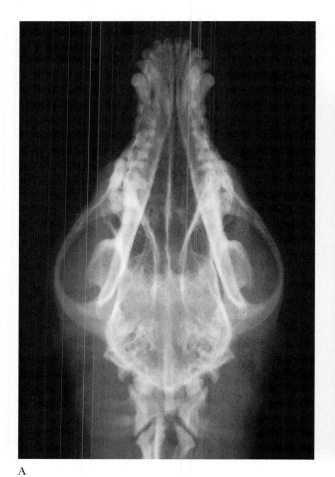

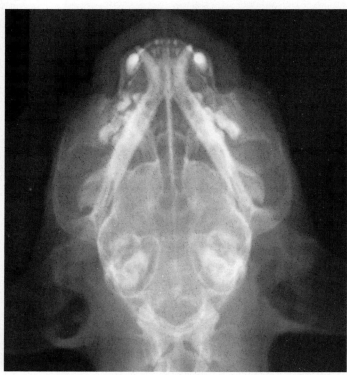

A

B

Figure 5–3. (A) Normal dorsoventral canine skull radiograph (B) Normal dorsoventral feline skull radiograph.

useful for evaluating the temporomandibular joints and osseous bullae. It may also be helpful in evaluating lesions of the temporal portion of the calvarium and horizontal ramus of the mandible.

OPEN-MOUTH LATERAL OBLIQUE VIEW

The open-mouth lateral oblique view has two variations. The first is used to evaluate the maxilla and maxillary dental arcade (Fig. 5–6 A&B). It is obtained by holding the mouth open with a mouth gag (speculum), tape, or other device; elevating the nose slightly so the maxilla is parallel to the film for its entire length; and rotating the skull around its long axis so that the uppermost mandible is rotated toward the dorsal portion of the skull. This rotation causes the up-side maxillary arcade (maxillary arcade farthest from the film) to be superimposed on the nasal passages and the down-side maxillary arcade (maxillary arcade nearest to the film) to be free from superimposition. Care should be taken to ensure that the tongue does not lie over the region of interest. The second variation of the open-mouth lateral oblique view is obtained by rotating the maxilla in the opposite direction. This is used to assess the mandible and mandibular dental arcade (Fig. 5–6 C&D). This view also requires that the mouth be open, the nose slightly elevated so that the mandible is parallel to the film for its entire length, and the skull rotated along its linear axis so that the down-side mandible is not superimposed by the other mandible or the maxilla. The degree of rotation varies with individuals and is best determined at the time of positioning. When making opposite obliques, the patient should be turned over rather than rotating the head dorsally for one view and ventrally for the other.

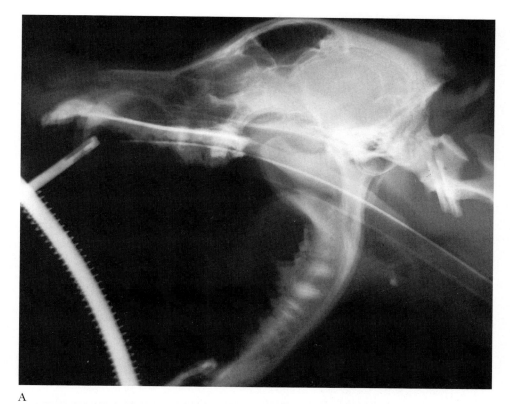

A

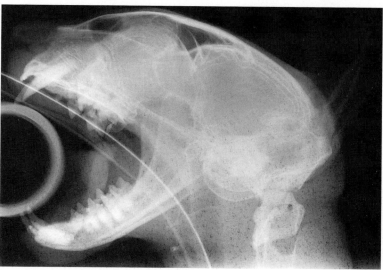

B

Figure 5–4. (A) Normal open-mouth lateral canine skull radiograph. (B) Normal open-mouth lateral feline skull radiograph.

INTRAORAL VENTRODORSAL AND DORSOVENTRAL VIEWS

The intraoral ventrodorsal view, used to evaluate the rostral teeth, is obtained by placing the patient in dorsal recumbency and then inserting either a cardboard or plastic film cassette or a nonscreen film into the mouth. When possible, the tongue should be positioned below the x-ray film or cassette. The tube should be angled slightly toward the caudal part of the animal. The degree of angulation should be estimated for each individual; the goal is to have the x-ray beam strike the roots of the mandibular incisors at a 90° angle. This view is helpful in evaluating the mandibular symphysis, incisors, and canine teeth. The intraoral dorsoventral view is obtained in a similar manner, except the animal is placed in ventral recumbency and

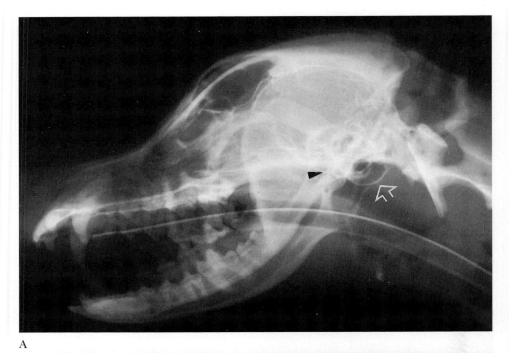

A

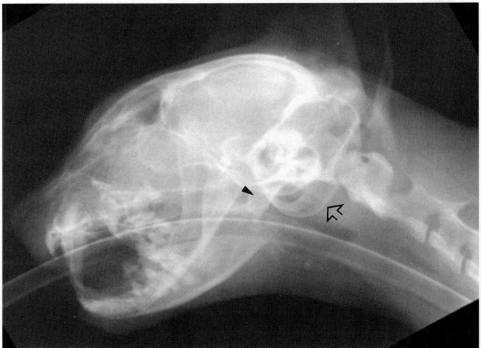

B

Figure 5–5. (A) Normal right lateral oblique (dog in right lateral recumbency) skull radiograph. The left temporomandibular joint (*black arrowhead*) and left osseous bulla (*open white arrow*) are isolated. (B) Normal lateral oblique (cat in right lateral recumbency) skull radiograph. The left temporomandibular joint (*black arrowhead*) and left osseous bulla (*open black arrow*) are isolated.

the x-ray beam is directed through the incisive bone. This view provides information on the incisive bone, the incisors, and the maxillary canine teeth (Fig. 5–7).

OPEN-MOUTH VENTRODORSAL VIEW

The open-mouth ventrodorsal view is essential for complete evaluation of the nasal cavity and frontal sinuses, and is obtained by positioning the animal in dorsal re-

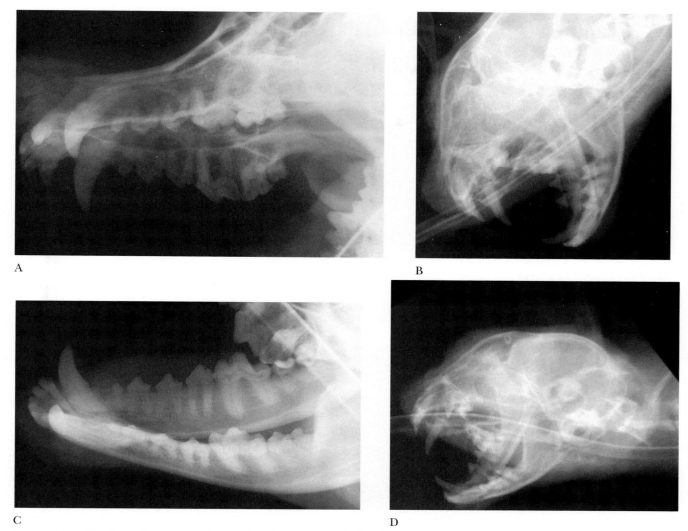

A

B

C

D

Figure 5–6. (A) Normal open-mouth lateral oblique canine skull radiograph isolating the maxilla. (B) Normal open-mouth lateral oblique feline skull radiograph isolating the maxilla. (C) Normal open-mouth lateral oblique canine skull radiograph isolating the mandible. (D) Normal open-mouth lateral oblique feline skull radiograph isolating the mandible.

cumbency in the same position required for the standard ventrodorsal view. The maxilla is taped down parallel to the x-ray table or cassette, and the mouth is held open as widely as possible by a mouth gag or tape (Fig. 5–8). The tongue and endotracheal tube are secured to the mandibles. The x-ray tube is angled in a rostroventral to caudodorsal direction aiming toward the caudal portion of the skull. The x-ray beam should strike the palate so that the mandible does not cast a shadow upon the nasal passages. The amount of angulation needed (approximately 20°) will vary and is best determined at the time of exposure. This view is most useful for evaluating the nasal cavity and the maxillary teeth. In brachycephalic dogs, an oblique projection made with the dog in dorsal recumbency with the mouth closed, and the x-ray beam angled 30° from caudoventral to rostrodorsal has been recommended for evaluation of the nasal cavity.[1]

FRONTAL VIEW

The frontal view is obtained by placing the patient in dorsal recumbency with the head flexed into a position perpendicular to the spine. The angle of the x-ray beam or degree to which the head is flexed varies with the shape of the skull and prominence of the frontal sinuses. Alignment of the frontal sinuses relative to the x-ray

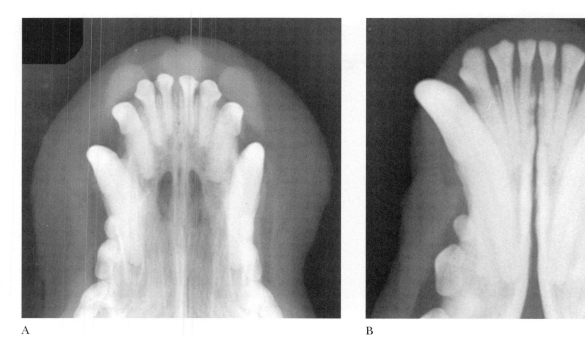

A

B

Figure 5–7. (A) Normal open-mouth view of the canine incisive bone. (B) Normal open-mouth view of the canine mandibular symphysis.

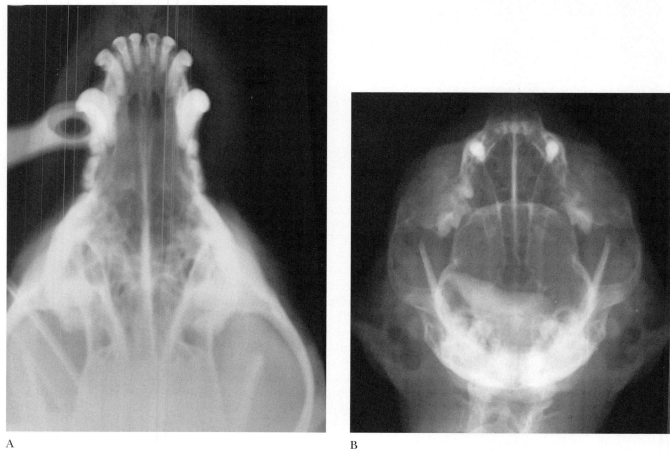

A

B

Figure 5–8. (A) Normal open-mouth ventrodorsal canine skull radiograph. (B) Normal open-mouth ventrodorsal feline skull radiograph.

beam should not result in their superimposition over the other structures (Fig. 5–9). This may not be possible in some breeds (chihuahua, Yorkshire terrier, etc.) with very small frontal sinuses. This view is particularly useful in evaluating the frontal si-

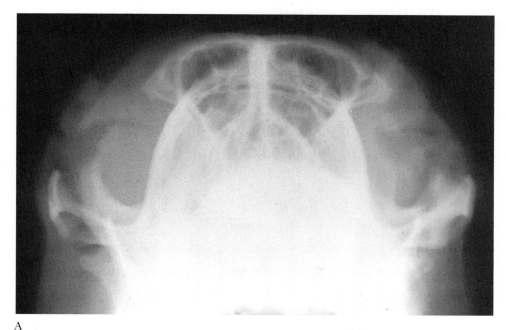

A

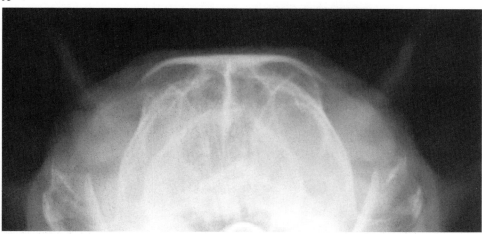

B

Figure 5–9. (A) Normal frontal view of the canine skull. (B) Normal frontal view of the feline skull.

nuses and foramen magnum. If properly positioned, this view permits comparison of the right and left sides.

OPEN-MOUTH FRONTAL VIEW

The open-mouth frontal view is obtained in a manner similar to the standard frontal view. The difference is that the mouth is held open as widely as possible and aligned so that the central ray of the x-ray beam bisects the angle between the mandible and maxilla (Fig. 5–10). The tongue and endotracheal tube should be secured on the midline between the mandibles. This view is particularly useful in evaluating the osseous bullae and odontoid process (dens) of C2.

MODIFIED OCCIPITAL VIEW

The modified occipital view is obtained by placing the animal in dorsal recumbency, tipping the patient's nose 10° down (toward the sternum) from the vertical, and

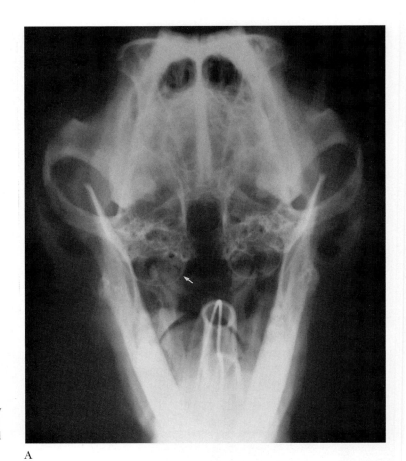

A

Figure 5–10. (A) Normal open-mouth frontal view of the canine skull. The osseous bullae (*white arrow*) are easily identified. (B) Normal open-mouth frontal view of the feline skull.

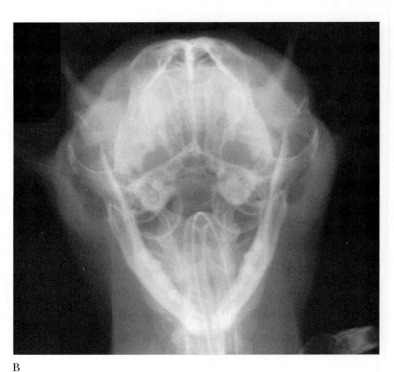

B

angling the x-ray beam at 30° caudally (toward the sternum) so that it strikes the patient just caudal to the frontal sinuses (Fig. 5–11).[2] This view is helpful in evaluating the lateral aspects of the calvarium, the foramen magnum, and the odontoid process of C2.

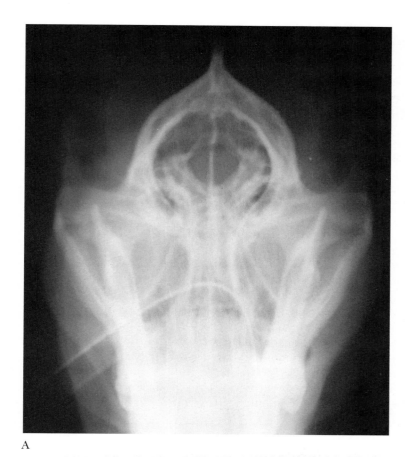

A

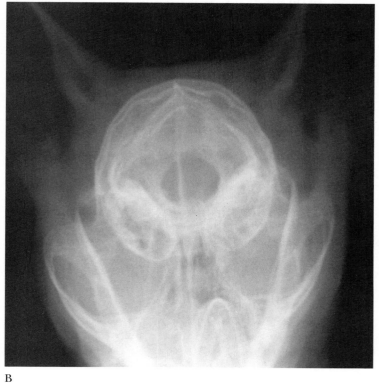

B

Figure 5–11. (A) Normal modified occipital view of the canine skull. (B) Normal modified occipital view of the feline skull.

DENTAL RADIOGRAPHY

Dental radiographs are recommended any time a dental abnormality is observed at the time of physical examination or if there is excessive bleeding during an oral examination.[3] Examples include evaluation of show dogs for missing or unerupted teeth, evaluation of older dogs with periodontal bleeding, evaluation of dogs with facial swelling or nasal discharge, evaluation of gingival masses, postoperative evaluation for the presence of retained tooth fragments or fractures, and evaluating patients for endodontics or periodontics.

Radiographs of the teeth can be obtained with regular x-ray equipment, and although dental x-ray machines are sometimes recommended, the purchase of an x-ray machine specifically for dental radiography is rarely necessary. Nonscreen dental film is often used, and the results obtained are better than those obtained with screen film and cassettes. If examination of the entire maxillary and/or mandibular arcade is desired, a single radiograph is sufficient when detail screens and film are used. Six or more views are required when nonscreen dental films are used.

Obtaining radiographs of the teeth often is a challenge because of the limited space within the oral cavity and the problems in identifying specific teeth when oblique views of the skull are used. Dental film designed for intraoral use in humans can be adapted for use in the dog. The bisection technique is recommended for dental radiography in the dog, especially when radiographs of the maxillary teeth are desired. This technique requires directing the primary x-ray beam perpendicular to the bisection of an angle formed by the dental x-ray film and the axis of the tooth.[3–5] In the parallel technique, the x-ray film is parallel to the long axis of the tooth, and the x-ray beam is perpendicular to the tooth. The technique can be used for some of the mandibular teeth. The dental x-ray film is held in place with stainless steel wire. The wire is secured to the teeth on either side of the tooth of interest.

NORMAL ANATOMY OF RADIOGRAPHIC SIGNIFICANCE

The anatomy of the normal skull is complex; however, the bilateral symmetry of the skull is helpful when evaluating radiographs because in many instances the opposite side may be used for comparison. Evaluation of the skull using a regional or topographic approach is recommended. In this manner, it is relatively easy to ensure full evaluation of the image. The system this text uses considers the following regions separately: (1) nasal passages and sinuses; (2) calvarium; (3) base of skull, middle ear, temporomandibular joints; (4) mandible; and (5) teeth.

NASAL PASSAGES AND SINUSES

The nasal passages of the dog and cat consist of several parts. Radiographically, the planum nasale at the rostral aspect is apparent as a soft tissue density with the air passages clearly demarcated. Further caudally, the nasal passages are evident as air-filled structures within the area surrounded by the maxilla and nasal bones. The fine, delicate bone densities of the conchae and turbinates will be seen clearly. Two fine, parallel radiodense lines, which bisect the nasal passages into left and right sides, will be seen on the open-mouth ventrodorsal and intraoral views. This is the vomer, which supports the cartilaginous nasal septum.[6] The nasal cavity terminates in the nasopharynx ventrally, the frontal bones of the calvarium caudally, and the frontal sinuses dorsally.[6] The maxillary sinuses are rarely visible as a specific structure; however, they are located immediately rostral to the frontal sinuses dorsal and medial to the fourth upper premolar. They appear as small, vaguely triangular-shaped, air-dense structures. These are not seen in cats and smaller breed dogs. Among dog breeds, the frontal sinuses vary considerably in size and shape. The smaller breeds have small to nearly nonexistent frontal sinuses that appear as small, inverted pyramid-shaped, air-dense structures just rostral to the dorsal part of the frontal bones. In cats and larger breed dogs, the frontal sinuses are relatively large, air-filled structures that are divided by one or more bony pillars.

CALVARIUM

The calvarium comprises the frontal, temporal, parietal, and occipital bones as well as the bones of the base of the skull. In dogs, the shape of the calvarium varies greatly with the breed. In some breeds (e.g., pit bull), the dorsal part of the skull may be remarkably thick (up to several centimeters). In other breeds (e.g., Chihuahua), the dorsal part may be very thin and the entire skull appears dome shaped. The sutures may be apparent in very young animals. In some toy breeds, these remain open throughout the animal's life. Normally there are irregularities in the bony density of the calvarium. These irregularities are caused by the jugae, which are bony protrusions of the skull into the spaces (sulci) between the gyri of the brain. Vascular channels, appearing as straight or branching, relatively radiolucent lines with fine sclerotic (radiodense) borders, may be visible on the lateral view of the calvarium.

The occipital crest is the dorsal-most portion of occipital bone and is seen on the lateral view as a bony projection extending caudally dorsal to the 1st cervical vertebra. The size of this projection varies among breeds. The occipital condyles are in the midventral portion of the occipital bone, and are seen routinely on both the ventrodorsal and lateral views as smooth rounded projections extending caudally from the occipital bone. Their articular surfaces should appear smooth and regular. The foramen magnum is centered between the occipital condyles and is oval or triangular in shape with smooth and regular borders. The foramen magnum is best seen on the modified occipital or open-mouth frontal views. On the modified occipital view, the impression in the skull for the vermis of the cerebellum may be seen as a slightly less dense part of the skull projecting dorsally from the dorsal aspect of the foramen magnum.

BASE OF THE SKULL, MIDDLE EARS, TEMPOROMANDIBULAR JOINTS

With the exceptions of the jugular processes, osseous bullae, and temporomandibular joints, the remaining structures of the base of the skull are difficult to assess radiographically. The jugular processes are small, smooth bordered, triangular-shaped bony projections of the occipital bone extending laterally from each side of the skull just caudal to the osseous bullae. On the ventrodorsal view, the osseous bullae are normally round, thin-walled, air-filled bony structures; the air-filled external ear canals are seen extending laterally from the osseous bullae. The lateral oblique views of the osseous bullae reveal smooth, thin-walled air-containing bony structures. Immediately dorsal, medial, and rostral to the osseous bullae are the petrous temporal bones. These are identified easily by their extreme bony density. The temporomandibular joints are rostral to the osseous bullae. They consist of the condyloid processes of the mandibles and the mandibular fossa of the temporal bone near the base of the zygomatic arch. The temporomandibular joints are seen on the dorsoventral view as a thin radiolucent line between the wide based triangular-shaped mandibular condyloid processes and the matching shape of the articular surface of the zygomatic bone. The surfaces are smooth and regular. Only a small portion of the mandibular condyle should extend rostral to the mandibular fossa. On the lateral and lateral oblique views, the articulation appears as a crescent-shaped radiolucency between the round- to oval-shaped mandibular condyloid processes and the semilunar cup shape of the articular portion of the mandibular fossa. These articular surfaces should be smooth and regular.

The zygomatic arches are laterally directed arches of bone that arise from the base of the skull at the temporal bone. The zygomatic arches extend cranially to meet the zygomatic bones, which fuse rostrally with the maxillae. The zygomatic arches are made up of two bones (the zygomatic bone rostrally and the zygomatic process of the temporal bone caudally). These two bones join in the middle of the zygomatic arch with a long, slightly oblique suture that has the zygomatic bone extending dorsal and rostral to the zygomatic portion of the temporal bone. This suture usually is apparent in young animals as a radiolucent line but it is rarely apparent in the adult.

MANDIBLE

The mandible consists of right and left portions that are united rostrally at the mandibular symphysis. Each half of the mandible may be divided into two major portions: the horizontal body and the vertical ramus. The ramus has three processes: (1) the most dorsal is the coronoid process, which is a relatively large, thin piece of bone that forms the dorsal-most portion of the vertical ramus; (2) the condyloid or articular process is the mandibular portion of the temporomandibular joint; (3) the most ventral is the angular process, which is a short, tubular bony protrusion directed caudally from the mandible. The vertical ramus does not contain teeth. The body of the mandible extends from the ramus rostrally to the mandibular symphysis. The body has a roughly tubular shape with a curve toward the midline in the rostral portion. On the lateral view, the mandibular canal is seen as an area of relative radiolucency ventral to the tooth roots running the length of the mandibular body. Cortical defects at the rostral end of the canal (the mental foramina) and at the caudal end of the canal (the mandibular foramen) may be identified. The mandibular canal contains the mandibular artery and vein and the mandibular alveolar nerve.

TEETH

The teeth are present in the incisive bones, mandible, and maxillae. In the adult dog, they are present in the formula (I3/3, C1/1, PM4/4, M2/3).[7] In the puppy, the dental formula is (I3/3, C1/1, PM3/3). In the adult cat, the dental formula is I3/3, C1/1, PM3/2, and M1/1. In the dog, the incisors are small, each having one major tubercle and a single root. The mandibular and maxillary canine teeth are very large, curved, and have more than half of their length as a root. In the maxilla, the 1st premolar is a simple tooth having a single small root. It erupts at approximately 4 or 5 months of age and is not replaced by a "permanent" tooth. The 2nd and 3rd premolars are fairly large; each has two roots. The 4th premolar, the carnassial tooth, is the largest maxillary tooth and has three roots. There are two rostral roots with the larger of the two located slightly lateral to the smaller root. There is a large single caudal root. The 1st and 2nd molars are much smaller than the 4th premolar and each have three roots. The lingual root is smaller than the vestibular roots. In the mandible, the 1st, 2nd, and 3rd premolars are very similar to those of the maxilla. The 4th premolar is slightly larger than the two preceding premolars and has two roots. The 1st mandibular molar is the largest tooth of the lower jaw. It also has a cranial and a caudal root. The 2nd molar is much smaller and also has two roots. The 3rd molar is a relatively small tooth with a single, simple root.

Each tooth has a covering of very radiodense enamel that surrounds the dentin and pulp canal. In young animals, the pulp canal is large. The size of the pulp canal and the amount of bone surrounding the roots of the tooth reduces gradually throughout the life of the animal as a normal aging phenomenon.[8,9] The apex of each root is open. Each tooth is embedded in a bony socket (the alveolus) and held in place by a relatively radiolucent dental ligament. The cortex of the alveolus, which appears radiographically as a thin, dense line known as the lamina dura dentes, is immediately adjacent to the dental ligament. Beyond this cortex the bone takes on the appearance of normal trabecular bone.

SPECIAL TECHNIQUES FOR EVALUATION OF THE SKULL

Several special procedures have been described which evaluate various anatomic structures of the skull. These include the cranial sinus venogram,[10] sialography,[11] orbital cone studies,[12] selective arteriography,[13] pneumoencephalography,[14] dacryocystorhinography,[15] positive-contrast rhinography, [16,17] and cisternography.[18,19] While some of these procedures are useful, their applicability is limited and most have been replaced by ultrasound, CT, MRI. Therefore, we will limit our discussion predominantly to radiography and ultrasound with brief discussions of CT and MRI.

ULTRASOUND OF THE SKULL

Ultrasound is of limited value in examining the skull. The most frequent structures evaluated are the eye and orbit.[20-24] When an open fontanelle is present, the brain can be examined using ultrasound.[25-28] In dogs with closed sutures, normal intracranial anatomy has been described with access to the brain provided by craniotomy.[25]

The eye is examined easily using high frequency transducers placed directly on the cornea.[20-22] Although the eye can be examined through the eyelid, direct corneal contact results in a superior image and is not damaging to the eye. An offset (fluid-filled or tissue-dense structure positioned between the transducer and the eye) can be used if examination of the aqueous chamber is important. Many of the high frequency transducers have reduced the contact artifact that interferes with the image of the aqueous chamber and therefore an offset is not always needed. Topical anesthetic and sterile lubricant are used for the ultrasound examination. Sedation is required in a few cases, but manual restraint is sufficient for most examinations. Most animals do not resent placement of the transducer directly on the anesthetized cornea. Although ultrasound gel is a non-irritant, it is a good practice to flush the eye with sterile saline after the ocular examination.

Both longitudinal and transverse planes are used for the ultrasound examination. The anatomy of the aqueous chamber, lens, iris, vitreous chamber, and retina can be demonstrated. A hyperechoic dot usually is seen on both the anterior and the posterior surfaces of the lens capsule. The lens, aqueous, and vitreous should be anechoic. In older dogs, echogenic debris may be observed within the vitreous chamber. This appears to be a normal finding. The optic disc may be identified in some dogs as an indentation in the posterior aspect of the globe. The normal retina is not identified.

The retrobulbar structures may also be examined through the globe,[23] although the extraocular muscles cannot be differentiated and the optic nerve cannot be traced. In addition, retrobulbar structures may be evaluated by placing the transducer on the dorsolateral aspect of the orbit posterior to the eye. Some ultrasonographers prefer the corneal contact method for examining the retrobulbar space, however we believe that the dorsolateral view is superior.

The open fontanelle at the frontoparietal suture has been used as an acoustic window in dogs from birth to 3 or 4 weeks of age. Ultrasound examination of the brain has been performed in older dogs with open fontanelles and in dogs with closed sutures through a craniotomy. Both transverse and longitudinal scans may be obtained and the detailed anatomy of the brain has been described. Dimensions of the lateral ventricle could be measured; however, the 3rd and 4th ventricles could not be identified in normal neonatal dogs. A maximum height of the lateral ventricle of 0.15 cm was reported for both neonatal and adult dogs. Lateral ventricles with heights greater than 0.35 cm were considered enlarged. Others have related the dorsoventral dimension of the lateral ventricle to the overall dorsoventral dimension of the brain. The dorsoventral dimension of the lateral ventricle should be 14% or less than the dorsoventral diameter of the brain.[25-28]

The lateral ventricles normally appear as slit-like anechoic areas. The 3rd ventricle may be identified depending on its size. It will be located on the midline and appears as an oval central anechoic area, with a surrounding thin hyperechoic region, which represents the choroid plexus.

COMPUTED TOMOGRAPHY AND MAGNETIC RESONANCE IMAGING

Both CT and MRI have been used for evaluation of the head. Most of the studies have involved brain lesions, but a few studies have focused on the orbit and nasal cavity. Both techniques produce cross sectional images of the head, and the information gained from the studies is superior to that obtained with most other imaging methods. The major limitations are the availability of the equipment and the expense of the examination. Most institutions or referral centers have access to these techniques. Anesthesia or sedation is usually required for both CT and MRI.

ABNORMAL FINDINGS

CALVARIUM

Neoplasia

Tumors of the calvarium are uncommon. Tumors of the nasal passage may invade through the cribriform plate and result in damage to the brain. CT and MRI are superior to radiography for detecting invasion into the cribriform plate.[29] A primary bone tumor, such as osteosarcoma, may arise from the calvarium usually producing a bone-dense mass. A tumor that is seen most often in large breed dogs and occasionally in cats arising from the aponeurosis adjacent to the calvarium has been called calcifying aponeurotic fibroma, juvenile aponeurotic fibroma, cartilage analogue of fibromatosis, ossifying fibroma, multilobular osteoma, multilobular chondroma, multilobular osteochondrosarcoma, multilobular osteosarcoma, and chondroma rodens.[30] This lesion is well-defined and densely calcified with a lobulated pattern. Varying degrees of destruction of the adjacent bone may be present (Fig. 5–12). The tumor has also been reported to involve the frontal bone, mandible, maxilla, and orbit.[31] Chondrosarcoma will usually have an irregular pattern of calcification. In cats, meningioma may cause a thickening of the calvarium adjacent to the tumor (Fig. 5–13). Dilation of the meningeal arteries may cause enlarged vascular impressions on the surface of the bone. The calvarial thickening has not been reported in dogs with meningioma. Meningioma may also produce destruction of the calvarium (Fig. 5–14). Other reported changes include mineralization of the mass and increased size of the middle meningeal artery.[32] Multiple myeloma may produce multifocal lytic areas in the calvarium that lack sclerotic borders. However, in dogs and cats with myeloma, it is more common to see these changes involving the appendicular skeleton or spine.

Tumors of the base of the skull are uncommon and usually are primary bone tumors (Fig. 5–15). These may be lytic or productive and are often difficult to perceive. Lesions involving the osseous bullae usually are not primary bone tumors but more

Figure 5–12. A 1-year-old male mixed breed dog had a hard palpable mass involving the right parietal area. The modified occipital view revealed a bone-dense mass that extends both laterally (*open white arrow*) and medially (*open black arrow*) from the right parietal bone. The pattern of calcification is dense and laminar. Differential diagnoses include osteoma, osteosarcoma, chondrosarcoma, other primary bone tumor, or metastatic tumor. **Diagnosis:** Osteoma.

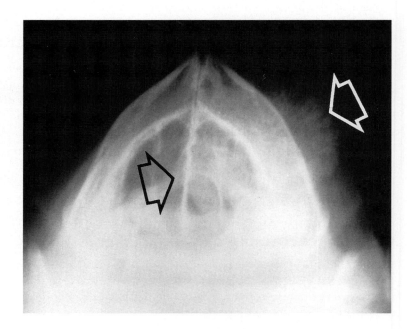

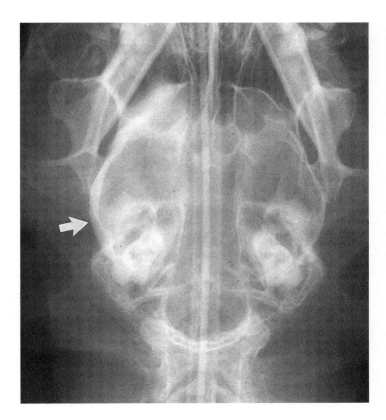

Figure 5–13. A 6-year-old neutered female domestic short-haired cat with lethargy and a marked change to an aggressive behavior. There is hyperostosis: bony thickening of the right side of the calvarium (*white arrow*). There is an overall increased density on the right calvarium when compared to the left calvarium. **Diagnosis:** Meningioma. (From Lawson C, Burk RL, Prata RG. Cerebral meningioma in the cat: Diagnosis and surgical treatment of 10 cases. JAAHA 1984;20:333. Reproduced with permission.)

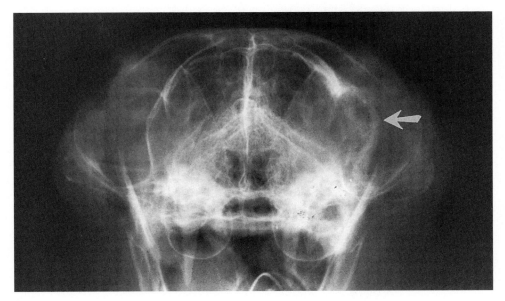

Figure 5–14. A 12-year-old neutered female domestic short-haired cat with circling to the left and a behavior change to increased aggression. The frontal view revealed destruction of the left frontal bone with expansion laterally (*white arrow*). There is a small area of hyperostosis at the junction of the lytic process with the less affected bone dorsally. Differential diagnoses include primary bone tumor, invasive meningioma, or metastatic tumor. **Diagnosis:** Meningioma. (From Lawson C, Burk RL, Prata RG. Cerebral meningioma in the cat: Diagnosis and surgical treatment of 10 cases. JAAHA 1984;20:333. Reproduced with permission.)

often arise from the lining of the bulla. Squamous cell carcinomas may affect the bullae and may completely destroy the osseous bulla, petrous temporal bone, and other bony structures that surround the external and middle ear. A stippled pattern of soft tissue mineralization is often seen in conjunction with squamous cell carcinoma. This helps discriminate between destruction of the bulla secondary to tumor and the changes that may be present secondary to previous bulla osteotomy.

Soft tissue tumors of the ear canal may be evident as a soft tissue density obliterating the normally air-filled ear canal. These may also enlarge and invade the area of the osseous bullae (Fig. 5–16).

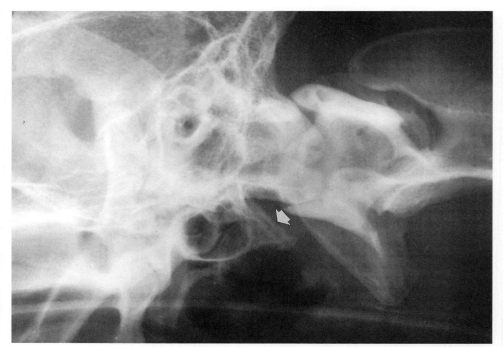

A

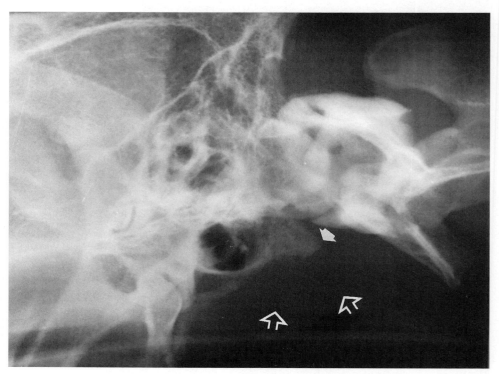

B

Figure 5–15. A 9-year-old male German shepherd dog with apparent neck pain. Meticulous physical examination revealed that pain could be elicited by deep palpation of the base of the skull behind the right ear. (A) The right lateral oblique view revealed that the left middle ear and jugular process (*white arrow*) were normal. There is minimal soft tissue in this area. (B) The left lateral oblique view revealed a normal middle ear. The jugular process (*solid white arrow*) has irregular cortical surfaces, and irregularly round calcifications are seen over the process. There is a large soft tissue mass (*open white arrows*) associated with the area. Differential diagnoses include primary bone tumor, soft tissue tumor affecting adjacent bone, metastatic neoplasia, or infection. **Diagnosis:** Osteosarcoma arising from the jugular process.

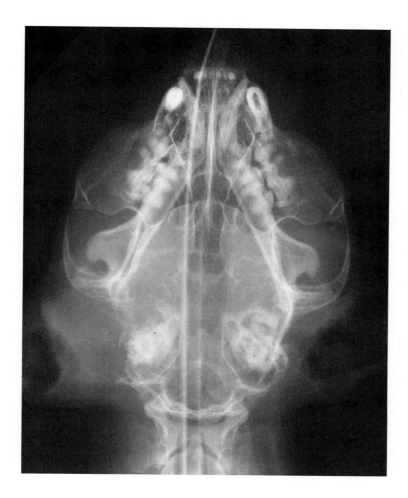

Figure 5–16. A 13-year-old male Siamese cat with a swelling about the base of the right ear. The ventrodorsal view revealed obliteration of the ear canal by a tissue-dense mass as well as destruction of the right temporal and parietal bones. Differential diagnoses include primary bone tumor, squamous cell carcinoma of the ear canal, mucinous gland adenocarcinoma of the ear canal, or metastatic neoplasia. **Diagnosis:** Mucinous gland adenocarcinoma.

Tumors of the zygomatic arch are usually primary bone tumors and lytic and/or productive lesions may be seen (Fig. 5–17).

The most common neoplastic lesions affecting the mandible and maxilla are squamous cell carcinoma, epulis, fibrosarcoma, and melanoma. Many of these tumors arise from the tissues around the teeth. While the tumors may displace teeth, they rarely cause tooth loss. Malignant tumors are more likely to cause irregular or poorly marginated bony destruction, while benign tumors more often result in smooth, distinctly marginated bony destruction.[33] Squamous cell carcinoma usually causes lysis, and frequently the soft tissue mass contains a pattern of punctate soft tissue calcifications (Fig. 5–18). Those melanomas that involve bone usually result in a smoothly bordered lytic lesion positioned eccentrically on the bone. Epulis, a tumor arising from the connective tissue of the gums, usually presents as a soft tissue mass that may or may not contain dystrophic calcification (Fig. 5–19). Adamantinoma, a tumor arising from tooth elements, usually is cystic and appears radiographically as multiloculated radiolucent areas within the bone. Mineral densities or areas of bony proliferation may be present within the expansile lesion (Fig. 5–20). Osteosarcomas are uncommon, but do occur. They are predominately lytic in appearance, but may have a productive component.

Trauma

Trauma to the calvarium can cause permanent or transitory neurologic changes without overt fractures. In those cases in which there is radiographically apparent bony damage, the most common finding is a linear defect in the bone with minimal displacement of fracture fragments (Fig. 5–21). It is important to differentiate vascular channels that create relatively smooth lucencies with sclerotic borders and

Figure 5–17. An 8-year-old male collie with a swelling involving the left side of the face. The slightly oblique ventrodorsal view revealed destruction of the cortex of the maxilla and production of new bone within the associated soft tissue mass. The periosteum has been elevated from its normal location, and a Codman's triangle is seen (*white arrow*). Differential diagnoses include primary neoplasia (e.g., osteosarcoma, chondrosarcoma, squamous cell carcinoma), metastatic neoplasia, or infection. **Diagnosis:** Squamous cell carcinoma.

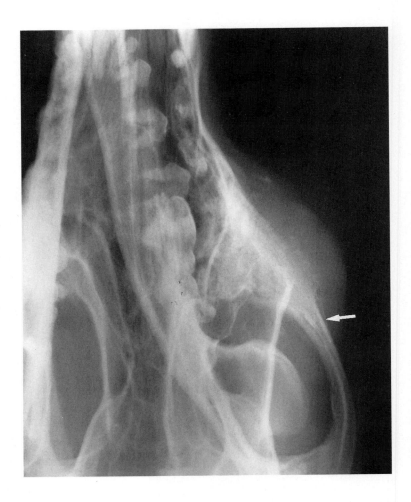

branching patterns from the more irregular fracture lines. Skull fracture fragments may be depressed into the brain. This is most common with fractures of the dorsal or lateral portions of the skull. Although radiography is rarely needed for evaluation of skull fractures, identification of these depression fractures is important.

Fractures of the base of the skull, middle ear, and temporomandibular joints may be difficult to assess. If fractures of the osseous bullae are present, the fragments may be displaced into their lumen. Fractures of the temporomandibular joints are uncommon, but may occur in association with luxations. Luxations of the temporomandibular joints may be best noted on the lateral obliques or dorsoventral views. The luxation will be apparent because of the loss or distortion of the normally smooth semilunar shape of the joint space or positioning of the condyloid process cranially or caudodorsal to the mandibular fossa of the temporal bone (Fig. 5–22). In cats, temporomandibular joint injury should be suspected when dental malocclusion is present with or without mandibular symphyseal separation. Fractures of the retroarticular process, mandibular fossa, zygomatic portion of the temporal bone, and condylar process of the mandible are seen in association with temporomandibular joint luxation in cats.[34] Subluxations are very difficult to evaluate. Although fractures affecting the temporomandibular joints usually involve the mandible (condyloid process), fractures of the temporal bone may also occur. Fractures in this region also are particularly difficult to demonstrate and multiple oblique projections may be required.

The zygomatic processes are susceptible to fracture and are readily evaluated. These usually involve the most lateral portion of the zygomatic arch but may involve other sites as well.

The mandible is quite susceptible to fracture in cases of head trauma. Usually it is

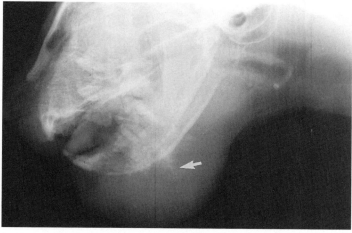

A

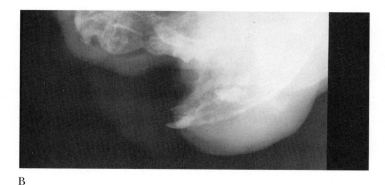

B

Figure 5–18. A 16-year-old male domestic short-haired cat with a large mass involving the rostral part of the right mandible. (A) The lateral radiograph revealed a large tissue-dense mass that contains spicules of tumor bone (*white arrow*). There is some lysis of the mandibular cortex. (B) The right lateral oblique radiograph revealed more evidence of mandibular lysis. Differential diagnoses include squamous cell carcinoma, primary bone tumor, or infection. **Diagnosis:** Squamous cell carcinoma.

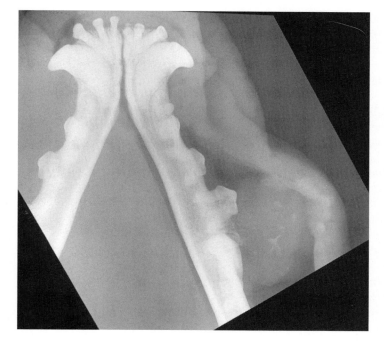

Figure 5–19. A 10-year-old male cockapoo had been excessively salivating for 3 weeks. Oral examination revealed a mass involving the left mandibular gingiva. The open-mouth ventrodorsal view revealed a tissue-dense mass associated with the left mandible at the level of the fourth premolar and first molar. There were areas of calcification within the mass. No evidence of bony destruction of the mandible was noted. Differential diagnoses include epulis, squamous cell carcinoma, melanoma, fibrosarcoma, or other soft tissue tumor. **Diagnosis:** Epulis.

easy to assess the extent of the fracture by using the open-mouth oblique and ventrodorsal views. Fractures most commonly affect the body (Fig. 5–23). Malalignment of the mandible or maxillae may be the first indication of the presence of a fracture.

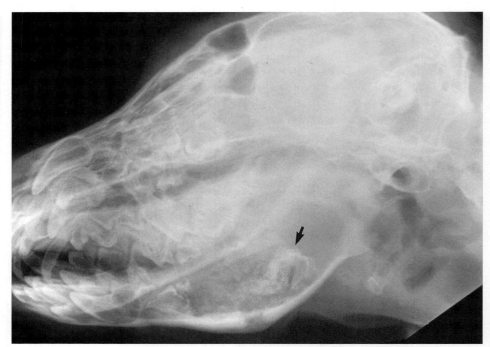

Figure 5–20. A 3-month-old male Labrador retriever with an enlarged left mandible. The oblique lateral view revealed a markedly expanded body of the mandible. The revealed body was relatively radiolucent in its center but contained some highly dense tooth-like structures (*black arrow*) which were poorly formed. **Diagnosis:** Adamantinoma.

If the fracture occurs through the mandibular symphysis, an intraoral film may be useful in establishing the diagnosis. Although the mandibular symphysis normally is completely bridged with bone, in some animals the union may be fibrous. A radiographic diagnosis of mandibular symphyseal separation or fracture should only be made when there is malalignment of the fragments. Fortunately, this area is examined easily and the diagnosis can be made clinically. When assessing mandibular fractures, it is important to look at the tooth roots to determine if they are involved. Tooth fragments may need to be removed at the time of the fracture repair. The teeth are also often used as anchors for wires when the fracture is repaired and tooth root fractures can affect the type of repair. Occasionally, a patient will present with fracture of the mandible without a history of significant trauma. In these instances, pathologic fracture secondary to periapical abscesses, hyperparathyroidism, or tumor may be present. The presence of bony proliferation or lysis at the site of an acute fracture suggests that the fracture is pathologic.

ULTRASOUND EVALUATION OF HEAD TRAUMA

Ultrasound may be used to evaluate the integrity of the brain when a skull fracture has produced a bony defect. The fracture fragment may be evident as a hyperechoic structure with distant shadowing. Intracranial hemorrhage may produce hypoechoic or hyperechoic areas within the brain depending on the duration of the hemorrhage. Brain abscess may develop secondary to trauma, and this may be recognized as a hypoechoic, poorly defined lesion within the brain (Fig. 5–24). Because abscess and hematoma have similar appearances, a fine-needle aspirate would be required to make a definitive diagnosis.

OSTEOARTHRITIS

Degenerative joint disease of the temporomandibular joints is seen occasionally. It may occur as a normal aging change or may be secondary to previous fracture or

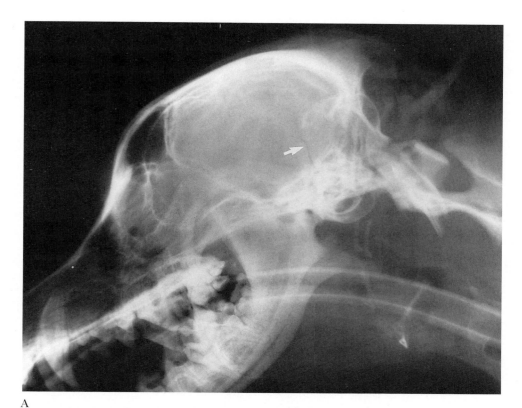

A

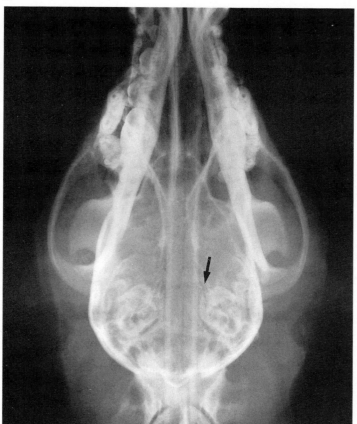

B

Figure 5–21. A 1-year-old male miniature poodle had been hit by a car the day this was taken. The dog was laterally recumbent and had a rotary nystagmus. (A) The lateral radiograph revealed a fine linear radiolucency extending dorsally from near the base of the ear (*white arrow*). (B) The ventrodorsal view revealed a fine linear radiolucency centered on the midline and extending to the left (*white arrow*). **Diagnosis:** Nondisplaced fracture of the basisphenoid and left temporal bones.

luxation. With temporomandibular degenerative joint disease, the subchondral bone will appear irregular, periarticular osteophytes may be present, and the joint space appears narrowed (see Figure 5–25).

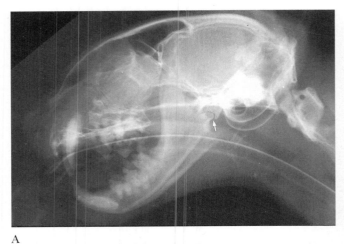

A

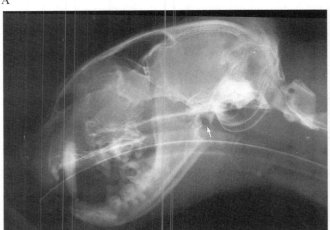

B

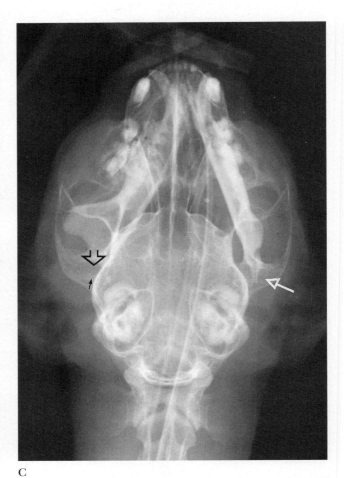

C

Figure 5–22. A 3-year-old domestic short-haired cat had been hit by a car 3 days prior to examination. The owner had noticed that the cat had not been eating since the accident. Physical examination revealed the cat's strong reluctance to open its mouth. (A) The right lateral oblique view revealed that the left temporomandibular joint is normal (*white arrow*). (B) The left lateral oblique revealed that the right temporomandibular joint was luxated because the condyloid process of the mandible was not present in the mandibular fossa of the temporal bone (*white arrow*). (C) The dorsoventral view revealed a normal left temporomandibular joint (*open white arrow*). The condyloid process of the right mandible (*open black arrow*) was displaced rostrally from its normal position in the mandibular fossa of the temporal bone (*small black arrow*). **Diagnosis:** Right temporomandibular joint luxation.

MISCELLANEOUS DISEASES

Otitis Externa and Otitis Media (Bulla Osteitis)

The external ear canals are common sites of infection. The normal air-filled external ear canal may be obliterated due to soft tissue proliferation or exudate within the ear canal. Dystrophic calcification of the external ear canals may occur in association with chronic otitis externa (see Fig. 5–25). This may be evident as well-defined, evenly mineralized or patchy, irregularly mineralized structures that conform to the shape of the external ear cartilages. Unless the radiograph is examined carefully, these calcifications may be misinterpreted as bony lesions arising from the skull.

Otitis externa may extend and result in otitis media with the development of exudate in the middle ear. This will be evident radiographically as an increased opacity of the bulla. If only one bulla is affected, the difference between the air-dense normal bulla and the tissue-dense affected bulla will be readily recognized (Fig. 5–26). There is a normal variation in density of the bulla among different breeds, and if the condition is bilateral, recognizing the radiographic changes may be diffi-

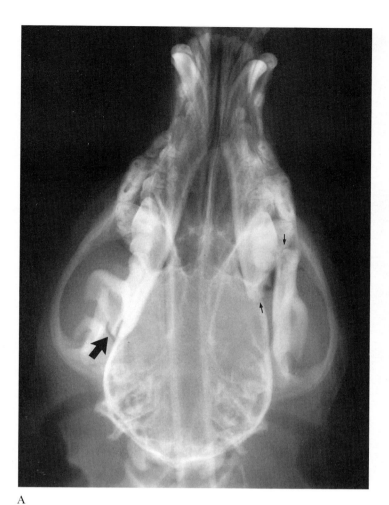

A

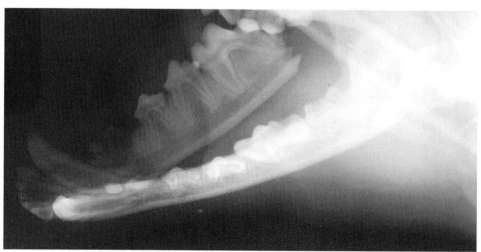

B

Figure 5–23. A 1-year-old female collie that had been hit by a car. Physical examination revealed a fractured mandible. (A) A ventrodorsal view revealed a fracture through the mid-part of the left mandibular body (*small black arrows*). There is also a fracture through the ramus of the right mandible (*large black arrow*). (B) The left open-mouth oblique view, isolating the mandible, revealed the fracture through the body just caudal to the first molar (carnassial tooth) and involving the caudal surface of the alveolus for the caudal root. **Diagnosis:** Fractured left mandible.

cult. The apparent density of the bulla also is affected by positioning and radiographic technique. Malpositioned or improperly exposed radiographs can create or mask the radiographic changes. Thickening of the wall of the osseous bulla and sclerosis of the petrous temporal bone may be identified especially in chronic cases. The radiographic changes must always be correlated with the clinical signs, because the radiographic changes usually persist even though the clinical signs may resolve.

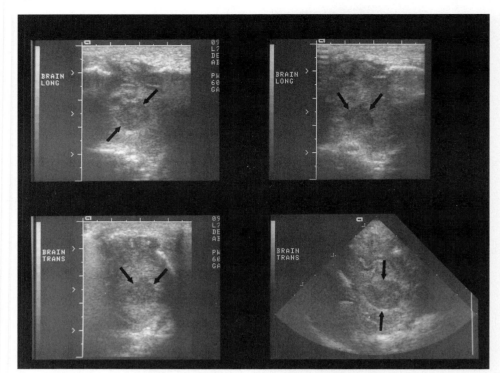

Figure 5–24. Longitudinal and transverse sonograms of the brain of a 2-year-old male dachs-hund with a history of having been attacked by a larger dog 2 weeks previously. There was a depression in the calvarium and a history of intermittent seizures. A poorly-defined hypoechoic lesion (*arrows*) is identified within the brain. This represents brain abscess. An ultrasound-guided aspirate of the lesion was obtained and purulent material was removed. **Diagnosis:** Brain abscess.

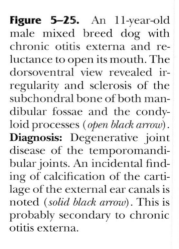

Figure 5–25. An 11-year-old male mixed breed dog with chronic otitis externa and re-luctance to open its mouth. The dorsoventral view revealed ir-regularity and sclerosis of the subchondral bone of both man-dibular fossae and the condy-loid processes (*open black arrow*). **Diagnosis:** Degenerative joint disease of the temporomandi-bular joints. An incidental find-ing of calcification of the carti-lage of the external ear canals is noted (*solid black arrow*). This is probably secondary to chronic otitis externa.

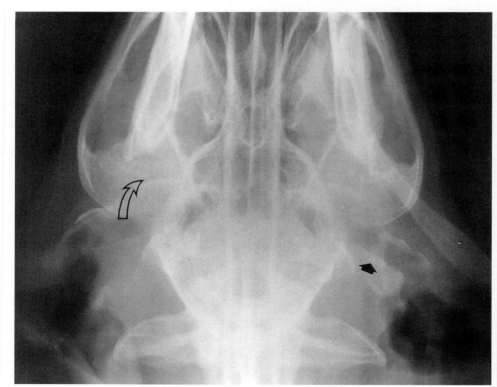

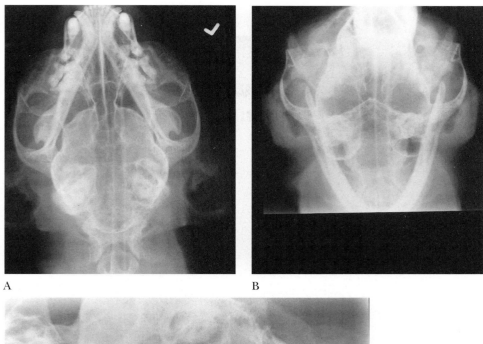

A

B

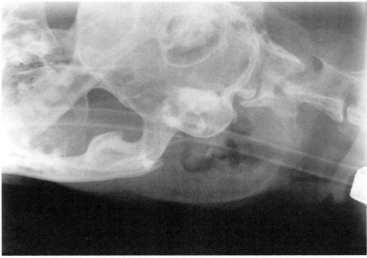

C

Figure 5–26. A 5-year-old neutered male domestic short-haired cat with circling and a head tilt to the right. (A) The ventrodorsal view revealed marked sclerosis of the right middle and internal ear. (B) The open-mouth frontal view confirmed the finding of increased density of the right middle ear. There was apparent thickening of the right osseous bulla. (C) The oblique view that isolated the right bulla demonstrated its thickening and increased density. (D) The opposite oblique view showing the normal left middle and internal ear. **Diagnosis:** Otitis media and interna of the right ear.

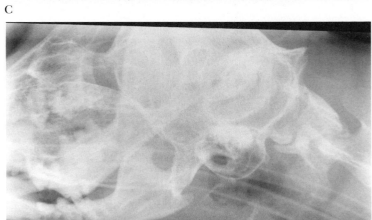

D

Therefore, radiographic changes may be more severe in the clinically normal, as opposed to the clinically affected, side.

Para-aural abscesses may result from chronic external ear infections.[35] These may

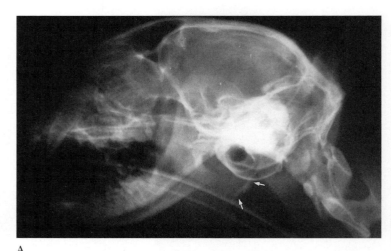

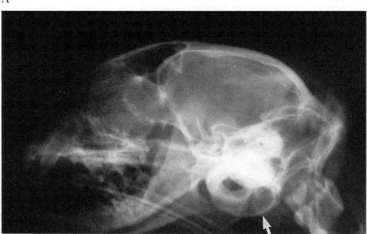

Figure 5–27. A 3-year-old female short-haired cat with a head tilt. (A) The left lateral oblique view revealed a normal right osseous bulla which contained air. A prominent soft tissue mass was noted in the pharynx (*white arrows*). (B) The right lateral oblique view revealed a slightly thickened irregular left osseous bulla (*white arrow*) that contained tissue density. **Diagnosis:** Aural-pharyngeal polyp.

A

B

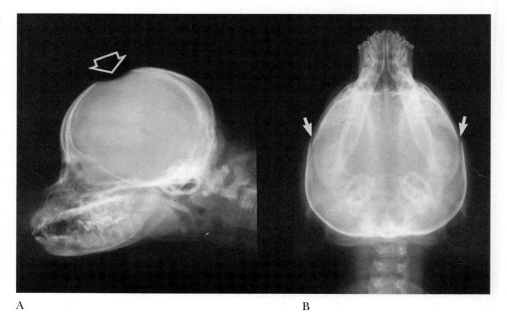

A   B

Figure 5–28. A 3-month-old female poodle with depression, lateral strabismus, and occasional seizures. (A) The lateral radiograph revealed a large bony defect (*open white arrow*) dorsally (a large open fontanelle), marked doming of the skull, and a near homogeneous density over the skull indicating obliteration of the normal juga. (B) The ventrodorsal view revealed open cranial sutures (*white arrows*), thinning of the lateral bones of the calvarium, and frontal bones. **Diagnosis:** Severe hydrocephalus.

produce sclerosis of the petrous temporal bone and thickening of the bulla secondary to the soft tissue infection.

Nasopharyngeal Polyp

In young cats, an inflammatory polyp may develop from the middle ear and extend into the pharynx through the auditory (eustachian) tube (Fig. 5–27).[36] This usually produces increased density and thickening of the osseous bulla. The soft tissue mass may be identified within the nasopharynx. The clinical signs usually are related to upper respiratory obstruction, and the mass usually is visible within the external ear canal or nasopharynx. Therefore, it is not difficult to recognize that the increased density of the bulla is secondary to the polyp and not due to otitis media.

Hydrocephalus

In severe hydrocephalus there may be a smooth, homogenous appearance to the calvarium as a result of the flattening of the jugae and thinning of the calvarial bones. The shape of the skull may be markedly domed, and the frontal bones may bulge cranially. An open fontanelle and/or open sutures may be noted (Fig. 5–28). In adult onset hydrocephalus, which occurs after the skull is well-ossified, bony changes usually are not visible. To confirm the diagnosis of hydrocephalus when bony changes are absent, ventriculography, CT, ultrasonography, or MRI may be needed.

Ultrasound can be used to confirm the diagnosis of hydrocephalus and is easily performed if an open fontanelle is present. The ventricles can be identified and their size evaluated. Normal ventricles should not exceed 0.35 cm or 14% of the ventrodorsal dimension of the brain.[25,27,28] Measurements between 0.15 cm and 0.35 cm are suggestive of hydrocephalus.[26] The ventricles are easily identified in both transverse and longitudinal planes. They appear as anechoic crescent-shaped structures (Figs. 5–29, 5–30, and 5–31). In severe hydrocephalus, the 3rd and 4th ventricles can be identified as an oval or linear anechoic structure located on the ventral midline.

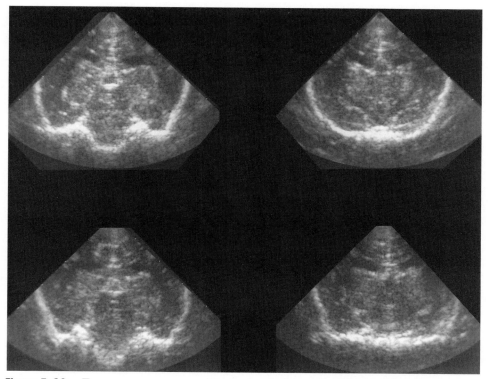

Figure 5–29. Transverse sonograms of the brain of a 5-month-old male chihuahua with a history of vomiting and diarrhea of 1 week's duration. The lateral ventricles are mildly dilated. This represents mild hydrocephalus, which is not unusual in a dog of this breed. **Diagnosis:** Mild hydrocephalus.

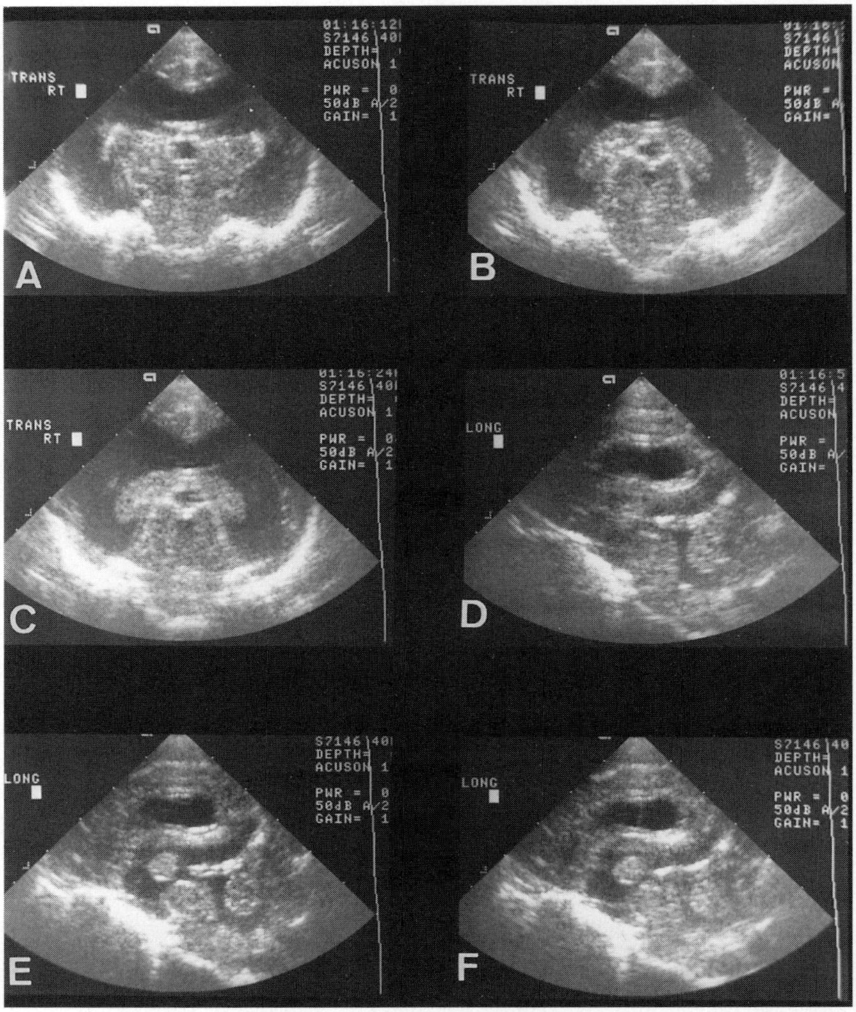

Figure 5–30. Transverse (A,B,&C) and longitudinal (D,E,&F) sonograms of the brain of a 1-year-old male Chihuahua with a history of acute quadriparesis. The lateral, third, and fourth ventricles are moderately distended. **Diagnosis:** Hydrocephalus.

When the fontanelle is large, the examination is easy. No correlation between fontanelle size and degree of hydrocephalus has been determined. There was no correlation between ventricular size and severity of clinical signs. In most instances, the cause of the ventricular enlargement cannot be determined by ultrasound examination.[25] Although the brain can be examined through a craniotomy, this is not recommended because the diagnosis can be made using CT or MRI, which are noninvasive techniques.

Lissencephaly

Lissencephaly, a congenital brain disorder in which the brain does not have normal convolutions (sulci and gyri), may be detected radiographically because the calvarium lacks the normal convolutional markings. Although rare, this condition produces a radiographic appearance similar to that of hydrocephalus.

Occipital Dysplasia

Occipital dysplasia is a morphologic variation in which the margin of the foramen magnum is extended dorsally.[37] This produces a foramen magnum that is enlarged, elongated, or pear shaped. In severe cases, this may result in a foramen magnum large enough to allow cerebellar herniation. The radiographic appearance is readily observed using the modified occipital view (Fig. 5–32). A potential pitfall is misinterpreting the impression of the vermis in the occipital bone as evidence of occipital dysplasia. Even when a foramen magnum malformation is present, there is almost always a fibrous band covering the bony defect preventing cerebellar herni-

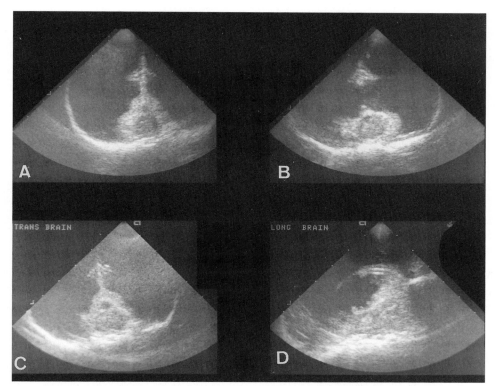

Figure 5–31. Transverse (A,B,&C) and longitudinal (D) sonograms of the brain of a 6-month-old male dachshund with a history of seizures for the previous 2 days. The lateral ventricles are markedly dilated. A small amount of residual neural tissue remains in the ventral calvarium. **Diagnosis:** Severe hydrocephalus.

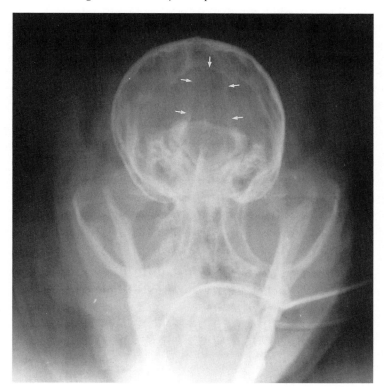

Figure 5–32. A 5-year-old Maltese cat that had cervical pain. On cervical radiographs, a suspicious appearance to the occiput was noted. The modified occipital view revealed a large bony defect extending dorsally from where the normal roof of the foramen would be expected (*white arrows*). **Diagnosis:** Asymptomatic occipital dysplasia (a cervical disc extrusion was responsible for the clinical signs).

ation.[38] The clinical significance of occipital dysplasia is not established. In a study of 80 Pekingese skulls, the shape of the foramen magnum varied from ovoid to rectangular and all but two had a dorsal notch.[38] Most dogs with occipital dysplasia are also hydrocephalic, and the clinical signs are probably related to the hydrocephalus rather than to the foramen magnum conformation.

Acromegaly

Acromegaly has been reported in cats in association with diabetes mellitus and pituitary adenoma.[39] Thickening of the bony ridges of the calvarium, mandibular prognathism, and spondylosis deformans have been described in these cats. Osteoarthritis of the shoulder, elbow, carpus, stifle, and digits also is present. CT scans were performed on six cats and the pituitary tumor was demonstrated in five. Mild to moderate cardiomegaly was observed on thoracic radiographs, and thickening of the left ventricular free wall and interventricular septum were demonstrated by echocardiography. Pulmonary edema, ascites, and pleural effusion were observed in those cats that progressed to heart failure. In acromegalic dogs, no abnormalities were noted in survey radiographs of the appendicular skeleton.[40] Soft tissue swelling was observed ventral to the pharynx. This abnormality was reversible and disappeared post treatment.

Mucopolysaccharidosis

An exaggerated brachycephalic appearance to the skull and a widened maxilla have been reported as features of mucopolysaccharidosis in cats.[41–44] The disease has been reported in Siamese and domestic short-haired cats. Abnormal nasal turbinate development and aplasia or hypoplasia of the frontal and sphenoid sinuses have been described. The nasal and ethmoid turbinates are short and tortuous. The vertebrae are wide and asymmetric with irregular epiphyses present when the cat is young. Widened wedge-shaped disc spaces and periarticular osteophytes also are present. Coxofemoral joint subluxation with femoral head remodeling is also observed in this disease. There is decreased bone density with thin cortices and a coarse trabecular pattern. Degenerative joint disease is present, with the changes being more severe in the hips and shoulders when compared to the stifles or tarsi. There is hypoplasia of the hyoid bones and hypoplasia or fragmentation of the odontoid process of the 2nd cervical vertebra. Fragmentation or abnormal ossification of the patella was observed. The radiographic diagnosis usually is made after examination of vertebral or pelvic radiographs rather than skull radiographs.

In dogs, the changes are similar with facial deformity and brachygnathism. Narrowed intervertebral disc spaces, cervical disc prolapse, vertebral articular facet irregularities, subluxation of vertebral bodies, and subchondral bone lysis with narrow joint spaces were reported.[45]

Craniomandibular Osteopathy

This condition affects young dogs, primarily the highland terriers (Scottish, Cairn, West Highland white). It has been reported infrequently in a large range of other breeds (e.g., Great Danes, Labrador retrievers, Boston terriers, Doberman pinchers).[46,47] In West Highland white terriers, the disease has been shown to be an autosomal recessive trait.[48] The primary radiographic change is the presence of palisading periosteal new bone involving the mandible and increased width and density of the tympanic bulla and the frontal, parietal, and temporal bones (Fig. 5–33). The bony proliferation is most often symmetrical; however, unilateral involvement has been observed. The bone lesions usually are self-limiting with regression of the lesions occurring after skeletal maturity is reached. Some dogs may not survive because they are unable to open their mouths to eat. As the disease regresses, the new bone will remodel and have smooth margins with the residual change appearing as particularly thick mandibular cortices. In some affected dogs, the condition is not limited to the skull and involvement of the appendicular skeleton has been described. The bony lesions consist of a metaphyseal periosteal proliferation, which extends into the diaphysis. The physis is not affected, and the metaphyseal lucencies seen in hypertrophic osteodystrophy are not observed in this disease. This permits discrimination between the lesions of the appendicular skeleton that were observed

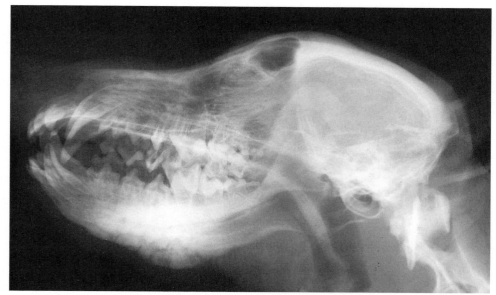

Figure 5–33. A 6-month-old male Scottish terrier with swelling of both mandibles. The lateral radiograph revealed a large amount of palisading periosteal new bone formation involving the bodies of both mandibles. **Diagnosis:** Craniomandibular osteopathy.

with hypertrophic osteodystrophy and those seen with craniomandibular osteopathy. The abnormal metaphyseal bony proliferation may result in an angular limb deformity similar to that of hypertrophic osteodystrophy. The lesion of the appendicular skeleton regresses in a manner similar to that of the skull.

Temporomandibular Subluxation (Dysplasia)

This condition has been associated with chronic intermittent open-mouth locking of the temporomandibular joint in the dog and cat.[49-51] Radiographic changes include an abnormally shaped temporomandibular joint space; flattened mandibular condyles; small, flat mandibular fossae; and an enlarged, hypoplastic or missing retroglenoid process. In some patients, the temporomandibular joint conformation may appear normal. When the jaw is locked open, the abnormal temporomandibular joint subluxates and the jaw shifts to the opposite side, which becomes locked. Locking of the jaw may also occur secondary to trauma without evidence of preexisting joint abnormality.

Thickening of the Osseous Tentorium Cerebelli

The tentorium cerebelli is a thin bony protrusion extending rostrally from the dorsal part of the occipital bone and from the dorsal caudal portions of the parietal bones dividing the cerebellum and brain stem from the cerebrum (caudal fossa from the cranial fossa). On occasion, radiographic changes may be noted. With marked hydrocephalus the size of this structure may be markedly diminished. Tumors also may affect the tentorial process causing either destruction or production of bone (Fig. 5–34). Thickening or enlargement of the tentorium may be observed, especially in cats. The significance of this finding is not known.

Metabolic Diseases

Metabolic diseases that affect calcium metabolism, such as primary, secondary, and tertiary hyperparathyroidism, or others, may be evaluated radiographically. The mandible is a convenient site for this evaluation because these conditions may cause a generalized loss of density in the lamina dura dentes, which is the cortical bone of the tooth alveolus.[52] In more advanced disease, there may be a generalized demineralization of the entire skull. The enamel of the teeth is one of the last areas

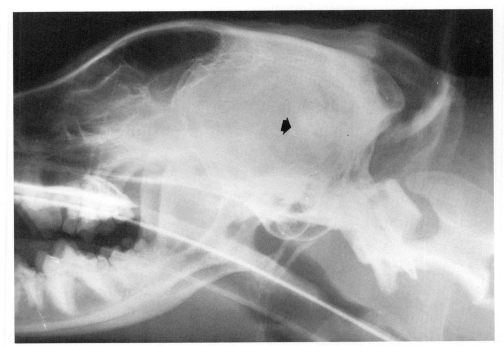

Figure 5–34. A 9-year-old female golden retriever with seizures for 2 months. The lateral radiograph revealed an irregularly round calcified density replacing the normally linear osseous tentorium cerebelli (*black arrow*). This was confirmed on the ventrodorsal view as well. Differential diagnoses include primary bone tumor, meningioma, or metastatic tumor. **Diagnosis:** Osteosarcoma.

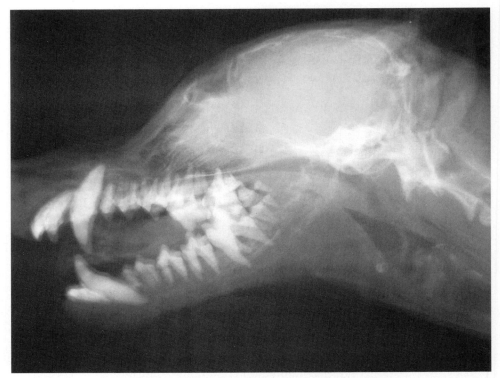

Figure 5–35. A 12-year-old male mixed breed dog with polyuria and polydipsia for 9 months and vomiting for 2 weeks. The lateral view of the skull reveals a severely osteoporotic skull. The teeth appear to be floating in soft tissue rather than anchored in the normal bone of the jaw. Laboratory data revealed severe azotemia. **Diagnosis:** Renal secondary hyperparathyroidism.

to be depleted of calcium; therefore, the appearance of teeth floating in soft tissue develops (Fig. 5–35).

NASAL PASSAGES AND SINUSES

Many diseases that affect the nasal passages and sinuses can present with radiographically apparent changes.[53-55] These include allergic, parasitic, bacterial, fungal, traumatic, foreign body, and neoplastic diseases. Parasitic causes include *Capillaria*,[56] *Eucoleus*,[57] *Baylisascaris*, *Linguatula*,[58] and *Pneumonyssus*.[59] Fungal causes include *Aspergillus*, *Cryptococcus*, *Penicillium*, *Rhinosporidium*,[60] and *Actinomyces*. Many different neoplasms may occur within the nasal cavity. Adenocarcinoma is the most common tumor of the nasal cavity. Fibrosarcoma and chondrosarcoma also are frequently seen. Lymphosarcoma, mastocytoma, meningioma, melanoma, transmissible venereal tumor, squamous cell carcinoma, and osteosarcoma are among the many different tumor types reported.[61-65] The radiographic findings are rarely specific for a tumor type.

Radiographic evaluation of the nasal cavity is performed to identify the location and extent of the lesion that is producing the patient's clinical signs. In many cases, a definitive diagnosis cannot be made based on the radiographic appearance of the lesion. This often happens when the lesion is localized to a small portion of the nasal cavity or when a non-specific finding, such as an increase in soft tissue density, is the only abnormality detected. In these cases, radiography is still useful because it provides guidance for rhinoscopy or biopsy.

When evaluating the nasal passages, the presence or absence of soft tissue density, masses, or radiopaque foreign objects should be noted. The absence or presence and extent of turbinate destruction should be evaluated. The overlying frontal bone and maxilla should be examined for bony destruction or overlying soft tissue masses. The radiograph should be evaluated for evidence of extension of the lesion into the frontal sinus or into the calvarium. The teeth should be examined carefully for evidence of tooth root abscess, and bones should be examined for fractures. Absence of the fine trabecular pattern within the nasal cavity may be caused by accumulation of fluid or soft tissue within the nasal cavity. The fluid may be inflammatory or hemorrhagic, and the soft tissue may be associated with rhinitis or neoplasia. Accumulation of fluid within the nasal cavity will cause some blurring of the normal parallel pattern of the nasal conchae.[66] Loss of the larger bony turbinates usually indicates bone destruction from tumor invasion or necrosis from fungal or chronic bacterial infection. Loss of the turbinate pattern, especially in the ethmoid turbinates, is caused by destruction of the conchae, which is most often associated with tumor or fungal rhinitis.

Rhinitis and Sinusitis

Rhinitis and sinusitis of bacterial origin may produce minimal, marked, or no radiographic changes. The presence of a tissue density within the normally air-filled nasal passages or paranasal sinuses may occur because of the presence of exudate (Fig. 5–36). This density obscures the normally apparent fine bone pattern formed by the turbinates. In many cases of rhinitis, the frontal sinuses will also contain exudate. This increases their radiographic density from air- to tissue-dense. In unilateral nasal disease, comparison to the uninvolved side facilitates detection of increased opacity. In bilateral disease, detecting increased opacity is more difficult. A triad of maladies (sinusitis, situs inversus, and bronchiectasis) known as Kartagener's syndrome has been reported in the dog.[67] Rhinitis, pneumonia, and defective neutrophil function has been reported in the Doberman.[68] When rhinitis is secondary to nonmetallic foreign material in the nasal passages, the exudate usually obscures the outline of the foreign body. Rhinitis may result from extension of infection around a tooth root (periapical abscess) into the nasal passages. In this situation, the radiographic signs of a periapical abscess (decreased density around the tooth root) will be evident in addition to the increased nasal passage density. In most patients

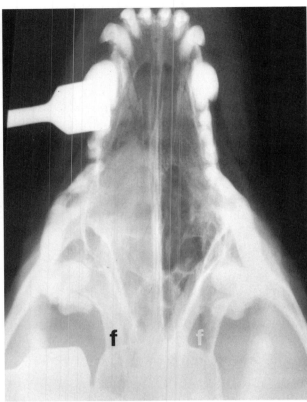

A

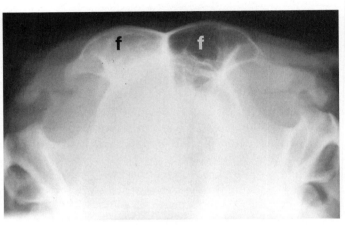

B

Figure 5–36. An 11-year-old male mixed breed dog with exudate from the right nostril for 3 weeks. (A) The open-mouth ventrodorsal view revealed a homogeneous tissue density involving the caudal half of the right nasal passage. The vomer was intact and no evidence of bony destruction was present. The areas of the right frontal sinuses that are not superimposed over the nasal passages (*black f*) also revealed tissue density as compared with the left side (*white f*). (B) The frontal sinus view revealed the tissue density in the right frontal sinus (*black f*) as compared to the normal left side (*white f*). Differential diagnoses include rhinitis/sinusitis or neoplasia. **Diagnosis:** Rhinitis and sinusitis of the right nasal passages and sinuses.

with bacterial rhinitis, the nasal turbinates appear normal because the exudate drains to the outside and does not accumulate in the nasal cavity. Obstruction to drainage will result in fluid accumulation within the nasal passages and will obliterate some of the fine turbinate pattern. In chronic cases, destruction or obliteration of the larger turbinates may be observed. Fungal rhinitis may present with radiographic changes that are similar to those observed in association with bacterial rhinitis; however, marked bone destruction with minimal exudate is more common, especially in chronic cases. Destruction of the turbinates occurs and the vomer or nasal bones may be partially or completely destroyed. The destroyed turbinate is not replaced with soft tissue, resulting in a pattern that has been described as hyperlucent nasal passages (Fig. 5–37).[55] Bilateral destructive rhinitis, which does not destroy or deviate the vomer, is more typical of fungal rhinitis than neoplasia.

Rhinitis and sinusitis of allergic and/or parasitic origin rarely produce radiographic changes. Although turbinate destruction was reported in association with *Capillaria* sinusitis, this amount of turbinate destruction is unusual.[32]

Neoplasia

Neoplasia involving the nasal passages may present with accumulation of tissue density within the normally air-filled nasal passages. These radiographic changes are similar to those observed with bacterial or fungal infection. In many cases of neoplasia, there is invasion into the nasal bones, maxillae, or frontal sinuses with bony destruction.[53–55,62] Destruction of the maxilla or frontal bone with extension of the soft tissue mass outside the nasal cavity is more typical of nasal tumor than destructive (fungal) rhinitis. Occasionally, new bone formation may be present within the nasal cavity. A pattern of punctate, stippled, or globular calcification may be observed in nasal chondrosarcoma. However, because several tumor types occur in the nasal cavity and most have no unique radiographic characteristic, it is only rarely possible to suggest a specific cell type.[53–55,62] Deviation or destruction of the vomer with the pres-

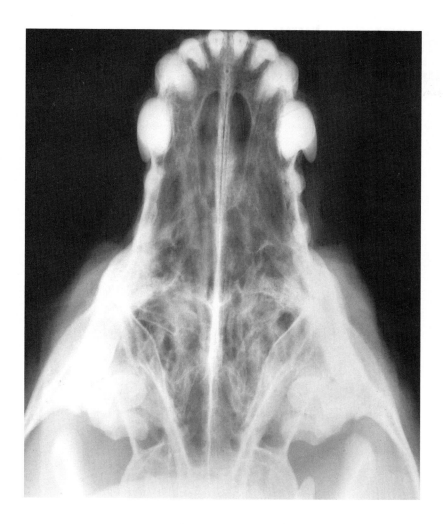

Figure 5–37. A 6-year-old female cocker spaniel with nasal discharge for several months. The open-mouth ventrodorsal radiograph revealed a moderate decrease in the prominence of the intranasal bony structures—this gives the appearance of hyperlucency. The present bony structures appear thickened and coarse. Differential diagnoses include fungal rhinitis or neoplasia. **Diagnosis:** Nasal aspergillosis.

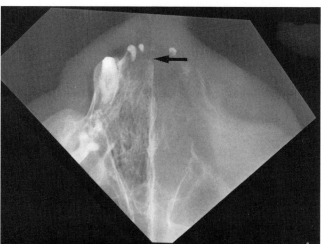

Figure 5–38. A 6-year-old Havana brown cat with bilateral nasal discharge for 3 weeks. The open-mouth ventrodorsal view revealed obliteration of air passages in the left planum nasale. There is an overall increased tissue density in the left nasal passages. All incisive and maxillary teeth are absent except for the second incisor. The vomer, which is normally apparent to the level of the rostral border of the incisive bones, has been destroyed in its most rostral aspect (*white arrow*). Differential diagnoses include nasal neoplasia or infection. **Diagnosis:** Nasal fibrous histiocytoma.

ence of tissue density in the nasal passages strongly suggests the presence of a neoplasm (Fig. 5–38). Destructive (fungal) rhinitis may also cause destruction of the vomer; however, when a tumor is present the tissue density within the nasal cavity will be contiguous at the site of vomer destruction. In destructive rhinitis, the erosion or deviation of the vomer may be present without an adjacent soft tissue density or mass. Erosion or destruction of the cribriform plate or frontal bones suggests a probable diagnosis of nasal adenocarcinoma with extension of tumor into the cranial vault (Fig. 5–39). Detecting the erosion may be difficult unless it is extensive. Computed or linear tomography and MRI are more sensitive in detecting small erosions, and these studies can be performed in addition to the radiographs if extension of the tumor into the cranial vault is suspected. Affected animals may present with seizures or other primary neurologic signs rather than showing signs of nasal disease.[64] Nasal tumors may also penetrate the nasal and maxillary bones resulting in a mass dorsal to the nasal passages (Fig. 5–40). In some cases, the tumor may penetrate the maxilla and extend to the retrobulbar space causing exophthalmos; this may be the clinical feature that is first noticed by the owner. The presence of soft tissue density within the frontal sinuses in animals with nasal cavity tumors rarely indicates the presence of tumor within the frontal sinus. The opacity usually results from obstruction to normal sinus drainage.

Nasal Hemorrhage

Nasal hemorrhage may occur as a result of bleeding diatheses, trauma, or vascular erosion caused by infection or neoplasia. The resulting tissue density in the nasal passages (one or both) is indistinguishable from the radiographic pattern that results from exudate accumulation or from neoplastic involvement without turbinate destruction. In most patients with nasal hemorrhage there is little accumulation of blood within the nasal cavity and the turbinates will appear normal.

Trauma

Fractures of the maxilla are the most common sequelae to nasal cavity trauma. Fracture fragments may be minimally displaced and may be evident as lucent lines within

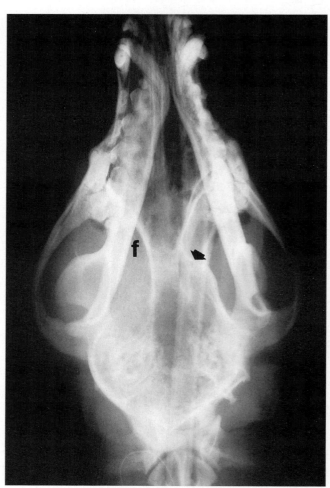

Figure 5–39. A 4-year-old male West Highland white terrier with occasional seizures for 2 months. The ventrodorsal radiograph revealed a tissue density in the caudal portion of the right nasal passages and frontal sinus (*f*). Scrutiny, i.e., comparison of the presence of the left frontal bone (*arrow*) with the opposite side, revealed lysis of the right frontal bone suggesting tumor penetration into the cranial vault. Differential diagnoses include nasal neoplasia or cranial neoplasia. **Diagnosis:** Nasal adenocarcinoma with extension into the cranial vault.

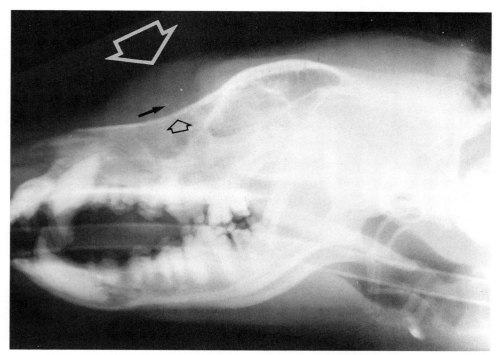

Figure 5–40. An 11-year-old male German shepherd dog with a soft tissue mass rostral to and involving the right eye. The lateral radiograph revealed a large tissue density mass in the area cranial to the eyes (*open white arrow*). Scrutiny revealed some loss of bone density in the maxillae (*open black arrow*) and a fine linear periosteal response dorsal to the maxillae (small white arrow). Differential diagnoses include nasal tumor with extension, primary bone tumor of the maxilla, or metastatic neoplasia. **Diagnosis:** Nasal adenocarcinoma with extension through the maxillae.

the bone. Displaced fractures may overlap and produce a radiodense rather than a radiolucent line. If the fracture completely encircles the nasal passages there may be complete detachment of the nose from the remainder of the skull. With fractures of the frontal sinuses, the fragments may be depressed into the sinuses. These may form sequestra and removal of the fragment may become necessary. All fractures into the sinuses should be considered open because they communicate with the outside. Tooth root involvement should be identified at the time of the initial injury because periapical abscessation could develop. Hemorrhage may accompany the fracture producing a soft tissue density within the nasal cavity or frontal sinus. Complete evaluation of nasal cavity fractures often requires multiple oblique views.

Foreign Bodies

Radiopaque foreign bodies, such as wires, bullets, or metal fragments, are easily detected. Bone-dense foreign objects, such as chicken bones, may be more difficult to detect because of the overlying shadows of the skull bones. Radiolucent foreign objects, such as grass, straw, or plant awns, cannot be detected on noncontrast radiographs. They may produce no radiographic changes if the exudate drains completely, may produce a soft tissue density if the exudate accumulates or if there is a focal granulomatous reaction, or (rarely) may cause turbinate destruction. The radiographic changes are unilateral unless the foreign body has migrated or been iatrogenically displaced from one side to the other. Endoscopy may be helpful in identifying the foreign object. Flushing the nasal cavity with saline may dislodge a foreign body.

Computed Tomography and Magnetic Resonance Imaging

CT is extremely valuable for the assessment of lesions of the nasal cavity.[69–71] The dorsal imaging plane has been recommended as being more accurate for assessing lesions within the cribriform plate when compared to the transverse plane.[72] CT has been shown to be more sensitive and more accurate than either radiography or linear tomography for detecting lesions of the cribriform plate.[29] CT has been compared to radiography for the evaluation of nasal tumors.[73] Although CT was more accurate in delineating tumor extent and in documenting tumor extension into adjacent structures, such as the palate and the cranial cavity, the tumor could be identified correctly on the radiographs. CT is useful for tumor staging and planning of radiation therapy or surgery. Destruction of ethmoids, extension of soft tissue into the retrobulbar area, destruction of the maxilla or nasal bone, or hyperostosis of the maxilla were identified in CT scans of dogs with nasal tumors.[70] In CT scans obtained following intravenous contrast injection, patchy areas of increased density (possibly due to contrast enhancement) were observed. Infection resulted in cavitating lesions, which thickened and distorted the turbinates.[71] No single finding or combination of findings was specific for tumor. MRI produces similar information. The soft tissue changes are better defined with MRI, and the bony lesions are better defined with CT. The extent of the tumor mass within the nasal cavity, the presence of exudate within the frontal sinus, and spread of the tumor to the brain are all easily identified with MRI.

TEETH

Inflammation and Infection

There are changes in the teeth and surrounding alveolar bone that should be recognized in order to distinguish normal aging changes from dental disease. The size of the pulp cavity is large in young animals and becomes small and nearly disappears in old dogs. Reabsorption of alveolar bone both vertically (along the tooth axis) and horizontally (along the axis of the mandible or maxilla) is a common finding in older dogs. Hypercementosis or deposition of excessive amounts of secondary cementum on the tooth roots resulting in root thickening and bulbous apical enlargement of the tooth roots is an uncommon but normal aging change.[9]

The most common problems that affect teeth result from inflammation and infection. Periodontal disease is common and may cause focal or generalized loss of

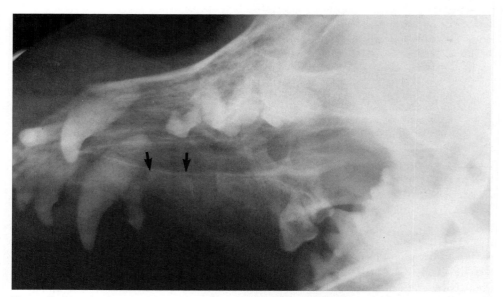

Figure 5–41. An 8-year-old male cocker spaniel with halitosis. Physical examination revealed active gingivitis. The lateral oblique radiograph isolated the left maxilla and revealed resorption of alveolar bone from the area around the first premolar and the area of absence of the second, third, and fourth premolars. Close scrutiny revealed the presence of root tips embedded in the bone where the teeth were missing. There are indistinct zones of lysis around these roots (*black arrows*) indicating the presence of active infection. **Diagnosis:** Gingivitis and osteomyelitis.

alveolar bone. In most instances, the radiograph underestimates the extent of the bony lesion. Periodontal disease is classified in five stages based on the degree of clinical and radiographic changes. Stages I and II have no radiographic changes. In stage III the alveolar crest becomes indistinct and rounded. In stage IV there is destruction of bone between the tooth roots. Further loss of bone is indicative of stage V disease.[3] The margins of the bone usually are smooth and regular with normal cortical density. Gingivitis may occur secondary to the presence of tooth root fragments retained from inadequate tooth extraction or fracturing of teeth below the gum line (Fig. 5–41). Untreated or chronic gingivitis predisposes to periodontitis, which is inflammation of the soft tissue structures adjacent to and supporting the teeth. This condition results in inflammation of the periodontal ligament, which causes resorption of the walls of the alveolus, destruction of the periodontal ligament and adjacent bone, and ultimately results in the loosening of the tooth (Fig. 5–42). In some instances of chronic infection, there may be partial resorption of the tooth root and/or enlargement of the bony alveolus (Fig. 5–43). Another manifestation of infection is abscess formation at the tip of the tooth root—the periapical abscess. This is radiographically seen as a focal loss of bone density with variable degrees of sclerosis at the borders of the lesion (Fig. 5–44). In severe cases there may be extension

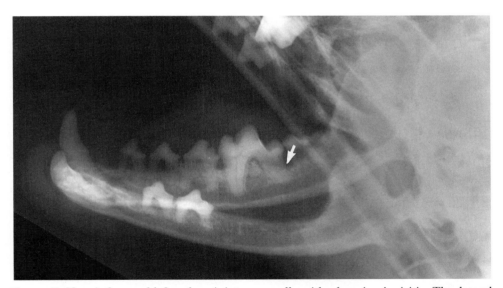

Figure 5–42. A 6-year-old female miniature poodle with chronic gingivitis. The lateral oblique radiograph, isolating the right mandible, revealed generalized resorption of bone from the mandible. This is particularly prominent between the teeth and around the roots (*white arrow*). **Diagnosis:** Gingivitis and periodontitis.

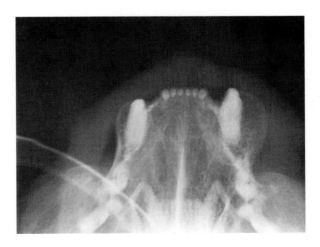

Figure 5–43. A 7-year-old female domestic short-haired cat with a swelling around the root of the left canine tooth. The open-mouth ventrodorsal view revealed a large bony mass involving the maxilla in the area of the alveolus for the canine tooth root. The left canine tooth is displaced cranially and the root is shortened. These findings are consistent with chronic infection within the alveolus. **Diagnosis:** Chronic infection causing lysis of the root tip and expansion of the alveolar bone of the left canine tooth.

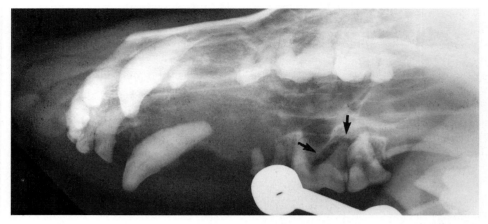

Figure 5–44. A 9-year-old neutered female cocker spaniel with reluctance to eat and drooling for 3 weeks. The lateral oblique radiograph, isolating the right maxilla, revealed a large area of bony lysis involving the maxilla from the canine tooth to the fourth premolar. It also revealed a focal area of lysis around the caudal root of the fourth premolar (*black arrows*). Differential diagnoses for the major lesion include squamous cell carcinoma, primary bone tumor, melanoma, or metastatic tumor. **Diagnosis:** Squamous cell carcinoma of the rostral maxilla and periapical abscess of the caudal root of the fourth premolar.

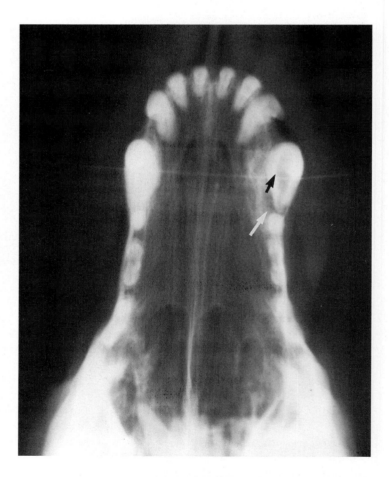

Figure 5–45. A 5-year-old female German shepherd dog with excessive salivation. The open-mouth ventrodorsal view revealed an enlarged pulp canal of the left canine tooth (*black arrow*) when compared with the right canine tooth. The tooth alveolus is also slightly enlarged (*white arrow*). The adhesive tape that was used in positioning is also seen. Differential diagnoses include infection or neoplasia. **Diagnosis:** Pulpal and periapical abscess. (Radiograph courtesy of Dr. A. Karmin, Bellerose Animal Hospital, Bellerose, NY).

of the infection into the nasal cavity or spread of infection diffusely into the supporting bone. A less common manifestation of infection is the pulp abscess, where infection is contained within the pulp cavity of the tooth. This is seen radiographically as an enlarged pulp cavity (Fig. 5–45). Necrosis of the pulp cavity may produce a dense, bony reaction adjacent to the apex of the tooth root. This has been referred to as condensing osteitis.[3]

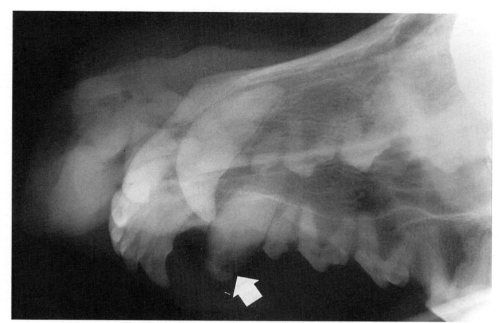

Figure 5–46. A 6-year-old male cocker spaniel with a fractured canine tooth was examined for consideration of restorative dentistry. The lateral oblique view, isolating the left maxilla, revealed the fractured crown of the left canine tooth (*white arrow*). There was no evidence of lysis of the root canal or periodontal or periapical areas. **Diagnosis:** Fractured left maxillary canine tooth crown without complication.

Although uncommon in dogs and cats, dental cavities (caries) appear more often than usually believed in cats. Unlike those seen in humans, which usually affect the crown of the tooth, caries in cats usually occur at the junction of the gum and tooth or slightly below the gum line.[74] Dental caries will appear as small radiolucent defects in the enamel. Defects in the teeth may also be present due to trauma in which part or all of the crown fractures (Fig. 5–46). These defects may predispose to periapical abscess formation. Tooth fractures may also occur below the gum line.

ULTRASOUND OF OCULAR ABNORMALITIES

Ultrasound is not needed in most animals with an ocular abnormality because the lesion can be seen with an ophthalmoscope. When the cornea or lens is opaque, ultrasound can be used to examine the eye.[20,21,24] Even when a mass can be seen during an ocular examination, an ultrasound examination is still useful because it provides information about the structures behind the mass and will more completely define the posterior extent of the mass (Fig. 5–47).

Foreign objects within the eye can be detected despite the presence of hemorrhage or inflammation, which would interfere with a direct examination. These objects usually are hyperechoic and have distant shadowing. Radiopaque foreign objects can be detected radiographically, however defining their exact position within the globe is difficult. The ultrasound examination will locate the exact position of the foreign body and will indicate whether it is in the globe or retrobulbar. Eye injury secondary to foreign body penetration can be evaluated (Fig. 5–48).

Masses that arise from the iris can be identified during an ultrasound examination and their extent can be defined. Most masses are heteroechoic and fixed in position. Iris and ciliary cysts are either attached to the iris or ciliary body or floating in the anterior chamber and usually can be detected during an ocular examination.[75] These cysts are filled with fluid and have a thin wall. Most cysts can be differentiated from tumors during the physical examination because the cysts can be transilluminated while the tumors are opaque. Cysts that are associated with the posterior surface of the iris may be more difficult to differentiate from tumors and, therefore, ultrasound

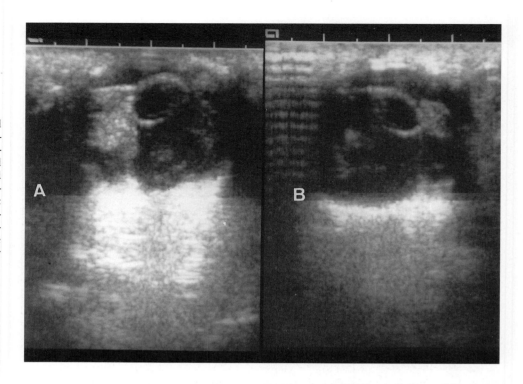

Figure 5–47. Longitudinal (A) and transverse (B) sonograms of the right eye of a 10-year-old castrated male pit bull who presented with uveitis and glaucoma of 1 month's duration. There is a heteroechoic mass noted dorsal (A) and lateral (B) to the lens. This represents a tumor arising from the ciliary body. **Diagnosis:** Ciliary carcinoma.

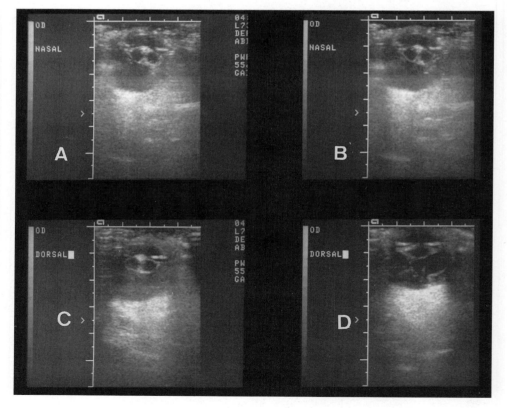

Figure 5–48. Longitudinal (A&B) and transverse (C&D) sonograms of the right eye of an 8-year-old male cocker spaniel with a history of perforating ocular injury that occurred 1 week previously. There are hyperechoic lesions involving the anterior and posterior portions of the lens. These lesions appear to touch in the central portion of the lens. These represent scars from perforation of the lens secondary to a penetrating ocular foreign body. A shotgun pellet was identified radiographically in the retrobulbar tissues. **Diagnosis:** Scar in the lens secondary to penetrating foreign body.

can be used to identify the anechoic cystic nature of these lesions. Blood clots or cellular debris may also be present within the eye. They may be less well defined than tumors or granulomas and may move during the ultrasound examination. These lesions are often heteroechoic. They may be fixed in position, making discrimination among organized hematoma, granuloma, and tumor impossible.

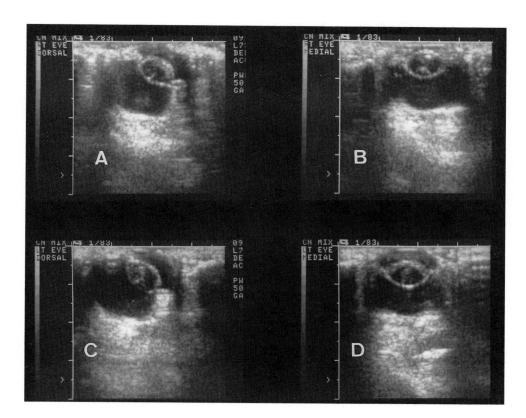

Figure 5–49. Transverse (A& C) and longitudinal (B&D) sonograms of the right (A&B) and left (C&D) eyes of a 10-year-old male mixed breed dog with a history of bilateral cataracts and asymmetrical ERG's. The lenses are echogenic with prominent lens capsules. This is indicative of bilateral cataracts. There is no evidence of retinal detachment. **Diagnosis:** Cataracts.

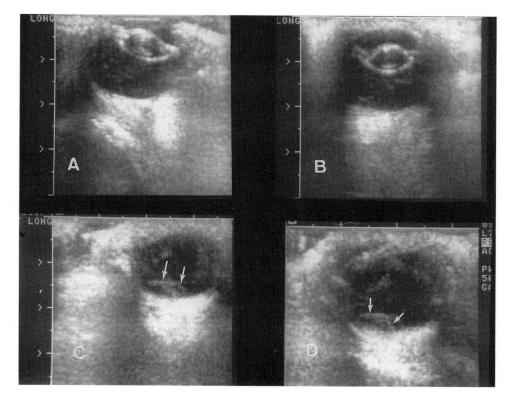

Figure 5–50. Longitudinal sonograms of the left eye of an 11-year-old female mixed breed dog who presented for preoperative evaluation of bilateral cataracts. The lens capsule is thickened and there is increased echogenicity in the lens. There is nonstructured echogenic material within the vitreous chamber. A curvilinear echogenic structure is located in the caudal medial aspect of the vitreous (*arrows*). This represents a small retinal detachment. **Diagnosis:** Retinal detachment, vitreal debris or degeneration, cataract.

The lens can be examined using ultrasound. Although this is rarely required for evaluating cataracts, it is important to examine the eye for retinal detachment prior to cataract removal.[24] A mature cataract will result in a lens that is highly echogenic, and the internal echoes from the cataract will be seen (Figs. 5–49 and 5–50). With hypermature cataracts the lens may appear thinner than normal. Luxation of the lens may also be detected (Fig. 5–51).

Retinal detachment can be detected during an ultrasound examination of the eye. A thin, echogenic line will be seen separated from the surface of the globe. The line often assumes a "sea gull" or "V" shape, with the point of the "V" attached at the optic disc. Incomplete retinal detachment may appear as a curved echogenic line separated from the globe. The detached retina may move slightly or float within the vitreous (Fig. 5–52). The space behind the retina may be anechoic, hypoechoic, or filled with echogenic cells. The major differentials for retinal detachment are the presence of a vitreous membrane or fibrous strands within the vitreous. A vitreal

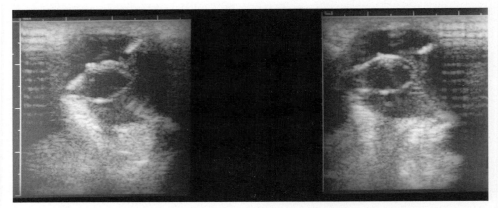

Figure 5–51. Transverse sonograms of the right eye of a 3-year-old spayed female cat with a history of glaucoma and uveitis of 2 week's duration. The eye is enlarged and the lens is luxated posteriorly. **Diagnosis:** Luxation of the lens, glaucoma.

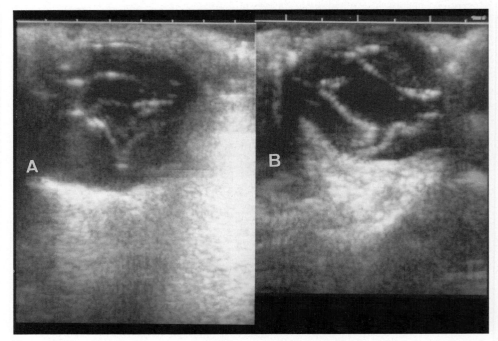

Figure 5–52. Transverse sonograms of the eyes of a 5-year-old mixed breed male dog who presented for evaluation of glaucoma (A), and of a 3-year-old spayed female mixed breed dog who presented for evaluation of cataract with poor light response (B). A curvilinear echogenic structure is visible in the vitreous chambers in both dogs. This structure can be traced caudally to the region of the optic disc. This represents a detached retina. **Diagnosis:** Retinal detachment.

membrane is a hyperechoic linear structure that may be seen in the vitreous chamber but does not attach to the globe at the optic disc. Fibrous strands may occur following intraocular hemorrhage. These can be distinguished from retinal detachment because they rarely attach at the optic disc.

Asteroid hyalosis may produce multiple echoes within the vitreous chamber (Fig. 5–53). Vitreous degeneration produces multiple echogenic lines or areas within the vitreous.

ULTRASOUND OF THE RETROBULBAR AREA

Ultrasound is useful for examining the retrobulbar area.[23] The exam may be performed by placing the transducer on the cornea and imaging the retrobulbar area through the eye. The transducer may also be positioned dorsal to the zygomatic arch and caudal to the eye to examine the retrobulbar area directly. Both transverse and longitudinal planes should be used. The area behind the eye usually is uniformly heteroechoic. Lesions may be hyperechoic or hypoechoic and diffuse or well defined. Distinction between tumor and inflammation is difficult.[23] Both tumors and abscesses may be well- or poorly defined (Figs. 5–53 and 5–54). Deformity of the globe may be identified. In addition to permitting identification of the mass, an ultrasound examination also helps guide needle aspiration or biopsy.[23]

Retrobulbar foreign bodies can be identified. They usually are hyperechoic and have shadowing deep to them. Hypoechoic zones may be identified if there is inflammation or abscess formation around the foreign body.

COMPUTED TOMOGRAPHY AND MAGNETIC RESONANCE OF THE ORBIT

CT has been used to evaluate the orbital structures of the dog. The infraorbital fat contrasts with the extraocular muscles and nerves and intracranial extension of an

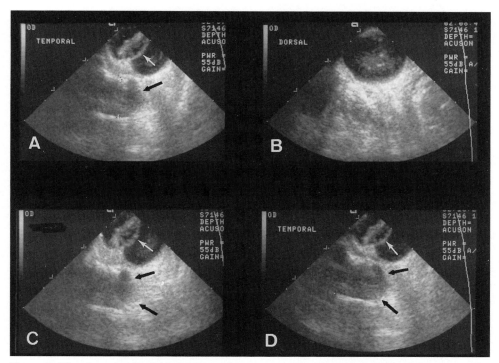

Figure 5–53. Longitudinal (A,C,&D) and transverse (B) sonograms of the right eye of a 12-year-old spayed female mixed breed dog with a history of exophthalmos and retrobulbar swelling of 3 week's duration. There is a hypoechoic irregularly shaped mass in the retrobulbar space (*black arrows*). This represents a retrobulbar tumor or abscess. There is irregularly shaped echogenic material in the vitreous chamber (*white arrows*). This is indicative of asteroid hyalosis. **Diagnosis:** Retrobulbar carcinoma.

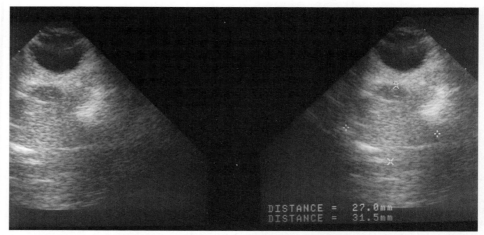

Figure 5–54. Longitudinal sonograms of the left eye of a 7-year-old male English Springer spaniel with a history of conjunctivitis and buphthalmos. There is an irregularly shaped hypoechoic mass in the retrobulbar space. This may represent a tumor or abscess. **Diagnosis:** Retrobulbar squamous cell carcinoma.

orbital mass can be detected easily.[76,77] MRI also can be used for examination of the eye and orbit. Good anatomic detail is produced. Ultrasound is less expensive, more readily available, and provides similar information. These techniques are all superior to contrast orbitography.

COMPUTED TOMOGRAPHY AND MAGNETIC RESONANCE IMAGING OF THE BRAIN

The brain can be evaluated using either CT or MRI. Technique selection is based mainly on availability, however MRI usually is preferred for evaluation of the human brain. There are many references describing both techniques and these should be consulted if imaging of the brain is desired.[78–81] High contrast landmarks, such as cerebrospinal fluid and bony structures, are important in identifying brain structures using CT. CT is useful in identifying neoplastic and inflammatory brain diseases in dogs and cats.[81] It provides information relative to lesion size, location, and character and defines the relationship between brain lesions and normal structures of the calvarium. Similar changes were noted in tumors and inflammatory lesions. These changes included enlargement or asymmetry of the ventricles, midline shift of the falx, edema, focal changes in opacity of the brain (both pre- and post-contrast administration), periventricular contrast enhancement, and ring-like enhancement of brain lesions. Only one of the inflammatory lesions described was multifocal.

MRI provides more anatomic information regarding the brain. Differentiation between white and gray matter is superior in MRI when compared to CT. Differentiation between neoplastic and inflammatory lesions is difficult.

Radiographic contrast often is administered during the CT examination, and paramagnetic contrast agents are used during MRI exams to enhance identification of lesions. Both radiographic contrast and paramagnetic contrast agents can cross a disrupted blood-brain barrier and this will increase the visibility of many lesions.

Quantitative CT, which utilizes radiographic contrast and quantitates the rate of contrast accumulation and washout, has been used in order to differentiate between inflammatory and neoplastic brain lesions. The value of this technique is questionable.[82,83]

REFERENCES

1. Kus SP, Morgan JP. Radiography of the canine head. Optimal positioning with respect to skull type. Vet Radiol 1985;26:196.

2. Burk RL, Corwin LA, Zimmerman D. Use of a modified occipital view for radiographic examination of the skull. VMSAC 1978;73:460.
3. Bellows J. Radiographic signs and diagnosis of dental disease. Semin Vet Med Surg 1993;8:138.
4. Emily PE. Intraoral radiology. VCNA 1986;2:801.
5. SanRoman F, Llorens MP, Pena MT, Garcia FA, Prandi D. Dental radiography in the dog with a conventional x-ray device. Vet Radiol 1990;31:235.
6. Harvey CE. The nasal septum of the dog: Is it visible radiographically? Vet Radiol 1979;20:88.
7. Evans HE, Christensen GC. Miller's anatomy of the dog. 2nd ed. Philadelphia: WB Saunders Co, 1979.
8. Zontine WJ. Dental radiographic technique and interpretation. VCNA 1974;4:741.
9. Morgan JP, Miyabayashi T. Dental radiology: Aging changes in permanent teeth of beagle dogs. JSAP 1991;32:11.
10. Oliver JE. Cranial sinus venography in the dog. JAVRS 1969;10:66.
11. Harvey CE. Sialography in the dog. JAVRS 1969;10:18.
12. Munger RJ, Ackerman N. Retrobulbar injections in the dog: A comparison of three techniques. JAAHA 1978;14:490.
13. Dorn AS. A Standard technique for canine cerebral angiography. JAVMA 1972;161:12.
14. Gillette EL, Thrall DE, Lebel JE. Carlson's veterinary radiology. Philadelphia: Lea and Febiger, 1977.
15. Ticer JW. Radiographic technique in veterinary practice. 2nd ed. Philadelphia: WB Saunders Co, 1984.
16. Goring RL, Ticer JW, Gross TL, Ackerman N. Positive-contrast rhinography. A technique for radiographic evaluation of the nasal cavity, nasal pharynx, and paranasal sinuses in the dog. Vet Radiol 1984;25:98.
17. Goring RL, Ticer JW, Ackerman N, Gross TL. Contrast rhinography in the radiographic evaluation of diseases affecting the nasal cavity, nasopharynx, and paranasal sinuses in the dog. Vet Radiol 1984;25:106.
18. Voorhout G. Cisternography combined with linear tomography for visualization of the pituitary gland in healthy dogs. Vet Radiol 1990;31:68.
19. Voorhout G, Rijnberk A. Cisternography combined with linear tomography for visualization of pituitary lesions in dogs with pituitary-dependent hyperadrenocorticism. Vet Radiol 1990;31:74.
20. Hager DA, Dziezyc J, Millichamp NJ. Two-dimensional real-time ocular ultrasonography in the dog: Technique and normal anatomy. Vet Radiol 1987;28:60.
21. Dziezyc J, Hager DA, Millichamp NJ. Two-dimensional real-time ocular ultrasonography in the diagnosis of ocular lesions in dogs. AAHA 1987;23:501.
22. Dziezyc J, Hager DA. Ocular ultrasonography in veterinary medicine. Semin Vet Med Surg 1988;3:1.
23. Morgan R. Ultrasonography of retrobulbar diseases of the dog and cat. JAAHA 1989;25:393.
24. van der Woerdt A, Wilkie DA, Myer W. Ultrasonographic abnormalities in the eyes of dogs with cataracts: 147 cases (1986–1992). JAVMA 1993;203;838.
25. Hudson JA, Cartee RE, Simpson ST, Buxton DF. Ultrasonographic anatomy of the canine brain. Vet Radiol 1989;30:13.
26. Hudson JA, Simpson ST, Buxton DF, Cartee RE, Steiss JE. Ultrasonographic diagnosis of canine hydrocephalus. Vet Radiol 1990;31:50.
27. Spaulding KA, Sharp NJH. Ultrasonographic imaging of the lateral cerebral ventricles in the dog. Vet Radiol 1990;31:59.
28. Hudson JA, Simpson ST, Cox NR, Buxton DF. Ultrasonographic examination of the normal canine neonatal brain. Vet Radiol 1991;32:50.
29. Berry CR, Koblik PD. Evaluation of survey radiography, linear tomography, and computed tomography for detecting experimental lesions of the cribriform plate in dogs. Vet Radiol 1990;31:146.
30. Straw RC, LeCouteur RA, Powers BE, Winthrow SJ. Multilobular osteochondrosarcoma of the canine skull: 16 cases (1978–1988). JAVMA 1989;195:1764.
31. Groff JM, Murphy CJ, Pool RR, Koblik P, Bellhorn R. Orbital multilobular tumor of bone in a dog. JSAP 1992;33:587.
32. Lawson C, Burk RL, Prata RG. Cerebral meningioma in the cat: Diagnosis and surgical treatment of ten cases. JAAHA 1984;20:333.
33. Frew DG, Dobson JM. Radiological assessment of 50 cases of incisive or maxillary neoplasia in the dog. JSAP 1992;33:11.
34. Ticer JW, Spencer CP. Injury of the feline temporomandibular joint: Radiographic signs. Vet Radiol 1978;19:146.
35. Lane JG, Watkins PE. Para-aural abscess in the dog and cat. JSAP 1986;27:521.
36. Bradley RL. Selected oral, pharyngeal, and upper respiratory conditions in the cat: Oral tumors, nasopharyngeal and middle ear polyps, and chronic rhinitis and sinusitis. VCNA 1984;14:1173.
37. Parker AJ, Park RD. Occipital dysplasia in the dog. JAAHA 1974;10:520.
38. Simoens P, Poels P, Lauwers H. Morphometric analysis of the foramen magnum in Pekingese dogs. AJVR 1994;55:34.
39. Peterson ME, Taylor RS, Greco DS, Nelson RW, Randolph JF, Foodman MS, Moroff SD, et al. Acromegaly in 14 cats. JVIM 1990;4:192.
40. Eigenmann JE, Venker-van Haagen AJ. Progesterone-induced and spontaneous canine acromegaly due a reversible growth hormone over production: Clinical picture and pathogenesis. JAAHA 1981;17:813.
41. Crowell KR, et al. Muccopolysaccharidosis in a cat. JAVMA 1976;169:334.
42. Langweiler M, Haskins ME, Jezyk PF. Mucopolysaccharidosis in a litter of cats. JAAHA 1978;14:748.
43. Haskins ME, Jezyk PF, Desnick RJ, McDonough SK, Patterson DF. Mucopolysaccharidosis in a domestic cat—A disease distinct from that seen in the siamese cat. JAVMA 1979;175:384.
44. Konde LJ, Thrall MA, Gasper P, Dial SM, McBiles K, Colgan S, Haskins M. Radiographically visualized skeletal changes associated with mucopolysaccharidosis VI in cats. Vet Radiol 1987;28:223.

45. Shull RM, Walker MA. Radiographic findings in a canine model of mucopolysaccharidosis I changes associated with bone marrow transplantation. Invest Radiol 1988;23:124.
46. Riser WH, Parkes LJ, Shirer JF. Canine craniomandibular osteopathy. JAVRS 1967;8:23.
47. Morgan JP. Radiology in veterinary orthopedics. Philadelphia: Lea and Febiger, 1972.
48. Padgett GA, Mostosky UV. Animal model: The mode of inheritance of craniomandibular osteopathy in west highland white terrier dogs. Am J Med Genet 1986;25:9.
49. Robbins G, Grandage J. Temporomandibular joint dysplasia and open-mouth jaw locking in the dog. JAVMA 1977;171:1072.
50. Lantz GC, Cantwell HD. Intermittent open-mouth lower jaw locking in five dogs. JAVMA 1986;188:1403.
51. Hazelwinkel HA, Koole R, Voorhout G. Mandibular coronoid process displacement: Signs, causes, treatment. VCOT 1993;6:29.
52. McNeel SV. Radiology of the skull and cervical spine. VCNA 1982;12:259.
53. Morgan JP, Suter PF, O'Brien TR, Park RD. Tumors of the nasal cavity of the dog. A radiographic study. JAVRS 1972;13:18.
54. Gibbs C, Lane JG, Denny HR. Radiological features of intranasal lesions in the dog: A review of 100 cases. JSAP 1979;20:515.
55. Harvey CE, Biery DN, Morello J, O'Brien JA. Chronic nasal disease in the dog: Its radiographic diagnosis. Vet Radiol 1979;20:91.
56. King RR, Greiner EC, Ackerman N, Woodard JC. Nasal capillariasis in a dog. JAAHA 1990;26:381.
57. Campbell BG, Little MD. Identification of the eggs of a nematode (*Eucoleus boehmi*) from the nasal mucosa of North American dogs. JAVMA 1991;198:1520.
58. Blagburn BL, et al. Canine linguatulosis. Canine Pract 1983;10:54.
59. Bedford PG. Diseases of the nose and throat. In: Ettinger SJ, ed. Textbook of veterinary internal medicine. Philadelphia: WB Saunders Co, 1989.
60. Allison N, Willard MD, Bentinck-Smith J, Davis K. Nasal rhinosporidiosis in two dogs. JAVMA 1986;188:869.
61. Norris AM. Intranasal neoplasms in the dog. JAAHA 1979;15:231.
62. Madewell BR, Priester WA, Gillette EL, et al. Neoplasms of the nasal passage and paranasal sinuses in domestic animals as reported by 13 veterinary colleges. AJVR 1976;37:851.
63. Beck ER, Winthrow SJ. Tumors of the canine nasal cavity. VCNA 1985;15:521.
64. Smith MO, Turrel JM, Bailey CS, Cain GR. Neurologic abnormalities as the predominant signs of neoplasia of the nasal cavity in dogs and cats: Seven cases (1973–1986). JAVMA 1989;195:242.
65. Cox NR, Brawner WR, Powers RD, Wright JC. Tumors of the nose and paranasal sinuses in cats: 32 cases with comparison to a national database (1977–1987). JAAHA 1991;27:339.
66. Schmidt M, Voorhout G. Radiography of the canine nasal cavity: Significance of the presence or absence of the trabecular pattern. Vet Radiol Ultrasound 1992;33:83.
67. Stowater JL. Kartagener's syndrome in a dog. JAVRS 1976;17:174.
68. Breitschwerdt EB, Brown TT, DeBuysscher EV, Andersen BR, Thrall DE, Hager E, Ananaba G, et al. Rhinitis, pneumonia, and defective neutrophil function in the doberman pincher. AJVR 1987;48:1054.
69. Burk RL. Computed tomographic anatomy of the canine nasal passages. Vet Radiol Ultrasound 1992;33:170.
70. Burk RL. Computed tomographic imaging of nasal disease in 100 dogs. Vet Radiol Ultrasound 1992;33:177.
71. Codner EC, Lurus AG, Miller JB, Gavin PR, Gallina A, Barbee D. Comparison of computed tomography with radiography as a noninvasive diagnostic technique for chronic nasal disease in dogs. JAVMA 1993;202;1106.
72. Koblik PD, Berry CR. Dorsal plane computed tomographic imaging of the ethmoid region to evaluate chronic nasal disease in the dog. Vet Radiol 1990;31:92.
73. Thrall DE, Robertson ID, McLeod DA, Heidner GL, Hoopes PJ, Page RL. A comparison of radiographic and computed tomographic findings in 31 dogs with malignant nasal cavity tumors. Vet Radiol 1989;30:59.
74. Tholen MA. Concepts in veterinary dentistry. Edwardsville: Veterinary Medicine Publishing Co, 1983.
75. Corcoran KA, Koch SA. Uveal cysts in dogs: 28 cases (1989–1991). JAVMA 1993;203:545.
76. Fike JR, LeCouteur RA, Cann CE. Anatomy of the canine orbital region. Multiplanar imaging by CT. Vet Radiol 1984;25:32.
77. LeCouteur RA, Fike JR, Scagliotti RH, Cann CE. Computed tomography of orbital tumors in the dog. JAVMA 1982;180:910.
78. Fike JR, LeCouteur RA, Cann CE. Anatomy of the brain using high resolution computed tomography. Vet Radiol 1981;22:236.
79. LeCouteur RA, Fike JR, Cann CE, Pedoria VG. Computed tomography of brain tumors in the caudal fossa of the dog. Vet Radiol 1981;22:6.
80. Fike JR, LeCouteur RA, Cann CE, Pflugfelder CM. Computerized tomography of brain tumors of the rostral and middle fossas in the dog. AJVR 1981;42:274.
81. Plummer SB, Wheeler SJ, Thrall DE, Kornegay JN. Computed tomography of primary inflammatory brain disorders in dogs and cats. Vet Radiol Ultrasound 1992;33:307.
82. Fike JR, Cann CE, Beringer WH. Quantitative evaluation of the canine brain using computed tomography. J Comput Assist Tomogr 1982;6:325.
83. Fike JR, Cann CA, Turowski K, Higgins RJ, Turrel JM. Differentiation of neoplastic from non-neoplastic lesions in dog brain using quantitative CT. Vet Radiol 1986;27:121.

Chapter Six

THE SPINE

SURVEY RADIOGRAPHIC TECHNIQUES

Radiography of the spine requires precise positioning; therefore, the patient should be anesthetized. However, when fracture, dislocation, or diskopondylitis is suspected, dorsoventral and lateral survey radiographs may be attempted without anesthesia. In these situations, some degree of malpositioning may be tolerated because the expected lesions usually are not subtle.

Because the x-ray beam diverges, there will be geometric distortion of the disc spaces that are farther away from the central x-ray beam. This change is more apparent when large films are used, because there is greater divergence at the edge of the radiation field. Using smaller cassettes and centering over the area of interest is important, especially when evaluation of disc space width is a primary concern. It is less important when surveying the spine for a site of infection, such as diskopondylitis, or when evaluating the spine for possible fractures.

CERVICAL SPINE

Radiography of the cervical spine requires careful positioning. For a true lateral view, the animal's nose should be slightly elevated and the mandibles should be supported so that they are positioned parallel to the film. As the midcervical area tends to sag toward the film when the animal is in lateral recumbency, a radiolucent material (i.e., roll cotton or foam sponge) must be put under the neck at the level of C4–C7. Similar material should be placed between the forelimbs and beneath the sternum to prevent rotation. The position of the neck should be neutral (i.e., the position it naturally assumes when the animal is anesthetized).

The ventrodorsal view should be taken when the cervical vertebrae are aligned with the thoracic vertebrae. The body should be in perfect ventrodorsal alignment with no tilting to either side. When radiographing the cranial cervical vertebrae for the dorsoventral radiograph, a vertical x-ray beam perpendicular to the table top is used. When radiographing the caudal cervical vertebrae, the x-ray beam should be angled from caudoventral to craniodorsal in order to project the intervertebral disc spaces properly.[1] Muscle spasm may prevent proper positioning; however, diazepam, administered intravenously at a dose of 0.25 mg/kg, will usually relieve the muscle spasm.

An oblique lateral view of the cervical spine is sometimes useful. For this radiographic view, the patient is positioned midway between the ventrodorsal and lateral view with the skull and spine in a straight line. This may be accomplished by elevating the sternum and skull by the means of a wedge-shaped foam sponge. The neural foramina of the "up" side (the left neural foramen on a right recumbent oblique view) will be superimposed over the vertebral bodies and not readily apparent.

THORACIC, THORACOLUMBAR, LUMBAR, AND SACROCOCCYGEAL SPINES

Lateral radiographs of the thoracic, thoracolumbar, lumbar, and sacral spine require external patient support. Because the torso tends to rotate, the ventral-most aspect of the chest becomes closer to the table and film than does the dorsal portion of the chest. To prevent this, a radiolucent material should be placed under the sternum to bring it up to the level of the thoracic vertebrae. In addition, the abdomen should be supported by placing lucent material under its ventral part, and the pelvis should be supported by placing a small amount of radiolucent material between the stifles, causing the femurs to be parallel to the table top.

The ventrodorsal views require the animal to be positioned so that the spine is in a straight line and the sternum is directly over the center of the vertebral column. This is most easily accomplished with sandbags or a Plexiglas cradle supporting the patient on each side of its body.

On occasion, it may be difficult to assess a change on the ventrodorsal view because of superimposed intestinal gas shadows. This may be partially overcome by using a prolonged exposure time and allowing the patient to breathe or mechanically ventilating the patient during the exposure. This will blur the image of the gas-containing structures and will allow the spine to be seen more clearly.

CONTRAST STUDIES

MYELOGRAPHY

A myelogram is performed to opacify the subarachnoid space and thereby delineate the spinal cord. Iohexol, a nonionic contrast material, currently is the most frequently used agent, although both iohexol and iopamidol appear to be equally effective.[2,3] Iohexol is used routinely at a concentration of 240 mg/ml and iopamidol is used at a concentration of 200 mg/ml, although concentrations varying from 180 to 300 mg/ml have been used. The contrast media may be introduced by injection into the subarachnoid space at either the cisterna magna or in the caudal lumbar spine. In most cases, a lumbar injection is performed although some individuals routinely perform cervical punctures. In cats, lumbar puncture was superior to cisternal puncture for evaluation of the thoracolumbar spine, and cisternal puncture was better for evaluation of the cervical spinal cord.[4] The volume of contrast required will vary with the area of interest and site of introduction. If a cervical puncture is used for evaluation of the cervical spinal cord, a dose of 0.3 ml/kg of body weight is recommended. If examination of the lumbar spinal cord also is desired, the contrast dose should be 0.5 ml/kg of body weight. If a lumbar puncture is used, the dose is 0.35 ml/kg body weight for the thoracolumbar region and 0.5 ml/kg for the cervical region. If the patient is grossly under- or overweight for the general body size, the dose should be based upon the ideal body weight. It is possible to influence the distribution of the contrast, which has a specific gravity slightly higher than normal cerebrospinal fluid (CSF), by positioning the patient so that gravity causes the contrast media to move to the area of interest. This can be accomplished by tilting the patient so that the area to which you wish the contrast to flow is dependent; however, in some cases this may require suspending the patient vertically for at least 5 to 10 minutes. In some instances, obstruction to contrast flow cannot be overcome by gravity.

Contrast injection into the subarachnoid space produces alterations in the CSF. These alterations include increased numbers of neutrophils, red blood cells, and total protein, pleocytosis, and a decrease in percentage of mononuclear cells. These changes usually disappear within 24 hours but can persist in some dogs for up to 72 hours.[5]

Because hazards and potential complications can occur, myelography must be performed with great care. Injections via a cisternal puncture risk cervical spinal cord injury. In animals with occipital dysplasia, the cerebellum may be displaced caudally and may be damaged as a result of the puncture. Injection of contrast media in the caudal lumbar subarachnoid space requires puncture of the spinal cord.[6] If performed at the L5–L6 space or at spaces more caudal to L6, there usually is no neurologic sequela. However, puncture cranial to L5–L6 carries a risk of iatrogenic spinal cord trauma.

During myelography, contrast may be injected into the central canal. This usually is an incidental finding; however, if the rate and quantity of contrast injected results in distension of the central canal, a transient exacerbation of the patient's clinical signs may occur.[7] Central canal filling is more likely to occur when the contrast is injected cranial to L5–L6 and when the contrast is injected into the ventral rather than the dorsal subarachnoid space.

If CSF puncture is successful, there are other risks and complications to consider. Bradycardia, arrhythmias, and apnea may occur during the contrast injection. These are unrelated to the amount of contrast or site of injection and are usually transient; however, careful monitoring of the patient during the contrast injection is essential. A major source of morbidity is the development of seizures in the patient when awakened from anesthesia. While this is much less common with nonionic contrast media, it remains a possible complication. Seizures are most often observed following cervical myelograms in large dogs and when the duration of anesthesia that follows the myelogram is short.[3] Most of the post-myelographic seizures can be controlled with valium but post-myelogram deaths have occurred. Other post-myelogram changes that can occur include hyperthermia, depression, and worsening of the original neurologic problem. Exacerbation of the neurologic signs may be due to the myelogram; however, the effects of positioning for the CSF puncture and for the radiographs has also been blamed.

Because of the possible myelographic complications the technique should be used cautiously. We recommend that it not be performed unless surgery or another definitive treatment is being considered. In those cases where a diagnosis might allow an owner to make a decision concerning the future for the pet, myelography is worth the risks.

LUMBAR SINUS VENOGRAPHY

Lumbar sinus venography is performed occasionally to evaluate structures within the lumbosacral spinal canal in patients suspected of having cauda equina compression. While several methods have been described, the easiest method is performed by placing a bone marrow needle into the body of L7 or one of the rostral caudal vertebrae.[8–10] When a caudal vertebra is used, a belly band may be placed tightly to occlude the caudal vena cava and to increase filling of the venous sinus. Contrast media injected through the needle then flows through the ventral venous sinuses allowing evaluation of their shape and integrity. This procedure requires careful technique and frequently is difficult to interpret. Extravasation of contrast into the epidural space or into the surrounding soft tissue may occur. This produces no adverse effect but makes interpretation of the study more difficult.[9]

EPIDUROGRAPHY

Epidurography has been advocated for evaluation of the cauda equina in animals suspected of having cauda equina compression. Nonionic contrast is injected directly into the epidural space, usually at the level of the caudal vertebra.[11,12] Irregular filling of the epidural space occurs, which makes it difficult to evaluate the radiographs. Some individuals have had a lot of experience performing and interpreting these studies, and in their hands the technique is useful. Similar information can be obtained by myelography, lumbar sinus venography, computed tomography (CT), and magnetic resonance imaging (MRI). The preference as to which technique is used is often based on availability of the equipment, personal experience, and training.

DISCOGRAPHY

Nonionic contrast material may be injected directly into the intervertebral disc space (using a 20- or 22-gauge spinal needle) to demonstrate prolapse of the intervertebral disc.[12] This technique requires fluoroscopic control of the injection, and although it can be useful, it is invasive, of limited value, and not often recommended. The procedure has been used for the evaluation of disc prolapse. Dorsal extension of the contrast material into the spinal canal or injection of more than 0.3 ml into the disc were considered evidence of disc prolapse.[12] Discography combined with epidurography was recommended for evaluation of dogs with cauda equina compression.

ULTRASOUND

Ultrasound is not often useful for evaluation of the vertebral column. The lumbar disc spaces can be identified during abdominal ultrasonography, however the value of this examination is limited. Ultrasound has been used to examine the spinal cord intraoperatively.[13] This examination has some value in determining the degree of spinal cord injury that is present following disc prolapse, fracture, or dislocation. Intraoperative ultrasound may also be valuable for identification and biopsy of intramedullary lesions, for evaluation of the central canal, and for evaluation of blood flow within the spinal cord.

COMPUTED TOMOGRAPHY AND MAGNETIC RESONANCE

Both computed tomography (CT) and magnetic resonance (MR) can be used for evaluation of the vertebral column. The vertebral and spinal cord anatomy can be demonstrated with cross sectional images providing extremely useful information. Anesthesia or sedation and careful positioning are mandatory. The time required to obtain the necessary knowledge, and the expense and availability of the equipment are the major limitations at this time.

CT may be used in conjunction with a myelogram to improve delineation of the subarachnoid space and spinal cord. A lower contrast concentration than that used for routine myelography should be injected because of the artifact associated with dense materials.

NORMAL ANATOMY OF RADIOGRAPHIC SIGNIFICANCE

GENERAL VERTEBRAL ANATOMY

All vertebrae have a basically similar structure. The ventral-most portion is the body, which is a tubular bony structure. The body has a dense cortex and a marrow cavity consisting of cancellous bone. The basivertebral veins run through the middle of the vertebral body producing a linear radiolucency. These veins connect the ventral venous sinuses on the dorsal surface of the vertebral body to the caudal vena cava. The transverse processes, which are bony projections that vary in size and orientation depending upon the specific vertebra, arise on the left and right sides of the vertebral bodies. Dorsal to the body are bony structures which combine to form the vertebral arch. These structures include the lamina, pedicles, and dorsal spinous process. The bony pedicles are the lateral walls of the spinal canal. These are composed of cortical bone and arise from the lateral-most part of the vertebral body. The pedicles have semilunar defects on their cranial and caudal borders which combine to form the intervertebral foramina through which the spinal nerves exit the spinal canal. The laminae that form the roof of the spinal canal connect the dorsal edges of the pedicles. Dorsal to the laminae is the spinous process, a laterally flattened bony extension that is centered on the midline and varies in size depending on the specific vertebra being described. At the junction of pedicles and laminae on the cranial and caudal aspects are paired articular processes, which articulate with those of the adjacent vertebra. Other bony processes (i.e., accessory and mammillary) and the costal foveae (for articulation with rib heads) are present on some vertebrae. All of the thoracic vertebrae have costal fovea. The mammillary processes (small, knob-like bony projections) begin with T2 or T3 and continue through all of the lumbar vertebrae. The accessory processes (small, tubular, caudally directed bony projections arising from the caudal aspect of the pedicles) begin with the midthoracic vertebrae and continue to L5 or L6.

Between almost all vertebrae (the exceptions being C1–C2 and the sacral vertebrae) is an intervertebral disc. This is composed of the annulus fibrosis (a perimeter of fibrous and fibrocartilaginous fibers arranged in concentric lamellae) and the nucleus pulposus (an eccentrically placed sphere of embryonic hyaline cartilage). The width of each disc space varies depending on which vertebrae it separates. The cervical disc spaces become gradually wider as they progress from C2 to C6. The thoracic disc spaces are narrower than the cervical disc spaces and are uniform in width to the level of T10 to T11. The disc spaces then widen gradually to the level of T13 to L1, at which point they are fairly consistent in width to the level of L7 to S1. The width of the L7–S1 disc spaces varies, but it may often be wider than the other disc spaces.

The normal spine of the dog and cat consists of seven cervical, thirteen thoracic, seven lumbar, three sacral, and a variable number of caudal vertebrae.

CERVICAL SPINE

The cervical vertebrae, except C1 and C2, have a similar shape (Fig. 6–1). C1 has a short, ovoid, tubular shape with prominent transverse processes. On the ventrodorsal view, these processes are relatively large and the lateral foramina, through which the spinal arteries course, are readily apparent. On the lateral view, C1 is shorter than the other vertebrae. On a well positioned lateral radiograph, the transverse processes are superimposed obscuring the odontoid process of C2. If the head is placed in an oblique position, the wings of C2 will be rotated. This position is particularly helpful when subluxation between C1 and C2 is suspected or when there is a lesion within the cranial portion of C2. The axis (C2) is the largest of the cervical vertebrae. The cranial-most aspect is the odontoid process (dens), which projects cranially from the body of C2 into the ventral portion of the spinal canal of C1. In the dog, the dorsal spinous process of C2 contains an area of relative radiolucency. There are no intervertebral discs between the skull and C1 or between C1 and C2. C3–C7 are all similarly shaped; however, the dorsal spinous processes become progressively larger from C3 to C7. The lateral processes become progressively larger and are projected more ventrally going from C3 to C6. C6 has large projections from the transverse process. C7 has smaller transverse processes than the preceding cervical vertebrae. The intervertebral disc spaces between the cervical vertebrae gradually increase in width from C2–C3 to C6–C7 and become narrow again at C7–T1. The normal cervical myelogram reveals that the cord is oval in cross section (it appears smaller in its dorsoventral dimension on the lateral view than it is in the left to right dimension on the ventrodorsal view) in the atlanto-occipital area through C1 and becomes circular in cross section (it appears to have equal dimensions in all views) as it passes into C2. The ventral dura is tightly juxtaposed to the dorsal border of the disc space at C2–C3. The roots of the spinal nerves frequently are seen as faint linear radiolucencies that sweep caudally to exit from the appropriate intervertebral foramen. The spinal cord increases in diameter as it passes through the C4 and C5 area and the cervical enlargement or brachial intumescence, which is that part of the cord where the nerve roots form the brachial plexus, is formed. Beyond C6, the cord reduces slightly in diameter as it passes into the thoracic vertebral canal.

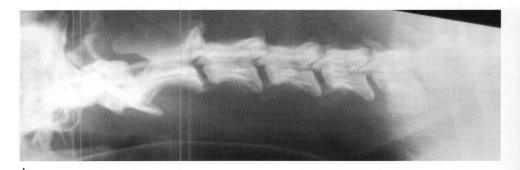

A

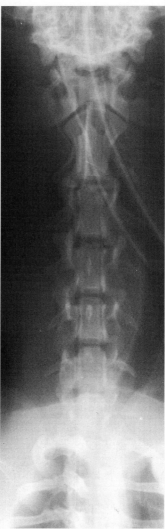

B

Figure 6–1. A 6-year-old male Labrador retriever. (A) The lateral view of the cervical spine was within normal limits. (B) The ventrodorsal myelogram of the cervical spine was within normal limits. (C) The survey lateral oblique view of the cervical spine was also normal. **Diagnosis:** Normal study.

C

THORACIC SPINE

The thoracic vertebrae are typified by short vertebral bodies, absence of transverse processes, articulations for the rib heads, and by relatively large dorsal spinous processes which gradually decrease in height from the cranial to the caudal thoracic vertebrae (Fig. 6–2). The intercapital ligament extends between the heads of the paired ribs and crosses over the dorsal surface of the intervertebral discs from T2–T11. The intervertebral disc spaces are relatively similar in size and shape with the exception of the disc space at the anticlinal space. The anticlinal space is the intervertebral disc space that is between the most caudal thoracic vertebra with a caudally directed dorsal spinous process and the most cranial thoracic vertebra with a cranially directed dorsal spinous process. This usually is at the T10–T11 intervertebral disc space but may vary by one space in different individuals. In the thoracic area, the spinal cord remains uniform in size and shape.

THORACOLUMBAR SPINE

Because the thoracolumbar junction is a common site for intervertebral disc problems, and because the entire lumbar spine cannot be properly imaged on one long view due to the divergence of the x-ray beam, the thoracolumbar spine should be radiographed separately. The caudal thoracic vertebrae have bodies that are similarly shaped to the more cranial thoracic vertebrae but the dorsal spinous processes will be shorter. The width of the disc spaces becomes progressively larger from the anticlinal vertebra caudally to the junction of T13–L1. The spinal cord in this region remains the same size and shape as in the more cranial thoracic areas.

LUMBAR SPINE

The lumbar vertebrae are all similar in size and shape (Fig. 6–3). The ventral margin of the third and fourth lumbar vertebral bodies often is poorly defined when viewed on the lateral radiograph. This is associated with the presence of a cartilage ridge which is present on these bodies and is related to the attachment of the diaphragmatic crura. Myelography of the lumbar cord reveals little change in size and shape from the caudal thoracic area until the cord begins to pass into the L4 spinal canal, at which point the cord diameter enlarges somewhat over the space of one or two vertebral segments. This is the lumbosacral enlargement or sacral intumescence, which is the portion of the spinal cord from which the nerves that form the sacral plexus arise. In the region of L5–L6, the spinal cord diminishes in diameter and the nerve roots that innervate the caudal structures continue caudally within the dural tube until they exit from the spinal canal. Caudal continuation of the nerve roots within the dural tube is known as the cauda equina. In smaller dogs, the spinal cord ends around L6–L7 while in larger dogs it terminates at L4–L5 or L5–L6.

SACROCAUDAL SPINE

The three sacral vertebrae are fused and articulate laterally with the ilia. The diameter of the spinal cord (actually the nerve roots contained within the dural tube) in

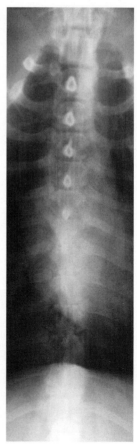

Figure 6–2. 6-year-old male Labrador retriever. (A&B) The spine and myelogram of the thoracic spine are within normal limits. **Diagnosis:** Normal study.

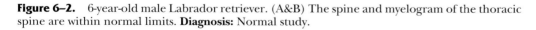

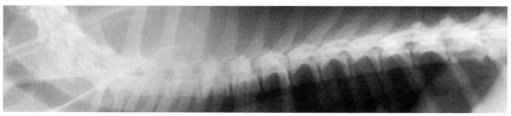

A

B

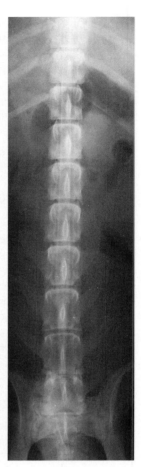

Figure 6–3. A 6-year-old male Labrador retriever. (A&B) The spine and myelogram of the lumbar spine are within normal limits. **Diagnosis:** Normal study.

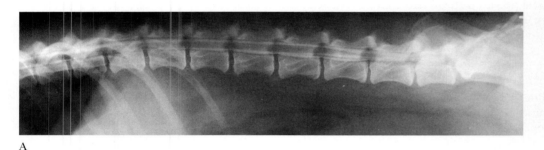

A

B

this region is very small. The dural tube adheres to the S1–S2 laminae and only individual nerve roots extend caudal to this region. In this region, the venous anatomy may be demonstrated by lumbar sinus venography. The dorsal vertebral sinuses will appear on the lateral view as small tubular structures which elevate slightly from the floor of the spinal canal at the intervertebral disc spaces. On the ventrodorsal view, the dorsal vertebral sinuses form arcs with the lateral-most deviation at the disc space and the two tubular structures nearly touching on the midline in the middle of each vertebral body.

The number of caudal vertebrae vary. The cranial-most vertebrae are complete and similar in shape to the lumbar vertebrae, although they are smaller in size. The distal vertebrae may be incomplete (missing pedicles and laminae). Small mineralized structures (hemal arches or hemal processes) may be evident ventral to the disc spaces between the caudal vertebrae. Myelography does not demonstrate the neural structures of this area.

ABNORMAL FINDINGS

Many abnormalities of the spine or spinal cord may be evident on carefully positioned and exposed survey radiographs. Because the survey radiograph does not demonstrate the spinal cord, the effect of a survey radiographic lesion on the spinal cord must be surmised. In many situations, the neurologic findings will indicate that the survey radiographic diagnosis is correct. However, in other instances, the neurologic findings may not completely correlate with the radiographic findings, or the radiographic changes may indicate more than one site of disease but may not indicate which is causing the neurologic abnormality. Additionally, the lesion causing the neurologic signs may not be apparent radiographically (e.g., some spinal cord tumors, fibrocartilaginous embolization of the spinal cord). Decisions concerning type and extent of surgery require precise neurologic evaluation as well as radiographic support. In those cases where correlation is inadequate or evaluation of the extent of the spinal cord lesion is needed, a myelogram is indicated.

METHOD OF EVALUATION

Evaluation of a spinal radiograph should be performed systematically. Positioning markedly affects the appearance of the vertebral bodies and should therefore be the first feature examined. Each vertebra should be evaluated for alteration in bony contour or density. The overall alignment of the spinal column should be assessed. The articular facets and the dorsal and transverse processes should be examined. The pedicles and lamina should be evaluated for density and symmetry between the left and right sides. The size and shape of the intervertebral foramina should be compared to the adjacent vertebra. The density of each intervertebral disc space should be evaluated and the width of the disc space should be compared to the adjacent disc spaces. If a myelogram is performed, it must be evaluated in a systematic manner. The contrast columns should be evaluated for any deviation in position or change in width. Also, the relatively radiolucent spinal cord should be evaluated for changes in size, shape, and position.

CLASSIFICATION OF MYELOGRAPHIC LESIONS

Myelographic abnormalities can be divided into intramedullary, extramedullary-intradural, and extradural patterns.[14]

Intramedullary

Intramedullary lesions (arising within the substance of the spinal cord) cause circumferential expansion and widening of the spinal cord. This results in a decreased width of the subarachnoid space on both lateral and ventrodorsal views (Fig. 6–4). This may occur as a result of spinal cord swelling due to edema or hemorrhage or may result from spinal cord neoplasia. Spinal cord tumors (either primary or metastatic), hemorrhage, or edema may produce focal cord swelling. If a long segment of the spinal cord (extending more than two or three vertebral bodies) is affected, the lesion is more likely due to hemorrhage or edema than tumor. Cord swelling may result from extradural lesions such as prolapsed intervertebral discs. In these cases, the intramedullary swelling may mask the extradural lesion.

Extramedullary-Intradural

Extramedullary-intradural lesions (arising within the dural tube but external to the substance of the spinal cord) result in widening of the cord in one view and deviation to the side on the other view (Fig. 6–5). The mass within the dural tube will be within the subarachnoid space or will impinge upon it and may be outlined by the contrast material. A "golf tee" appearance, caused by focal widening of the subarachnoid space and contrast displacement around the mass, may be identified. Extramedullary-intradural lesions may be due to tumors such as meningioma or neurofibroma. Rarely, a prolapsed intervertebral disc may penetrate the dura and produce an extramedullary-intradural lesion.

Extradural

Extradural lesions (arising external to the dural tube) will produce widening of the cord on one view and displacement away from the lesion with resultant compression of the spinal cord on the opposite view (Fig. 6–6). In rare instances, an extradural lesion will be distributed circumferentially around the spinal cord producing cord

Figure 6–4. A 4-year-old male Doberman pinscher with paraparesis. (A&B) There is circumferential expansion of the spinal cord with narrowing of the subarachnoid space at L3–L4 (*white arrows*). This finding, confirmed on both views, indicates an intramedullary mass. Differential diagnoses include neoplasia (ependymoma, glioma, or metastatic tumor), granuloma, hemorrhage, or disc extruded into the spinal cord. **Diagnosis:** Metastatic melanoma.

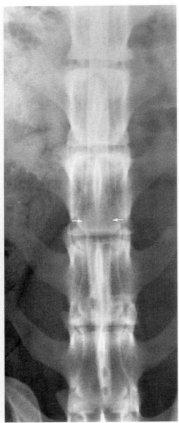

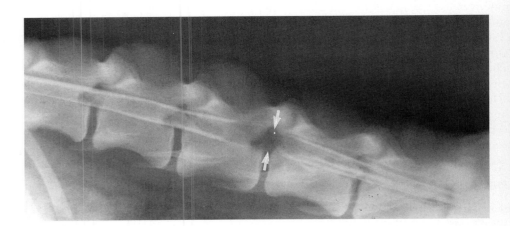

A
B

narrowing on both views. The most common extradural lesion is a prolapsed intervertebral disc. Tumors arising from the vertebral body, tumors arising from the dura, neurofibromas, and metastatic tumors may also produce extradural lesions.

CONGENITAL ANOMALIES

Transitional Vertebra

Vertebral body anomalies are readily recognizable and most cause no clinical signs. Transitional segments frequently are seen at the lumbosacral and thoracolumbar junctions. They are less common at the cervicothoracic junction. These transitional vertebral segments have characteristics of one portion of the vertebral column, yet when the vertebra are counted they belong in another segment. One of the most common of these anomalies is referred to as sacralization of L7 or lumbarization of S1 (Fig. 6–7).[15,16] In this anomaly, either L7 articulates with the ilia in a manner similar to the sacrum, or the first sacral segment will have transverse processes and may be distinctly separated from S2 and S3. The articulation between L7 or S1 and the ilium may be asymmetric with a transverse process on one side and a sacroiliac joint on the other. This asymmetry has no clinical significance, but it may interfere with symmetrical positioning of the pelvis for hip radiographs. A relationship between transitional lumbosacral vertebrae and hip dysplasia or cauda equina syndrome has been suggested.[16,17] The evidence for a cause and effect relationship is weak. Incomplete or transitional ribs involving T13 or L1 also are very common and are most often identified on the ventrodorsal view. The incomplete ribs are linear bony structures that may lack apparent rib heads but have a junction with the vertebral body similar to the lumbar transverse processes. The incomplete ribs extend beyond the normal length of the transverse processes but usually are shorter than normal ribs

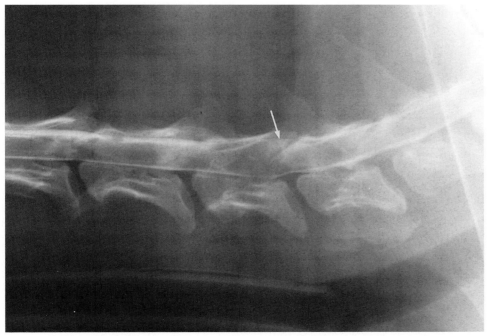

A

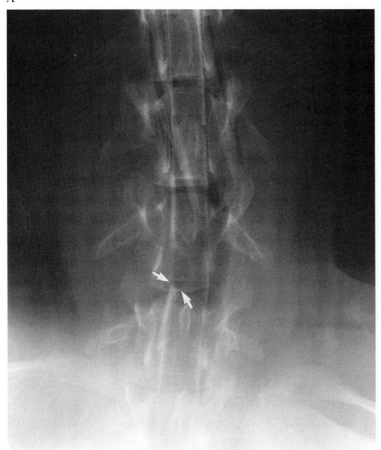

B

Figure 6–5. An 8-year-old male Old English sheep-dog with a non-weight-bearing lameness of the right forelimb. The dog would not touch the limb to the ground even at rest. Survey radiographs were normal. (A) The lateral myelogram revealed a narrowing of the subarachnoid space and enlargement of the spinal cord shadow at the C5–C6 region. There is a rim of contrast media extending ventral, which is due to the presence of an extramedullary-intradural mass (*white arrow*). (B) The ventrodorsal myelogram revealed displacement of the spinal cord to the left with narrowing of the left subarachnoid space. There is widening of the subarachnoid space on the right at this level with concave terminations ("golf tees") of this widening at the cranial and caudal aspects (*white arrows*). This indicates an extramedullary-intradural mass. Differential diagnoses include neurofibroma and meningioma. **Diagnosis:** Neurofibroma of the right sixth cervical nerve root.

and have a greater curvature than the normal lateral process (Fig. 6–8). A transitional vertebra may be seen at the cervicothoracic junction. This most often takes the form of ribs on C7. These ribs often are wider than normal ribs and frequently are fused with the first thoracic ribs distally.

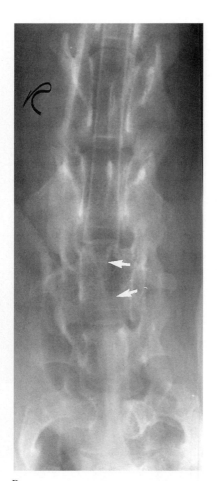

Figure 6–6. A 9-year-old male English pointer with a 4-week history of stumbling, and neck pain apparent on physical examination. (A) The lateral radiograph revealed lysis of the entire C6, most apparent in the pedicles and laminae. The myelogram revealed a ventral deflection of the dorsal subarachnoid space (*white arrow*). (B) The ventrodorsal view revealed loss of the left pedicle and deviation of the subarachnoid space to the right (*white arrows*) at C6. These findings indicate that the subarachnoid space is pushed in more than one direction by mass(es) external to the dural tube. This indicates a complex extradural mass. **Diagnosis:** Osteosarcoma of C6 with tumor mass in the left and dorsal portions of the extradural space.

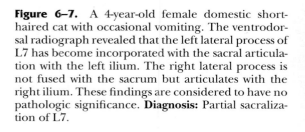

A

B

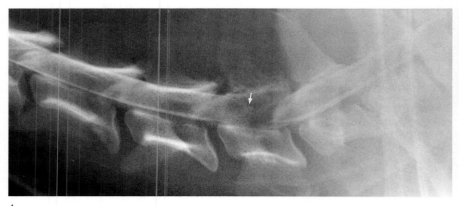

Figure 6–7. A 4-year-old female short-haired cat with occasional vomiting. The ventrodorsal radiograph revealed that the left lateral process of L7 has become incorporated with the sacral articulation with the left ilium. The right lateral process is not fused with the sacrum but articulates with the right ilium. These findings are considered to have no pathologic significance. **Diagnosis:** Partial sacralization of L7.

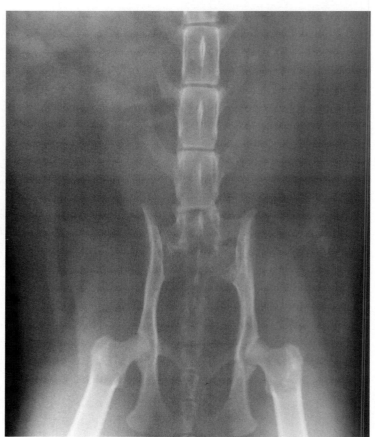

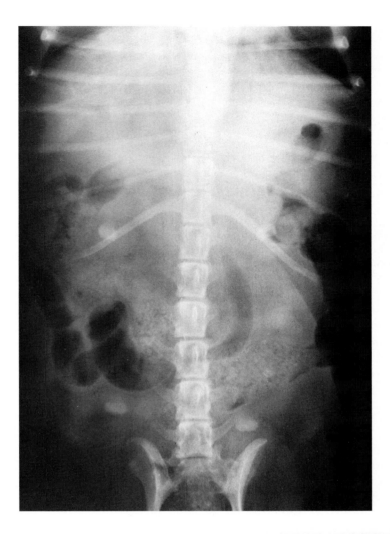

Figure 6–8. A 3-year-old female mixed breed dog with hematuria. The ventrodorsal radiograph revealed that the 13th thoracic vertebra has lateral processes with broad bases more similar to those seen in the lumbar spine than in the ribs. These findings are considered to have no pathologic significance. **Diagnosis:** Transitional ribs of T13.

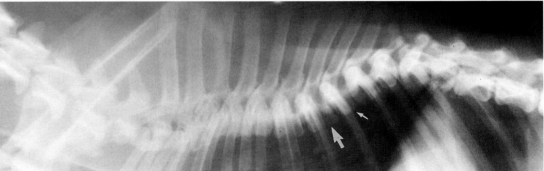

Figure 6–9. A 6-year-old male French bulldog with an acute onset of left-sided hemiplegia. The lateral thoracic spinal radiograph revealed hemivertebrae (*small white arrow*). These are readily apparent when compared with the more normal vertebrae (*large white arrow*). These findings were of no clinical significance. The dog's neurologic problem was due to a cervical disc extrusion. **Diagnosis:** Multiple hemivertebrae.

Hemivertebra

Hemivertebrae (vertebral bodies that are the result of incomplete formation and appear wedge-shaped) and butterfly vertebrae (vertebrae that are cleft in the sagittal plane) may be seen in any breed of dog but are common in brachycephalic or so-called "screw-tailed" breeds such as the English bulldog, Boston terrier, or pug (Fig. 6–9). These vertebral abnormalities usually are without clinical significance, how-

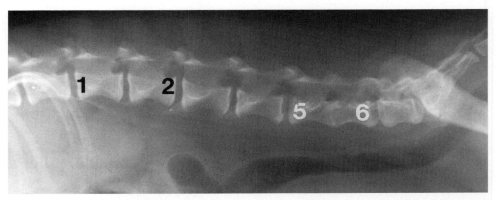

Figure 6–10. A 7-year-old male miniature poodle with occasional back pain. The lateral radiograph revealed absence of the intervertebral disc space between L5–L6 (*white numerals*) as well as an absence of the articular spaces of the dorsal components. The intervertebral disc space between L1–L2 (*black numerals*) was narrowed, the neural foramina diminished in size, and the space between the articular components dorsally are closer together than normal. **Diagnosis:** Block vertebrae of L5–L6 and intervertebral disc extrusion at L1–L2.

ever some instances of spinal cord compression associated with hemivertebra have been reported.[18–20] Trauma to the vertebral physis may cause a growth deformity that appears identical to a hemivertebra. This can be symptomatic if cord compression results from the abnormal growth of the vertebral body. A myelogram usually is required to determine if cord compression has occurred secondary to the vertebral deformity.[18]

Block Vertebra

Block vertebra refers to the congenital fusion of two or more adjacent vertebrae (Fig. 6–10). This anomaly usually has no pathologic significance, although a predisposition to herniation of intervertebral discs adjacent to the block vertebra has been suggested.[19,21] The dogs in those reports were chondrodystrophoid and therefore the relationship between the disc prolapse and the block vertebra may have been fortuitous. This abnormality usually results in a smooth bony union between adjacent vertebral bodies. The disc space may be completely absent or a portion of a disc space may be identified. Articular facets usually are still present, however joint fusion may be observed. The intervertebral foramen usually is malformed and may be absent. The block vertebra usually is equivalent in length to the two fused vertebral bodies, however abnormal angulation and shortening of the vertebra may be observed. Fusion of vertebral bodies may also occur as a result of trauma or infection (discospondylitis). If these lesions have healed completely, differentiation of an acquired block vertebra from a congenital lesion may be impossible.

Kyphosis and Scoliosis

Kyphosis (dorsal arching) and scoliosis (lateral bowing) are rarely observed in dogs and cats. Hemivertebrae may produce a kyphosis. Severe deformities of the vertebral bodies and articular facets may produce a kyphosis and scoliosis. Severe kyphosis and scoliosis has been reported in an Afghan hound and in a mixed breed dog.[21] The Afghan had an abnormal gait but no neurologic abnormalities.

Atlantoaxial Subluxation

Atlantoaxial luxations or subluxations may be congenital or traumatic.[22,23] The condition is most commonly observed in small and toy breeds, however other breeds may be affected.[24] The congenital condition results from a hypoplastic, un-united, or absent dens or from absence of the dorsal atlantoaxial membrane, apical ligament of the dens, or transverse atlantal ligament (Fig. 6–11). Trauma may cause disruption of the ligaments or fracture of the dens. On lateral cervical radiographs, the distance between the dorsal arch of C1 and the spinous process of C2 will be greater

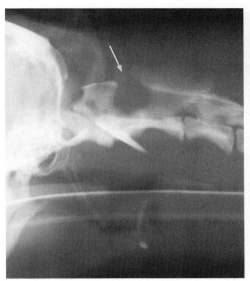 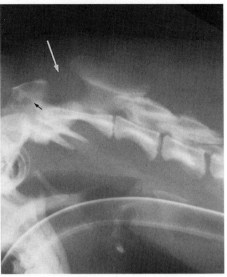

A   B

Figure 6–11.   A 3-year-old male Chihuahua with incoordination and neck pain. (A) The survey lateral view revealed a slightly greater than normal distance between the dorsal portions of caudal C1 and cranial C2 (*white arrow*). (B) The flexed lateral view demonstrates marked subluxation of C1–C2. Note the increased space between C1 and C2 (*white arrow*) and the decreased space within the spinal canal caused by the dorsal displacement of the odontoid process (*black arrow*). Fortunately, this examination did not render the patient permanently paraparetic. Studies of this area should include either an oblique lateral or *mild* flexion view if confirmation of a diagnosis is needed. **Diagnosis:** Atlantoaxial subluxation.

than normal. In normal small breed dogs, this distance should not exceed 2 to 3 mm. Flexion of the head will increase this distance in affected dogs. This maneuver should be performed cautiously, because spinal cord compression may result from aggressive manipulation of the head and neck especially when the dog is anesthetized and cannot protect itself. Anesthesia is recommended when radiographing a dog suspected of having atlantoaxial subluxation, because the patient may object to being radiographed and could therefore exacerbate its clinical signs. Oblique or frontal-occipital views may be required to demonstrate the lesion, especially when a fracture or un-united dens is present. Manipulation of the head and neck in patients with atlantoaxial subluxation must be performed cautiously, especially when the dens is present. Atlantoaxial subluxation has been reported in the cat.[25]

Occipitoatlantoaxial Malformation

Occipitoatlantoaxial malformation has been reported in dogs and cats.[26,27] The atlas is small and fused to the occipital bones. The axis is abnormally shaped with a dorsal spinous process, which is rounded on its cranial aspect with an absence of the dens. Atlantoaxial subluxation was demonstrated when the head was flexed and this is responsible for the animal's clinical signs.

Spina Bifida

Spina bifida is a condition with a midline cleft in the vertebral arch, which may involve one or several adjacent vertebra.[19] There may be two incomplete spinous processes or a complete absence of the spinous process. Paired bone densities may be seen on either side of the midline in the ventrodorsal view. These bone densities represent the un-united dorsal arch.[28] The condition may be totally asymptomatic or may be associated with other neurologic defects such as meningocele or meningomyelocele (Fig. 6–12). Myelography usually is required to identify those animals in which a neural tube defect is present. Spina bifida may occur at any level of the vertebral column, but is most often observed in the caudal lumbar or sacral spine. Some defects are associated with specific breeds, for example syringomyelia

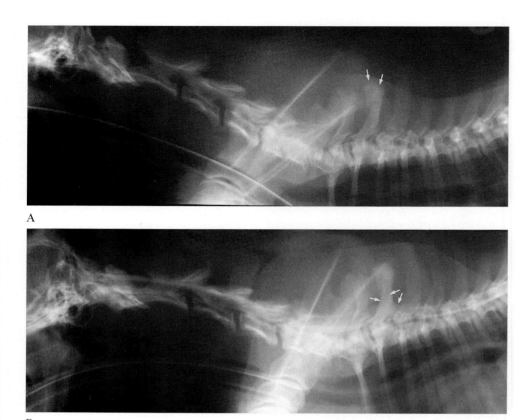

A

B

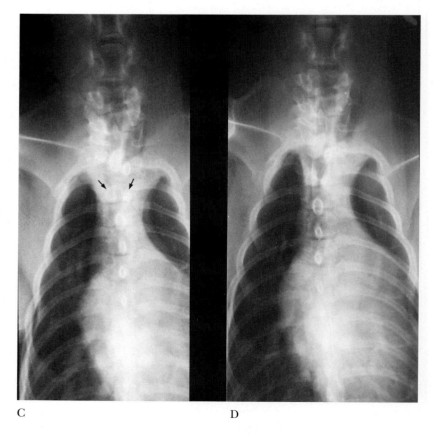

Figure 6–12. A 7-month-old male retriever with a draining fistula between the scapulae. (A&C) The survey radiographs revealed multiple congenital vertebral anomalies including a block vertebrae formation of C5, C6, and C7 as well as spina bifida of T1 and T2. The bilateral dorsal spinous processes are visible on both the lateral and ventrodorsal views (*arrows*). (B&D) The myelogram revealed that the subarachnoid space extends dorsally through the spinal defect and into the soft tissues (*white arrows*). The spinal cord also appears to be similarly affected. **Diagnosis:** Block vertebrae, spina bifida, and meningomyelocele.

C   D

and spinal dysraphism may cause gait problems in weimeraners.[19] Manx cats and brachycephalic dogs are predisposed to sacro-coccygeal deformities ranging from the presence of multiple hemivertebrae and/or spina bifida to sacral dysgenesis.[19,28–30] In some cases, these defects will have neurologic manifestations such as posterior paresis and urinary or fecal incontinence (Fig. 6–13).

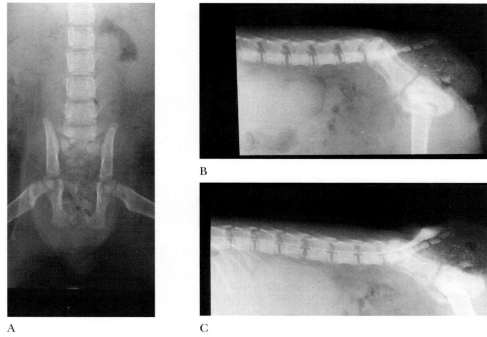

A   C

Figure 6–13. A 3-month-old male manx cat with rear limb ataxia. (A&B) The survey radiographs reveal partial agenesis of the sacrum and dorsal components of the proximal coccygeal vertebrae. (C) The myelogram revealed a dilated terminal subarachnoid space (meningocele) that is located in the soft tissues. **Diagnosis:** Multiple sacral anomalies associate with a Manx cat.

CERVICAL VERTEBRAL MALFORMATION (WOBBLER SYNDROME)

Cervical vertebral malformation, "wobbler syndrome," is most frequently seen in older Doberman pinschers and young great Danes, although dogs of any age and several different breeds may be affected.[31–35] The radiographic changes are slightly different in the young great Danes when compared to the older Dobermans. The clinical signs may be due to a number of anatomic abnormalities including intervertebral disc prolapse, hypertrophy of the vertebral ligaments (ligamentum flavum or dorsal longitudinal ligament), stenosis of the spinal canal, synovial proliferation associated with the spinal articular facets, enlargement of the articular facets, and malalignment of the vertebral bodies. In young dogs, malformation and malalignment of the vertebral bodies is the most common abnormality identified. The vertebral bodies are abnormally shaped, losing their normal rectangular conformation and becoming narrower ventrally. The cranioventral and caudoventral margins of the vertebral bodies become flattened. There is spondylosis deformans with bridging osteophytes forming between the adjacent vertebral bodies. The cranial orifice of the vertebrae may become narrowed, producing a wedge-shaped spinal canal.[31,32,35] The radiographic abnormalities most often affect the caudal cervical vertebrae (C5–C7); however, in severe cases the more cranial vertebral bodies may be affected. The joint spaces of the caudal cervical vertebrae have a more vertical orientation, which is similar to that of the thoracic vertebra rather than the oblique orientation typical of normal cervical articulations. In older dogs, remodeling of the vertebral bodies may be present to some extent, however the major radiographic findings are associated with intervertebral disc prolapse and ligamentous hypertrophy. On noncontrast radiographs, spondylosis deformans may be evident on the ventral aspect of the vertebral bodies. The intervertebral disc space may be narrowed or the disc may be calcified. There may be evidence of degenerative joint disease around the articular facets.[32,33] Myelography is required to document the site and extent of cord compression that is present.[36,37] Some authors believe that myelography is mandatory before surgery.[33] This is especially important because more than one

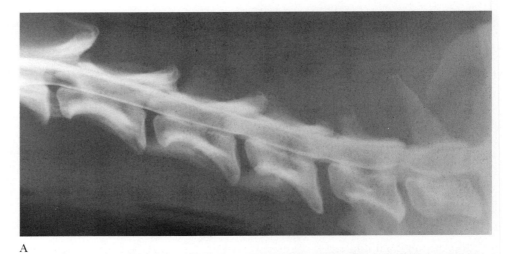

A

Figure 6–14. A 1-year-old male Doberman pinscher with incoordination. (A) The lateral cervical myelogram, taken with the neck in a neutral position, revealed a moderate sized ventral extradural mass at C6–C7 consistent with either disc protrusion or hypertrophy of the dorsal longitudinal ligament. (B) The lateral cervical myelogram, taken with the neck extended, revealed an increase in size of the C6–C7 extradural mass (*white arrow*) as well as a dorsal extradural mass at C4–C5 consistent with hypertrophy of the ligamentum flavum (*black arrow*). (C) The lateral cervical myelogram, taken with the neck flexed, showed a slight decrease in size of the C6–C7 ventral extradural mass (*white arrow*) and complete resolution of the dorsal extradural mass at C4–C5 (*black arrow*). **Diagnosis:** "Wobbler syndrome."

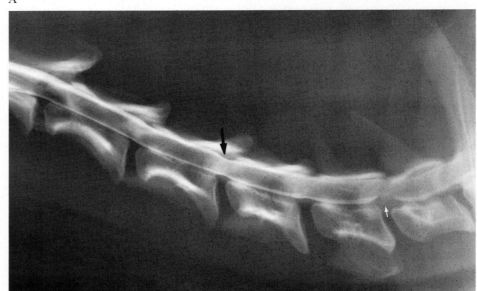

B

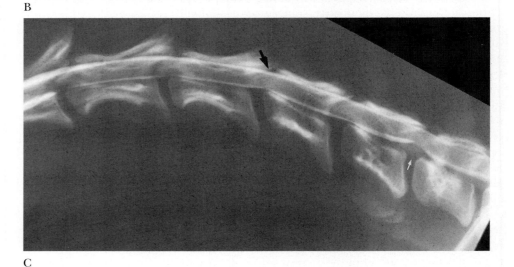

C

site of compression is common and the compression may be dorsal, lateral, ventral, or a combination of these. Compression of the cord from the ventral surface usually is related to disc prolapse or hypertrophy of the dorsal longitudinal ligament. Compression from the dorsal surface is associated with hypertrophy of the ligamentum flavum. Compression from one or both sides may occur secondary to synovitis with thickening of the joint capsule. After the myelographic contrast has been injected, flexed, neutral, and hyperextended radiographs are helpful in defining the location and number of lesions and these radiographs should be obtained before surgery. Some authors recommend a neutral positioned radiograph with rostral-caudal traction applied to the head in order to determine if vertebral traction will reduce the degree of compression.[38] Others recommend against stress views fearing exacerbation of the dog's clinical signs.[33] All of these views are helpful in determining the surgical procedure that will be used to eliminate the spinal compression. We recommend that stress views be used judiciously.

The compression of the spinal cord that results from hypertrophy of the dorsal longitudinal ligament or ligamentum flavum is exacerbated by dorsiflexion of the neck and usually is minimized by ventral flexion (Fig. 6–14). Mild traction of the neck may reduce the severity of spinal cord compression. Spondylolisthesis (subluxation of the vertebrae) has been used as a synonym for cervical vertebral malformation. Although a mild degree of vertebral subluxation does occur with neck flexion (especially in the younger dogs with vertebral malformation), this term is not accurate.[36,37] Flexion or extension studies should be done with extreme caution to avoid iatrogenic spinal cord injury (Figs. 6–15 and 6–16).

CT has been recommended for evaluation of dogs suspected of having cervical vertebral malformation.[39] The dog is positioned in sternal recumbency with the forelimbs retracted caudally. A myelogram may be performed concurrently with the CT scan; however, a reduced dose of contrast is recommended because of the artifact created on the CT scan due to the presence of the contrast material (blooming artifact).

DEGENERATIVE DISEASE

Spondylosis Deformans

Spondylosis deformans is the most common degenerative disease that affects the spinal column. This produces a partial or complete bony bridge between the caudal aspect of one vertebral body and the cranial aspect of the adjacent vertebral body

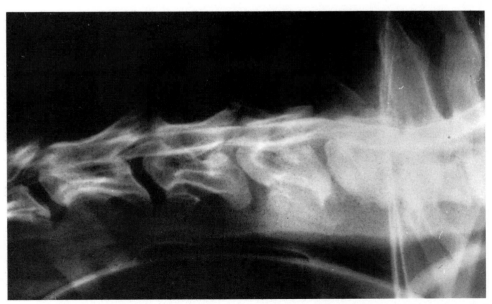

Figure 6–15. A 2-year-old male Great Dane with severe incoordination. The lateral cervical myelogram with the neck in mild flexion revealed sclerosis and remodeling of the bodies of C6 and C7 as well as subluxation and compression of the spinal cord at that site. **Diagnosis:** Spondylolisthesis.

Figure 6–16. A 2-year-old male Great Dane with incoordination of all four limbs. (A&B) The ventrodorsal myelograms reveal multiple sites of lateral compression of the subarachnoid space and spinal cord at C5–C6 and C6–C7 (*white arrows*). These changes signify the presence of extradural masses. **Diagnosis:** Extradural compression of the spinal cord at C5–C6 and C6–C7 due to hypertrophy of joint capsules and periarticular osteophytes affecting the synovial joints of these areas.

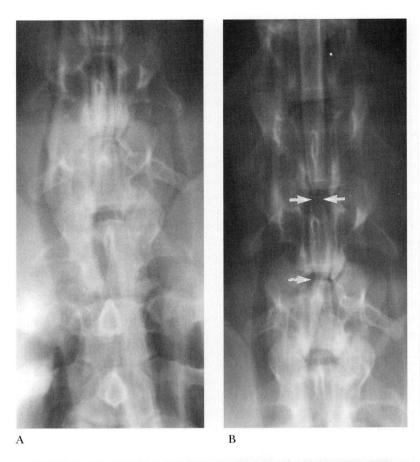

A

B

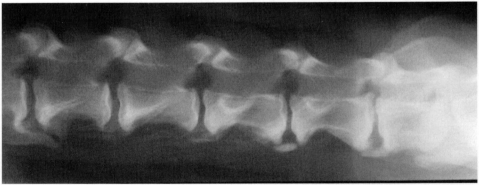

A

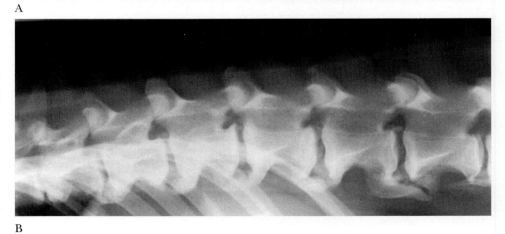

B

Figure 6-17. A 12-year-old male mixed breed dog with occasional vomiting. (A&B) Lateral radiographs revealed moderate bony bridging at several intervertebral spaces. These sites are not considered to be active sites of disease. **Diagnosis:** Spondylosis.

(Fig. 6–17).[40,41] The bony proliferation, while frequently present on the ventral and lateral surfaces of the vertebral bodies, rarely is present on the dorsal portion and therefore rarely encroaches upon the spinal cord or on the nerve root. Thus, spondylosis almost never has clinical ramifications. In rare cases, the amount of spondylosis may become extensive and close scrutiny of these animals will reveal some stiffness (Fig. 6–18). Spondylosis may be seen at necropsy in dogs as young as 6 months of age, but is usually a disease of older large breed dogs. The ossification may start from one vertebra and grow toward the other, may start on both and meet in the middle, may start in the middle and progress in both directions, or may present with any combination of these variations. Spondylosis may result in complete spinal fusion. Some mechanical interference with normal activity may result but in most cases the bony lesion does not produce clinical signs. Narrowing of the intervertebral disc space may occur secondary to spondylosis, but in most cases the disc is not prolapsed. Spondylosis may also occur secondary to chronic disc prolapse. The distinction between these two conditions usually is based on the amount of spondylosis that is present. If only one disc space is affected and there is no evidence of spondylosis at other sites, then the lesion most likely is primary disc degeneration with secondary spondylosis. If there is extensive spondylosis with only one narrowed disc space, then the lesion most likely is primarily spondylosis deformans with secondary disc degeneration. If clinical signs are present, a myelogram is needed to document or rule out disc prolapse.

Degenerative Joint Disease

Arthritis of the articular facets of the spine may be seen. This may result in the production of periarticular osteophytes with irregularity of the articular facets and loss of the normal joint space (Fig. 6–19). The clinical significance of this radiographic change is unknown, and unless the osteophytes are so large that they impinge upon the spinal cord the changes are most likely incidental findings.

Dural Ossification

Occasionally, a fine linear calcified density will be noted on the edge of the dural tube. This represents ossification of the dura and is rarely of clinical significance (Fig. 6–20).[42] The thin, linear mineral opacity may extend continuously along several vertebral bodies. Its position and length help discriminate this lesion from mineralization of the annulus fibrosis or dorsal longitudinal ligament. This lesion usually is observed in older large breed dogs and is more common in the caudal cervical and midlumbar regions.

INTERVERTEBRAL DISC DISEASE

Prolapse of intervertebral disc material into the spinal canal may impinge upon the spinal cord or the spinal nerve roots and produce neurologic signs. Degenerative

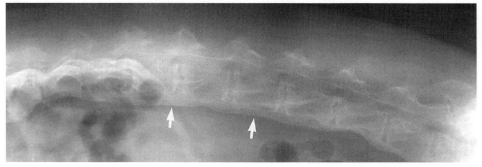

Figure 6–18. A 13-year-old neutered female mixed breed dog with vomiting and constipation. There is marked, smoothly bordered bony bridging between the lumbar vertebrae (*white arrows*). **Diagnosis:** Severe spondylosis.

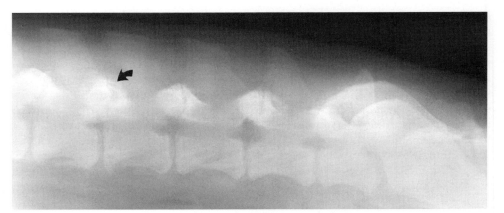

Figure 6–19. A 9-year-old male Great Dane with fever, rear limb ataxia, and a palpably enlarged prostate. There is a moderately enlarged prostate as well as irregular subchondral bone margins and periarticular osteophytosis of the articular facets of the lumbar spine. **Diagnosis:** Lumbar spine articular degenerative joint disease and prostatomegaly. The dog's clinical signs resolved after castration and antibiotic therapy.

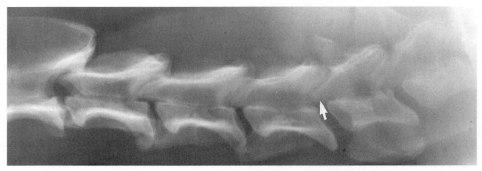

Figure 6–20. A 6-year-old neutered female Weimaraner with tetraparesis. A fine linear calcification, which runs parallel to the spinal cord (*white arrow*), is present dorsal to the floor of the vertebrae. Differential diagnoses include calcification of the dura or dorsal longitudinal ligament. **Diagnosis:** Dural calcification.

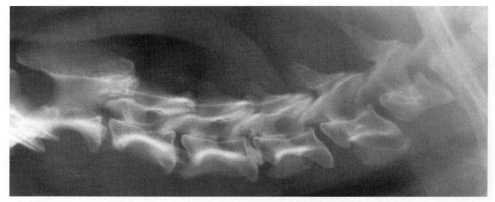

Figure 6–21. A 9-year-old female beagle with neck pain. The lateral cervical radiograph revealed a calcified intervertebral disc at C4–C5. Scrutiny revealed that the disc tapered dorsally and that some material had extruded into the spinal canal. **Diagnosis:** C4–C5 intervertebral disc calcification and extrusion.

changes within the disc predispose it to prolapse. Calcification of the intervertebral disc is a radiographically apparent sign of disc degeneration (Fig. 6–21). The disc may calcify centrally or at the rim. All or a portion of the mineralized material may remain in the disc space, may prolapse dorsally into the spinal canal, or (less fre-

THE SPINE ■ 603

quently) may prolapse ventrally or laterally. Prolapse of disc material is indicated radiographically by: (1) narrowing of the intervertebral disc space (the disc space may be uniformly narrowed or may be asymmetrically narrowed or "wedge shaped"), (2) narrowing of the space between the paired cranial and caudal articular facets, (3) decreased size or a change in shape of the neural foramen, (4) increased density in the area of the neural foramen, and (5) presence of calcified disc material within the spinal canal (Fig. 6–22). When most of the disc spaces contain mineralized disc material, the presence of an empty disc space (one without mineralized material) may be an indication of disc prolapse. In rare cases the disc material may extrude laterally or dorsolaterally into the area where the spinal nerve root passes through the neural foramen. In these cases, the disc material is apparent radiographically only on lateral oblique views of the spine (Fig. 6–23).[43] Disc material may prolapse ventrally; however, this is extremely uncommon and is usually ignored because it does not cause clinical signs.

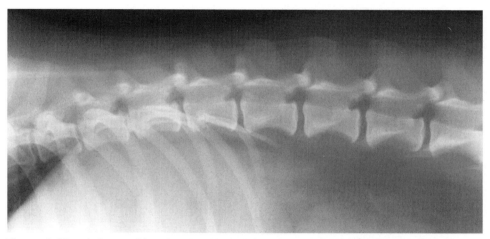

Figure 6–22. A 6-year-old male mixed breed dog with acute paraparesis and pain over the thoracolumbar spine. The lateral radiograph revealed narrowing of the disc space as compared to those spaces immediately cranial and caudal to this site. There appears to be a decreased space between the articular facets at T12–T13 when compared to those adjacent to it. Increased density is suggested in the area of the neural foramen at this site. **Diagnosis:** Acute intervertebral disc prolapse at T12–T13.

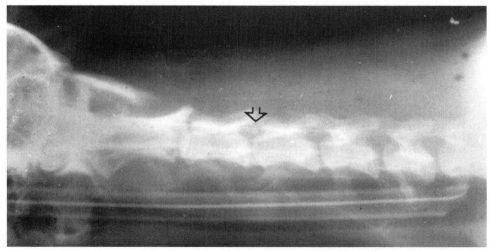

Figure 6–23. A 7-year-old male mixed breed dog with right forelimb lameness. The dog would hold the limb off the ground at rest. The left recumbent lateral oblique view of a cervical myelogram revealed increased density in the neural foramen at C3–C4 (*open black arrow*). This was best appreciated when compared to the other neural foramina. **Diagnosis:** Intraforaminal intervertebral disc extrusion at C3–C4.

Accurate determination of the site of intervertebral disc protrusion on survey radiographs is possible in 70% to 75% of affected dogs.[44,45] When the clinical signs and the radiographic changes are inconsistent, more than one possible site of disc prolapse is identified on the survey radiograph, or documentation of the exact site of the prolapsed disc material is desired, a myelogram is indicated. Myelography can determine the site of the disc prolapse accurately in 97% of the patients.[45] Myelographically, the disc prolapse will produce signs of an extradural mass. If there is spinal cord swelling or hemorrhage associated with the disc prolapse, there may be myelographic signs of an intramedullary lesion. The disc material may be located on the ventral midline of the spinal canal displacing the contrast column dorsally in a single line over the mass (Fig. 6–24). If the disc material is ventral and slightly off the midline of the spinal canal, the myelogram will show a double line effect (Fig. 6–25). In some cases, the disc material will extrude into a completely lateral position within the spinal canal; this results in displacement of the spinal cord away from the disc on the ventrodorsal myelogram and results in widening of the spinal cord on the lateral view (Fig. 6–26). In rare cases, a disc extrusion occurs with such force that it penetrates the dura and lodges within the spinal cord. In these cases, either a swollen spinal cord suggestive of an intramedullary lesion or an extramedullary intradural lesion may be observed on the myelogram (Fig. 6–27). Oblique radiographs are helpful when the disc material is located ventrolateral to the spinal cord.[43,45] In some cases a disc extrusion will cause ascending/descending myelomalacia (or hematomyelia). This may result in a normal myelogram, but usually produces a swollen

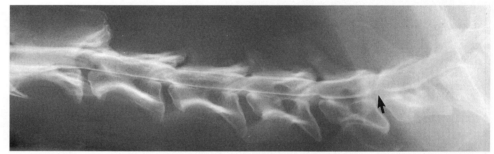

Figure 6–24. A 7-year-old female mixed breed dog with neck pain. The lateral cervical myelogram revealed a small ventral extradural mass at C5–C6 and a larger mass at C6–C7 (*black arrow*). Because only one contrast column is seen, there is indication that the mass is on the midline. **Diagnosis:** Intervertebral disc protrusion C5–C6 and C6–C7.

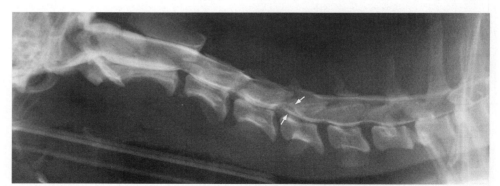

Figure 6–25. A 5-year-old male Maltese with neck pain and mild left lateralizing tetraparesis. The dorsal subarachnoid space is narrowed. A ventral extradural mass is at C4–C5. Close examination revealed there are two apparent ventral contrast columns, one of which is a great deal more elevated than the other. This results from extrusion of disc material slightly to one side of the midline but not enough to be considered truly lateral in location. Incidental findings of slight disc protrusion at C5–C6 and C6–C7 as well as slight hypertrophy of the ligamenta flavum at C3–C4 and C4–C5 are noted. **Diagnosis:** Disc extrusion at C4–C5.

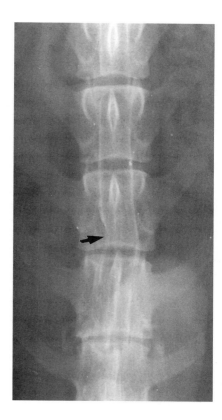

Figure 6–26. A 5-year-old male beagle with paraparesis that is more profound on the right. The ventrodorsal view of a lumbar myelogram revealed a right lateral extradural mass (*black arrow*) that displaced the spinal cord to the left at the L4–L5 disc space. Differential diagnoses include a disc extrusion or extradural tumor. **Diagnosis:** Right lateral disc extrusion at L4–L5.

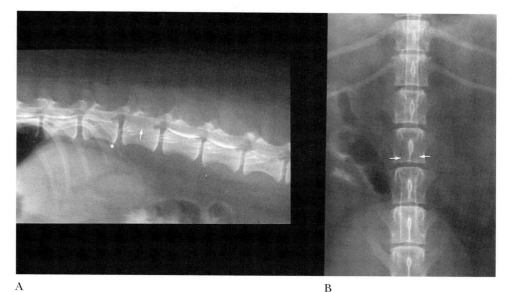

A   B

Figure 6–27. A 13-year-old neutered female miniature dachshund with acute paraparesis. (A) The lateral myelogram revealed an enlargement of the subarachnoid space immediately cranial to L2–L3 (*white arrow*). (B) The ventrodorsal myelogram revealed mild swelling of the spinal cord at this site (*white arrows*). These findings suggest a forceful extrusion of disc material into the spinal cord substance at this site. Other differential diagnoses include neoplasia or granuloma. **Diagnosis:** Extrusion of the L2–L3 intervertebral disc into the substance of the spinal cord.

spinal cord with contrast media intermixed within the neural tissue. Extruding disc material may rupture a vertebral venous sinus and cause extradural hemorrhage. This will cause the spinal cord to be compressed by a relatively lengthy dorsal extradural mass, which may be more on one side (right or left) than the other (Fig. 6–28). In cases where disc degeneration is chronic, there may be narrowing of the disc space and sclerosis of the adjacent vertebral body segments as well as spondylosis. The myelogram may demonstrate slight elevation of the contrast column over the prolapsed disc. The dorsal and lateral contrast columns may remain normal or may be slightly narrowed. The diameter of the spinal cord remains unchanged. These changes are often seen with Type II disc prolapse, which is more common in

Figure 6–28. A 4-year-old male chow chow that had run away was discovered by its owners as having acute paraparesis. (A) The lateral myelogram revealed narrowing of the T12–T13 disc space and facets, a decrease size of the neural foramina, a ventral extradural mass at T12–T13, and a dorsal extradural mass (displacement of the dorsal subarachnoid space ventrally) from T11 to L2 (*white arrow*). (B) The ventrodorsal view revealed a right-sided extradural mass effect from T12 to L3 which pushes the right subarachnoid space to the left (*white arrow*). The dorsal lateral mass effect extended over a space of more than two vertebral bodies strongly suggests extradural hemorrhage. **Diagnosis:** Suspected traumatic disc extrusion at T12–T13 with laceration of the right lumbar dorsal vertebral venous sinus.

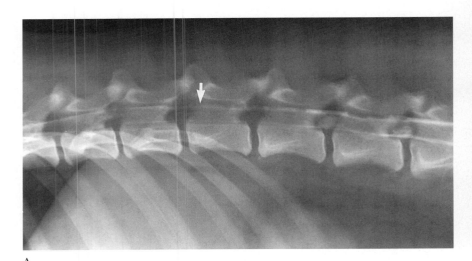

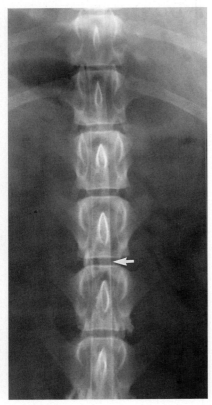

A
B

older large breed dogs. A narrowed disc space may return to its normal width after the disc prolapse. The mechanism by which this occurs is unknown.

Post fenestration, the width of the intervertebral disc space decreases. Spondylosis occurs 1 to 4 years after disc fenestration.[46]

INFECTION

Diskospondylitis

Diskospondylitis (intradiscal osteomyelitis) is an infection of the intervertebral disc and adjacent vertebral endplates.[47–50] The earliest radiographic change is decreased density within the vertebral endplate with loss of the densely calcified cortical border of the vertebral body. The disease progresses to lysis of the vertebral endplates and subsequently the bodies, with sclerosis or bony proliferation following the bony lysis. In some lesions, the disc space becomes widened and irregular and in others collapse of the disc space is observed. A sequestrum may be identified at the vertebral endplate. Several disc spaces are often involved, however the severity of the lesion usually varies at different sites. In the resolution phase disc space collapse, sclerosis, spondylosis, and sometimes fusion of the vertebral bodies occurs (Fig. 6–29). Resolution of the bony lesion lags behind the resolution of the clinical signs. The lesion may appear active radiographically with increased bony lysis or proliferation and new lesions observed despite resolution of the clinical signs.[51] Some reports have stressed the role of *Brucella sp.* in these infections, but other bacteria such as *Staphylococcus aureus*, *Corynebacterium diphtheriae*, and *Escherichia coli* are apparently more common.[48–53] *Aspergillus* has also been incriminated in discospondylitis. The infection usually is hematogenous in origin, although direct extension from a soft tissue infection and migrating foreign bodies have been incriminated.[47]

Spondylitis

Spondylitis (vertebral osteomyelitis) is infection of the vertebral body. The radiographic changes are typified by marked periosteal new bone formation primarily

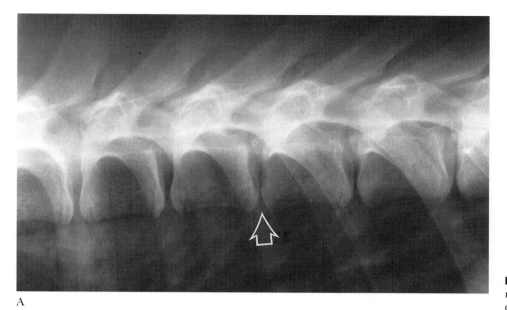

A

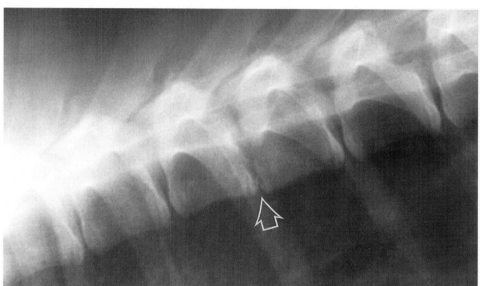

B

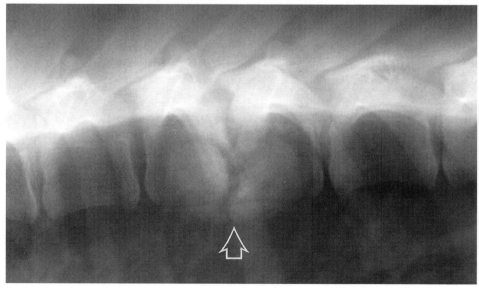

C

Figure 6–29. A 4-month-old male Irish wolfhound with pain over the midthoracic spine. (A) The initial lateral radiograph revealed a moderate decrease in the density of the cranial endplate of T8 as well as a slight decrease in the width of the T7–T8 intervertebral disc space (*open white arrow*). (B) Four weeks later there was marked destruction of the vertebral endplates at the T7–T8 interspace as well as significant collapse of the disc space (*open white arrow*). (C) Fourteen weeks after the first radiograph there was complete collapse of the disc space and marked periosteal new bone formation around the T7–T8 interspace (*open white arrow*). This series demonstrates the progression of intradiscal osteomyelitis (diskospondylitis) from very early in the clinical presentation to the resolution phase. **Diagnosis:** Intradiscal osteomyelitis of T7–T8.

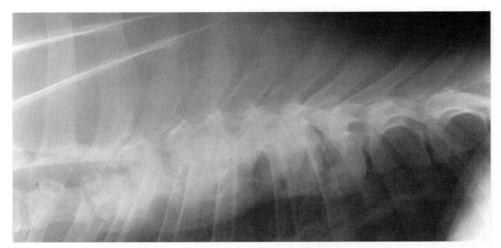

Figure 6–30. A 1-year-old female Doberman pinscher with midthoracic pain. On the lateral radiograph there is marked periosteal new bone formation involving the vertebral bodies of T2–T8. Also seen is the loss of definitive vertebral shape, decreased vertebral body density, and possible compression fractures. Because of the several contiguous vertebral bodies involved, infection, rather than neoplasia, is strongly suggested. **Diagnosis:** Infectious spondylitis of T2–T8.

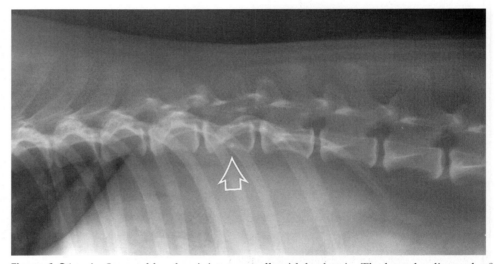

Figure 6–31. An 8-year-old male miniature poodle with back pain. The lateral radiograph of the thoracolumbar spine revealed marked loss of bone density of T12 (*white arrow*). Differential diagnoses include primary or metastatic neoplasms or an unusual infectious process. **Diagnosis:** Osteosarcoma of T12.

involving the midportion of the vertebral body. Bone lysis usually is minor compared to the proliferative response (Fig. 6–30). Spread to adjacent vertebral bodies is common. This may be caused by many types of organisms including bacteria, fungi, or protozoa.[54–56] In some areas of the western United States, the most common cause is plant awn migration through the respiratory tract and along the crura of the diaphragm. The second and third lumbar vertebrae are frequently involved in these cases.

Neoplasia

Primary and Metastatic Neoplasms

Both primary and metastatic tumors may affect the vertebral column. Primary tumors may originate in the bone or in the neural tissue.[57,58] While some tumor types have relatively specific patterns of radiographic change, no type is pathognomonic and biopsy is needed to reach a specific diagnosis. Although the majority of primary and metastatic spinal tumors are lytic, many are proliferative or a combination of lytic and proliferative (Fig. 6–31). A paravertebral soft tissue mass may be visible.[58] Disc space collapse occurs in a small number of both primary and metastatic vertebral tumors. Primary tumors usually are localized to one vertebral body; however, they may spread to adjacent vertebrae. Osteochondroma or multiple cartilaginous exostoses may produce well-defined bony masses. These are most often found in the vertebral column but also may occur on the ribs, long bones, and pelvis.[59] Metastatic tumors frequently involve more than one vertebral body. Any portion of the vertebra may be involved. Prostatic, bladder, urethral, mammary, and perianal neoplasia may metastasize to the lumbar, sacral, or caudal vertebrae. In these cases periosteal new bone formation or bony lysis may be observed. The ventral aspects of the 5th through 7th lumbar vertebral bodies are most often affected (Fig. 6–32). The bony proliferation may occur in association with tumor spread to the sublumbar (iliac) lymph nodes with no histological evidence of tumor within the vertebral bodies themselves. Multiple myeloma typically presents with multiple lytic, well-circumscribed bony lesions that do not have sclerotic borders (Fig. 6–33). In a few multiple myeloma cases a diffuse loss of bone density will be seen (Fig. 6–34). Multiple myeloma may also produce solitary or multiple, destructive and proliferative lesions

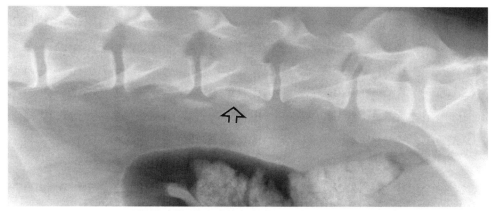

Figure 6–32. A 9-year-old male mixed breed dog with dyschezia. The lateral radiograph of the caudal lumbar spine revealed "fluffy" periosteal new bone formation affecting the ventral aspects of L7, L6, and L5 (*open black arrow*). Differential diagnoses include metastatic neoplasia of the prostate or other perineal organ or infection. **Diagnosis:** Metastatic prostatic adenocarcinoma.

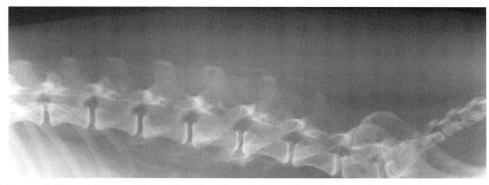

Figure 6–33. A 9-year-old female mixed breed dog with polyuria and polydipsia. There are multiple focal lytic areas without sclerosis in the lumbar vertebrae, particularly in the laminae and dorsal spinous processes. Differential diagnoses include multiple myeloma or metastatic neoplasia. **Diagnosis:** Multiple myeloma.

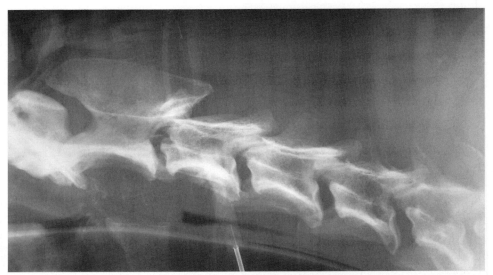

Figure 6–34. A 10-year-old male German shepherd dog with polyuria and polydipsia. There is diffuse osteopenia of the cervical vertebrae. Differential diagnoses include hyperparathyroidism (primary or secondary), hyperadrenocorticism, multiple myeloma, or hyperthyroidism. **Diagnosis:** Multiple myeloma.

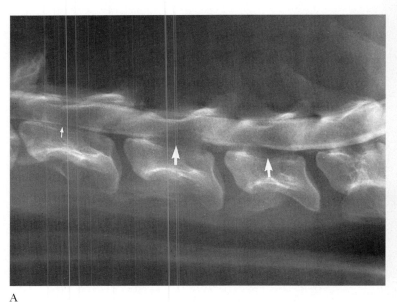

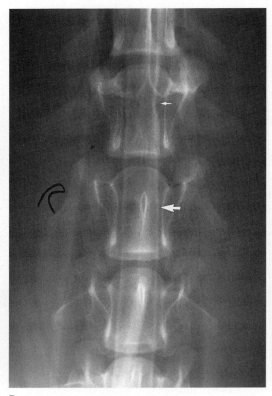

A

B

Figure 6–35. An 8-year-old male Siberian husky with a slow onset of tetraparesis. (A) The lateral myelogram revealed ventral extradural masses centered in the bodies of C4 and C5 (*large white arrows*). The spinal cord at C3 appears enlarged in the dorsoventral aspect due to a lateral extradural mass (*small white arrow*). (B) The ventrodorsal view revealed a left lateral extradural mass at C3 (*small white arrow*) and ventral extradural masses at C4 and C5 causing the cord to appear widened at these sites (*large white arrow*). Differential diagnoses include any of the multifocal extradural masses. The most likely is metastasis to the internal vertebral venous plexus (dorsal venous vertebral sinuses). **Diagnosis:** Renal carcinoma metastasis to the cervical internal vertebral venous plexus.

similar to those observed with other vertebral neoplasms. Lymphoma may also produce multicentric proliferative or destructive lesions.[60] Epidural tumors may occur and may produce erosions of the pedicle or arch but usually produce no bony changes and must be documented by myelography.

Tumors may metastasize to the spinal canal without involving the vertebral body or the spinal cord. These tumors usually exhibit no survey radiographic changes and can only be identified by myelography. They will appear as extradural lesions (Fig. 6–35).

Spinal Cord and Nerve Root Tumors

Neoplasia of the spinal cord or spinal nerves may have some subtle survey radiographic changes but most are difficult to diagnose without myelography.[61] Survey radiographs may reveal enlarged neural foramina or erosion of the pedicles or laminae. An enlarged neural foramen may be apparent on either the ventrodorsal or lateral view (Fig. 6–36). Comparison with the adjacent neural foramina is helpful in recognizing this abnormality. Erosion of a pedicle, best seen on the ventrodorsal view, appears as a loss of the sclerotic border medial to the pedicle, particularly as compared with those pedicles cranial and caudal to it (Fig. 6–37). Careful positioning is essential for recognition of this change. Overlying gas or ingesta may mimic or obscure this radiographic abnormality. Erosion of the laminae is manifested as a loss of the sclerotic border of the ventral-most part of the roof of the spinal canal (Fig. 6–38). This should also be compared with the appearance of those vertebrae that are cranial and caudal to the affected one. Tumors of the spinal cord may present with an extramedullary-intradural myelographic pattern, which may be seen with either neurofibromas or meningiomas. They may also present with an intramedullary myelographic pattern such as that seen with ependymoma or metastasis.

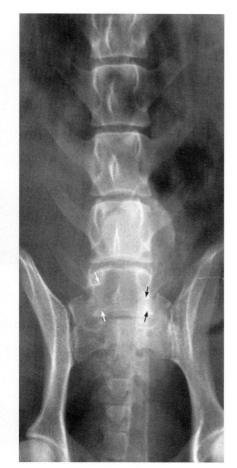

Figure 6–36. An 8-year-old male miniature schnauzer holding up and refusing to use the right hind limb. (A) On the lateral view there is a smooth bordered enlargement of the neural foramen of L7 (*black arrow*). (B) The ventrodorsal view revealed that the right L7 neural foramen is enlarged (*white arrows*) when compared to the contralateral foramen (*black arrows*). Differential diagnoses include neurofibroma, meningioma, or metastatic tumor. **Diagnosis:** Neurofibroma of the right seventh lumbar nerve.

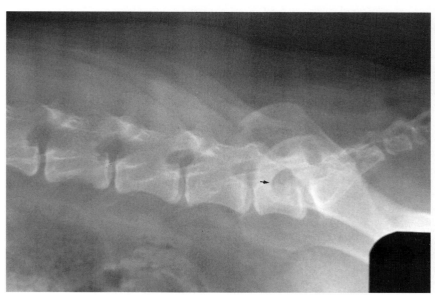

A

B

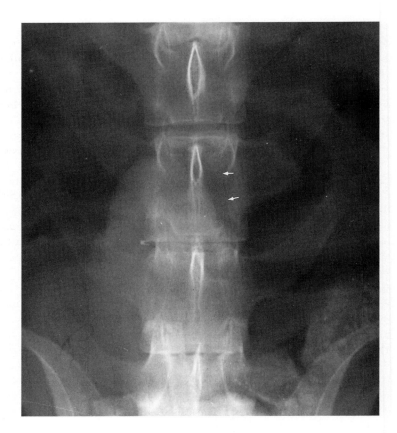

Figure 6–37. A 9-year-old male spitz with paraparesis which was worse on the right. The ventrodorsal view revealed a loss of the cortical line of the right pedicle of L5. The left pedicle is present but less apparent than usual (*white arrows*). Differential diagnoses include neoplasms of the spine, spinal cord, or meninges. **Diagnosis:** Osteosarcoma of L5.

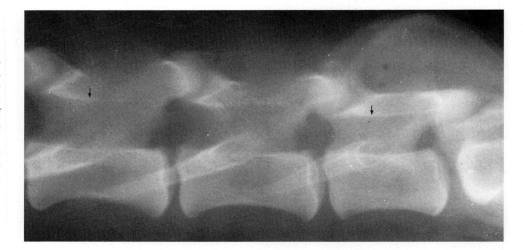

Figure 6–38. A 5-year-old male Samoyed with slowly progressive paraparesis. The lateral view of the caudal lumbar spine revealed erosion of the laminae (roof) of the arch of L6. The normal cortical line is clearly seen in L5 and L7 (*black arrows*). Differential diagnoses include primary spinal cord tumors or primary or metastatic neoplasia of the vertebral body. **Diagnosis:** Ependymoma.

OSTEOCHONDROSIS

Osteochondrosis of the spine is rare. Lesions that resemble osteochondrosis have been reported in association with cervical vertebral malformation.[62] Whether these lesions are primary and cause the clinical signs or are secondary to the cervical vertebral malformation is unknown. The lesions appear similar to osteochondrosis histologically; however, they may be the result of degenerative joint disease and may not be the same as osteochondrosis in the appendicular skeleton. A lesion that resembles osteochondrosis has also been reported in the sacrum, predominantly in German shepherd dogs.[63] This lesion was identified in older dogs with cauda equina compression and in younger dogs without cauda equina compression. A radiolucent defect was identified in the dorsal aspect of the cranial endplate of S1—there was endplate sclerosis and one or more bone densities were identified on the ventral midline of the spinal canal. In older dogs that also had other degenerative changes, such as spondylosis and degenerative joint disease of the articular facets, cauda equina compression was documented myelographically. The bone densities appeared to be attached to the intervertebral disc and were identified histologically as hyaline cartilage with a bone center. In affected immature dogs, the cartilaginous mass appeared histologically to be associated with the sacral physis.

CAUDA EQUINA SYNDROME

Some animals may develop entrapment of one or more of the terminal lumbar nerve roots (cauda equina). There may be no radiographic changes, however survey radiographic findings, such as sclerosis, vertebral malalignment, and/or spondylosis of the lumbosacral articulation, may be identified.[64,65] Flexion and extension radiographs of the lumbosacral junction may be helpful in identifying malalignment or instability, but these changes may be present without cauda equina compression because the compression usually is associated with ligamentum flavum or dorsal longitudinal ligament hypertrophy or disc prolapse.[66] Measurements of the lumbosacral angle have not been useful in separating symptomatic from asymptomatic dogs.[67] Definitive diagnosis requires either myelography, lumbar sinus venography, epidurography, discography, CT, or MRI. [8–11,67–75] Myelography with lateral radiographs that are obtained with the lumbosacral junction flexed and extended can be used to demonstrate cauda equina compression in those dogs in which the dural sac extends beyond the lumbosacral junction. This examination was successful in 80% of the dogs in one study.[69] Although compression of the cauda equina could be observed when the lumbosacral joint was flexed, the compression was most often demonstrated when the lumbosacral joint was extended. Some normal variation in the appearance of the dural sac was described.[69] The normal vertebral sinus venogram shows the sinuses in the sacral and caudal lumbar area. When the venogram is abnormal, the sinus may be displaced laterally and/or dorsally. Occasionally, the sinus will be blocked and there will be a lack of opacification (Fig. 6–39). Epidurography may demonstrate the prolapsed disc as a filling defect along the floor of the spinal canal. In an experimental study, epidurography was better than myelography or venography but demonstrated an injected silicon mass in only 41% of the dogs.[71] Both false-positives and false-negatives may occur.[72] CT and MRI will demonstrate the soft tissue mass and loss of the epidural fat. MRI is superior to the other techniques because it demonstrates the neural structures more completely.[74]

METABOLIC DISEASES

Metabolic disease may be reflected in the spine by overall loss of bone density and the appearance of relatively sclerotic vertebral endplates.[76] This can be due to hyperparathyroidism (either primary or secondary), hyperadrenalcorticism, osteoporosis due to immobility, multiple myeloma, or other causes. The loss of bone mineral usually is not a problem but may rarely predispose to spinal fracture (Fig. 6–40). The spine of apparently normal older cats frequently appears osteopenic (Fig. 6–41). A metabolic disorder that results in vertebral changes is mucopolysaccharidosis in the cat. This may cause osteopenia, agenesis of the odontoid process, widening of the intervertebral disc spaces, and shortening of the vertebral bodies.[77] A diet that is overly rich in vitamin A can produce proliferative changes involving the arches and lateral bodies of the cervical vertebrae.[78] Lead poisoning has been reported to cause metaphyseal sclerosis of the vertebral bodies.[78] Osteopetrosis may affect the vertebral bodies as well as the appendicular skeleton. This is discussed in Chapter 4.

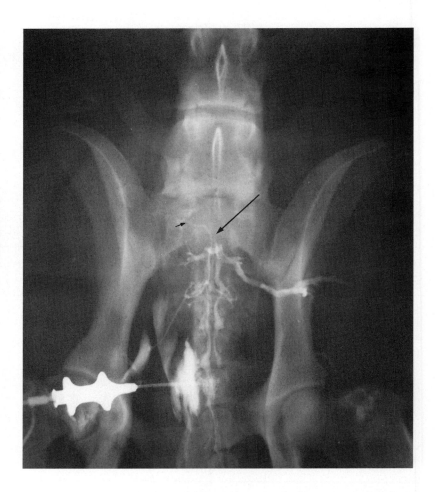

Figure 6–39. A 6-year-old male Labrador retriever with tail biting for 8 weeks. On the lateral view the lumbar sinus venogram revealed the opacified sinuses from C3 to the lumbosacral junction. On the ventrodorsal view the right dorsal lumbar sinus is obstructed at L7–S1 (*small black arrow*) and the left dorsal lumbar sinus is blocked slightly caudal to this level (*long black arrow*). Differential diagnoses include disc extrusion, hypertrophy of dorsal longitudinal ligament, degenerative joint disease with periarticular osteophytes encroaching upon the spinal canal, and fibrous adhesions within the spinal canal from unknown causes. **Diagnosis:** L7–S1 Disc extrusion.

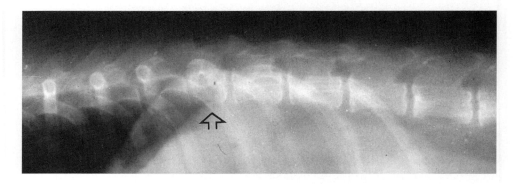

Figure 6–40. A 9-year-old female mixed breed dog with polyuria and polydipsia for 3 months and acute back pain. The lateral radiograph of the thoracolumbar spine revealed a decrease in length of both the body and arch components of T11 as well as a generalized osteopenia. Differential diagnoses for the osteopenia include hyperadrenocorticism, primary or secondary hyperparathyroidism, or nutritional deficiencies. **Diagnosis:** Pathologic impaction fracture of T11 due to primary hyperparathyroidism.

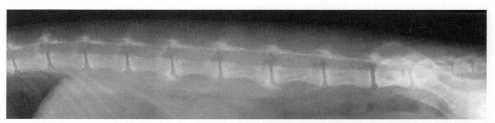

Figure 6–41. A 10-year-old male domestic short-haired cat with hematuria. The spine revealed diffuse osteopenia. While many differential diagnoses should be considered the most common is senile osteopenia of unknown etiology. **Diagnosis:** Senile osteopenia.

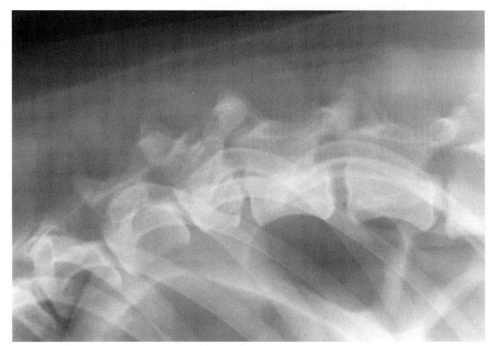

A

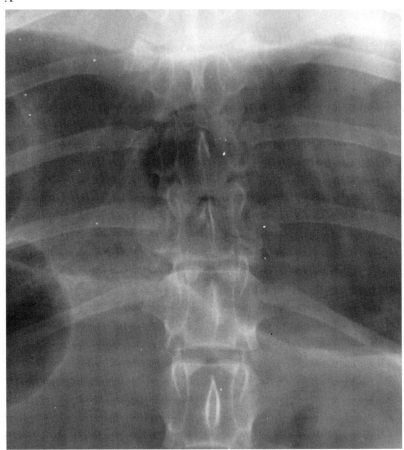

B

Figure 6–42. An 8-year-old male Labrador retriever that was hit by a car. The dog has acute paraparesis and hyperpathia of the thoracolumbar region. (A) The lateral radiograph revealed shortening of the vertebral body and slight malalignment with the neighboring vertebrae. The dorsal components of the spine are normal. (B) The ventrodorsal view revealed shortening of the vertebral body. **Diagnosis:** Traumatic impaction (compression) fracture of T12.

TRAUMA

Fractures

Spinal trauma may cause fractures or soft tissues injuries. The most frequent site of injury in cats is the sacral spine, while in dogs the lumbar spine is affected slightly

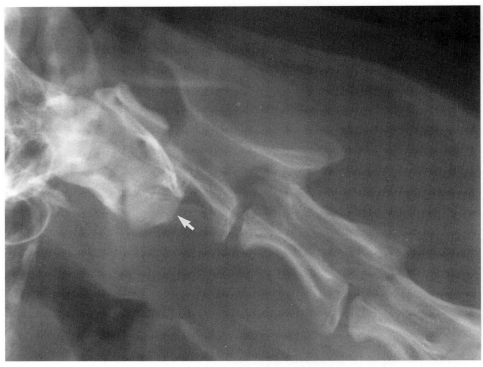

A

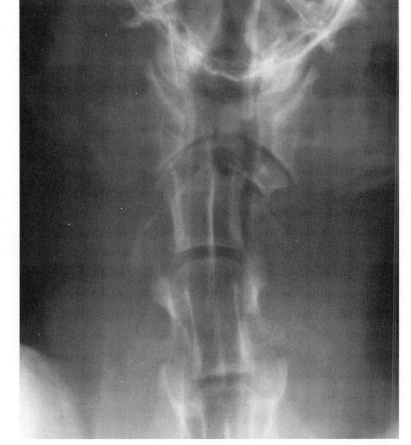

B

Figure 6–43. A 3-year-old male Doberman pinscher that was hit by a car. (A) The lateral view of the cervical spine revealed a fracture through the base of the odontoid process (*white arrow*) with cranial and dorsal displacement of the caudal fragment. (B) The ventrodorsal view revealed some foreshortening of C2. The dog was treated by conservative management and developed no long-term neurologic signs. **Diagnosis:** Shearing fracture of C2.

more frequently than the sacral and thoracic spine.[79] Fractures most frequently occur through the vertebral body. Injury to more than one vertebra, especially adjacent vertebral segments, is not uncommon particularly in the lumbosacral area. It is difficult to determine the extent of the spinal cord injury based solely on the radiographic appearance of the fracture, because the nature of the fracture and the level at which it occurs influence the neurologic signs. As a general rule, displacement of the fragments more than one-half the diameter of the spinal canal is indicative of a severe spinal cord injury. One categorization of spinal fractures is by the type of force that caused the fracture (impaction, avulsion, shearing, bursting, or rotation); another method classifies the fractures according to the manner in which the force is applied (rotation, hyperflexion, or hyperextension). The factors that are most important for treatment decisions are the displacement and stability of the fracture fragments.

The most common cause of impaction (compression) fractures is trauma. This usually results in a shortened vertebral body with the pedicles and laminae unaffected (Fig. 6–42). Comparison with adjacent vertebral bodies is helpful in recognizing a compression fracture, because the alteration in trabecular pattern that accompanies the fracture may be subtle. Some systemic diseases (primary or secondary hyperparathyroidism, hyperadrenocorticism), infection, and neoplasia may weaken

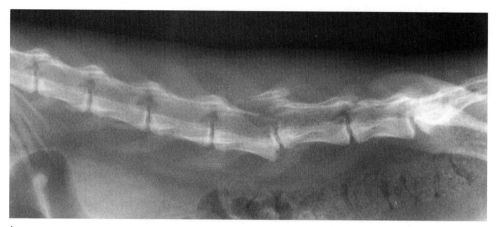

A

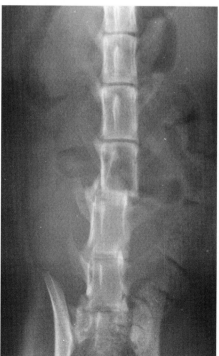

B

Figure 6–44. A 1-year-old female domestic short-haired cat that was hit by a car. (A) The lateral radiograph revealed fractures of the pedicles and laminae of the caudal portion of L5. There is an avulsion fracture of the caudal endplate of L5. (B) The ventrodorsal view revealed malalignment at L5–L6 and displacement to the left of the dorsal fragments. **Diagnosis:** Extensional injury fractures of L5.

the bony structures of the vertebrae and predispose them to compression fractures. This usually results in compression of both the vertebral body and the more dorsal structures (pedicles and laminae) (see Fig. 6–40).

Avulsion and shearing fractures commonly are seen as a result of trauma. A straight shearing force may cause fracture through the entire vertebra (Fig. 6–43). Extensional trauma usually results in avulsion fractures of the ventral spinal components and shearing fractures of dorsal spinal components (Fig. 6–44). In flexional trauma, the ventral vertebral body components will experience shearing forces and the dorsal components will experience avulsive forces (Fig. 6–45).

Bursting fractures are caused by a massive force such as that caused by a gunshot wound to a vertebral body. This results in complete dispersion of the vertebral fragments (Fig. 6–46). This type of fracture is uncommon.

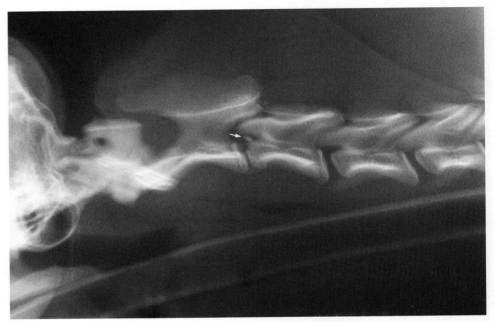

Figure 6–45. An 8-month-old male cocker spaniel that had been hit by a car. The lateral cervical radiograph revealed an avulsion fracture of the dorsal part of the cranial endplate of C3 which was displaced dorsally. **Diagnosis:** Flexional injury-fracture of C3.

Figure 6–46. A 3-year-old pit bull that had been shot. (A) The bullet fragments are clearly visible. The caudal half of the arch of C2 has been shattered. (B) The ventrodorsal view revealed multiple fragments of C2, particularly on the left side. **Diagnosis:** Bursting fracture of C2 due to gunshot wound.

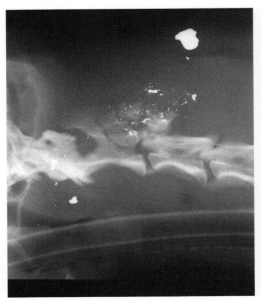

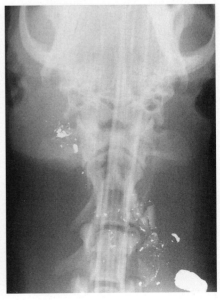

A

B

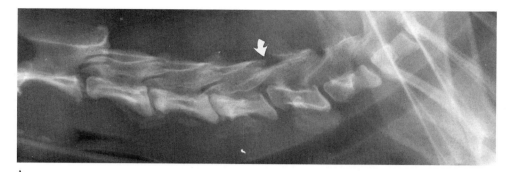

A

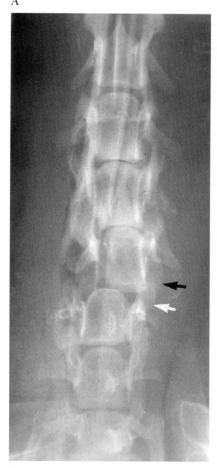

B

Figure 6–47. A 12-year-old male poodle hit by a car. The dog has tetraparesis and neck pain. (A) On the lateral view there is apparent subluxation at C5–C6 (*white arrow*). (B) On the ventrodorsal view there is rightward displacement of C6 relative to C5. Careful examination revealed that the left articular facet of C6 (*white arrow*) is displaced toward and locked to the right of the articular facet of C5 (*black arrow*). There is incidental evidence of chronic cervical intervertebral disc disease with narrowing of the disc spaces and sclerosis of the adjacent endplates at C3–C4, and C4–C5. **Diagnosis:** Rotational injury at C5–C6 with locked facets.

Dislocations

Trauma may bring rotational or complex forces to bear upon the spine. Subluxation or luxation of the spine may occur with the dorsal facets of one vertebra malaligned with those of the vertebra immediately cranial to it (Fig. 6–47). Articular facet fractures may occur concurrently with luxation or subluxation, and careful examination of the radiograph may be required to identify these small fragments. When traumatic vertebral body luxation is present, concurrent vertebral body fractures are more common than articular facet fractures.[79] A widened disc space may be the only radiographic change identified when subluxation of the vertebral bodies has occurred. On a ventrodorsal radiograph, an abrupt change in alignment of the dorsal spinous processes may be observed. It is difficult to predict the severity of the neurologic injury from the radiographic changes that are present. Myelography may be helpful in determining the extent of the neurologic injury, however a normal myelogram may be present despite severe myelomalacia.

Intervertebral Disc Prolapse

Intervertebral disc prolapse may occur as a result of trauma. Approximately 10% of dogs with spinal trauma have disc herniation.[79] A narrowed intervertebral disc, alteration in contour and size of the intervertebral foramen, and collapse of the interarcuate space may be observed. Myelography may be required to evaluate the extent of the spinal cord injury.

REFERENCES

1. Ticer JW. Radiographic technique in small animal practice. Philadelphia: WB Saunders Co, 1975.
2. Allan GS, Wood AKW. Iohexol myelography in the dog. Vet Radiol 1988;29:78.
3. Widmer WR, Blevins WE, Jakovljevic S, Teclaw RF, Han CM, Hurd CD. Iohexol and iopamidol myelography in the dog: Clinical trial comparing adverse effects and myelographic quality. Vet Radiol Ultrasound 1992;33:327.
4. Pardo AD, Morgan JP. Myelography in the cat: A comparison of cisternal versus lumbar puncture using metrizamide. Vet Radiol 1988;29:89.
5. Carakostas MC, Gossett KA, Watters JW, MacWilliams PS. Effects of metrizamide myelography on cerebrospinal fluid analysis in the dog. Vet Radiol 1983;24:267.
6. Tilmant L, Ackerman N, Spencer CP. Mechanical aspects of subarachnoid space punctures in the dog. Vet Radiol 1984;25:227.
7. Kirberger RM, Wrigley RH. Myelography in the dog: Review of patients with contrast medium in the central canal. Vet Radiol Ultrasound 1993;34:253.
8. McNeel SV, Morgan JP. Intraosseous vertebral venography: A technique for examination of the canine lumbosacral junction. JAVRS 1978;19:168.
9. Blevins WE. Transosseous vertebral venography: A diagnostic aid in lumbosacral disease. Vet Radiol 1980;21:50.
10. Koblik PD, Suter PF. Lumbosacral vertebral sinus venography via transjugular catheterization in the dog. Vet Radiol 1981;22:69.
11. Barthez PY, Morgan JP, Lipsitz D. Discography and epidurography for evaluation of the lumbosacral junction in dogs with cauda equina syndrome. Vet Radiol Ultrasound 1994;35:152.
12. Feeney DA, Wise M. Epidurography in the normal dog: Technique and radiographic findings. Vet Radiol 1981;22:35.
13. Nakamiyama,M. Intraoperative spinal ultrasonography in dogs: Normal findings and case-history reports. Vet Radiol Ultrasound 1993;34:264.
14. Prata RG. Diagnosis of spinal tumors in the dog. VCNA 1977;7:165.
15. Larsen JS. Lumbosacral transitional vertebra in the dog. JAVRS 1977;18:76.
16. Morgan JP, Bahr A, Franti CE, Bailey CS. Lumbosacral transitional vertebra as a predisposing cause of cauda equina syndrome in German shepherd dogs: 161 cases (1987–1990). JAVMA 1993;202:1877.
17. Morgan JP, Rosenblatt L. Canine hip dysplasia: Significance of pelvic and sacral attachment. Cal Vet 1987;1:12.
18. Parker AJ, Park RD. Clinical signs associated with hemivertebra in three dogs. Canine Pract 1974;3:34.
19. Bailey CS. An embryological approach to the clinical significance of congenital vertebral and spinal cord abnormalities. JAAHA 1975;11:426.
20. Knecht CD, Blevins WE, Raffe MR. Stenosis of the thoracic spinal canal in English bulldogs. JAAHA 1979;15:181.
21. Bagley RS, Forrest LJ, Cauzinille L, Hopkins AL, Kornegay JN. Cervical vertebral fusion and concurrent intervertebral disc extrusion in four dogs. Vet Radiol Ultrasound 1993;34:336.
22. Hurov L. Congenital atlantoaxial malformation and acute subluxation in a mature basset hound—surgical treatment by wire stabilization. JAAHA 1979;15:177.
23. Cook JR, Oliver JE. Atlantoaxial luxation in the dog. Comp Cont Ed 1981;3:242.
24. Parker AJ, Park RD. Cervical kyphosis in an Afghan hound. JAVMA 1973;162:953.
25. Shelton SB, Bellah J, Chrisman C, McMullen D. Hypoplasia of the odontoid process and secondary atlantoaxial luxation in a Siamese cat. PVN 1991;2:209.
26. Watson AG. Congenital occipito-atlantoaxial malformation (OAAM) in a dog. Anat Histol Embryol 1979;8:187.
27. Watson AG. Congenital occipito-atlantoaxial malformation in a cat. Comp Cont Ed 1985;7:245.
28. Parker AJ, Park RD, Byerly CS, Stowater JL. Spina bifida and protrusion of spinal cord tissue in a dog. JAVMA 1973;163:158.
29. Kitchen H, Murray RE, Cockrell BY. Spina bifida, sacral dysgenesis and myelocele. Am J Pathol 1972;68:203.
30. Leipold HW, Huston K, Blauch B, Guffy MM. Congenital defects of the caudal vertebral column and spinal cord in manx cats. JAVMA 1974;164:520.
31. Wright F, Rest JR, Palmer AC. Ataxia of the great dane caused by stenosis of the cervical vertebral canal: Comparison with similar conditions in the basset hound, doberman pinscher, ridgeback and the thoroughbred horse. Vet Rec 1973;92:1.
32. Trotter EJ, deLahunta A, Geary JC, Brasmer TH. Caudal cervical vertebral malformation-malarticulation in great danes and doberman pinschers. JAVMA 1976;168:917.
33. Chambers JN, Betts CW. Caudal cervical spondylopathy in the dog: A review of 20 cases and the literature. JAAHA 1977;13:571.
34. Hurov LI. Treatment of cervical vertebral instability in the dog. JAVMA 1979;175:278.

35. Raffe MR, Knecht CD. Cervical vertebral malformation—A review of 36 cases. JAAHA 1980;16:881.
36. Parker AJ, Park RD, Henry JD. Cervical vertebral instability associated with cervical disc disease in two dogs. JAVMA 1973;163:1369.
37. Parker AJ, Park RD, Cusick PK, Small E, Jeffers CB. Cervical vertebral instability in the dog. JAVMA 1973;163:71.
38. Ellison GW, Seim HB, Clemmons RM. Distracted cervical spinal fusion for management of caudal cervical spondylomyelopathy in large breed dogs. JAVMA 1988;193:447.
39. Sharp NJH, Wheeler SJ, Cofone M. Radiological evaluation of "wobbler" syndrome—Caudal cervical spondylomyelopathy. JSAP 1992;33:491.
40. Morgan JP. Spondylosis deformans in the dog: Its radiographic appearance. JAVRS 1967;8:17.
41. Morgan JP, Ljunggren GL, Read R. Spondylosis deformans (vertebral osteophytosis) in the dog: A radiographic study from England, Sweden and USA. JSAP 1967;8:57.
42. Morgan JP. Spinal dural ossification in the dog: Incidence and distribution based on a radiographic study. JAVRS 1969;10:43.
43. Felts JF, Prata RG. Cervical disc disease in the dog: Intraforaminal and lateral extrusions. JAAHA 1983;19:755.
44. Brown NO, Helphrey ML, Prata RG. Thoracolumbar disc disease in the dog: A retrospective analysis of 1897 cases. JAAHA 1977;13:665.
45. Kirberger RM, Roos CJ, Lubbe AM. The radiological diagnosis of thoracolumbar disc disease in the dachshund. Vet Radiol Ultrasound 1992;33:255.
46. Dallman MJ, Moon ML, Giovannitti-Jensen. Comparison of the width of the intervertebral disc space and radiographic changes before and after intervertebral disc fenestration in dogs. AJVR 1991;52:140.
47. Hurov L, Troy G, Turnwald G. Diskospondylitis in the dog: 27 cases. JAVMA 1978;173:275.
48. Kornegay JN, Barber DL, Earley TD. Cranial thoracic diskospondylitis in two dogs. JAVMA 1979;174:192.
49. Kornegay JN, Barber DL. Diskospondylitis in dogs. JAVMA 1980;177:337.
50. Johnson RG, Prata RG. Intradiscal osteomyelitis: A conservative approach. JAAHA 1983;19:743.
51. Kerwin SC, Lewis DD, Hribernik TN, Partington B, Hosgood G, Eilts BE. Diskospondylitis associated with *Brucella canis* infection in dogs: 14 cases (1980–1991). JAVMA 1992;201:1253.
52. Henderson RA, Hoerlein BF, Kramer TT, Meyer ME. Discospondylitis in three dogs infected with *Brucella canis*. JAVMA 1974;165:451.
53. Turnwald GH, Shires PK, Turk MAM, Cox HU, Pechman RD, Kearney MT, Hugh-Jones ME, et al. Diskospondylitis in a kennel of dogs: Clinicopathologic findings. JAVMA 1986;188:178.
54. Patnaik AK, Liu S-K, Wilkins RJ, et al. Paeciliomycosis in a dog. JAVMA 1972;161:806.
55. Turrel JM, Pool RR. Bone lesions in 4 dogs with visceral leishmaniasis. Vet Radiol 1982;23:243.
56. Barton CL, Russo EA, Craig TM, Green RW. Canine hepatozoonosis: A retrospective study of 15 naturally occurring cases. JAAHA 1985;21:125.
57. Wright JA, Bell DA, Clayton-Jones DG. The clinical and radiological features associated with spinal tumors in thirty dogs. JSAP 1979;20:461.
58. Morgan JP, Ackerman N, Bailey CS, Pool RR. Vertebral tumors in the dog: A clinical, radiologic, and pathologic study of 61 primary and secondary lesions. Vet Radiol 1980;21:197.
59. Santen DR, Payne JT, Pace LW, Kroll RA, Johnson GC. Thoracolumbar vertebral osteochondroma in a young dog. JAVMA 1991;199:1054.
60. Turner JL, Luttgen PJ, VanGundy TE, Roenigk WJ, Hightower D, Frelier PF. Multicentric osseous lymphoma with spinal extradural involvement in a dog. JAVMA 1992;200:196.
61. Zaki FA, Prata RG, Hurvitz AI, Kay WJ. Primary tumors of the spinal cord and meninges in six dogs. JAVMA 1975;166:511.
62. Olsson SS. Osteochondrosis in the dog. In: Kirk RW, ed. Current veterinary therapy VI. Philadelphia: WB Saunders Co, 1977;880.
63. Lang J, Hani H, Schawalder P. A sacral lesion resembling osteochondrosis in the German shepherd dog. Vet Radiol Ultrasound 1992;33:69.
64. Oliver JE, Selcer RR, Simpson S. Cauda equina compression from lumbosacral malarticulation and malformation in the dog. JAVMA 1978;173:207.
65. Tarvin G, Prata RG. Lumbosacral stenosis in dogs. JAVMA 1980;177:154.
66. Berzon JL, Dueland R. Cauda equina syndrome: Pathophysiology and report of seven cases. JAAHA 1979;15:635.
67. Wright JA. Spondylosis deformans of the lumbo-sacral joint in dogs. JSAP 1980;21:45.
68. Selcer BA, Chambers JN, Schewnsen K, Mahaffey MB. Epidurography as a diagnostic aid in canine lumbosacral compressive disease: 47 cases (1981–1986). Vet Comp Orthop Trauma 1988;2:97.
69. Lang J. Flexion-extension myelography of the canine cauda equina. Vet Radiol 1988;29:242.
70. Denny HR, Gibbs C, Holt PE. The diagnosis and treatment of cauda equina lesions in the dog. JSAP 1982;23:425.
71. Hathcock JT, Pechman RD, Dillon AR, Knecht CD, Braund KG. Comparison of three radiographic contrast procedures in the evaluation of the canine lumbosacral spinal canal. Vet Radiol 1988;29:4.
72. Sisson AF, LeCouteur RA, Ingram JT, Park RD, Child G. Diagnosis of cauda equina abnormalities by using electromyography, discography, and epidurography in dogs. JVIM 1992;6:253.
73. Morgan JP, Bailey CS. Cauda equina syndrome in the dog: Radiographic evaluation. JSAP 1990;31:69.
74. deHaan JJ, Shelton SB, Ackerman N. Magnetic resonance imaging in the diagnosis of degenerative lumbosacral stenosis in four dogs. Vet Surg 1993;22:1.
75. Chambers JN, Selcer BA, Butler TW, Oliver JE, Brown J. A comparison of computed tomography to epidurography for the diagnosis of suspected compressive lesions at the lumbosacral junction in dogs. Prog Vet Neurol 1994;5:30.
76. Ticer JW. Roentgen signs of endocrine disease. VCNA 1977;7:465.

77. Haskins ME, Jezyk PF, Desniak RJ, et al. Mucopolysaccharidosis in a domestic short haired cat: A disease distinct from that seen in the Siamese cat. JAVMA 1979;175:384.
78. Morgan JP. Radiology in veterinary orthopedics. Philadelphia: Lea and Febiger, 1972.
79. Feeney DA, Oliver JE. Blunt spinal trauma in the dog and cat: Insight into radiographic lesions. JAAHA 1980;16;885.

INDEX OF FIGURE LEGENDS

INDEX

Page numbers in *italics* refer to radiographs; numbers in **boldface** refer to sonograms; numbers followed by the letter t refer to tables.